Treatment of the Seriously Obese Patient

Treatment of the Seriously Obese Patient

Edited by
THOMAS A. WADDEN, PhD
THEODORE B. VANITALLIE, MD

Foreword by Per Björntorp, MD, PhD

THE GUILFORD PRESS
New York   London

© 1992 The Guilford Press
A Division of Guilford Publications, Inc.
72 Spring Street, New York, NY 10012

All rights reserved

No part of this book may be reproduced, stored in a retrieval system, or transmitted, in any form or by any means, electronic, mechanical, photocopying, microfilming, recording, or otherwise, without written permission from the Publisher.

Printed in the United States of America

This book is printed on acid-free paper.

Last digit is print number: 9 8 7 6 5 4 3 2 1

Library of Congress Cataloging-in-Publication Data

Treatment of the seriously obese patient / edited by Thomas A. Wadden, Theodore B. VanItallie.
    p.   cm.
  Includes bibliographical references and index.
  ISBN 0-89862-879-2
  1. Obesity—Treatment. I. Wadden, Thomas A. II. VanItallie, Theodore B., 1919-   .
  [DNLM: 1. Caloric Intake. 2. Diet, Reducing. 3. Obesity—diet therapy. 4. Weight Loss. WD 210 T7864]
RC628.T697 1992
616.3'9806—dc20
DNLM/DLC
for Library of Congress   92-1459
                                                                    CIP

*To my mother and late father,
with deepest love and appreciation.*
T. A. W.

To Sallie.
T. B. V. I.

Contributors

Richard L. Atkinson, MD, Division of Clinical Nutrition, Department of Internal Medicine, Eastern Virginia Medical School, Norfolk, Virginia; Research Service, Department of Veterans Affairs Medical Center, Hampton, Virginia

Susan J. Bartlett, MEd, Obesity Research Group, Department of Psychiatry, University of Pennsylvania School of Medicine, Philadelphia, Pennsylvania

Per Björntorp, MD, PhD, Department of Medicine, Sahlgren's Hospital, University of Göteberg, Göteberg, Sweden

George L. Blackburn, MD, PhD, Center for Study of Nutrition and Medicine, New England Deaconess Hospital, Boston, Massachusetts; Department of Surgery, Harvard Medical School, Boston, Massachusetts

Kelly D. Brownell, PhD, Department of Psychology and Yale Center for Eating and Weight Disorders, Yale University, New Haven, Connecticut

Gary D. Foster, MS, Obesity Research Group, Department of Psychiatry, University of Pennsylvania School of Medicine, Philadelphia, Pennsylvania

Kenneth R. Fox, PhD, School of Education, University of Exeter, Exeter, England; Physical Education Association Research Centre, Exeter, England

Bernard Guy-Grand, MD, Service de Médecine et Nutrition, Hôtel Dieu de Paris, Paris, France

Steven B. Heymsfield, MD, Obesity Research Center, St. Luke's–Roosevelt Hospital Center, New York, New York; Department of Medicine, College of Physicians and Surgeons, Columbia University, New York, New York

Prasoon Jain, MD, Fellow in Endocrinology, Diabetes, and Nutrition, and Obesity Research Center, St. Luke's–Roosevelt Hospital Center, New York, New York

Mark P. Jarrell, PhD, Weight Management Center, Department of Psychiatry and Behavioral Sciences, Medical University of South Carolina, Charleston, South Carolina

Janet Jasper, BA, Philadelphia, Pennsylvania

Beatrice S. Kanders, EdD, MPH, RD, Center for Study of Nutrition and Medicine, New England Deaconess Hospital, Boston, Massachusetts; Department of Surgery, Harvard Medical School, Boston, Massachusetts

John G. Kral, MD, PhD, Department of Surgery, State University of New York Health Science Center at Brooklyn, Brooklyn, New York

Kathleen A. Letizia, BA, Obesity Research Group, University of Pennsylvania School of Medicine, Philadelphia, Pennsylvania

Edward A. Lew, AM, FSA, Retired Vice President and Actuary, Metropolitan Life Insurance Company; Past President, Society of Actuaries

Suzanne McNulty, MS, RD, Marymount College, Tarrytown, New York

Patrick Mahlen O'Neil, PhD, Weight Management Center, Department of Psychiatry and Behavioral Sciences, Medical University of South Carolina, Charleston, South Carolina

Oscar Ortiz, MD, Obesity Research Center, St. Luke's–Roosevelt Hospital Center, New York, New York

Michael G. Perri, PhD, Department of Clinical and Health Psychology, University of Florida, Gainesville, Florida

F. Xavier Pi-Sunyer, MD, Division of Endocrinology, Diabetes, and Nutrition, and Obesity Research Center, St. Luke's–Roosevelt Hospital Center, New York, New York; Department of Medicine, College of Physicians and Surgeons, Columbia University, New York, New York

Eric Ravussin, PhD, Visiting Scientist, Clinical Diabetes and Nutrition Section, National Institute of Diabetes and Digestive and Kidney Diseases, National Institutes of Health, Phoenix, Arizona

Albert J. Stunkard, MD, Department of Psychiatry, University of Pennsylvania School of Medicine, Philadelphia, Pennsylvania

Boyd A. Swinburn, MB, ChB, FRACP, Medical Research Council Research Fellow, Department of Community Health, University of Auckland School of Medicine, Auckland, New Zealand

Theodore B. VanItallie, MD, Obesity Research Center, St. Luke's–Roosevelt Hospital Center, New York, New York; Department of Medicine, College of Physicians and Surgeons, Columbia University, New York, New York

Thomas A. Wadden, PhD, Department of Psychology and Center for Health and Behavior, Syracuse University, Syracuse, New York

Masako Waki, MD, Obesity Research Center, St. Luke's–Roosevelt Hospital Center, New York, New York

Rena R. Wing, PhD, Department of Psychiatry, University of Pittsburgh, Western Psychiatric Institute and Clinic, Pittsburgh, Pennsylvania

Mei-Uih Yang, PhD, Obesity Research Center, St. Luke's–Roosevelt Hospital Center, New York, New York

Eleanor A. Young, PhD, RD, LD, Department of Medicine, University of Texas Health Science Center at San Antonio, San Antonio, Texas

Foreword

The problem with the treatment of the seriously obese patient is not mainly a technical one; the question is, in my opinion, why this therapy constitutes such a problem in the more general sense. All therapists in this field know the scenario. There is a massive need for weight reduction in both the United States and Europe. Recent World Health Organization data from certain parts of Europe show alarming incidence figures of up to 25% obesity. Many victims of this disorder suffer from their condition, both physically and mentally, and seek help. The enthusiasm during early phases of treatment and the happiness of people when achieving desirable weight demonstrate how eager most patients are to be rid of their excess fat. But yet, there are many failures, both during ongoing therapy and frequently in the posttreatment period, with the challenging but often less motivating problem of maintaining body weight at a lower level. In fact, in a majority of severely obese patients, failures of this sort are the rule rather than the exception.

The problem then is, why is obesity treatment so difficult in practice when it is so easy in theory, and so strongly desired by patients? Recent work has shown the powerful impact of genetic factors, but not the mechanisms through which these factors are expressed. Whatever the agency responsible, it is no doubt a strong force that acts to impede any long-term change of the body weight equilibrium, either upwards or downwards. There is of course no basic reason for despair; the genes do not produce obesity in the absence of an environment that fosters a positive energy balance, in the same way as scurvy does not develop without a severe deficiency of ascorbic acid.

The therapeutic difficulties and failures, in combination with the widespread need and desire for treatment, have unfortunately provided a playground for a plethora of remedies without documented effects. In fact, such remedies rarely if ever have a sound theoretical basis in science. Unhappy, disappointed patients are easily trapped by promises of quick and easy cure. Quick and easy, however, are terms that more appropriately describe the profits of entrepreneurs in this unsound business.

This excellent book has collected the viewpoints on the most important problems in the treatment of seriously obese patients, written by experienced researchers and therapists in the field. The title is well chosen in that it focuses on the seriously obese patient. This means not only the severely obese patient in the restricted sense of kilograms or pounds, but also the moderately obese or less obese patient with cardiovascular and diabetes risk. It seems to be frequently forgotten that insulin resistance, established diabetes, hypertension, and hyperlipidemia are all improved by weight reduction, long before an ideal or normal body weight has been reached.

In my view, the most urgent research problem in this area is to try to find the factor(s) that prevent weight maintenance after weight loss. Information in this area is still mainly, or even only, descriptive and provides little if any guidance for future research. Virtually everyone is able to mobilize and burn the triglyceride stored in adipose tissue, to any desired level, provided drastic enough measures are taken. To dispose of body fat is thus not the problem. What we badly need to know is why it is so difficult to prevent the "replenishment" of triglyceride in adipocytes following significant weight loss.

PER BJÖRNTORP

Preface

These are confusing times for obese individuals. Conventional wisdom has long held that they should try to lose weight to prevent or control medical complications of their obesity. In a period, however, as brief as the 3 years since we began planning this volume, a number of developments have led the public, the media, and some investigators to question the wisdom of weight reduction efforts.

Congressional hearings initiated in March 1990 by Representative Ron Wyden of Oregon charged America's weight loss industry with fraud and deception. Commercial programs could provide few data to support claims of long-term weight loss. On the contrary, several former clients of such programs testified that they had regained most or all of their lost weight within 1 to 5 years, an unsurprising assertion, entirely consistent with findings from research trials. In addition, a number of people declared that they had developed complications, most notably gallstones, while participating in weight loss programs. One result of this ferment was a class-action suit against a leading commercial program.

A study published in the *New England Journal of Medicine* in the summer of 1991 raised additional concerns. It suggested that cycles of weight loss and regain increase an individual's risk of cardiovascular morbidity and mortality. Further investigation is needed to reach a definitive conclusion, but these findings certainly made some individuals hesitate before undertaking yet another round of weight reduction.

The title of the present volume, *Treatment of the Seriously Obese Patient*, implicitly conveys our view concerning whether obese individuals should undertake weight reduction. We support those who seek to relax the overriding preoccupation with weight and shape which today afflicts females as young as 8 and as old as 80. It drives many to weight loss programs in hopes of losing 5 or 10 pounds and achieving weights that are often below desirable goals. On the other hand, we are alarmed by those practitioners who would discourage individuals who are seriously obese from attempting to lose weight. Results of the Nurses' Health Study, published in 1990 in the *New England Journal of Medicine*, leave little doubt that significant obesity is health and life threatening. Women 30% or more overweight had a threefold greater risk of illness and death from coronary heart disease than did women of optimal weight. These and similar findings lead us to believe that persons who are 30% or more overweight should seek weight reduction. Individuals with obesity-related risk factors may need treatment even if they are less than 30% overweight. Patients should, however, be given greater assistance with the difficult task of maintaining weight loss than they typically have been in the past.

The Present Volume

The present volume is edited by a clinical psychologist (T.A.W.) and a physician who specializes in internal medicine (T.B.V.I.), and includes contributors from fields ranging from clinical nutrition to exercise physiology. This diverse perspective reflects findings that obesity is a heterogeneous disorder that results from genetic, metabolic, behavioral, and other influences. Our choice of contributors also reflects our belief that the treatment of the seriously obese individual frequently requires a multidisciplinary team—a physician to care for the patient's health, a dietitian to provide nutritional counseling, an exercise specialist to design a program of physical activity, and a psychologist or similar professional to help the patient meet the emotional and behavioral challenges of weight control. We note that there have been no research studies comparing the effectiveness of such multidisciplinary care with that provided by a single practitioner. Moreover, health professionals in traditional outpatient practice may not have the capacity to assemble a full, multidisciplinary team. Experience tells us, however, that the more they attempt to meet the diverse needs of the seriously obese, the more favorable the outcome they can expect.

This volume is intended primarily for practitioners, although we hope that researchers also will find it of value. The principal treatment approach described is delivered by a multidisciplinary team and incorporates the short-term use of a very low calorie diet (VLCD). Three points deserve comment here, the first of which is that all obese individuals should be treated by a conventional reducing diet of 1000–1500 kilocalories (kcal) prior to their being considered for a more restrictive regimen. Second, there is no consensus concerning the optimal energy content of VLCDs. We recently showed that an 800-kcal/day diet produced weight losses that were only slightly smaller than those achieved with a diet providing half as many calories. We believe that the success of these diets may be more attributable to their use of portion- and calorie-controlled servings, which facilitate adherence, than to the severity of their energy restriction. Third, the general treatment principles described in this volume are applicable to the care of all seriously obese individuals, whether their obesity is managed primarily by behavioral, dietary, pharmacological, or surgical means.

Plan of the Book

This volume is divided into five parts. The first, entitled "Introduction and Overview," opens with a chapter by VanItallie and Lew which provides guidelines to help practitioners assess the health and mortality risks of overweight patients. In particular, the chapter addresses the problem of integrating information about such important risk-modifying factors as pattern of regional fat distribution with more quantitative data obtained from major population studies concerning the relationship of excess weight to morbidity and mortality risks. The next chapter, by Stunkard, presents a classification of obesity and an overview of current therapies, ranging from behavior modification to surgery. Stunkard focuses primarily upon the treatment of mildly obese individuals (30% or less overweight), whereas Wadden and Bartlett, in the third chapter of this section, discuss the treatment of the seriously obese by VLCD. Their chapter provides a summary of research findings for treatment by behavior modification combined with both VLCDs and conventional reducing diets.

The following part, "Biological Response to Caloric Restriction," contains five chapters that should be of particular interest to researchers. The first, authored by Yang and VanItallie, describes methods of measuring body composition in the obese and the changes that occur in fat and fat-free mass during therapeutic weight loss. Particular attention is devoted to the important relationship between the macronutrient composition of the diet and the retention of fat-free mass. The next chapter, by Young, reviews the animal literature on caloric restriction, body composition, and organ function. The use of animal models was prompted in large measure by efforts to explain the fatal cardiac arrhythmias that occurred in obese women and men who consumed liquid protein diets in 1976–1977. The following chapter, by Heymsfield and colleagues, provides a thorough review of these fatalities, as well as an analysis of the effects of obesity on cardiac function and structure. Ravussin and Swinburn examine in the next chapter the very topical issue of the effects on energy expenditure of dieting and weight loss. They conclude that caloric restriction has few long-term effects on resting metabolic rate. Pi-Sunyer, in the final chapter of this section, similarly concludes that exercise has few significant effects on resting metabolic rate in the obese. Of particular interest is the finding that the obese, unlike their lean counterparts, do not compensate for increased physical activity by consuming sufficient calories to remain in energy equilibrium.

The three chapters in the third part of the book examine the "Health Consequences of Therapeutic Weight Loss." In the first chapter, Kanders and Blackburn summarize recent literature that suggests that a reduction in initial weight of as little as 10% is frequently sufficient to improve or control the adverse health effects of obesity. This finding suggests that seriously obese patients and those who treat them can often select more modest weight loss goals, as compared with the traditional recommendation of attaining ideal weight. Wing's chapter, which follows, examines the potentially unique advantages of using VLCDs with obese Type II diabetics. Even with partial weight regain 1 year after therapy, patients treated by a VLCD still showed improved glycemic control. O'Neil and Jarrell discuss in their chapter the psychological status of obese individuals and changes that can be anticipated with weight loss. They also examine the very timely issue of binge eating in the obese and provide recommendations for further research in this area.

The fourth part reviews the "Clinical Use of Very Low Calorie Diets" in the context of treatment by a multidisciplinary team. Practitioners should welcome the six chapters that comprise this section because they describe the "how to" of treatment. The lead chapter, by Atkinson, a physician, discusses the initial medical evaluation, guidelines for monitoring patients throughout treatment, and the management of any dieting-related side effects. In the chapter that follows, Wadden and Foster, both psychologists, describe the initial psychosocial evaluation of patients and then review behavioral interventions employed in a typical course of therapy. McNulty, a nutritionist and registered dietitian, examines in her chapter the criteria for selecting an appropriately low calorie diet, methods of managing the refeeding period, and means to facilitate patients' long-term consumption of a nutritionally adequate low fat diet. Fox, an exercise physiologist, reviews the many health benefits of physical activity and discusses the special exercise needs of the seriously obese. In the following chapter, Wadden and Letizia review the literature on predictors of weight loss and attrition from therapy, with the goal of identifying patients least likely to be successful. The final chapter of this section is perhaps its most notable. In it, Jasper, a former patient, describes her experiences in losing weight in a combined program of VLCD and lifestyle modification. Her account will increase practitioners' sensitivities to the challenges that patients confront daily in their efforts to manage their weight.

The book's final part examines the critical issue of "Maintenance of Weight Loss and Alternative Therapies" for the seriously obese. Brownell addresses the question of how best to interpret long-term follow-up data on the treatment of obesity, given the paucity of experimental data on persons who do not receive or refuse therapy. He also presents a theoretical model for relapse prevention. In the chapter that follows, Perri summarizes the results of six studies in which he investigated methods to facilitate maintenance of weight loss. Patient–practitioner contact following treatment emerges as one of the best predictors of long-term weight control. Guy-Grand's chapter on the pharmacological treatment of obesity summarizes findings on the serotonergic agents, which have been a topic of great interest in recent years. He proposes that such drugs be used on a chronic basis to manage obesity, in a manner similar to the pharmacological treatment of hypertension or diabetes. In the final chapter of the book, Kral provides an overview of surgical interventions for massively obese individuals (100% or more overweight) who have failed to reduce using more conservative approaches. The results presented in this chapter (and at a recent National Institutes of Health Consensus Development Conference) indicate that surgery, although not without its hazards and complications, is of long-term benefit to a majority of such individuals.

We hope that the many contributions that comprise this volume will provide practitioners with new approaches to the treatment of their seriously obese patients, as well as a better understanding of the nature of their patients' ongoing struggle with weight. Neither we, nor our contributors, are aware of any easy solutions to the problem presented by significant obesity. Nevertheless, we hope that this volume will contribute to efforts to control this disorder.

Acknowledgments

This volume would never have appeared if it were not for Mickey Stunkard, our dear friend and colleague who introduced us over a decade ago and fostered collaboration between our respective laboratories at the University of Pennsylvania and St. Luke's–Roosevelt Hospital. Mickey's enduring enthusiasm for obesity research is matched only by the generosity and strength of his friendship.

We count many of the contributors among our closest friends and colleagues and thank all of them for the very scholarly and thought-provoking chapters they provided. In particular, we thank our former respective colleagues at the University of Pennsylvania's Obesity Research Group and at the Obesity Research Center located at St. Luke's–Roosevelt Hospital Center and Rockefeller University.

A Research Scientist Development Award (to T.A.W.) from the National Institute of Mental Health facilitated our collaboration on this volume. We thank the NIMH and other public and private agencies for their generous support of our research.

We acknowledge Susan Bartlett for her superb editorial assistance, as we do Kathy Letizia and Jean Weimer. This volume would not have been completed in as timely a fashion without their assistance.

We thank Seymour Weingarten, Editor-in-Chief of The Guilford Press, for so generously supporting this effort and Judith Grauman, his associate, for handling in so congenial and helpful a manner the innumerable details involved in producing this book. Marie Sprayberry is acknowledged for her excellent work in copyediting.

And, finally, we thank Jan and Sallie for their love, support, and understanding.

THOMAS A. WADDEN
THEODORE B. VANITALLIE

Contents

PART ONE. INTRODUCTION AND OVERVIEW

1. Assessment of Morbidity and Mortality Risk in the Overweight Patient   3
   Theodore B. VanItallie and Edward A. Lew

2. An Overview of Current Treatments for Obesity   33
   Albert J. Stunkard

3. Very Low Calorie Diets: An Overview and Appraisal   44
   Thomas A. Wadden and Susan J. Bartlett

PART TWO. BIOLOGICAL RESPONSE TO CALORIC RESTRICTION

4. Effect of Energy Restriction on Body Composition and Nitrogen Balance in Obese Individuals   83
   Mei-Uih Yang and Theodore B. VanItallie

5. Marked Caloric Restriction and Organ Response in Normal-Weight and Obese Experimental Animals   107
   Eleanor A. Young

6. Cardiac Structure and Function in Markedly Obese Patients before and after Weight Loss   136
   Steven B. Heymsfield, Prasoon Jain, Oscar Ortiz, and Masako Waki

7. Effect of Caloric Restriction and Weight Loss on Energy Expenditure   163
   Eric Ravussin and Boyd A. Swinburn

8. The Effects of Increased Physical Activity on Food Intake, Metabolic Rate, and Health Risks in Obese Individuals   190
   F. Xavier Pi-Sunyer

PART THREE. HEALTH CONSEQUENCES OF THERAPEUTIC WEIGHT LOSS

9. Reducing Primary Risk Factors by Therapeutic Weight Loss 213
   Beatrice S. Kanders and George L. Blackburn

10. Very Low Calorie Diets in the Treatment of Type II Diabetes: Psychological and Physiological Effects 231
    Rena R. Wing

11. Psychological Aspects of Obesity and Dieting 252
    Patrick Mahlen O'Neil and Mark P. Jarrell

PART FOUR. CLINICAL USE OF VERY LOW CALORIE DIETS

12. Medical Evaluation and Monitoring of Patients Treated by Severe Caloric Restriction 273
    Richard L. Atkinson

13. Behavioral Assessment and Treatment of Markedly Obese Patients 290
    Thomas A. Wadden and Gary D. Foster

14. Nutritional Counseling during Severe Caloric Restriction and Weight Maintenance 331
    Suzanne McNulty

15. A Clinical Approach to Exercise in the Markedly Obese 354
    Kenneth R. Fox

16. Predictors of Attrition and Weight Loss in Patients Treated by Moderate and Severe Caloric Restriction 383
    Thomas A. Wadden and Kathleen A. Letizia

17. The Challenge of Weight Control: A Personal View 411
    Janet Jasper

PART FIVE. MAINTENANCE OF WEIGHT LOSS AND ALTERNATIVE THERAPIES

18. Relapse and the Treatment of Obesity 437
    Kelly D. Brownell

19. Improving Maintenance of Weight Loss Following Treatment
by Diet and Lifestyle Modification   456
Michael G. Perri

20. Long-Term Pharmacological Treatment of Obesity   478
Bernard Guy-Grand

21. Surgical Treatment of Obesity   496
John G. Kral

INDEX   507

PART ONE

INTRODUCTION AND OVERVIEW

1

Assessment of Morbidity and Mortality Risk in the Overweight Patient

THEODORE B. VANITALLIE
EDWARD A. LEW

Many epidemiological studies, prospective, cross-sectional, and retrospective, have investigated the relationship between relative weight on the one hand and future health status and life expectancy on the other. For the most part, such studies have shown quite clearly that the risk of developing certain health problems and of having a shortened lifespan is significantly higher among overweight individuals than it is among nonoverweight people of the same sex, race, age, and socioeconomic status. Moreover, the magnitude of risk increases, sometimes in accelerating fashion, as overweight becomes more and more severe (VanItallie & Lew, 1990).

Although physicians are generally aware of the relationship between overweight and an enhanced risk of illness and premature death, their ability to categorize overweight patients according to magnitude of risk has been hampered by the fact that the relevant epidemiological information, for the most part, has not been translated into clinically useful terms. In this regard, the quantitative aspects of the relationship between overweight and various health risks have not been given sufficient attention. Also, the clinical significance of values for indices such as "mortality ratio" (MR) has remained obscure. For example, it is not clear to physicians how a particular value for MR relates to life expectancy at any given age.

Physicians have been told that the probability of developing certain health problems is higher among persons with upper body (abdominal) obesity than among persons with lower body (femoral–gluteal) obesity (Vague, 1991). However, it is not evident how great these risks can be; nor, in any given patient, is it clear how one can reconcile the contribution of degree of severity of overweight to overall health risk with that of the pattern of regional fat distribution (see Table 1.1).

Finally, physicians do not have a clear understanding of the possible modifying effects of sex, age, duration of overweight, and genetic factors on health risk in overweight patients. In this chapter, we attempt to address these

TABLE 1.1. Anthropometric Indices Associated with Overweight-Related Risk Factors

Index	Description
Relative weight (RW)	Weight relative to some standard of weight for some height. RW (%) = actual weight ÷ optimal (or, in some cases, average) weight for the same height × 100.
Body mass index (BMI)	Body weight normalized for height. The most commonly used BMI is Quetelet's index (Quetelet, 1869), calculated by dividing body weight in kilograms by the square of the height in meters (kg/m^2).
Body composition	In the two-compartment model of body composition, various methods are used to estimate the body's content of fat-free mass (FFM) and body fat mass (BFM).
Pattern of regional fat distribution	Two different patterns of regional fat distribution distribution are commonly identified: (1) "upper body" or "abdominal" obesity; and (2) "lower body" or "femoral-gluteal" obesity. These two patterns are usually distinguished by inspection or by the waist-to-hips (waist–hip) circumference ratio (WHR).

issues with the goal of providing practitioners with frames of reference, however imperfect, that will enable them to categorize overweight patients in terms of their degree of risk of dying or of developing certain overweight-related illnesses.

Anthropometric Indices of Overweight and Obesity

To estimate morbidity and mortality risk in an overweight patient, a physician needs to be familiar with the various anthropometric indices or markers associated with excessive weight that are believed to identify or predict health and/or mortality risk. These indices are listed and briefly described in Table 1.1.

Relative Weight

"Relative weight" (RW) is an index that was widely used until a decade or so ago, after which it became increasingly supplanted by the "body mass index" (BMI). RW was used in conjunction with weight–height tables of various kinds, most notably the Metropolitan Life Insurance Company (Met Life) tables of recommended weights for heights published in 1942 (tables of "ideal" weights); 1959 (tables of "desirable" weights); and 1983 (1983 Met Life tables) (Simopoulos & VanItallie, 1984). When one is attempting to interpret values for RW (and for derivatives of RW, such as "excess weight," percentage of "ideal" or "desirable" weight, etc.), it is essential that the source of the "standard" weight for height be identified. For example, the value for RW can change materially if "average" rather than "optimal" weight is used in the calculation.

Body Mass Index

Because the calculation of RW requires frequent recourse to complicated tables of height and weight, it has been found less burdensome and time-consuming to use the BMI to assess weight status. As noted in Table 1.1, the BMI is an index of body mass that is normalized for height. Use of the BMI greatly simplifies the task of estimating the extent to which a given patient's height-normalized weight (kg/m^2) deviates from some reference value or range of values (Benn, 1971; Keys, Fidanza, Karvonen, Kimura, & Taylor, 1972).

Body Composition

The term "overweight" refers to weight in excess of some standard or norm. The diagnosis of overweight requires (1) information about a patient's weight and height, and (2) a suitable reference table that will permit one to judge whether (and by how much) the patient's weight for height or BMI exceeds a given norm. On the other hand, such terms as "obesity," "adiposity," and "corpulence" clearly refer to an excessive body fat content, not simply overweight. Degree of fatness can be estimated anthropometrically, by underwater weighing (hydrodensitometry), and by measurement of body electrical conductivity or impedance (see Yang & VanItallie, Chapter 4, this volume). However, the point stressed here is that overweight and obesity are two different bodily attributes (VanItallie, 1985). Although most overweight people are also obese, it is possible to be obese without being overweight (i.e., sedentary individuals with a small muscle mass) and overweight without being obese (i.e., body builders and certain athletes).[1]

The degree of fatness of an individual is usually described in terms of body fat mass (BFM) and expressed as a percentage of body weight—that is, BFM (kg) ÷ body weight (kg) × 100. Although this method for expressing fatness has the advantage of simplicity, it has distinct limitations when applied to situations in which body composition is changing, as occurs during therapeutic weight loss or during muscle building. In such instances, fat-free mass (FFM) and BFM may be changing at different rates and, on occasion, in opposite directions. Hence, expressing either or both of them as a percentage of total body weight can create serious problems of interpretation (VanItallie, Yang, Heymsfield, Funk, & Boileau, 1990).

---

[1] Despite these valid distinctions, most workers in the field tend to use the terms "overweight" and "obesity" interchangeably. This practice is reluctantly followed in the present chapter.

Pattern of Regional Fat Distribution

In 1914, a study of mortality among insured men showed that an abdominal girth greater than that of the expanded chest was associated with increased mortality risk. Indeed, the relative mortality of those with large abdominal girth was greater than the already heavy mortality found to exist among the general population of those of corresponding weight (for a discussion, see VanItallie & Lew, 1990). Some three decades later, Jean Vague (1947) codified the differences that usually occur in distribution of subcutaneous fat between obese men and women, and called attention to the significance for health status of these differences. As he pointed out, the male (android) type of obesity is characterized by the predominance of excess subcutaneous fat in the upper half of the body: nape, neck, cheeks, shoulders, and upper half of the abdomen. This pattern corresponds to what is currently called "upper body" or "abdominal" obesity. In contrast, in the female (gynoid) form of obesity, most commonly found in women, excess fat predominates in the lower half of the body (hips, buttocks, thighs, and lower half of the abdomen). In current parlance, this pattern corresponds to "lower body" or "femoral–gluteal" obesity. As Vague emphasized, the clinical importance of making a distinction between these two forms of obesity arises from the fact that android obesity, whether it occurs in men or women, is associated with an enhanced risk of developing non-insulin-dependent diabetes mellitus (NIDDM), atherosclerosis, and hyperuricemia, as well as other diseases and metabolic abnormalities (Table 1.2). In contrast, patients with gynoid obesity appear to have a far lower risk of developing metabolic and cardiovascular complications (Vague, 1956).

In 1984, Larsson et al. reported the results of a prospective study of risk factors for ischemic heart disease (IHD) in 792 Swedish men born in 1913 and first examined in 1967. Thirteen years later, the baseline findings were reviewed in relation to the number of men who had subsequently developed IHD, who had had a stroke, or who had died from any cause. Surprisingly, none of the usual indices of obesity, such as BMI, skinfold thickness measurements, or simple waist circumference, showed a significant correlation with any of the three end points. However, the waist–hip circumference ratio (WHR) showed a significant association with the occurrence of IHD ($p = .04$) and stroke ($p = .002$). The risk ratio for the highest versus lowest quintile for WHR was 2.5 for IHD, 5.9 for stroke, and 1.7 for death.

In a separate report, Lapidus et al. (1984) described the results of a prospective study of the relation of subcutaneous fat distribution to risk of cardiovascular disease (CVD) and death in 1462 Swedish women aged 38 to 60. In this population, a significant positive association was found between WHR and the 12-year incidence of myocardial infarction, angina pectoris, stroke, and sudden death. Indeed, of all the anthropometric variables studied, WHR correlated best with the end points under consideration.

From the clinical standpoint, the WHR is a convenient objective method for estimating pattern of regional fat distribution. A WHR equal to or greater

TABLE 1.2. Some Diseases or Metabolic Abnormalities Linked to Upper Body (Abdominal) Obesity

Atherogenic lipid profile
High fibrinogen levels
Insulin resistance
Hyperinsulinemia
Glucose intolerance
Non-insulin-dependent diabetes mellitus (NIDDM)
Premature coronary heart disease
Stroke
Sudden death
Angina pectoris
Congestive heart failure
Hypertension
Gallbladder disease
Gout
Obstructive sleep apnea
Breast cancer (in postmenopausal women)
Uric acid nephrolithiasis
Arthrosis
Menstrual abnormalities

Note. Adapted, with additions, from Larsson (1989).

than 1.0 in men (0.8 in women) is considered by some investigators to indicate a degree of upper body obesity sufficiently pronounced to warrant considerable concern about the associated health risks (Björntorp, 1987).

Terminology of Risk

From the standpoint of the physician, the terminology of health and mortality risk often seems recondite; hence, some of the more commonly used expressions are briefly discussed as follows.

Mortality Rate

In technical literature, the probability of death is denoted by q and is calculated as the quotient of the number of deaths recorded over a period of time (customarily a year) divided by the number of subjects at the beginning of the study. The mortality rate is usually calculated as the quotient of the number of deaths over a period of time divided by the average number of subjects exposed to the risk of death over that period. It is usually designated by m. Sometimes the question arises as to how the "lost to follow-up" are to be counted; commonly, the subjects lost to follow-up are included for half the period involved.

Mortality Ratio

The MR is the quotient of the probability of death (q) in the population under study divided by the corresponding probability of death calculated from the experience in a defined population that may be regarded as an appropriate standard for judging normal mortality levels; it is generally denoted by (q'). Frequently, the mortality rate (m) is used instead of the probability of death (q), and it is compared with the mortality rate in the standard population (m').

When one is examining an overweight population specified in terms of RW, the subjects may be studied separately by sex, age groups, time elapsed, and other categories (overall health status, socioeconomic level, smoking habits, etc.) By way of illustration, if the mortality rate in a segment of the overweight population is 5 per 1000 over a year's time, and that of a corresponding standard population is 2.5 per 1000, then the MR for this segment of the overweight population would be 2 or 200%. Usually the quotient is multiplied by 100 to provide a percentage value. Thus,

$$\text{MR} = 100 \times \left\{ \frac{q \text{ or } m \text{ in particular segment of study}}{q' \text{ or } m' \text{ in corresponding segment of standard population}} \right.$$

"MR" and "relative mortality" have the same meaning and have been used interchangeably.

Excess Death Rate

The excess death rate (EDR) is the difference between the probability of death (q) (or the mortality rate [m]) in the population under study and the corresponding probabilities of death (q') (or mortality rate [m']) in the standard population. The EDR may be expressed as an absolute number per 1000 per year, such as $q - q'$ (or $m - m'$) or as a percentage, such as $100 \times (q - q')/q'$ (or $100 \times [m - m']/m'$). Thus, if the probability of death in the population under study (q) is 10 per 1000, and the corresponding probability in the standard population (q') is 5 per 1000, then the EDR would be 5 per 1000 or 100%.

To sum up, EDR is calculated either as $q - q'$ or $m - m'$ in absolute terms, or as MR in population under study minus MR in standard population in relative terms.

Morbidity Rates

Morbidity rates are expressed in terms of either incidence rates or prevalence rates. Incidence rates are calculated as the quotient of new morbid events reported over a period of time (customarily a year) divided by the average number of subjects exposed to the risk of morbidity over that period, not including the subjects who had already succumbed to morbidity. Incidence rates are in effect strictly analogous to death rates, in mathematical form.

Prevalence rates are calculated as the quotient of existing subjects with a morbid condition divided by the total number of subjects in the population under study. For instance, if the prevalence of hypertension among overweight individuals aged 20–45 is 56 per 1000, but 10 per 1000 among corresponding nonoverweight individuals in the same population, then the relative prevalence is 5.6. From the relative prevalence, one can obtain an understanding in quantitative terms of the extent to which possession of a particular risk attribute such as overweight enhances the risk of becoming hypertensive, diabetic, or ischemic.

Attributable Risk

Attributable risk may be defined as the maximum proportion of a particular disease (or group of diseases) that may be attributed to a particular cause. For instance, in a prospective study of obesity and coronary heart disease (CHD) in women (Manson et al., 1990), it was found that the adjusted rate of nonfatal and fatal CHD combined was 32 per 100,000 person-years in the leanest weight grouping and 106 per 100,000 person-years in the most obese grouping. The excess incidence of coronary events was therefore 74 per 100,000 person-years; in other words, the maximum proportion of coronary events that might be attributed to excess weight was 70%.

Sources of Information about Risk

The principal sources of information on mortality according to weight are (1) a series of large-scale investigations of the mortality among insured lives, culminating in the so-called Build Study 1979 (Society of Actuaries and the Association of Life Insurance Medical Directors of America, 1980), which covered 4 million persons traced from 1954 through 1972; and (2) a study of 750,000 persons who answered questionnaires from the American Cancer Society in 1959–1960 and were traced from 1960 through 1973 (Lew & Garfinkel, 1979).

Both investigations dealt overwhelmingly with middle-class men and women who at time of entry into the studies were in ostensibly good health. To draw well-founded conclusions about the effects on mortality of various degrees of overweight, it is necessary to exclude from such a study persons who are hypertensive, diabetic, or suffering from heart disease, in order that the results may reflect only the excess mortality attributable to overweight. Persons with these and other serious impairments are subject to distinctly higher-than-average mortality, and it is essential that their effects not obscure the effects of overweight alone. Then, too, men and women at the lower socioeconomic levels likewise experience increased mortality, and a high proportion of such persons in a study may make it difficult to evaluate the effects of overweight as such.

Because excess mortality in overweight individuals may not manifest itself until 10 or more years have elapsed, it is important that mortality studies of overweight extend over longer periods of time. Virtually all of the mortality investigations of insured lives according to degree of overweight have covered 20 or more years of experience (VanItallie & Lew, 1990).

Although numerous other, lesser studies of the effects of overweight on mortality have been carried out, many have been of short duration or have not excluded persons in impaired health, and some have been heavily weighted with persons at the lower socioeconomic levels. Studies of overweight limited to persons who are actively at work in occupations where reasonably high standards of health must be met reflect the selection of healthier lives at entry into the occupation, as well as the selection for continuing employment, which removes persons disabled or in poor health from the active list. This is known as "the healthy worker effect."

Until recently, most investigations of the effects on mortality of various degrees of overweight have not distinguished between smokers and nonsmokers. In the United States, the two most notable exceptions have been the American Cancer Society's study (Lew & Garfinkel, 1979) and the Framingham Heart Study's 26-year follow-up (Garrison, Feinleib, Castelli, & McNamara, 1983).

Categories of Risk Associated with Overweight

The risks associated with overweight fall under two major headings—mortality and morbidity. These two categories are considered separately.

Mortality Risk

Because of the pioneering work of the Actuarial Society of America and the Association of Life Insurance Medical Directors (1912), it is now widely recognized that overweight is associated with an increased risk of premature death—a risk that can be quantified (VanItallie & Lew, 1990). Indeed, when various confounding effects such as smoking, occult illness, and duration of period of observation are controlled for, there remains a direct positive relationship between an increasing BMI and MR. In the Framingham Heart Study, for example, the risk of death within 26 years increased by 1% per extra pound for ages 30 to 49 and by 2% per extra pound for ages 50 to 62 (Garrison et al., 1983).

As mentioned earlier, it is important that physicians understand how to translate indices such as MR into concepts that patients are able to comprehend and relate to everyday experience. Moreover, it needs to be kept in mind that published values for MRs exhibited by overweight men and women are derived from studies of varying sample sizes and durations, in which data were collected under different circumstances and on populations that often were quite different from one another. Indeed, a number of serious methodological limitations (some of which are discussed below) have been identified in most of the major epidemiological studies that have addressed the issue of body weight and longevity; hence, both the ability to generalize and the internal validity of many of these studies have been questioned (VanItallie & Lew, 1990; Manson, Stampfer, Hennekens, & Willett, 1987).

Nevertheless, most of the major studies have been well conducted and have yielded results that are to some extent both consonant and generalizable. Thus, from the available information it is possible to derive a tentative "mortality-optimal" BMI range, and also to characterize in approximate fashion the relationship between an increasing BMI and mortality risk.

In examining mortality findings, one has to bear in mind that such data can refer to what is called "all-cause (AC) mortality," "CVD mortality," "NIDDM mortality," "cancer mortality," and so on. Thus, in the same population, one may be able to demonstrate that while overweight is associated with an enhanced CVD mortality, it is also associated with a reduced mortality from certain types of cancer, which may simply reflect competitive causes of death (see Figure 1.1).

Mortality-Optimal Body Mass Index

Table 1.3 lists the findings of three studies conducted in the United States that provide information bearing on AC mortality-optimal BMI in nonsmoking men and women of all ages. In studies in which the BMI was not utilized as an index, data on RW have been translated into BMI units. In terms of AC mortality, "optimal" refers to that BMI range associated with the lowest AC MRs.

As Table 1.3 shows, for nonsmoking men, the lower end of the "optimal" BMI range is 19.8–22, while the upper end varies between 20.9 and 24.0 kg/m^2. For nonsmoking women, the lower end of the optimal BMI range is 18.8–21.5, while the upper end varies between 20.9 and 23.4 kg/m^2.

As indicated above, these ranges are based on AC mortality. If one were concerned about death from CVD or from cancer, the optimal ranges might be different. As emphasized by Rissanen et al. (1989), the nature of the relation of BMI to AC mortality is strongly influenced by the age distribution and mortality pattern of the population under examination. In their words, "Where cardiovascular deaths predominate, the contribution of overweight to overall mortality is substantial, but the impact of overweight may be concealed when noncardiovascular causes predominate" (p. 787). Also, compared to mortality-optimal BMI ranges, morbidity-optimal ones are often more restrictive.

Most longitudinal studies concerned with the relationship of relative weight to patterns of mortality have shown that AC mortality-optimal BMI

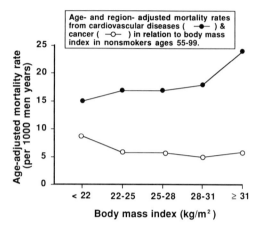

FIGURE 1.1. Relation of body mass index (BMI) to mortality rates from cardiovascular diseases (CVD) and cancer among nonsmoking Finnish men aged 55–99. In contrast to the level mortality rate from cancer, the CVD rate rises as BMI increases. The data are from Rissanen et al. (1989).

ranges tend to be somewhat higher in the older age categories. In the Finnish study of weight and mortality (Rissanen et al., 1989), the lowest segment of the J-shaped curve, denoting the AC mortality-optimal BMI range (defined by the authors as the range of the BMIs associated with MRs of 1.0 or less), shifts to the right after age 54. On the other hand, in the recently published report on BMI and patterns of mortality among Seventh-Day Adventist men (Lindsted, Tonstad, & Kuzma, 1991), there was no evidence for a J-shaped relationship between BMI and mortality. Although the protective effect associated with the lowest BMI quintile (<22.3 kg/m^2) decreased slightly with increasing age for

TABLE 1.3. All-Cause (AC) Mortality-Optimal BMI Ranges for Nonsmoking Men and Women of All Ages (Studies Conducted in the United States)

Study	Author(s)	Number of subjects[a]	Duration of study	AC mortality-optimal BMI (kg/m^2) ranges
American Cancer Society study	Lew & Garfinkel (1979)	336,442 men 410,060 women	13 years 13 years	19.8–22.1 18.8–20.9
Framingham Heart Study	Garrison et al. (1983)	2,252 men 2,818 women	26 years 26 years	22.0–24.0 21.5–23.4
Seventh-Day Adventist study[b]	Lindsted et al. (1991)	8,828 men	26 years	<22.3

[a]Nonsmoking study subjects were drawn from overall numbers of men and women who participated.

[b]Because of their distinctive lifestyle, Seventh-Day Adventists constitute a highly selected population with a significantly lower mortality than the general population.

AC mortality, this quintile continued to be associated with an optimal MR between the ages of 50 and 90 years.

Disease-Specific Mortality

As regards disease-specific mortality, a number of epidemiological studies have demonstrated a nearly linear increase in mortality from CVD with increments in BMI among both men and women. The Finnish study (Rissanen et al., 1989) disclosed such a relationship between BMI and CVD; in contrast, the mortality rate from cancer among Finnish men did not rise as BMI increased (Figure 1.1).

In the American Cancer Society study conducted on 750,000 men and women (Lew & Garfinkel, 1979), a 13-year follow-up disclosed that CHD was the major factor in the higher mortality of overweight individuals. Mortality was 55% higher among those whose RWs were 30–40% heavier than average (with BMIs ranging from about 30 to 34), and about 100% higher in those more than 40% overweight (BMI > 34 kg/m^2).

Cancer mortality was increased only among those who were 40% or more overweight. In the American Cancer Society study, the principal sites of excess cancer mortality among men were cancer of the colon and rectum. Among severely overweight women, the major causes of excess cancer mortality were cancer of the gallbladder and biliary passages, breast, cervix, endometrium, and ovary.

The highest disease-specific MRs among overweight individuals of both sexes were caused by diabetes. For men who were 40% or more above average weight for height (BMI > 35 kg/m^2), the ratio was greater than 500%; for women 40% or more above average weight (BMI > 33 kg/m^2), the ratio was about 800%.

Cerebrovascular disease mortality was significantly elevated among overweight men and women. Among men who were 40% or more above average weight (BMI > 35 kg/m^2), the cerebrovascular MR was 225%. For similarly overweight women, the cerebrovascular MR was 150%.

Morbidity Risk

The second National Health and Nutrition Examination Survey (NHANES II), conducted during 1976–1980, revealed that, based on prevalence findings, overweight adults (namely, those with a BMI at or above the 85th percentile of a reference population of U.S. men and nonpregnant women 20–29 years of age[2]) are subject to a significantly enhanced risk of developing hypertension, diabetes, and hypercholesterolemia (VanItallie, 1985). As shown in Table 1.4,

---

[2]By this criterion, men with a BMI > 27.8 kg/m^2 and women with a BMI > 27.3 kg/m^2 were considered to be overweight (VanItallie, 1985).

TABLE 1.4. Relative Risk Ratios for Overweight American Adults

	Age ranges		
	20–74	20–44	45–74
Hypertension	2.9	5.6	1.9
Diabetes mellitus	2.9	3.8	2.1
Hypercholesterolemia	1.5	2.1	1.1

Note. "Relative risk ratio" is the prevalence of a health problem among overweight persons divided by prevalence of the same problem among nonoverweight persons in the same population and within the same age range. From data reported in VanItallie (1985).

the relative risk of hypertension for overweight American adults aged 20 to 75 years was 2.9. Interestingly, among overweight adults aged 20 to 45 years, the relative risk of having hypertension was 5.6. In contrast, among overweight Americans aged 45 to 75 years, the relative risk of having hypertension was only twice that for nonoverweight people within the same age category.

As the table indicates, among overweight Americans aged 20 to 45 years, the relative (prevalence) risk of having NIDDM was 3.8, while that of having an elevated cholesterol level was 2.1.

Hypertension, NIDDM, and hypercholesterolemia are risk factors or risk attributes closely associated with the overweight condition. However, because many overweight/obese individuals do not exhibit these risk factors, efforts have been made to identify other chacteristics of overweight individuals that can predict risk of subsequent illness and premature death with enhanced sensitivity and specificity. As mentioned earlier, there is evidence suggesting that the presence of a particular pattern of regional fat distribution—namely, upper body or abdominal obesity—is a better predictor than BMI alone of hypertension, hyperlipidemia, and NIDDM. It also appears that the body's content of visceral fat ("visceral obesity") may prove to be an even better predictor than pattern of regional fat distribution of metabolic complications of overweight (Fujioka, Matsuzawa, Tokunaga, & Tarui, 1987; Despres et al., 1990). Unfortunately, at the present time, there is insufficient information about the extent to which pattern of regional fat distribution (as inferred from WHR) is superior to BMI or to skinfold thickness measures as a predictor of a variety of health risks.

Grundy and Barnett (1990) have proposed that "overnutrition" produces clinical disease ". . . only in individuals who already possess a metabolic weakness or 'defect' in a given system. In the absence of such underlying defects, overnutrition or obesity is well tolerated" (p. 645). If their view is correct, then one of the reasons why certain overweight individuals do not develop obesity-related risk factors such as hypertension, diabetes, or hyperlipidemia is that they do not suffer from the latent metabolic insufficiencies that would render them vulnerable to the stresses imposed by obesity.

Cardiovascular Disease

Almost all prospective studies concerned with the relation between overweight and present or subsequent health status have clearly shown that overweight individuals have an increased risk of developing premature heart disease. This should not come as any surprise, inasmuch as hypertension, diabetes, and hypercholesteremia, more commonly found among the overweight, are important risk factors for CHD.

Findings from the Framingham Heart Study, representing the results of a 26-year follow-up, have disclosed that men and women who were 10% or more overweight by 1959 Met Life standards (BMI = 24.4 kg/m^2 or more) when they entered the study had an increased risk in later life of developing premature CVD (Hubert, Feinleib, McNamara, & Castelli, 1983). Thus, the Framingham Study indicates that even a modest degree of overweight in early adult life can significantly increase the risk of developing heart disease in middle age and subsequently. In a recently reported prospective study of obesity and risk of CHD in women, Manson et al. (1990) found that for increasing levels of current BMI (<21, 21-<23, 23-<25, 25-<29, and 29 + kg/m^2), age- and cigarette-smoking-adjusted relative risks of combined nonfatal myocardial infarction and fatal CHD were 1.0, 1.3, 1.3, 1.8, and 3.3, respectively. Thus, during 8 years of follow-up of participants in the so-called Nurses' Cohort Study of 115,886 U.S. women who were 30 to 55 years of age and free of diagnosed CHD, stroke, and cancer in 1976, it was determined that even mild to moderate overweight is associated with an increase in CHD risk in middle-aged women.

Non-Insulin-Dependent Diabetes Mellitus

NIDDM is a disease in its own right, as well as being a risk factor for other health problems (the same can be said for hypertension and some types of hyperlipidemia). About 70% to 80% of NIDDM patients are overweight; moreover, up to 60% of severely overweight individuals eventually develop NIDDM (Grundy & Barnett, 1990). Studies of identical twins have shown that genetic factors are involved in the pathogenesis of NIDDM (Barnett, Eff, & Leslie, 1981). Postulated inherited metabolic derangements that could contribute, singly or in combination, to the development of NIDDM include (1) peripheral insulin resistance (Prager, Wallace, & Olefsky, 1986); (2) inadequate insulin secretion by pancreatic beta cells (insufficient to permit normal glucose disposal) (Ward, Bolgiano, McKnight, Halter, & Porte, 1984); and (3) overproduction of glucose by the liver (Glauber, Wallace, & Bretchel, 1987).

Grundy and Barnett (1990) point out that, in individuals who are genetically prone to NIDDM, a high calorie diet and an increasing burden of depot fat "may tip the balance toward overt diabetes" (pp. 672–673). As Grundy and Barnett (1990) suggest, possible mechanisms by which a chronically positive energy balance and excessive fat stores could compromise further an already vulnerable glucose metabolism include (1) accentuation of peripheral resistance (in muscle as well as in fat cells); (2) overload of metabolic disposal systems by diet-derived substrates; and (3) paradoxical reduction in insulin secretion, possibly mediated by prolonged hyperglycemia (perhaps via glycosylation damage to islet cells).

The point to be made here is that patients with a family history of NIDDM may be especially vulnerable to the diabetogenic effect of overweight. In contrast, individuals without such a family history may be relatively resistant to this overweight-related complication. Yet, however appealing it may be, the foregoing explanation of how environmental and genetic factors can interact in the pathogenesis of NIDDM needs to be reconciled with the growing body of evidence that patients with visceral obesity are especially likely to develop diabetes (Fujimoto, Newell-Morris, & Shuman, 1991). Inasmuch as pattern of regional fat distribution also may be in part inherited (Bouchard et al., 1990), it is unclear at present where the genetic factors that determine the vulnerability of certain patients to obesity-precipitated or obesity-exacerbated NIDDM predominate.

It is noteworthy that members of certain races (e.g., Native Americans, Hispanics) are especially susceptible to developing both obesity and diabetes. If diabetes rates among white Americans are used as the benchmark, the relative risk of developing diabetes among the Pima Indians in the American Southwest is almost 11-fold (U.S. Department of Health and Human Services, 1986). This extraordinarily high incidence of NIDDM is closely related to the Pimas' remarkable predisposition to become obese. It has been theorized that Native Americans (who for many millenia lived as hunters and gatherers) developed by natural selection a genetic trait (or traits) for efficient energy conservation (a "thrifty genotype") that was advantageous to survival under conditions of chronic food scarcity (Neel, 1962).

Hypertension

Obesity can cause or aggravate hypertension, as suggested by the fact that in many instances, the successful treatment of obesity (even without a reduction in salt intake) will result in blood pressure normalization among previously hypertensive individuals. Indeed, about 48% of hypertension among white members of the U.S. population has been attributed to obesity (Tyroler, Heyden, & Hames, 1975).

The mechanisms by which obesity might promote hypertension have been widely discussed and studied. Possible mechanisms to explain the association of obesity and hypertension include elevated cardiac output; increased body sodium as a result of hyperinsulinemia or abnormal aldosterone–renin relationships; and neuroendocrine abnormalities arising from increased noradrenergic activity or opiate suppression (Dustan, 1983). It is also possible that on occasion, the peripheral insulin resistance associated with obesity may interfere with potassium uptake by smooth muscle cells, thereby enhancing vascular tone (DeFronzo, 1988). Such increased tone, combined with an increased cardiac output, could cause an elevation of blood pressure (Grundy & Barnett, 1990).

Many obese individuals are not hypertensive; this fact suggests that in some people, blood pressure is especially responsive to the effects of worsening adiposity, an increasing BMI (which could include enlargement of the FFM), or an increasing accumulation of visceral fat. It is conceivable that nonobese, nonhypertensive individuals with a family history of high blood pressure have an enhanced risk of becoming hypertensive as they acquire excess weight. Although firm evidence to support this notion is lacking, it would seem especially prudent for individuals who are at risk of becoming hypertensive—for example, those with borderline hypertension, with gestational hypertension, with a family history of hypertension, or with a tendency to deposit excess fat in the upper segment—to avoid becoming overweight.

Cholesterol Gallstones

As Bennion and Grundy (1978) have emphasized, obesity is a potent risk factor for the development of cholesterol gallstones. It is now well established that obesity is associated with enhancement of biliary secretion of cholesterol. (Estrogenic hormones also appear to increase the rate of cholesterol transfer into the bile.) However, despite the finding that synthesis of cholesterol in the body is directly related to body weight (Bennion & Grundy, 1975), many obese persons do not develop gallstones. As suggested by Grundy and Barnett (1990), other contributing factors also may have to be present before gallstones can develop. Among these factors is a possible defect in bile acid metabolism. The resulting decrease in hepatic excretion of bile acids, particularly in combination with an increased secretion of biliary cholesterol, gives rise to supersaturated or "lithogenic" bile (Grundy, Metzger, & Adler, 1972). But for actual lithogenesis to occur, such supersaturated bile may further require the presence of crystals that can serve as a nidus for stone formation. As reported by Holzbach, Marsh, Olszewski, and Holan (1973), some people can maintain a supersaturated bile and yet not develop gallstones. These individuals rarely if ever have cholesterol crystals in their bile. In contrast, it is usually possible to demonstrate crystals in the bile of individuals who are known to be gallstone formers (Sedaghat & Grundy, 1980). Grundy and Barnett (1990) have hypothesized that "crystal formers" may lack a key protein that helps maintain cholesterol in solution (Holzbach et al., 1984).

For the purposes of this chapter, the importance of the foregoing information lies in the suggestion that obesity may promote cholesterol gallstone formation in a metabolically vulnerable subset of the population by virtue of enhancement of biliary secretion of cholesterol. Unfortunately, knowledge that such metabolic susceptibility may exist does not help physicians identify susceptible patients prospectively. Yet it seems likely that obesity superadded to other risk factors, such as pregnancy, femaleness, treatment with certain drugs (e.g., clofibrate or estrogen), a family history of cholelithiasis, or membership in a gallstone-prone race (e.g., Pima Indian), could be responsible for precipitating (in several senses) cholesterol cholelithiasis.

Other Obesity-Related Health Problems

There are many other health disorders and problems that may be caused or made worse by obesity (VanItallie, 1979). Some of these are listed by system in Table 1.5.

People with coronary atherosclerosis are more likely to have angina pectoris if they are also overweight. In some instances, the angina can be ameliorated by some degree of weight reduction. Individuals who are overweight and have left ventricular hypertrophy are more likely than the nonoverweight to exhibit frequent ventricular premature contractions. Such ectopy may contribute to the increased incidence of sudden death observed among the obese (Messerli, Nunez, Ventura, & Snyder, 1987).

In people with underlying heart disease, obesity increases the risk of developing congestive heart failure. Obese individuals are more likely than the nonobese to experience a variety of problems arising from venous stasis—notably, varicose veins in the lower extremities, hemorrhoids, and thromboembolic disease.

Most patients who develop obstructive sleep apnea are obese, hypertensive men who eventually develop cardiovascular abnormalities. Unfortunately, weight reduction in obese patients with sleep apnea may result in only limited and variable improvement of the condition; nevertheless, a serious effort should be made to help such patients lose weight (Kales, Vela-Bueno, & Kales, 1987).

Overweight people have an enhanced risk of having hyperuricemia and of developing gout.

Severely obese people are likely to have numerous skin problems, such as intertrigo and acanthosis nigricans. If they already have osteoarthritis of the weight-bearing joints, the arthritic symptoms are aggravated by obesity, which also shifts the body's center of gravity and thereby puts undue stress on the joints and muscles of the lower extremities and the lower back.

Women who are overweight are prone to menstrual problems; moreover, if they become pregnant, the pregnancy is more likely to terminate with a stillbirth.

The physical agility of severely obese individuals is often impaired, and when they fall, the resulting injury is more severe.

The presence of marked obesity may interfere with the physical examination conducted by the physician; thus, important diagnoses may be missed or delayed. When obese patients are subjected to surgery and anesthesia, the risk of complications from these procedures is enhanced.

Estimation of Health and Mortality Risk in the Overweight Patient

Explaining the Concept of Relative Risk to the Patient

One way of explaining the concept of mortality and/or morbidity risk to an overweight patient is in terms of some sort of relative risk ratio. Such a ratio could be described as involving comparison of the patient's actuarial risk of dying (or of developing an illness such as NIDDM) with the estimated risk that same patient would carry if he or she were not overweight. Thus, one might tell an otherwise healthy white female patient aged 40–49, with a BMI of 32.9 kg/m^2 or greater, that her risk of dying over some specified period of time would be approximately double that of a woman who was just like her except for having a BMI of 23.5 kg/m^2.

This is by no means the same thing as implying that death is imminent. Perhaps a better way of communicating the concept of health risk is by analogy with airline safety records. If airline A consistently has an accident rate double that of an otherwise comparable carrier (airline B), one would prefer to fly by airline B. In either case, the predicted risk of having an accident is small, but it is substantially lower in airline B.

In Table 1.6, magnitude of decrease in life expectancy in relation to MR is shown for middle-aged men with various risk attributes, including severe overweight. Note that, as the men get older, the ratio of the decrease in life expectancy to MR increases. If one were to express these decreases in life expectancy as percentages of remaining life expectancy rather than in years, the values for such percentages would rise substantially with advancing age.

The assessment of risk in any given patient can never be better than an estimate or an "educated guess." Risk ratios are usually derived from epidemiological studies that have all sorts of limitations and imperfections. Yet the results of a number of large or lengthy morbidity and mortality investigations have been sufficiently consonant to generate confidence in their approximate validity.

Calculating Relative Risk

When attempting to estimate the extra burden of risk placed on a patient by the presence of some degree of overweight, the physician must take into account such modifying factors as the duration of the overweight; the patient's race; personal health habits (use of cigarettes and ethanol); overall health status; physical activity level; family history of relevant illness; the presence of

TABLE 1.5. Some Health Disorders and Other Problems Thought to Be Caused or Exacerbated by Obesity

Heart
    Premature coronary heart disease
    Left ventricular hypertrophy
    Angina pectoris
    Sudden death (ventricular arrhythmia)
    Congestive heart failure

Vascular system
    Hypertension
    Stroke (cerebral infarction and/or hemorrhage)
    Venous stasis (with lower extremity edema, varicose veins, hemorrhoids, thromboembolic disease involving lower extremities and inferior vena cava)

Respiratory system
    Obstructive sleep apnea
    Pickwickian syndrome (alveolar hypoventilation)
    Secondary polycythemia
    Right ventricular hypertrophy (sometimes leading to failure)

Hepatobiliary system
    Cholelithiasis and cholecystitis
    Hepatic steatosis

Hormonal and metabolic functions
    Diabetes mellitus (insulin-independent)
    Gout (hyperuricemia)
    Hyperlipidemias (hypertriglyceridemia and hypercholesterolemia)

Kidney
    Proteinuria and, in very severe obesity, nephrosis
    Renal vein thrombosis

Skin
    Striae
    Acanthosis nigricans (benign type)
    Hirsutism
    Intertrigo
    Plantar callus
    Multiple papillomas

Joints, muscles, and connective tissue
    Osteoarthritis of knees
    Bone spurs of the heel
    Osteoarthrosis of spine (in women)
    Aggravation of pre-existing postural faults

Neoplasia
    Among women: increased risk of cancer of endometrium, breast, cervix, ovary, gallbladder, and biliary passages
    Among men: increased risk of cancer of colon, rectum, and prostate

Reproductive and sexual function
    Impaired obstetric performance (increased risk of toxemia, hypertension, and diabetes mellitus during pregnancy; prolonged labor; need for cesarean section more frequent)
    Irregular menstruation and frequent anovulatory cycles
    Reduced fertility

TABLE 1.5. (continued)

Psychosocial function
Impairment of self-image with feelings of inferiority
Social isolation
Subject to social, economic, and other types of discrimination
Susceptibility to psychoneuroses
Loss of mobility
Increased employee absenteeism
Miscellaneous
Increased surgical and anesthetic risks
Reduced physical agility and increased accident proneness
Interference with diagnosis of other disorders

Note. Adapted from "Obesity: Adverse Effects on Health and Longevity" (p. 2275) by T. B. VanItallie, 1979, *American Journal of Clinical Nutrition, 32,* 2723-2733. Copyright 1979 by American Society for Clinical Nutrition, Inc. Adapted by permission.

obesity-related risk factors such as hypertension, hyperlipidemia (including high density lipoprotein [HDL] cholesterol status), or NIDDM; and the regional pattern of fat distribution.

One practical method for dealing with some of these modifying factors is to incorporate them into the risk assessment after an MR or morbidity ratio has been provisionally determined on the basis of BMI, sex, and age. However, one has to be aware that the value obtained for a relative risk ratio is critically dependent on the nature of the reference population. For example, if the "average" BMI of a source population is used as the denominator, the relative risk ratio will be lower than it would be if the overall source population were divided into BMI quintiles, with quintile V being compared with quintile I. Also, since "optimal" BMI is generally lower than average BMI, the use of

TABLE 1.6. Mortality Ratios and Decreases in Life Expectancy among Middle-Aged Men with Various Risk Attributes

	MR (%)			Decrease in life expectancy (yr)		
Risk attribute	Age: 45	55	60	Age: 45	55	60
Severe overweight (150% of average)	200	175	150	2.0	2.0	2.0
Hypertension (148-157/88-97)	200	175	175	2.0	2.0	4.0
Diabetes mellitus (treated with oral agents)	200	200	175	1.5	2.0	4.0
Organic apical systolic murmur	200	200	—	1.5	2.5	—

Note. Based on mortality experience of otherwise healthy insured lives studied between 1954 and 1974. Data from Lew and Gajewski (1990).

optimal BMI in calcuating risk ratios would shift upward the range of numerical values for such ratios.

Some Factors That Modify the Risk Calculation

Duration of Follow-Up

As shown in the Build Study 1979 (Society of Actuaries and the Association of Life Insurance Medical Directors of America, 1980) and other investigations (Rabkin, Mathewson, & Hsu, 1977; Hubert et al., 1983), the morbidity ratios and MRs exhibited by overweight men and women tend to increase with the duration of follow-up. Thus, in the Build Study 1979, men with BMIs of 29.2–31.8 had a mortality ratio of 106% during the first 5 years. With a duration of 16–22 years, the ratio rose to 131%.

Confounding Effect of Cigarette Smoking

Nonoverweight people are more likely than overweight people to smoke cigarettes, the ratio being about 1.3 among white American men and women (Higgins & D'Agostino, 1991). Thus, in mortality investigations (e.g., the Build Study 1979) that lack information permitting a distinction to be made between smokers and nonsmokers, the true relative mortality of the overweight is further understated, owing to the extra health risk incurred by the margin of nonoverweight versus overweight smokers in the study population.

Risk in Relation to Age

Morbidity ratios and MRs also may be affected by age. As shown in Table 1.4, the relative risks of developing hypertension, diabetes, or hypercholesterolemia are substantially lower in overweight Americans aged 45 to 75 than in comparably overweight Americans aged 20 to 45 (VanItallie, 1985). This observation does not necessarily mean that the accumulation of years somehow protects people from the adverse affects of overweight. The findings shown in the table must also be considered in light of the abundant evidence that as people get older, they are increasingly likely to develop health problems such as hypertension and diabetes in the absence of overt overweight.

When one examines the MRs exhibited by overweight individuals in different age categories, these ratios tend to diminish as people get older, as indicated by the findings of the American Cancer Society study (Lew & Garfinkel, 1979) (see Figure 1.2). When one is attempting to analyze the relationship of advancing age to relative mortality, it is preferable to use data such as those generated by the American Cancer Society study rather than rely on mortality data based on life insurance policies. One problem with life insurance data is that, as people get older, their ability to pass a life insurance medical examination decreases. Indeed, the rejection rate of people purchasing

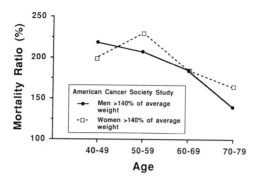

FIGURE 1.2. Diminution of MRs with advancing age among overweight men and women, as reported in the American Cancer Society study. The data are from Lew (1985).

life insurance at ages 60 and older may run from 10% to 25%, as compared with about 2% for all ages combined. Clearly, middle-aged and elderly individuals who have been accepted for life insurance cannot be considered representative of the population at large (Lew, 1977). As one example, 65-year-old men accepted for standard life insurance have recently exhibited death rates of only about 19 per 1000, as compared with about 27 per 1000 among corresponding white men in the general population (Society of Actuaries, 1982).

In the Finnish study (Rissanen et al,, 1989), when cigarette smoking was adjusted for, men with BMIs of 31.0–33.9 kg/m² exhibited the following AC MRs (based on a reference BMI of 22.0–24.9 kg/m²): 130% for those 25–44 years of age; 120% for those 45–54; 110% for those 55–64; 110% for those 65–74; and 120% for those 75 and older. CVD MRs in this same cohort were as follows: 100% for those 25–44 years of age; 160% for those 45–54; 130% for those 55–64; 120% for those 65–74; and 100% for those 75 and older. AC and CVD MRs in severely overweight Finnish men (BMI > 34.0) in relation to age are shown in Figure 1.3.

Stature

A great deal of evidence has accumulated that in humans, genotype is a major determinant of stature. As far back as the turn of the century, Galton (1886a, 1886b) and Pearson (1903) described a very high correlation between the heights of sons and fathers. On the other hand, a host of investigations conducted over the years have shown conclusively that certain environmental influences, particularly a diet chronically restricted in energy content, can significantly hinder normal growth and thereby prevent an individual from realizing his or her genetic potential as regards stature (Johnson, 1979).

Mortality investigations of large numbers of persons according to height are more recent. In the Build and Blood Pressure Study 1959 (Society of Actuaries, 1959), which covered 4 million insured lives, it was found that the

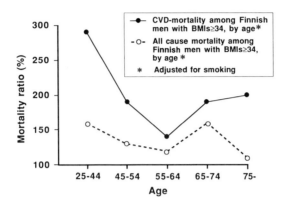

FIGURE 1.3. Comparison of all-cause (AC) mortality with CVD mortality in severely overweight Finnish men (BMI > 34 kg/m^2) by age. The data are from Rissanen et al. (1989).

death rates from all causes among men 40 and older were about 10% higher among those under 160 cm (5 feet, 3 inches) in height than among those 170 cm (5 feet, 7 inches) and taller. In the equally large Build Study 1979, the differential was smaller, being on the order of 5%.

In the monumental study conducted by Waaler (1984), the mortality experience of 1.7 million Norwegians (involving over 18 million observation-years) was related to their height and weight measurements taken during compulsory mass examinations for tuberculosis between 1963 and 1975. The observation period used in the survey covered the years 1963–1979, during which 176,574 deaths occurred.

The Norwegian study showed that for both sexes and for all ages, there was a clear reduction in mortality as height increased. Waaler found that among women 40–44 years of age, the mortality rate was halved when height increased from 145–149 cm (4 feet, 9 inches to 4 feet, 11 inches) to 165–169 cm (5 feet, 5 inches to 5 feet, 6½ inches). For men, the mortality rate was halved when height increased from 150–155 cm (4 feet, 11 inches to 5 feet, 1 inch) to 185–189 cm (6 feet, 1 inch to 6 feet, 2½ inches). The excess mortality associated with short stature was to a considerable degree attributable to obstructive lung diseases, tuberculosis, and stomach and lung cancer. Accordingly, Waaler suggested that the negative association of body height and mortality might result in large part from a past socioeconomic history marked by poverty, chronic ill health, a poor diet, or an unhealthy lifestyle.

Although the association between height and mortality in the Norwegian study is striking, Waaler (1984) cautioned: ". . . one should remember that there are relatively few individuals who are so short that they have a marked excess mortality" (p. 17). As he pointed out, 50% excess risk owing to short stature was observed in only 2–8% of the Norwegian cohort, depending on age and sex.

Based on data collected during the Physicians' Health Study, an ongoing survey of over 22,000 doctors, Hebert et al. (1991) recently reported that male physicians 170 cm (5 feet, 7 inches) or shorter had experienced significantly more heart attacks than those 185 cm (6 feet, 1 inch) and taller. (Incidentally, overweight was more prevalent among the short than among the tall physicians.) After Hebert et al. had adjusted for high cholesterol levels, smoking, diabetes, elevated blood pressure, parental history of heart attack, alcohol use, exercise frequency, age, and prophylactic use of aspirin, they still found about a 60% higher risk of first heart attack among the shortest compared to the tallest men.

More curious are the findings of a number of investigators about the incidence of cancer in short and tall men. In 1988, Albanes, Jones, Schatzkin, Micozzi, and Taylor reported on the relationship between adult stature and cancer incidence using data from the first National Health and Nutrition Examination Survey (NHANES I), conducted in 1971–1974 (National Center for Health Statistics, 1979), and its follow-up study (Madans et al., 1986). Albanes et al. (1988) found that among 12,554 participants, there was a significant lowering in the relative risk of all-sites cancer among men in the shortest quartile of stature as compared to taller men, and a lesser reduction in risk among women in the shortest quartile of stature compared to taller women. Among short women, the reduced risk was restricted primarily to cancer of the breast and colon/rectum.

The findings of the American Cancer Society study on adult stature and risk of cancer (Lew, 1988), as well as those of the Build Study 1979 (Lew, 1988), are consonant with the observations of Albanes et al. (1988). However, the decreases in cancer mortality among short men as compared to tall men disclosed by these two studies (Lew, 1988) were smaller than those described by Albanes and colleagues. Data available from the Build Study 1979 (Lew, 1988) also indicate the possibility that the increased relative risk of developing cancer exhibited by tall men may be augmented by overweight.

The basis for the relationship between stature and risk of cancer is presently unclear. Two facts may be relevant. First (as mentioned earlier), it is widely recognized by nutrition scientists that retardation of linear growth (resulting in shorter stature) is a frequent response to prolonged caloric privation during maturation (Johnson, 1979). Second, animal experiments have repeatedly shown that cancer arises less frequently and is usually harder to induce in chronically underfed rodents than in rodents maintained on an *ad libitum* diet (Tannenbaum, 1947; Albanes, 1987; Rogers & Longnecker, 1988).

Pattern of Fat Distribution

Several longitudinal studies have now shown that the presence of upper body obesity enhances the risk of CHD exhibited by the overweight (Larsson, 1991). In the Framingham Heart Study, the 34-year incidence of CHD for men and women was examined in relation to subscapular skinfold thickness, taken to be an index of upper body or truncal obesity (Higgins & D'Agostino, 1991).

Within each tertile of BMI, the risk of CHD rose along with increasing subscapular skinfold thickness. In the Honolulu Heart Program, involving the study of about 8000 men of Japanese ancestry, a 12-year follow-up showed that within each BMI tertile, CHD risk was approximately doubled in the highest versus the lowest tertile of subscapular skinfold (Donahue, Abbott, Bloom, Reed, & Yano, 1987).

In their study of men born in 1913, Larsson et al. (1984) found that within each tertile of BMI, the risk of CHD was almost doubled in those with the highest compared to the lowest WHR. Accordng to Larsson et al., the highest risk was found for "lean men" with a high WHR. When follow-up of this cohort was extended to 18 years, the WHR was no longer a risk factor for CHD (Larsson, 1991). Thus, it seemed that as this group of subjects approached the age of 70, pattern of regional fat distribution rapidly lost its value as a predictor of CHD. Yet, according to Larsson (1991), the importance of upper body (abdominal) obesity is almost as great as that of the other major risk factors for CHD, such as smoking, hypertension, and hypercholesterolemia. In the study of men born in 1913, about 20% of CHD cases were regarded by Larsson et al. (1984) as being attributable to an increased WHR above tertile limit I (WHR > 0.9).

Analysis of Morbidity and Mortality Data

The commonest approach to survival analysis is to focus on mortality at a critical period, such as at the end of 5 or 10 years, and to consider a number of explanatory variables. Dependence on explanatory variables—treatments, characteristics of individuals, or specific outside influences—requires some formulation of the relationships between the variables considered and the outcome observed. This formulation is usually expressed in the form of mathematical models.

The so-called "proportional hazards model" is among the most widely used in the study of the relationships between death rates and explanatory variables. As regards analysis of morbidity data, the proportional hazards model can be used to assess the independent effect of overweight/obesity on the risk of CHD (for example) in the presence of other risk factors, such as cigarette smoking or excessive ethanol consumption. Those interested in this or other mathematical models should refer to books or papers dealing with analysis of survival data (see Cox & Oakes, 1984; Lee, 1980).

The Obesity Workup: Risk-Related Considerations

In the assessment of health and mortality risks in a patient who is overweight, the physician must first of all rely on the results of an obesity-oriented medical history and physical examination, as well as suitable laboratory tests. From the

TABLE 1.7. The Obesity Workup: Some Risk-Oriented Considerations

Weight history: age of onset, duration, severity of overweight
Family history of overweight
Family history of obesity-relevant health problems (see Tables 1.2 and 1.5)
Personal history of obesity-relevant health problems
Race (Native American, Hispanic, African-American, etc.)
BMI (kg/m^2)
Pattern of regional fat distribution (WHR; subscapular skinfold thickness)
Body fat content as determined by a body composition method
Presence on physical examination of one or more obesity-relevant health problems
Laboratory evidence of obesity-relevant health problems
Assessment of overall health status: Is the patient in ostensibly good health?

medical examination, the physician can then arrive at a diagnosis that takes into account considerations such as those listed in Table 1.7. A sample diagnosis of this kind could be formulated along the following lines:

> Severe obesity (BMI = 34) of the upper body type (WHR = 1.2) in a 45-year-old man. The obesity had its onset immediately prior to adolescence and has been most severe since age 40. Obesity-relevant problems disclosed by the medical examination include hypertension (180/100 mm Hg); moderate elevation of LDL cholesterol (136–160 mg/dl) and reduction of HDL cholesterol (30–40 mg/dl); and a history of substernal discomfort during moderate physical exertion. Fasting blood glucose and resting electrocardiogram are within normal limits.

Once an obesity-oriented diagnosis has been assembled, the physician can proceed with a risk assessment based on information generated about the patient, considered in the light of available epidemiological evidence that relates risk to such markers as BMI and pattern of regional fat distribution.

If the BMI were the only factor to be considered in risk assessment of the overweight patient, the job would be relatively easy; however, as we have seen, the relation between BMI and risk may be subject to material modification by a variety of other factors, including sex, age, duration of overweight, pattern of fat distribution, general health status (in "ostensibly good health"), and the presence of certain putative metabolic "weaknesses."

Most of the information available to us about the relation of overweight to health and mortality risk has been derived from studies that used either RW or BMI as the index of overweight. Hence, in the present analysis of overweight in relation to risk, the BMI (which can be derived from RW) is used whenever possible as the point of departure. (In the future, another marker such as visceral obesity may take primacy.)

Estimation of Relative Risk in the Individual Patient

In order to obtain a common basis for comparing the findings of different mortality and morbidity investigations, we have translated the RW data reported in the American Cancer Society study (Lew & Garfinkel, 1979; Lew, 1985) into BMI values. BMI ranges associated with the lowest mortality experience for each sex have been designated "AC mortality-optimal" and assigned an MR of 100%. MRs in excess of 100%, associated with higher BMIs, have been recalculated using this new benchmark.

Figure 1.4 shows the adjusted MRs for men and women associated with various BMIs for all ages combined. For reasons mentioned earlier, these ratios understate somewhat the true relative mortality of overweight. In assessing the overweight patient, the physician can use Figure 1.4 to make a preliminary rating of the patient's mortality risk. However, it then becomes necessary to consider how other factors might worsen or mitigate the risk. Although the effect of these "modifiers" on risk (either singly or in aggregate) cannot be quantified, given our present state of knowledge, there is abundant evidence to indicate that they should always be taken into account when a risk assessment of the patient is being made.

Some of the more important risk-modifying factors are shown in Table 1.8, together with an indication of the direction in which each would be expected to displace the risk ratio. It seems reasonable to suggest that for any given BMI in excess of the AC mortality-optimal range, a patient's mortality risk is likely to be increased by the presence of one of the augmenting factors shown in the table. Indeed, it is probable that the risk will rise in some proportion to the number of such factors present. Conversely, if the patient

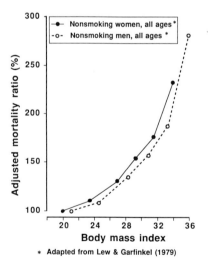

FIGURE 1.4. MRs in relation to BMI of nonsmoking men and women of all ages who participated in the American Cancer Society study (Lew & Garfinkel, 1979). In this figure, relative weights reported in the study have been translated into BMIs, and MRs in relation to relative weight (Lew, 1985) have been recalculated, with the lowest MR for each relative weight category assigned a value of 100%.

Risk Assessment in the Overweight Patient

TABLE 1.8. Some Modifiers of BMI-Associated Morbidity and/or Mortality Risk

Abaters	Augmenters
Lower body (femoral–gluteal) fat distribution pattern	Upper body (abdominal) fat distribution pattern
Ostensibly good health	Impaired health
Absence of obesity-related risk factors	Presence of one or more obesity-related risk factors
Middle-aged or elderly	Young adult (20–45 years of age)
Female	Male
Absence of a family history of obesity-relevant illness	Presence of a family history of obesity-relevant illness
Obesity of brief duration	Obesity of prolonged duration
Membership in a race not known to be vulnerable to obesity-associated health problems	Membership in a race known to be vulnerable to obesity-associated health problems (e.g., NIDDM vulnerability in obese Pima Indians).
Above normal stature	Below normal stature

exhibits a preponderance of abating factors, the risk should be correspondingly reduced.

How can the physician use the kind of information shown in Figure 1.4 and Table 1.8 to arrive at a clinical judgment? As one example, prompt treatment to reduce body fat content is indicated in a 35-year-old male patient with a BMI of 34 kg/m^2 who has been severely overweight for 15 years; has a family history of diabetes; and is found to have a WHR of 1.2 (marked abdominal obesity), together with mild hypertension and borderline glucose intolerance.

In contrast, fat reduction treatment is not a high priority (and may not even be warranted) in a 35-year-old female patient in ostensibly good health with a BMI of 34 kg/m^2, who has been severely overweight for 5 years; has no family history of obesity-relevant illness; and is found to have a WHR of 0.6 (femoral–gluteal obesity), normal systolic and diastolic blood pressures, normal glucose–insulin tolerance, a nonatherogenic serum lipid profile, and no clinical evidence of other obesity-related health problems.

References

Actuarial Society of America and the Association of Life Insurance Medical Directors. (1912). *The medical–actuarial mortality investigation* (Vols. I–V). New York: Authors.
Albanes, D. (1987). Total calories, body weight, and tumor incidence in mice. *Cancer Research, 47*, 1987–1992.
Albanes, D., Jones, D. Y., Schatzkin, A., Micozzi, M. S., & Taylor, P. R. (1988). Adult stature and risk of cancer. *Cancer Research, 48*, 1658–1662.

Barnett, A. H., Eff, C., & Leslie, R. D. G. (1981). Diabetes in identical twins. *Diabetologia, 20*, 87-93.

Benn, R. T. (1971). Some mathematical properties of weight-for-height indices used as measures of adiposity. *British Journal of Preventive and Social Medicine, 25*, 42-50.

Bennion, L. J., & Grundy, S. M. (1975). Effects of obesity and caloric intake on biliary lipid metabolism in men. *Journal of Clinical Investigation, 56*, 996-1011.

Bennion, L. J., & Grundy, S. M. (1978). Risk factors for the development of cholelithiasis in man. *New England Journal of Medicine, 299*, 1161-1167, 1221-1227.

Björntorp, P. (1987). Classification of obese patients and complications related to the distribution of surplus fat. *American Journal of Clinical Nutrition, 45*, 1120-1125.

Bouchard, C., Tremblay, A., Despres, J. P., Nadeau, A., Lupien, P. J., Theriault, G., Dussault, J., Moorjani, S., Pinault, S., & Fournier, G. (1990). The response to long-term overfeeding in identical twins. *New England Journal of Medicine, 322*, 1477-1482.

Cox, D. R., & Oakes, D. (1984). *Analysis of survival data*. London: Chapman & Hall.

DeFronzo, R. A. (1988). Obesity is associated with impaired insulin-mediated potassium uptake. *Metabolism, 37*, 105-108.

Despres, J. P., Moorjani, S., Lupien, P. J., Tremblay, A., Nadeau, A., & Bouchard, C. (1990). Regional distribution of body fat, plasma lipoproteins, and cardiovascular disease. *Arteriosclerosis, 10*, 497-511.

Donahue, R. P., Abbott, R. D., Bloom, E., Reed, D. M., & Yano, K. (1987). Central obesity and coronary heart disease in men. *Lancet, i*, 821-824.

Dustan, H. P. (1983). Mechanisms of hypertension associated with obesity. *Annals of Internal Medicine, 98*(P. 2), 860-864.

Fujimoto, W. Y., Newell-Morris, L. L., & Shuman, W. P. (1991). Intra-abdominal fat and risk variables for non-insulin-dependent diabetes (NIDDM) and coronary heart disease in Japanese American women with android or gynoid fat patterning. In Y. Oomura, S. Tarui, S. Inoue, & T. Shimazu (Eds.), *Progress in obesity research 1990* (pp. 317-322). London: John Libbey.

Fujioka, S., Matsuzawa, Y., Tokunaga, K., & Tarui, S. (1987). Contribution of intraabdominal fat accumulation to the impairment of glucose and lipid metabolism in human obesity. *Metabolism, 36*, 54-59.

Galton, F. (1886a). Regression toward mediocrity in hereditary stature. *Journal of the Anthropological Institute, 15*, 246-263.

Galton, F. (1886b). Family likeness in stature. *Proceedings of the Royal Society in London, 40*, 42-73.

Garrison, R. J., Feinleib, M., Castelli, W. P., & McNamara, P. M. (1983). Cigarette smoking as a confounder of the relationship between relative weight and long term mortality in the Framingham Study. *Journal of the American Medical Association, 249*, 2199-2203.

Glauber, H., Wallace, P., & Bretchel, G. (1987). Effects of fasting on plasma glucose and prolonged tracer measurement of hepatic glucose output in NIDDM. *Diabetes, 36*, 1187-1194.

Grundy, S. M., & Barnett, J. P. (1990). Metabolic and health complications of obesity. In R. C. Bone (Ed.), *Disease-a-month* (Vol. 36, No. 12, pp. 643-731). St. Louis: C. V. Mosby-Year Book.

Grundy, S. M., Metzger, A. L., & Adler, R. D. (1972). Mechanisms of lithogenic bile formation in American Indian women with cholesterol gallstones. *Journal of Clinical Investigation, 51*, 3026-3043.

Hebert, P. R., Rich-Edwards, J. W., Manson, J. E., Ridker, P. M., Buring, J. E., & Hennekens, C. H. (1991). Height and risk of future myocardial infarctions. *Circulation, 84*(4), II-35.

Higgins, M., & D'Agostino, R. (1991). Obesity and cardiovascular disease. In Y. Oomura, S. Tarui, S. Inoue, & T. Shimazu (Eds.), *Progress in obesity research 1990* (pp. 375-379). London: John Libbey.

Holzbach, R. T., Kibe, A., Thiel, E., Howell, J. H., Marsh, M., & Hermann, R. E. (1984). Biliary proteins: Unique inhibitors of cholesterol crystal nucleation in human gallbladder bile. *Journal of Clinical Investigation, 73*, 35-45.

Holzbach, R. T., Marsh, M., Olszewski, M., & Holan, K. (1973). Cholesterol solubility in bile:

Evidence that supersaturated bile is frequent in healthy man. *Journal of Clinical Investigation, 52*, 1467-1479.
Hubert, H. B., Feinleib, M., McNamara, P. M., & Castelli, W. P. (1983). Obesity as an independent risk factor for cardiovascular disease: A 26-year follow-up of participants in the Framingham Heart Study. *Circulation, 67*(5), 968-977.
Johnson, F. E. (1979). Nutrition and growth. In F. E. Johnson, A. F. Roche, & C. Suzanne (Eds.), *Human physical growth and maturation: Methodologies and factors* (pp. 291-301). New York: Plenum Press.
Kales, A., Vela-Bueno, A., & Kales, J. D. (1987). Sleep disorders: Sleep apnea and narcolepsy. *Annals of Internal Medicine, 106*, 434-443.
Keys, A., Fidanza, F., Karvonen, M. J., Kimura, N., & Taylor, H. L. (1972). Indices of relative weight and obesity. *Journal of Chronic Diseases, 25*, 329-343.
Lapidus, L., Bengtsson, C., Larsson, B., Pennert, K., Rybo, E., & Sjöström, L. (1984). Distribution of adipose tissue and risk of cardiovascular disease and death: A 12-year follow-up of participants in the population study of 1462 women in Gothenburg, Sweden. *British Medical Journal, 289*, 1257-1261.
Larsson, B. (1989, Sept. 11-13). *Morbidity and mortality data—overview of prospective studies including fat distribution.* Abstract in National Institutes of Health Workshop "Basic and Clinical Aspects of Regional Fat Distribution," Bethesda, MD, p. 85.
Larsson, B. (1991). Obesity, fat distribution and cardiovascular disease. In Y. Oomura, S. Tarui, S. Inoue, & T. Shimazu (Eds.), *Progress in obesity research 1990* (pp. 375-379). London: John Libbey.
Larsson, B., Svardsudd, K., Welin, L., Whilhelmsen, L., Björntorp, P., & Tibblin, G. (1984). Abdominal adipose tissue distribution, obesity, and risk of cardiovascular disease and death: 13-year follow-up of participants in the study of 792 men born in 1913. *British Medical Journal, 288*, 1401-1404.
Lee, E. T. (1980). *Statistical methods for survival analysis.* Belmont, CA: Lifetime Learning.
Lew, E. A. (1977). Some observations on mortality studies. *Journal of the Institute of Actuaries, 104*, 221-225.
Lew, E. A. (1985). Mortality and weight: Insured lives and the American Cancer Society studies. *Annals of Internal Medicine, 103*(6, Pt. 2), 1024-1029.
Lew, E. A. (1988). [Mortality from cancer by height and weight derived from Build Study 1979 material.] Unpublished raw data.
Lew, E. A., & Gajewski, J. (Eds.). (1990). *Medical risks: Mortality trends by age and time elapsed.* New York: Praeger.
Lew, E. A., & Garfinkel, L. (1979). Variations in mortality by weight among 750,000 men and women. *Journal of Chronic Diseases, 32*, 563-576.
Lindsted, K., Tonstad, S., & Kuzma, J. W. (1991). Body mass index and patterns of mortality among Seventh-Day Adventist men. *International Journal of Obesity, 15*, 397-406.
Madans, J. H., Kleinman, J. C., Cox, C. S., Barbano, H. E., Feldman, J. J., Cohen, B., Finucane, F. F., & Coroni-Huntley, J. (1986). Ten years after NHANES I: Report of initial followup, 1982-84. *Public Health Reports, 101*, 465-473.
Manson, J. E., Colditz, G. A., Stampfer, M. J., Willett, W. C., Rosner, B., Momson, R. R., Speizer, F. E., & Hennekens, C. H. (1990). A prospective study of obesity and risk of coronary heart disease in women. *New England Journal of Medicine, 372*, 882-889.
Manson, J. E., Stampfer, M. J., Hennekens, C. H., & Willett, W. C. (1987). Body weight and longevity. A reassessment. *Journal of the American Medical Association, 257*, 353-358.
Messerli, F. H., Nunez, B. D., Ventura, H. O., & Snyder, D. W. (1987). Overweight and sudden death: Increased ventricular ectopy in cardiopathy of obesity. *Archives of Internal Medicine, 147*, 1725-1728.
National Center for Health Statistics. (1979, May). *Weight and height of adults 18-74 years of age: United States, 1971-74* (DHEW Publication No. PHS 79-1659, Vital and Health Statistics, Vol. 11, No. 211). Washington, DC: U.S. Government Printing Office.

Neel, J. V. (1962). Diabetes mellitus: A "thrifty" genotype rendered detrimental by "progress." *American Journal of Human Genetics, 14,* 353-362.

Pearson, K. (1903). Laws of inheritance in man. I. Inheritance and physical characteristics. *Biometrika, 2,* 357-462.

Prager, R., Wallace, P., & Olefsky, J. M. (1986). In vivo kinetics of insulin action on peripheral glucose disposal and hepatic glucose output in normal and obese subjects. *Journal of Clinical Investigation, 78,* 427-481.

Quetelet, L. A. J. (1869). *Physique sociale* (Vol. 2). Brussels: C. Muquardt.

Rabkin, S. W., Mathewson, F. A. L., & Hsu, P. H. (1977). Relation of body weight to development of ischemic heart disease in a cohort of young North American men after a 26-year observation period: The Manitoba Study. *American Journal of Cardiology, 39,* 452-458.

Rissanen, A., Heliovaara, M., Knekt, P., Aromaa, A., Reunanen, A., & Maatela, J. (1989). Weight and mortality in Finnish men. *Journal of Clinical Epidemiology, 42*(8), 781-789.

Rogers, A. E., & Longnecker, M. P. (1988). Dietary and nutritional influences on cancer: A review of epidemiologic and experimental data. *Laboratory Investigation, 59,* 729-759.

Sedaghat, A., & Grundy, S. M. (1980). Cholesterol crystals and the formation of cholesterol gallstones. *New England Journal of Medicine, 302,* 1274-1277.

Simopoulos, A., & VanItallie, T. B. (1984). Body weight, health, and longevity. *Annals of Internal Medicine, 100,* 285-295.

Society of Actuaries. (1959). *Build and Blood Pressure Study.* Chicago: Author.

Society of Actuaries. (1982). *Reports of mortality and morbidity experience.* Chicago: Author.

Society of Actuaries and the Association of Life Insurance Medical Directors of America. (1980). *Build Study 1979.* Boston: Authors.

Tannenbaum, A. (1947). Effects of varying caloric intake upon tumor incidence and tumor growth. *Annals of the New York Academy of Sciences, 49,* 5-18.

Tyroler, H. A., Heyden, S., & Hames, C. G. (1975). Weight and hypertension: Evans County studies of blacks and whites. In O. Paul (Ed.), *Epidemiology and control of hypertension* (pp. 177-205). New York: Grune & Stratton.

U.S. Department of Health and Human Services. (1986). *Report of the Secretary's Task Force on Black and Minority Health: Vol. 2. Cross-cutting issues in minority health; Vol. 7. Chemical dependency and diabetes.* Washington, DC: U.S. Government Printing Office.

Vague, J. (1947). La différenciation sexuelle, facteur déterminant des formes de l'obésité. *Presse Médicale, 55,* 339-340.

Vague, J. (1956). The degree of masculine differentiation of obesities: A factor determining predisposition to diabetes, atherosclerosis, gout, and uric calculous disease. *American Journal of Clinical Nutrition, 4,* 20-34.

Vague, J. (1991). *Obesities.* London: John Libbey.

VanItallie, T. B. (1979). Obesity: Adverse effects on health and longevity. *American Journal of Clinical Nutrition, 32,* 2723-2733.

VanItallie, T. B. (1985). Health implications of overweight and obesity in the United States. *Annals of Internal Medicine, 103*(6, Pt. 2), 983-988.

VanItallie, T. B., & Lew, E. A. (1990). Overweight and underweight. In E. A. Lew & J. Gajewski (Eds.), *Medical risks 1987: Mortality trends by age and time elapsed* (pp. 13.1-13.22). New York: Praeger.

VanItallie, T. B., Yang, M. U., Heymsfield, S. B., Funk, R. C., & Boileau, R. A. (1990). Height-normalized indices of the body's fat-free mass and fat mass: Potentially useful indicators of nutritional status. *American Journal of Clinical Nutrition, 52,* 953-959.

Waaler, H. T. (1984). Height, weight and mortality: The Norwegian experience. *Acta Medica Scandinavica* (Supple. 679), 1-56.

Ward, W. K., Bolgiano, D. C., McKnight, B., Halter, J. B., & Porte, D., Jr. (1984). Diminished B-cell secretory capacity in patients with noninsulin-dependent diabetes mellitus. *Journal of Clinical Investigation, 74,* 1318-1328.

2

An Overview of Current Treatments for Obesity

ALBERT J. STUNKARD

The basis for the treatment of obesity is simplicity itself: Reduce energy intake below energy output. All treatments for obesity have as their goal this one simple task. How they achieve it varies widely, and anyone approaching the treatment of obesity could be easily bewildered by the myriad of possibilities. Fortunately, a rationale for selecting among these possibilities is provided by a classification of obesity that is achieving increasing acceptance.

An ideal classification of disease derives from an understanding of etiology and pathogenesis, and we are far from such an understanding of human obesity. But for the purpose of selecting among treatments, such information is by no means necessary. A simple threefold classification based on nothing more than the severity of the obesity is perfectly adequate. It consists of "mild," "moderate," and "severe" obesity (Garrow, 1981; Stunkard, 1984).

The extent of overweight characterizing the three categories of obesity has been defined in the past by percentage overweight according to standard tables of height and weight, and I will follow this precedent here. Percentage overweight has the advantage of being readily appreciated by patients and practitioners. It has the disadvantage, however, of being vulnerable to arbitrary changes in the tables defining ideal or standard body weight, and what is moderate obesity on one day can become mild obesity overnight by the stroke of a pen. For these reasons, there is merit in defining the extent of overweight in terms of the body mass index (BMI = weight in kilograms/height in meters squared) rather than in terms of percentage overweight. There is, however, a disadvantage in defining overweight in terms of BMI. Most persons, including many practitioners, are not familiar with BMI units, making it difficult to appreciate the significance of the measure and use it for practical purposes. A potential solution to the problem of each measure—using them both—also has drawbacks. While percentage overweight increases linearly with increasing weight and height, BMI does not. The exponent in its denominator means that the BMI is relatively higher than percentage overweight for shorter persons and lower for tall persons. For this reason, the BMI values below are only approximately related to percentage overweight.

The three categories of obesity are characterized by percentages overweight of 20–40%, 41–100%, and more than 100%, respectively, corresponding approximately to respective BMIs of 27–30, 30.1–35, and more than 35. The lower limit, 20% overweight, or a BMI of 27 (and 25 for women), is selected on the basis of a National Institutes of Health Consensus Conference, which found that the risk to health begins when the body mass exceeds this threshold value and weight loss becomes medically indicated (VanItallie, 1985). Forty percent overweight, or a BMI of about 30, corresponds to an upward inflection in the mortality ratio and represents a point at which medical intervention becomes more strongly indicated (VanItallie, 1985). Overweight of 100% (BMI greater than 35), traditionally termed "morbid obesity," defines a level at which the risks of obesity appear to make surgical intervention a reasonable option—a judgment supported by years of experience (Mason, 1981).

The distribution of body weights in the general population is highly skewed, and the percentage of persons falling into the three categories varies greatly: 90% of obese persons are mildly obese, and no more than 0.5% are severely obese (National Center for Health Statistics [NCHS], 1983; Stunkard, 1984).

In earlier years, this classification of obesity was useful in selecting appropriate treatments, and it still is. It also served as the best estimate of risk to individuals. Thus, mild obesity was associated with the least risk, moderate obesity with greater risk, and severe obesity with the greatest risk. These estimates of risk still hold, particularly for the category of severe obesity, which confers increased risk on most (and greatly increased risk on some) severely obese persons. A measure that is stronger than extent of obesity in predicting its risks, however, has become apparent in recent years—the distribution of body fat (Seidell, Baky, DeBoer, Durenberg, & Hautvast, 1985). Upper body obesity is associated with a greatly increased risk of cardiovascular, metabolic, and other complications. Many, perhaps most, of these adverse effects are due to excess fat in the abdominal visceral depot (Ashwell, Cole, & Dixon, 1985). Furthermore, the benefits of weight loss extend to persons with upper body abdominal visceral obesity, reversing most of its ill effects. In Chapter 1 of this volume, VanItallie and Lew have described the implications of body fat distribution in greater detail.

How does this classification of obesity help us select among the different forms of treatment?

Severe Obesity

Table 2.1 indicates that surgery is the treatment of choice for severe obesity (Mason, 1981). Although severe obesity is an uncommon disorder, affecting no more than 0.5% of obese persons (and thus 0.13% of the general population), there are more than a million severely obese persons in the United States, and they are at high risk for many disorders. Among severely obese young men, for example, the mortality rate is 12 times that of young men of normal weight (Drenick, Bale, Seltzer, & Johnson, 1980). Severe obesity, regardless of body

TABLE 2.1. Proposed Classification of Obesity by Degree of Severity

Class	Percentage overweight	Body mass index (BMI)	Prevalence (among obese)	Treatment
Mild	20–40%	27–30	90%	"Conservative" therapy
Moderate	41–100%	30.1–35	9.5%	VLCD? and behavior therapy?
Severe	>100%	>35	0.5%	Surgery

Note. VLCD, very low calorie diet.

fat distribution, is associated with unequivocal medical complications in almost every person who suffers from it, and most of the complications are controlled or abolished by weight reduction. Weight reduction is thus strongly indicated for persons suffering from severe obesity. Gastric restriction, either by vertical banded gastroplasty or by gastric bypass surgery, is the treatment of choice (Mason, 1981). Although such surgery may be life-saving, especially when viewed from a long-term perspective, it is basically an elective procedure. In considering surgery, the patient should be helped to balance the undoubted risks of operation against its several benefits. In Chapter 21, Kral provides further information about the surgical treatment of severe obesity.

Moderate Obesity

Moderate obesity, characterized by a percentage overweight of 41–100% and a BMI of more than 30, afflicts 9% of obese persons (NCHS, 1983; Stunkard, 1984). In contrast to the clear choices for the treatment of severe and mild obesity, there is uncertainty about the optimal treatment for moderate obesity. The use of a very low calorie diet (VLCD) in combination with behavior modification has shown promise and is the topic of many of the chapters in this volume.

Mild Obesity

Mild obesity, characterized by a percentage overweight of 20–40% and a BMI of 27–30 for men and 25–30 for women, is by far the most common of the three levels of severity, affecting 90% of all obese persons (NCHS, 1983; Stunkard, 1984). Since mildly obese persons may suffer from upper body obesity, with its potentially serious complications, treatment can be very helpful for some persons. In contrast to moderate obesity, there exists a high degree of consensus as to the most effective (and the most cost-effective) form of treatment. Since it is not dealt with elsewhere in this volume, this treatment will be described briefly here.

Mild obesity is best managed by what may be called "conservative treatment" (Stunkard, 1987). Conservative treatments can be characterized in a negative sense as treatments other than surgery, VLCDs, pharmacotherapy, or instruments such as gastric balloons. They can be characterized in a positive sense by the rate of weight loss that they produce—approximately 1% of total body weight per week.

A more conventional measure of the rate of weight loss is kilograms per week, but this measure has two related disadvantages. First, it fails to take into account the different weight loss requirements of patients of differing body weight. Heavier persons can, and probably should, lose more weight than lighter persons, and it is awkward to specify in kilograms how much greater that rate should be for heavier or lighter persons. Second, weight loss per week is a measure that makes it difficult to compare weight losses of persons with widely varying weights. Even within the category of mild obesity, there is great variability in body weight, as exemplified by the difference between a tall man and a short woman with the same degree of overweight. The use of a percentage (i.e., the loss of 1% of body weight per week) simplifies the calculation of weight loss per week, lowers that rate as weight falls, and facilitates comparison of programs that treat different patient populations.

Conservative treatments for obesity can be characterized also in terms of the caloric deficits of the diets that they prescribe. It is probably wisest not to prescribe for all patients a diet with a fixed number of calories or a particular caloric deficit. Instead, following the precedent of using percentage of body weight to determine weight loss goals, diets of conservative treatments may be best characterized in terms of the energy required to maintain body weight. The optimal diet can then be calculated for each person: It should provide about 50% of maintenance requirements of that person and should rarely, if ever, fall below 40% of these requirements. Such a caloric deficit permits adequate loss of body fat while minimizing the loss of lean body mass. It also makes clear the desirability of measuring resting metabolic rate of patients prior to the initiation of treatment, to aid in calculating the desired caloric deficit.

Conservative treatments in the past have placed primary emphasis on one treatment modality—either diet, behavior modification, or medication. The past few years have seen a marked decrease in the use of medication and a salutary amalgamation of the best elements of dietary and behavioral treatments.

During the years immediately following the introduction of behavior therapy of obesity, major emphasis was placed upon changing food habits and eating behavior. Some of these measures, such as self-monitoring and stimulus control, went beyond the simple early goals of slowing eating and gaining control over eating behavior. For the most part, however, early behavioral programs were conducted in a setting of ideological purity that was derived from the original assumption that obesity resulted primarily from disordered eating behavior. It is now clear that obesity has far more extensive biological determinants and requires far more extensive treatment.

During the period when behavioral programs were developing, traditional programs continued their emphasis on diet, nutrition education, and physical activity. The two camps are now moving closer together, and programs that once were exclusively behavioral have increasingly incorporated features of traditional ones, while traditional programs have incorporated behavioral measures. Very few purely behavioral or purely nonbehavioral programs exist at the present time, and there is a growing consensus that the best treatment incorporates features of both kinds of programs. An interesting example of the amalgamation that is currently taking place is the use of behavioral methods to increase physical activity, a goal that had formerly been in the province of nonbehavioral programs. Similarly, efforts are currently being made to develop behavioral approaches to nutrition education, a modality that had formerly been in the domain of nonbehavioral programs. Table 2.2 provides a summary of the various methods currently comprising conservative treatments for obesity (Stunkard & Berthold, 1985). It is based upon the behaviors recommended in the five treatment manuals in widest use in 1985.

Most current treatment programs for obesity are conservative ones that consist of the three modalities of diet, physical activity, and behavior modification, designed to produce weight loss at a rate of 1% of body weight per week. Since they involve primarily the development of sound personal habits and of a healthy lifestyle, they pose little risk to participants and require little, if any, medical supervision. As a result, they can be provided at a modest cost, and cost is increasingly a factor in the evaluation of treatment programs for obesity.

The evaluation of treatment programs must assess not only their effectiveness, but also their costs in money and inconvenience. Even an effective treatment will be of only limited usefulness if its costs exceed its benefits. In recent years, this issue has been approached by preliminary cost-effectiveness analysis, utilizing two easily measured indices—the extent of weight loss and the financial costs of treatment. The ratio between costs and effectiveness permits a comparison among treatment programs.

Figure 2.1 shows the results of cost-effectiveness analysis of the treatments that were compared in a controlled clinical trial. This comparison utilized the cost to lose 1% of body weight, which is, as I have noted, approximately the weight lost during 1 week of conservative treatment. This trial compared conservative treatment with a VLCD used alone and with a VLCD used with conservative treatment. The cost to lose 1% of body weight was $19.62 for conservative treatment, $28.30 for VLCD alone, and $26.02 for a combination of the two methods. At the end of treatment, there was not a great deal of difference among the results of these three treatments. One year later, however, the differences among them in the regain of body weight were quite different. At this time, the cost for the conservative and combined treatment conditions had risen to $29.52 and $38.94, respectively. Because of the large regain in

TABLE 2.2. Behavioral Weight Loss Principles Described in Five Leading Treatment Manuals

Principles	Books citing	Principles	Books citing
1. STIMULUS CONTROL		3. REWARD	
A. Shopping		1. Solicit help from family and friends	5
1. Shop for food after eating	3	2. Help family and friends provide this help in the form of praise and material rewards	5
2. Shop from a list	3		
3. Avoid ready-to-eat foods	3	3. Utilize self-monitoring records as basis for rewards	5
4. Don't carry more cash than needed for shopping list	2	4. Plan specific rewards for specific behaviors (behavioral contracts)	3
B. Plans		4. SELF-MONITORING	
1. Plan to limit food intake	4	Keep diet diary that includes:	
2. Substitute exercise for snacking	4	1. Time and place of eating	5
3. Eat meals and snacks at scheduled times	3	2. Type and amount of food	5
4. Don't accept food offered by others	2	3. Who is present/How you feel	5
C. Activities		5. NUTRITION EDUCATION	
1. Store food out of sight	5	1. Use diet diary to identify problem areas	5
2. Eat all food in the same place	5	2. Make small changes that you can continue	5
3. Remove food from inappropriate storage areas in the house	5	3. Learn nutritional values of foods	5
4. Keep serving dishes off the table	4	4. Decrease fat intake; increase complex carbohydrates	4
5. Use smaller dishes and utensils	3		

6. Avoid being the food server
7. Leave the table immediately after eating
8. Don't save leftovers
D. Holidays and Parties
  1. Drink fewer alcoholic beverages — 2
  2. Plan eating habits before parties — 2
  3. Eat a low calorie snack before parties — 2
  4. Practice polite ways to decline food — 2
  5. Don't get discouraged by an occasional setback — 2

2. EATING BEHAVIOR
  1. Put fork down between mouthfuls — 4
  2. Chew thoroughly before swallowing — 4
  3. Prepare foods one portion at a time — 4
  4. Leave some food on the plate — 4
  5. Pause in the middle of the meal — 3
  6. Do nothing else while eating (read, watch television) — 3

6. PHYSICAL ACTIVITY
  A. Routine Activity
    1. Increase routine activity — 5
    2. Increase use of stairs — 5
    3. Keep a record of distance walked each day — 2
  B. Exercise
    1. Begin a very mild exercise program — 5
    2. Keep a record of daily exercise — 2
    3. Increase the exercise very gradually — 2

7. COGNITIVE RESTRUCTURING
  1. Avoid setting unreasonable goals — 4
  2. Think about progress, not shortcomings — 4
  3. Avoid imperatives like "always" and "never" — 4
  4. Counter negative thoughts with rational restatements — 4
  5. Set weight goals — 4

Note. From "What Is Behavior Therapy: A Very Short Description of Behavioral Weight Control" (p. 822) by A. J. Stunkard and H. C. Berthold, 1985, *American Journal of Clinical Nutrition, 41,* 821–823. Copyright 1985 by American Society for Clinical Nutrition, Inc. Reprinted by permission.

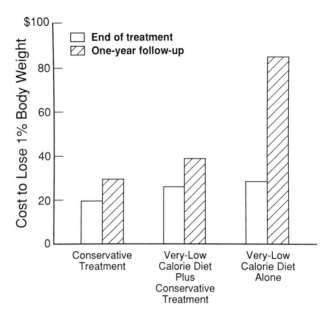

FIGURE 2.1. Cost-effectiveness of three forms of treatment for obesity. At the end of treatment, there were modest differences in the cost to lose 1% of body weight, while at 1-year follow-up the costs had risen, particularly in the group treated by very low calorie diet alone. From "Conservative Treatments for Obesity" (p. 1147) by A. J. Stunkard, 1987, *American Journal of Clinical Nutrition, 45*(Suppl.), 1142–1154. Copyright 1987 by American Society for Clinical Nutrition, Inc. Reprinted by permission.

weight of patients who had received the VLCD alone, however, the cost to lose 1% of body weight that was retained for 1 year had risen to $84.84.

Treatment Programs

The practitioner who seeks to refer a patient for treatment of obesity will find that medically sponsored programs are few and far between. Most of the treatment of obesity in the United States today is carried out by commercial organizations.

The shift in the treatment for obesity from medical auspices began at least 40 years ago with the rise of nonprofit self-help groups based to some degree on the model of Alcoholics Anonymous (Stunkard, Levine, & Fox, 1970). One of them, Overeaters Anonymous (OA), has adopted an addictive model of obesity and follows the Alcoholics Anonymous program in considerable detail. OA appears to be useful primarily to persons suffering from bulimia and is probably of limited size, although the nature of the organization precludes information about its size. A second early self-help group was Take Off Pounds Sensibly (TOPS), which has a less evangelistic approach than OA and relies heavily upon group support (and group sanctions). TOPS, which once counted more than 450,000 members, seems to be in a state of decline, with a greatly decreased membership.

As the feasibility of nonmedical group approaches to the management of obesity became apparent, commercial groups entered the picture. The first, and still the largest, is Weight Watchers. This group, now the prototype of commercial programs for the treatment of mild obesity, claims a yearly enrollment of

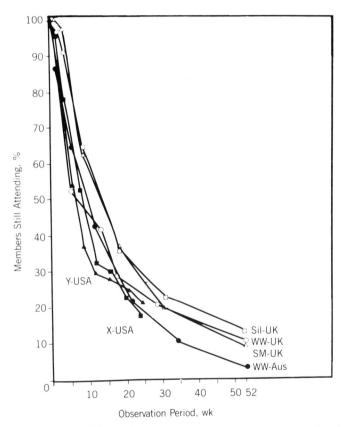

FIGURE 2.2. Life table of participants in six treatment programs under observation for up to 52 weeks showing dropout rates. Data from Nash, United States (X-USA); Volkmar, Stunkard, Woolston, and Bailey (Y-USA); Williams and Duncan, Weight Watchers, Australia (WW-AUS); Silhouette Slimming Club, United Kingdom (Sil-UK); Slimming Magazine, United Kingdom (SM-UK); and Weight Watchers, United Kingdom (WW-UK). From "High Attrition Rates in Commercial Weight Reduction Programs" (p. 427) by F. R. Volkmar, A. J. Stunkard, J. Woolston, and R. A. Bailey, 1981, *Archives of Internal Medicine, 141,* 426–428. Copyright 1981 by American Medical Association. Reprinted by permission.

3 million people. Over the years, Weight Watchers has evolved from its quasi-Alcoholics Anonymous origins to a conservative program of diet, physical activity, and behavior modification. There are few available data on the outcome of commercial weight loss programs. Nevertheless, it seems clear that, while they may be excellent in their overall conception, these programs suffer from flawed implementation. One result is an attrition rate that largely nullifies the benefits of the program. One study, for example, showed that 50% of people entering the program drop out within 6 weeks (Volkmar, Stunkard, Woolston, & Bailey, 1981).

Figure 2.2 illustrates the very high attrition rates of six commercial programs on three continents (Ashwell, 1978; Ashwell & Garrow, 1975). No matter how well conceived they are, programs that are not attended can hardly change behavior. It should be noted that the attrition rate in current academic programs of 26 weeks' duration is rarely more than 15%.

Commercial programs for the treatment of moderate obesity are conducted with medical supervision and are better implemented than those for the treatment of mild obesity. They are also much more expensive, as discussed by Wadden and Bartlett in Chapter 3 of this volume.

Summary and Conclusions

A simple classification of obesity has proven useful in selecting among the myriad of possible treatments of this disorder. The classification is a simple threefold one based upon the severity of the obesity—"mild," "moderate," and "severe."

The selection of patients for treatment of severe and moderate obesity is discussed elsewhere in this volume. The treatment of mild obesity involves primarily changes in lifestyle that affect food intake and physical activity. Most treatment programs for mild obesity are conducted under commercial auspices. There are few published results, and none is encouraging. In contrast, treatment of mild obesity in academic settings is far more effective (see Wadden & Bartlett, Chapter 3). The challenge is learning to transfer this treatment to commercial settings and to deliver it at an affordable cost.

References

Ashwell, M. (1978). Commercial weight loss groups. In G. Bray (Ed.), *Recent advances in obesity research: II. Proceedings of the Second International Congress on Obesity* (pp. 266–276). London: Newman.

Ashwell, M., Cole, T. J., & Dixon, A. K. (1985). New insight into the anthropometric classification of fat distribution shown by computed tomography. *British Medical Journal, 290*, 1692–1694.

Ashwell, M., & Garrow, J. S. (1975). A survey of three slimming and weight control organizations in the U.K. *Nutrition, 29*, 346–356.

Drenick, E. J., Bale, G. S., Seltzer, F., & Johnson, S. G. (1980). Excessive mortality and causes of death in morbidly obese men. *Journal of the American Medical Association, 243*, 443–445.

Garrow, J. S. (1981). *Treat obesity seriously: A clinical manual.* New York: Churchill Livingstone.

Mason, E. E. (1981). *Surgical treatment of obesity.* Philadelphia: W. B. Saunders.

National Center for Health Statistics (NCHS). (1983). *Obese and overweight adults in the United States* (VHS Publication No. 230, Series II). Washington, DC: U.S. Government Printing Office.

Seidell, J. C., Baky, J. C., DeBoer, E., Durenberg, P., & Hautvast, J. G. A. J. (1985). Fat distribution of over weight persons in relation to morbidity and subjective health. *International Journal of Obesity, 9*, 363–374.

Stunkard, A. J. (1984). The current status of treatment of obesity in adults. In A. J. Stunkard & E. Steller (Eds.), *Eating and its disorders* (pp. 157–174). New York: Raven Press.

Stunkard, A. J. (1987). Conservative treatments for obesity. *American Journal of Clinical Nutrition, 45*(Suppl.), 1142–1154.

Stunkard, A. J., & Berthold, H. C. (1985). What is behavior therapy: A very short description of behavioral weight control. *American Journal of Clinical Nutrition, 41*, 821–823.

Stunkard, A. J., Levine, H., & Fox, S. (1970). The management of obesity: Patient self-help and medical treatment. *Archives of Internal Medicine, 125*, 1067–1072.

VanItallie, T. B. (1985). Health implications of overweight and obesity in the United States. *Annals of Internal Medicine, 103*, 983–989.

Volkmar, F. R., Stunkard, A. J., Woolston, J., & Bailey, R. A. (1981). High attrition rates in commercial weight reduction programs. *Archives of Internal Medicine, 141*, 426–428.

3

Very Low Calorie Diets: An Overview and Appraisal

THOMAS A. WADDEN
SUSAN J. BARTLETT

In what was to become the most frequently cited review of the outcome of obesity therapy, Stunkard (1958) proclaimed: "Most obese persons will not stay in treatment. Of those who stay in treatment, most will not lose weight, and of those who lose weight, most will regain it" (p. 79). This pessimistic assessment was based in large measure upon findings from 100 consecutive outpatients treated by conventional reducing diets at a hospital nutrition clinic (Stunkard & McLaren-Hume, 1959). Only 12% of patients lost 20 pounds (9.09 kg) or more. A scant 6% maintained a comparable weight loss 1 year after treatment.

Given this outcome, it is not surprising that clinicians began in the late 1950s and early 1960s to explore more aggressive forms of therapy. Thus, just 1 year after Stunkard's review, Bloom (1959) reported that nine inpatients subjected to total fasting lost an average of 8.4 kg in 1 week. Additional investigations followed shortly and documented average weight losses of 15 to 23 kg, achieved in as few as 51 days (Drenick & Smith, 1964; Thomson, Runcie, & Miller, 1966). Poor maintenance of weight loss and adverse health consequences, including death (Spencer, 1968), led to the abandonment of total fasting, but not before two research teams had begun to explore the use of modified fasting using very low calorie diets (VLCDs) high in dietary protein (Apfelbaum, 1967; Bollinger, Lukert, Brown, Guevara, & Steinberg, 1966). By the mid-1970s, four prominent research teams were investigating the use of these diets, which by the late 1980s would be consumed by an estimated 12 to 15 million persons worldwide (Apfelbaum, 1967; Blackburn, Bistrian, & Flatt, 1975; Genuth, Castro, & Vertes, 1974; Howard, 1989; Howard & McLean Baird, 1977).

This chapter will briefly review the development and current status of VLCDs. We will examine the safety and efficacy of these diets and, where possible, compare their results with those produced by conventional reducing diets. We also will discuss issues pertinent to clinical practice and future research. This chapter updates our previous review of this literature (Wadden, Stunkard, & Brownell, 1983), to which the reader is referred for background information.

Very Low Calorie Diets: Definition and Development

There is no universally accepted definition of a VLCD. A group of American investigators suggested in 1979 that the term be reserved for diets providing less than 800 kilocalories (kcal) daily (Life Sciences Research Office, 1979). Advisory committees from various European nations, however, have proposed that VLCDs provide a minimum daily intake ranging from 330 to 900 kcal, with recommended amounts of protein ranging from 31 to 60 g daily (Munro & Stolarek, 1989). In the United Kingdom, a report recommended that VLCDs provide a minimum of 400 kcal and 40 g of protein daily for women, and 500 kcal and 50 g of protein daily for men (Committee on Medical Aspects of Food Policy, 1987).

The recommendations of the British report are noteworthy because of their explicit recognition that men typically have higher caloric requirements than women, and thus, to maintain adequate health while dieting, should receive more calories and protein than women. Moreover, the British report implicitly recognizes that the definition of a VLCD depends, in large measure, upon the size of the caloric deficit that the diet induces in a given individual. Thus, a 700-kcal/day diet induces a rather modest deficit of only 500 kcal/day in a very short but obese woman with a daily energy requirement of 1200 kcal. By contrast, the same diet induces a very substantial deficit of 2500 kcal/day in a tall, obese man with a daily energy requirement of 3200 kcal. The woman would be expected to lose only 0.45 kg (1 pound) a week, as compared to the man's loss of 2.27 kg (5 pounds) weekly.

Convenience probably led to defining VLCDs solely in terms of the number of kilocalories that they provide and to the practice of prescribing the same diet for persons of vastly different weights. It would appear, however, more appropriate to define a VLCD in relation to the patient who receives it and, ultimately, in terms of the size of the caloric deficit that it induces. Thus, Atkinson (Chapter 12, this volume) has suggested that a VLCD is one that provides less than 10 kcal/day per kilogram of ideal body weight (as compared with the norm of approximately 30 kcal/day). A more precise estimation of the expected caloric deficit would be achieved by defining a VLCD as one that provides 50% or less of the patient's daily resting energy expenditure (REE), as determined by indirect calorimetry (Feurer & Mullen, 1986). Thus, the woman described above might have an REE of 900 kcal/day, which, for her, would define a VLCD as one providing 450 kcal or fewer daily. The man's probable REE of 2500 kcal/day would define a VLCD as providing 1250 kcal or fewer daily, the equivalent of what is frequently considered a conventional reducing diet.

Development

The discussion above does not address the macronutrient composition of VLCDs, the development of which were largely guided by concerns for protein rather than calorie content. Researchers theorized that if 4 g of nitrogen were lost daily during total starvation, then this amount of nitrogen as dietary protein (25 g daily) might be sufficient to prevent losses of bodily protein (Wadden et al., 1983). Thus, Bollinger et al. (1966) reported that 40 to 60 g of protein daily were sufficient to produce nitrogen balance (suggesting the preservation of bodily protein) in 2 to 3 weeks.

Investigators generally agree that dietary protein is critical to the preservation of lean body mass and that the protein should be of high biological value, in contrast to that of notoriously poor quality used in the liquid protein diets of 1976–1977 (VanItallie, 1978). Thus, current diets provide protein from lean meat, fish, or fowl (served as food) or from egg and milk sources. In the latter case, the protein is powdered, mixed with vitamins and minerals, and finally hydrated (by the patient) to yield a liquid diet.

Beyond the consensus on the need for high quality protein, investigators disagree concerning the amount required or the optimal mix of protein and carbohydrate (Wadden et al., 1983). Blackburn and Bistrian reported that large amounts, approximately 75 g daily for men and 55 g for women, produced positive nitrogen balance in moderately obese patients within 2 to 3 weeks (Bistrian, Blackburn, & Stanbury, 1977; Blackburn et al., 1975). They call for 1.2 to 1.5 g of protein per kilogram of ideal body weight, based on findings that the greater the protein intake, the better the nitrogen retention (Bistrian, 1978; Blackburn et al., 1975). These investigators include only minimal amounts of carbohydrate in their diets, given findings that the isocaloric substitution of carbohydrate for protein decreased protein sparing (Blackburn, Flatt, Clowes, O'Donnell, & Hensle, 1973; Hoffer, Bistrian, Young, Blackburn, & Matthews, 1984).

By contrast, Howard and colleagues employed a diet that originally provided only 33 g of protein daily, with 44 g of carbohydrate (Howard, Grant, Edwards, Littlewood, & McLean Baird, 1978). These investigators contend that the inclusion of carbohydrate both prevents the hyperuricemia and electrolyte loss common to protein-only diets and spares lean body tissue (Howard, 1989; Howard et al., 1978). It should be noted, however, that patients who consumed this diet frequently remained in negative nitrogen balance 4 to 6 weeks after beginning treatment.

Commercial manufacturers of VLCDs have generally erred on the side of safety by providing in their formulas 50 to 90 g of protein daily and 30 g or more of carbohydrate. This is a prudent decision, but one, regrettably, that will not ensure that all patients achieve positive nitrogen balance within the first few weeks. This is because Yang and colleagues found that six obese male inpatients remained in negative nitrogen balance for at least 4 weeks, even on protein intakes of either 66 or 132 g per day (Yang, Barbosa-Saldivar, Pi-Sunyer, & VanItallie, 1981). Moreover, one patient failed to achieve positive balance during the 64-day study, despite consuming 66 g of protein daily, with 59 g of carbohydrate. Fisler and colleagues have reported similar findings (Fisler, Drenick, Blumfield, & Swendseid, 1982).

Body Composition and Weight Loss

Findings that patients may lose significant amounts of lean tissue—ranging from 2 to 7 kg in the Yang et al. (1981) and Fisler et al. (1982) studies—have alarmed investigators. The principal concern is that lean tissue could be lost from vital organs such as the heart, as was observed in persons who consumed the liquid protein diets (Heymsfield, Jain, Ortiz, & Waki, Chapter 6, this volume; Isner, Sours, Paris, Farrans, & Roberts, 1979; VanItallie, 1978). The vast majority of practitioners do not have the resources to measure nitrogen balance in their patients; even if they did, Nettleton and Hegsted (1975) have noted that overall changes in nitrogen balance are not sufficiently sensitive to detect changes in specific tissues. More sophisticated procedures, including magnetic resonance imaging, would be required to detect changes in lean tissue in the heart and other organs, thus making weight reduction by VLCD impractical if not unaffordable.

Fortunately, however, reductions in fat-free mass that occur with weight loss in markedly obese persons are likely to be benign in the vast majority of cases. This belief is based on findings that approximately 22% to 30% of the excess weight in the markedly obese consists of fat-free mass (Forbes, 1987; Foster et al., 1988; Webster, Hesp, & Garrow, 1984). As weight and fat increase, so does fat-free mass. Thus, Garrow (1981) has suggested that weight lost on a reducing diet may be comprised of as much as 25% fat-free mass, with the remainder from fat.

In studies in which patients lost approximately 20 kg by consuming VLCDs providing 400 to 800 kcal daily (with 50 to 90 g of protein), the percentage of the weight loss from fat-free mass ranged from approximately 15% to 25% (Barrows & Snook, 1987; Donnelly, Pronk, Jacobsen, Pronk, & Jakicic, 1991; Foster et al., 1992; Wadden, Foster, Letizia, & Mullen, 1990). Our most recent study revealed that only 14% of a 20.6-kg weight loss was derived from fat-free mass (Foster et al., 1992).

These findings compare very favorably with those reported for conventional reducing diets of 1000–1200 kcal/day. It is perhaps unknown to many practitioners that approximately 15% to 20% of the weight loss occurring with this approach consists of fat-free mass (Ballor, Katch, Becque, & Marks, 1988; Ballor, McCarthy, & Wilterdink, 1990; Weltman, Matter, & Stamford, 1980). The somewhat better preservation of fat-free mass associated with conventional reducing diets may be attributable to patients' losing smaller amounts of weight (typically 5 to 10 kg), as compared with losses on a VLCD. Thus, in examining diets providing 420, 660, and 800 kcal daily, we (Foster et al., 1992) found that the magnitude of the weight loss was the best predictor of reductions in fat-free mass, accounting for 42% of the variance. The caloric content of the diets per se (i.e., 420, 660, or 800 kcal/day) did not contribute significantly to the variance.

These findings suggest that practitioners should expect some loss of fat-free mass whenever a reducing diet is used, and that these losses will be acceptable in most cases. Caution, however, suggests that VLCDs should be limited to markedly obese persons (i.e., 30% or more overweight), who have been shown to spare lean body tissue more satisfactorily during caloric restriction than do lighter individuals (Forbes, 1987; Forbes & Drenick, 1979; VanItallie & Yang, 1977; Yang & VanItallie, Chapter 4, this volume). Moreover, heavier individuals are likely to have more fat and fat-free mass than are the mildly obese (Webster et al., 1984; Yang, 1988), which may provide an added measure of protection during weight loss (VanItallie & Yang, 1984).

Prudence also suggests that practitioners assess patients' body composition before treatment, using one of the methods described by Yang and VanItallie (Chapter 4, this volume). This assessment would identify persons with reduced fat-free mass and for whom a VLCD would therefore be inadvisable. The elderly are likely to display reduced fat-free mass, as are many individuals with chronic disability that limits their physical activity.

Clinical Use of Very Low Calorie Diets

Patient Selection

Most investigators believe that VLCDs should be restricted to persons 18 to 65 years old, who are a minimum of 30% or more overweight and have failed to lose weight with more conservative approaches (Bistrian, 1978; Genuth, 1979; Wadden et al., 1983). Reasons for the weight restriction include findings, as previously noted, of poor nitrogen retention in persons of lesser degrees of obesity, as well as the fact that mildly obese individuals can be successfully treated with safer and significantly less expensive approaches.

Several investigators, including Atkinson (Chapter 12, this volume), have described the goals and methods of the initial medical evaluation and the conditions that, if discovered, would contraindicate the use of a VLCD (Bistrian, 1978; Blackburn, Lynch, & Wong, 1986; Genuth, 1979). Contraindications include a recent myocardial infarction; a cardiac conduction disorder; a history of cerebrovascular, renal, or hepatic disease; cancer; Type I diabetes; and pregnancy. Behavioral and psychiatric contraindications include bulimia nervosa (i.e., binge eating followed by purging); significant depression, including bipolar disorder (i.e., manic–depressive illness); acute psychiatric disturbance; and substance abuse disorders, excluding cigarette smoking (Wadden & Foster, Chapter 13, this volume).

Course of Treatment

Treatment by VLCD is frequently delivered by a multidisciplinary team that includes a physician, behavioral psychologist, and dietitian (and frequently an exercise specialist). Multidisciplinary care is thought to be needed because of the diverse requirements of the medical and treatment protocols (Wadden, VanItallie, & Blackburn, 1990). Regrettably, however, no studies have been conducted to assess the safety and efficacy of treatment as delivered by a single practitioner (most likely a physician), as compared with delivery by a full or partial team composed of the above-listed professionals. This is an important issue, given the higher costs but possibly better long-term outcome associated with multidisciplinary care. The one study that indirectly addressed this issue showed that patients who received an intensive program of lifestyle modification in combination with a VLCD achieved better maintenance of weight loss than patients treated by diet alone (Wadden & Stunkard, 1986).

A typical course of treatment by VLCD includes four distinct phases: (1) introduction; (2) the VLCD; (3) refeeding; and (4) weight stabilization/maintenance.

Introduction

Many practitioners begin treatment with a 1- to 4-week introductory period in which patients consume a balanced-deficit diet of 1200 to 1500 kcal/day and prepare themselves and family members for the period of severe caloric restriction (Palgi et al., 1985; Wadden & Foster, Chapter 13, this volume). Patients may be asked to record their food intake and to increase their physical activity. Poor adherence to these behaviors may serve to identify persons at risk of nonadherence later in therapy (Bistrian & Hoffer, 1982; Lindner & Blackburn, 1976).

Very Low Calorie Diet

Introduction of the VLCD is associated with a large diuresis and weight losses that average 2 to 5 kg for the first 2 weeks. Thereafter, losses average 1 to 2 kg weekly for women and 1.5 to 2.5 kg for men. Weekly group counseling sessions assist patients in developing an exercise program and in adhering to the diet (Wadden & Foster, Chapter 13, this volume). Those who select a protein-sparing modified fast usually consume their diet (of lean meat, fish, and fowl) in three daily servings and take supplements that include a multivitamin capsule, 3 to 5 g of sodium chloride, and 2 to 3 g of potassium (Bistrian, 1978; Palgi et al., 1985). Patients who select a liquid diet usually consume five servings daily, which supply all vitamins and minerals (for which requirements have been established).

Regardless of the diet selected, patients are requested to drink at least 2 L of noncaloric fluid daily and to avoid consumption of all other foods. A majority of persons appear to achieve adequate adherence. In LaPorte and Stunkard's (1990) study of 76 patients who were prescribed a liquid diet for 10 weeks, 36% reported that they were fully adherent, and an additional 28% were judged to have good adherence (defined as consuming fewer than 3000 excess kcal during the 10 weeks). By contrast, 12% of patients were unable "to give up food" and discontinued treatment. In our most recent clinical trial, we observed adherence sufficient to produce a minimum weight loss of 10 kg in 100% of subjects (Foster et al., 1992).

Prudence suggests that patients be examined weekly by a physician or other health care professional while they consume the VLCD and refeeding diet, and that their electrolytes (and other laboratory values) be assessed at least every other week. As Atkinson (Chapter 12, this volume) has noted, however, there is no universally accepted schedule of medical supervision, and entirely satisfactory results have been reported with less intensive monitoring (Atkinson & Kaiser, 1981; Bistrian, 1978). Investigators, however, do agree that less intensive monitoring is sufficient following the refeeding period, when weight loss slows dramatically. Medical monitoring also probably does not need to be as intensive when higher calorie diets are prescribed, as discussed later.

Patients in controlled investigations have typically consumed VLCDs for 8 to 16 weeks, which we believe to be the appropriate duration for the majority of patients (Palgi et al., 1985; Sikand, Kondo, Foreyt, Jones, & Gotto, 1988; Wadden & Stunkard, 1986; Wing et al., 1991). Some investigators, however, have used the diets for 24 weeks or more with no apparent complications (Vertes, Genuth, & Hazelton, 1977). The length of time that a given patient should diet is dependent upon a number of factors, including the achievement of a satisfactory rate of weight loss, favorable medical findings, and the individual's initial weight. As noted earlier, heavier individuals generally have more fat-free mass (Yang, 1988; Yang & VanItallie, Chapter 4, this volume) and conserve nitrogen more satisfactorily while dieting than do less obese persons (Forbes & Drenick, 1979; VanItallie & Yang, 1977). Thus, under normal circumstances, they can apparently diet safely for longer periods than can the less obese. It is prudent, however, to increase energy intake as these patients lose large amounts of weight (VanItallie, 1988). Our recommended limit of 16 weeks is based upon the fact that there are no adequate studies of cardiac function beyond this point (Doherty et al., 1991).

Refeeding Period

Conventional foods are gradually reintroduced into the patient's diet during a 4- to 8-week period following the VLCD. If a liquid diet has been used, then lean meat, fish, and fowl are substituted as the protein servings. Fruits and vegetables, breads and cereals, and fats are then slowly introduced into the diet, in this order, to prevent an abrupt increase in fluid (Bistrian, 1978; Genuth, 1979). Refeeding following a protein-sparing modified fast follows a similar protocol.

The refeeding period presents an excellent time to instruct patients in the fundamentals of sound nutrition, as described by McNulty (Chapter 14, this volume). It also, however, may be a time of high anxiety for some patients who doubt their ability to control their food intake (Wadden & Foster, Chapter 13, this volume). We discuss later possible behavioral complications occurring during this period.

Weight Stabilization/Maintenance

Patients are instructed in methods of maintaining their weight losses during the last phase of treatment (Perri, Chapter 19, this volume; Wadden & Foster, Chapter 13, this volume). These include the modification of eating, exercise, dietary, and thinking habits. Patients are frequently encouraged to enroll in a formal program of weight loss maintenance. Regrettably, however, only 55% of patients in some of the best programs of which we are aware complete these four stages of treatment (Wadden, Foster, Letizia, & Stunkard, in press). Of these, we suspect that no more than one-third participate in a formal program of weight loss maintenance.

Safety of Very Low Calorie Diets

VLCDs appear to be safe when used by appropriate persons under careful medical supervision (Wadden et al., 1983; Wadden, VanItallie, & Blackburn, 1990). This record of safety stands in sharp contrast to the more than 60 fatalities associated with the consumption of "liquid protein diets" (Linn & Stuart, 1976), with which current VLCDs should not be confused. The safety of current diets is probably attributable to their provision of adequate amounts of high quality protein and to more stringent medical supervision of patients, the vast majority of whom are treated in hospital-based programs.

Cardiac Function

Evidence of the safety of current diets is provided by findings of no increase in cardiac abnormalities, as determined by 24-hour Holter monitoring (Amatruda, Richeson, Welle, Brodows, & Lockwood, 1988; Doherty et al., 1991; Phinney et al., 1983). In the longest study to date, which included use of a VLCD for 16 weeks, Doherty et al. (1991) actually observed a greater (though not statistically significant) incidence of premature ventricular beats in nondieting obese controls and in patients treated by a conventional 1200-kcal/day diet than in patients who received a VLCD. These findings point to the likelihood of observing occasional, minor cardiac abnormalities in any sample of otherwise healthy obese individuals.

Heymsfield et al. (Chapter 6, this volume) have provided an exhaustive review of the factors associated with sudden death in persons who consumed the 1976–1977 liquid protein diets. They have also examined factors contributing to the safety of current diets. Despite this apparent safety, we should note that it is impossible to rule out the chance of sudden death in persons who consume current VLCDs. Markedly obese persons are at increased risk of sudden death, which is independent of their efforts to lose weight by dieting (Isner et al., 1979; Sours et al., 1981). Thus, we are aware of several reports of sudden death in patients treated by current VLCDs, none of which, however, has been attributed to the diet or weight loss.

Complications and Symptoms

Consumption of a VLCD may be associated with several complications, described by Atkinson (Chapter 12, this volume), which require medical attention. These may include elevated uric acid, anemia, and gallstones, the last of which has received significant attention in recent years. Two controlled trials found that approximately 26% of persons treated by a VLCD developed gallstones, as detected by ultrasound (Broomfield et al., 1988; Liddle, Goldstein, & Saxton, 1989). Supersaturation of the biliary cholesterol and gallbladder stasis are two mechanisms believed responsible for this occurrence.

Further research is needed to determine the incidence of clinically significant gallstones occurring with weight loss by VLCDs as compared with conventional reducing diets. In the meantime, the risk of gallstones during a VLCD can be reduced by the use of diets that (1) provide sufficient protein and fat at one meal (i.e., 14 g of protein and 10 g of fat) to ensure gallbladder contraction; (2) limit weight loss to 2% or less per week; and (3) are used for 12 or fewer weeks (Honig & Blackburn, 1991; Kanders & Blackburn, Chapter 9, this volume).

Symptoms

Patients are likely to experience a number of symptoms in the first few days to weeks in which they consume a VLCD. These typically include fatigue, dizziness, muscle cramping, headache, gastrointestinal distress, and cold intolerance. In three separate investigations, however, our research team found that these symptoms were associated with only minimal discomfort and largely remitted when the VLCD was terminated (Foster et al., 1992; Wadden, Stunkard, Brownell, & Day, 1985; Wadden, Stunkard, Day, Gould, & Rubin, 1987). The two possible exceptions are complaints of dry skin and hair loss, which, though mild in magnitude, persisted in one study following termination of the VLCD (Foster et al., 1992). Continued observation, however, showed that both symptoms eventually remitted.

Hunger

One symptom that does not occur in the great majority of persons is hunger. Several controlled investigations have shown that patients report significantly less hunger and preoccupation with food when consuming a VLCD than when

Very Low Calorie Diets: An Overview

consuming a conventional 1200-kcal/day reducing diet (Foster et al., 1992; Rosen, Gross, Loew, & Sims, 1982; Wadden et al., 1985; Wadden et al., 1987) (see Figures 3.1 and 3.2). The reduction in hunger has been attributed to ketosis, which is marked on most VLCDs. Research findings, however, have not supported this hypothesis (Foster et al., 1992; Rosen et al., 1982). It is more than likely that the reductions in hunger and food cravings are related to the monotony and lesser palatability of VLCDs as compared with conventional reducing diets (Wadden et al., 1987).

Behavioral/Psychiatric Complications

Binge Eating

Approximately 25% to 70% of obese individuals who seek weight reduction therapy at research clinics report that they engage in binge eating for which they do not compensate by purging (Keefe, Wyshogrod, Weinberger, & Agras, 1984; Marcus, Wing, & Lamparski, 1985; Spitzer et al., in press). Anecdotal reports have suggested that treatment by VLCD may exacerbate binge eating in persons who present with this disorder and induce it in persons previously free of it (O'Neill, 1990). This possibility is suggested by findings that bingeing is almost invariably preceded by a period of severe dietary restriction, as associated with a VLCD (Polivy & Herman, 1985). Clinical observations suggest that the refeeding period is the time of greatest risk for patients, who are frequently anxious about their ability to resume consumption of conventional foods.

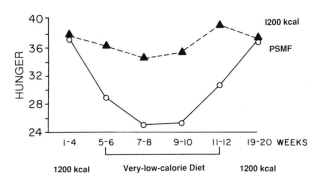

FIGURE 3.1. Comparison of reports of hunger in patients randomly assigned to a protein-sparing modified fast (PSMF) providing 400–500 kcal/day or to a 1200-kcal/day balanced-deficit diet. Consumption of the PSMF was limited to weeks 5–12. Higher scores indicate greater hunger (0 = "not at all hungry"; 80 = "as hungry as you have ever felt"). From "Less Food, Less Hunger: Reports of Appetite and Symptoms in a Controlled Study of a Protein Sparing Modified Fast" (p. 243) by T. A. Wadden, A. J. Stunkard, S. C. Day, C. Rubin, and R. A. Gould, 1987, *International Journal of Obesity, 11,* 239–249. Copyright 1987 by Macmillan Press Ltd. Reprinted by permission.

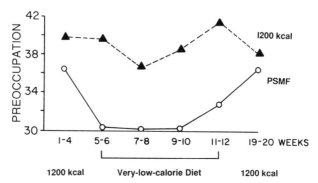

FIGURE 3.2. Comparison of reports of preoccupation with eating in patients randomly assigned to a PSMF providing 400–500 kcal/day or to a 1200-kcal/day balanced-deficit diet. Consumption of the PSMF was limited to weeks 5–12. Higher scores indicate greater preoccupation with eating (0 = "not at all preoccupied"; 80 = "constant preoccupation"). From "Less Food, Less Hunger: Reports of Appetite and Symptoms in a Controlled Study of a Protein Sparing Modified Fast" (p. 244) by T. A. Wadden, A. J. Stunkard, S. C. Day, C. Rubin, and R. A. Gould, 1987, *International Journal of Obesity, 11,* 239–249. Copyright 1987 by Macmillan Press Ltd. Reprinted by permission.

We are aware of only two studies in this area, neither of which provides adequate data concerning the relationship between VLCDs and binge eating. The first found that persons who consumed a VLCD reported no more dietary lapses during treatment than did those who consumed a 1200-kcal/day diet (Drapkin, Wing, Shiffman, Buchoff, & Grillo, 1991). The second showed that obese binge eaters displayed rates of attrition and weight loss comparable to those of nonbingers during treatment by VLCD and lifestyle modification (Wadden, Foster, & Letizia, in press). Binge eaters, however, were significantly more likely than nonbingers to discontinue treatment immediately following the refeeding period. Additional studies are needed to assess the occurrence of binge eating during and after weight reduction in persons with and without this disorder before treatment. In the meantime, interventions suggested by Telch, Agras, Rossiter, Wilfley, and Kenardy (1990) and Wadden and Foster (Chapter 13, this volume) may assist in the management of obese binge eaters.

Depression

Stunkard and Rush's (1974) review of the literature suggested that dieting was associated with depression, anxiety, and other untoward symptoms. This conclusion has not been supported by recent studies of obese individuals treated by behavior therapy combined with conventional reducing diets (Wing, Marcus, Epstein, & Kupfer, 1983) or VLCDs (O'Neil & Jarrell, Chapter 11, this volume; Wadden & Stunkard, 1986). Some patients may display transient increases in depression during weight loss (Wadden, Stunkard, & Smoller, 1986), but in the vast majority of cases we have observed, such increases have been attributable to adverse life events (such as the death of a loved one) or pre-existing psychiatric disturbance.

Metabolic Complications

Investigators have voiced concerns that cycles of weight loss and regain may permanently suppress metabolic rate, thus exacerbating efforts to control weight (Brownell, 1988; Brownell, Greenwood, Stellar, & Shrager, 1986). The gravest concerns have been expressed about VLCDs, which may be associated with reductions in resting metabolic rate (RMR) as great as 20% (Elliot, Goldberg, Kuehl, & Bennett, 1989). Our research team completed two long-term studies of the effects of dieting on RMR (Foster et al., 1990; Wadden, Foster, Letizia, & Mullen, 1990). Each showed that VLCDs were associated with marked reductions in RMR. When caloric restriction was terminated, however, RMR rose to a level appropriate for patients' new, reduced body weights (see Figure 3.3).

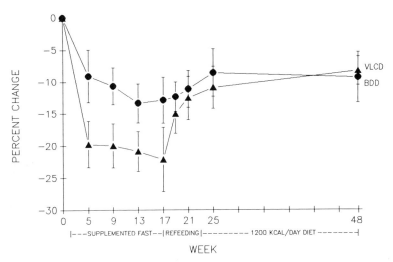

FIGURE 3.3. Percentage reduction in resting metabolic rate (RMR) in patients randomly assigned to a balanced-deficit diet (BDD) (circles) or to a very low calorie diet (VLCD) (triangles). The BDD patients consumed approximately 1200 kcal/day throughout treatment, while the VLCD patients consumed 420 kcal/day for 16 of the first 17 weeks, a refeeding diet for weeks 18 through 23, and a balanced-deficit diet providing 1200 to 1500 kcal/day for the remainder of treatment. Mean weight losses of the BDD patients at weeks 17 and 48 were 11.0 kg and 18.2 kg, respectively. Losses for the VLCD patients at weeks 17 and 48 were 23.1 kg and 21.6 kg, respectively. From "Long-Term Effects of Dieting on Resting Metabolic Rate in Obese Outpatients" (p. 710) by T. A. Wadden, G. D. Foster, K. A. Letizia, and J. L. Mullen, 1990, *Journal of the American Medical Association, 264*, 707–711. Copyright 1990 by American Medical Association. Reprinted by permission.

Ravussin and Swinburn (Chapter 7, this volume) have provided an exhaustive review of the effects of caloric restriction on the various components of total energy expenditure and have concluded that dieting does not adversely affect RMR. Wing (in press), in her review, also concluded similarly that "weight cycling has no consistent effect on metabolic variables, such as energy expenditure, ease of weight loss, or body fat."

Short-Term Efficacy of Very Low Calorie Diets

The popularity of VLCDs is attributable to the large, rapid weight losses that they produce. Table 3.1 presents the results of treatment for eight major studies published before 1983, and Tables 3.2 and 3.3 present the results of studies published after that time. These latter two tables include only those studies that had 50 or more patients and used diets providing fewer than 800 kcal/day. Thus, a number of relevant studies have not been included.

Short-Term Weight Losses

The data presented in Tables 3.1 and 3.2 indicate that persons treated by a VLCD for 12 to 16 weeks lose approximately 20 kg. Longer treatment is associated with larger weight losses, although the rate of weight loss appears to slow significantly after the first 12 weeks. Thus, women treated by Donnelly et al. (1991) for 12.8 weeks lost 20.5 kg, whereas those treated by Hovell et al. (1988) for 16 to 26 weeks lost only 4 kg more, for a total loss of 24.5 kg. Our research team observed a loss of 17.3 kg in women during the first 3 months of treatment by a 420-kcal/day diet (Wadden, Foster, & Letizia, 1990). This average monthly loss of 5.8 kg slowed to 3.1 kg, however, when the diet was extended to a fourth month, despite patients' remaining more than 50% overweight on average.

Poor dietary adherence (LaPorte & Stunkard, 1990), as well as a diet-induced reduction in metabolic rate (Wadden, Foster, Letizia, & Mullen, 1990), may contribute to the slower rate of weight loss over time. Regardless of the cause, we believe that it is hard to justify the increased costs and health risks associated with a VLCD when the monthly rate of weight loss falls below 4 kg.

Attrition

The large weight losses reported with VLCDs could result from selective attrition in which persons who respond poorly to treatment drop out, and their weight losses are not included in determining mean end-of-treatment losses.

TABLE 3.1. Summary Analysis of Eight Major Studies (to 1983) Using Very Low Calorie Diets

Reference	Subjects (n)[a]	Sex	Mean pretreatment weight (kg)	Mean age (yr)	Diet regimen	Mean treatment duration (wk)	Mean weight loss (kg)	Mean weight loss at follow-up (kg)[b]
Howard et al. (1978)	22	19 F, 3 M	107.8	—	Formula (protein, 31 g; carbohydrate, 44 g)	4	9.6	13.2 (seven subjects stayed on diet 6 wk)
	28 (22)	25 F, 3 M	96.3	—	Formula (same as above)	6	9.0	15.7 (six subjects stayed on diet 12 wk)
McLean Baird & Howard (1977)	38 (25)	30 F, 8 M	104.4	17–62 (range)	Formula (protein, 25 g; carbohydrate, 40 g)	8	13.8	12.2 kg (1 mo)
Atkinson & Kaiser (1981)	234	200 F, 34 M	104.5	37.9	Formula (protein, 1 g/kg ideal body weight; sucrose, 0.5 g/kg ideal body weight)	Maximum of 12 wk	18.7 (at 12 wk)	—
Tuck et al. (1981)	25	14 F, 11 M	103.9	40.7	Formula (OPTIFAST)	12	20.2	—
Lindner & Blackburn (1976)	67	57 F, 10 M	93.6	48	Formula (Hentex P-20; training in nutrition and behavior modification)	16.7	20.8	18.4 kg (12 mo); 14.5 (18–24 mo)

(*continued*)

TABLE 3.1. (continued)

Reference	Subjects (n)[a]	Sex	Mean pretreatment weight (kg)	Mean age (yr)	Diet regimen	Mean treatment duration (wk)	Mean weight loss (kg)	Mean weight loss at follow-up (kg)[b]
Palgi et al. (1985)	668	564 F, 104 M	98	38.5	Animal protein (protein, 1.5 g/kg ideal body weight; training in nutrition and behavior modification)	17	21	6.6 (216 subjects sampled at 4.5 yr)
Vertes et al. (1977)[c]	411	F	109.6	40	Formula (protein, 45 g; glucose, 30 g)	23.8	31.2	—
	119	M	136.6	40	Same as above	19.9	37.6	—
Genuth et al. (1978)	45 (28)	F	112.5	42	Formula (protein, 45 g; glucose, 30 g)	23	32.5	56% of total regained 50% of weight lost (22 mo)
	30 (19)	M	137.8	44	Same as above	19	41.1	—

Note. From "Very Low Calorie Diets: Their Efficacy, Safety, and Future" (p. 679) by T. A. Wadden, A. J. Stunkard, and K. D. Brownell, 1983, *Annals of Internal Medicine, 99,* 675–684. Copyright 1983 by American College of Physicians. Reprinted by permission.

[a] All subjects seen as outpatients except for 22 subjects in Howard et al. (1978). Subjects in Genuth et al. (1978) seen as inpatients for first week, but as outpatients thereafter. Number in parentheses is number of subjects after attrition.

[b] All follow-up weights calculated from pretreatment values.

[c] Data show mean weight loss for all patients, rather than percentage of patients meeting weight loss criteria as in original study.

TABLE 3.2. Summary Analysis of Five Major Studies Using Very Low Calorie Diets (1984–1991)

Reference	Subjects	Mean pretreatment weight (kg)	Mean age (yr)	Treatment regimen	Mean treatment duration (wk)	Mean weight loss (kg)	Mean weight loss at follow-up (kg)
Andersen et al. (1984)	50 F, 7 M (56; 53)	117.4[a]	34[a]	1. VLCD for 8 wk; 900 kcal/day for 2 wk; VLCD for 8 wk	26	22.0[a]	18 mo: 11 kg
				2. Gastroplasty + short-term VLCD	39	26.1[a]	18 mo: 18 kg
Donnelly et al. (1991)	69 F	102.5	N/A	1. VLCD alone	12.9	20.4	N/A
				2. VLCD + aerobic activity	12.9	21.4	
				3. VLCD + weight training	12.9	20.9	
				4. VLCD combined with aerobic activity + weight training	12.9	22.9	
Hovell et al. (1988)	402 F, 95 M (220)	152.1% of ideal weight	45.4	VLCD for 16–26 wk; 6 wk refeeding; BT for 16 wk minimum	22–32	F = 24.5 M = 28.8	30 mo: Regained 59% to 82% of initial excess weight
Kirschner et al. (1988)	4026 (F:M, 3.5:1) (3020)	F = 99.1 M = 123.6	40.8	VLCD	F = 14.1 M = 13.2	23.4	18 mo: 58% of M and 35% of F who remained in treatment at least 20 wk maintained within 4.5 kg of end-of-treatment loss (n = 966)
Pavlou et al. (1989)	160 M (110)	122% of ideal weight	41.9	1. 1000-kcal/day diet	8	7.1$_x$	Subjects who exercised maintained full end-of-treatment losses at 6 and 18 mo; those who did not exercise regained 60% and 90% of weight loss at these times, respectively
				2. 1000-kcal/day diet + exercise	8	12.0$_y$	
				3. 1000-kcal/day PSMF	8	10.6$_y$	
				4. 1000-kcal/day PSMF + exercise	8	12.5$_y$	
				5. 420-kcal/day VLCD	8	13.2$_y$	
				6. 420-kcal/day VLCD + exercise	8	12.3$_y$	
				7. 800-kcal/day VLCD	8	9.6$_x$	
				8. 800-kcal/day VLCD + exercise	8	12.1$_y$	

Note. Numbers in parentheses indicate number of persons remaining at the end of treatment and at successive follow-up evaluations. VLCD, very low calorie diet; BT, behavior therapy; PSMF, protein-sparing modified fast; N/A, not available. Dissimilar lowercase subscripts (i.e., $_x$, $_y$) indicate statistically significant differences between conditions.
[a]Median value reported.

Attrition does not appear to be a problem in research trials, in which it averages 15% to 20% (Andersen, Backer, Stokholm, & Quaade, 1984; Sikand et al., 1988; Wadden, Sternberg, Letizia, Stunkard, & Foster, 1989; Wing et al., 1991) (see Tables 3.2 and 3.3).

By contrast, attrition appears to be a significant problem in proprietary, hospital-based programs. Hovell et al. (1988) and Kirschner, Schneider, Ertel, and Gorman (1988) observed that 55% and 68% of their patients, respectively, did not complete treatment satisfactorily. Approximately 25% of the patients treated by Kirschner et al. (1988) discontinued therapy within the first 3 weeks, a fact that is not reflected in the mean weight loss of 23.4 kg reported in Table 3.2. These high attrition rates are consistent with those reported for proprietary programs that employ conventional 1200-kcal/day reducing diets (Ashwell, 1978; Feuerstein, Papciak, Shapiro, & Tannenbaum, 1989; Volkmar, Stunkard, Woolston, & Bailey, 1981).

Our research group (Wadden, Foster, Letizia, & Stunkard, in press) assessed attrition and end-of-treatment weight losses in 407 women who participated in a 26-week proprietary program that included 12 weeks of a VLCD (OPTIFAST Core Program, Sandoz Nutrition Corporation, Minneapolis, MN). Fifty-six percent of women completed the full course of treatment, at which time they achieved a mean weight loss of 22.0 kg. Women who discontinued treatment attended an average of 11.7 treatment sessions and lost a mean of 14.3 kg. Mean weight loss for the entire sample of 407 was 19.2 kg. These data show that even when attrition is fully accounted for, VLCDs are still associated with substantial weight losses.

Health Benefits

Weight losses associated with VLCDs are accompanied by substantial reductions in blood pressure, serum total cholesterol, and glucose levels (in Type II diabetics) (Wadden et al., 1983). These and other benefits are reviewed extensively by Kanders and Blackburn (Chapter 9, this volume) and Wing (Chapter 10, this volume) and are not examined further here.

Long-Term Efficacy of Very Low Calorie Diets

Few studies have reported the long-term results of treatment by VLCD. Fewer still have provided data that meet research standards. Thus, in many cases only a small percentage of patients who started treatment were followed up, and these were assessed at varying times. In addition, several investigators reported treatment outcome in terms of the percentage of weight loss or of excess weight that was regained. Such reporting makes comparison with other studies difficult.

The scarcity of long-term data reflects another shortcoming in this area—

a lack of randomized trials in which the efficacy of VLCDs has been compared with other approaches or with no treatment. This is a discouraging occurrence, given the millions of persons who have been treated by VLCDs. Table 3.3 presents the results of the four randomized trials of which we are aware that included at least a 1-year follow-up evaluation and reported weight losses in terms permitting comparison with other studies.

Long-Term Weight Losses

Three of the four studies shown in Table 3.3 found that patients treated by VLCD regained substantial amounts of weight in the first 1 to 2 years following therapy (Sikand et al., 1988; Wadden et al., 1989; Wing et al., 1991). Thus, Sikand et al. (1988) found at a 2-year follow-up that patients treated by diet alone regained a full 16.7 kg (95%) of their 17.5-kg loss. Those who received diet combined with an intensive exercise program did somewhat better, but still regained 12.7 kg (58%) of a 21.8-kg loss. Wing et al. (1991) observed similar findings in a 1-year follow-up evaluation of Type II diabetics treated by diet and lifestyle modification. Patients regained 10 kg (53%) of their 18.6-kg end-of-treatment loss.

Behavior Therapy

Our research team (Wadden et al., 1989) demonstrated that instruction in behavioral methods of weight control may facilitate maintenance of weight loss at 1-year follow-up. Thus, patients who received diet alone (without lifestyle modification) regained 8.4 kg (65%) of their 13.1-kg loss. By contrast, patients who received the VLCD combined with behavior therapy (i.e., combined treatment) regained only 6.2 kg (37%) of their 16.8-kg loss. In addition, 32% of the combined-treatment patients maintained their full end-of-treatment weight loss, as compared with only 5% of persons treated by diet alone.

The effects of behavior therapy, however, appear to be relatively short-lived, as revealed by findings of our 5-year follow-up. At this time, patients in both conditions had returned, on average, to their baseline weights (prior to treatment). There were some individual successes, including 27% of the combined-treatment patients and 11% of the diet-alone patients who maintained a weight loss of 5 kg or more. But the outcome for a majority of patients was clearly disappointing.

Findings of generally poor maintenance of weight loss observed in these three studies stand in sharp contrast to the excellent results reported by Miura, Arai, Tsukahara, Ohno, and Kideda (1989). This team of Japanese investigators found, as we did (Wadden et al., 1989), that behavior therapy significantly improved the maintenance of weight loss achieved by VLCD. They further found, however, that patients treated by the combination of VLCD and behavior therapy continued to lose weight from the end of treatment (mean

TABLE 3.3. Summary Analysis of Randomized Clinical Trials of Very Low Calorie Diets That Include Follow-Up Data

Reference	Subjects	Mean pretreatment weight (kg)	Mean age (yr)	Treatment regimen	Mean treatment duration (wk)	Mean weight loss (kg)	Mean weight loss at follow-up (kg)
Miura et al. (1989)	46 F, 24 M	148% of ideal weight	35.4	1. VLCD for 4–8 wk followed by conventional diet	16	8.6	1 yr: 5.0 2 yr: 4.1
				2. BT + conventional diet	16	4.5	1 yr: 5.5 2 yr: 5.8
				3. BT + VLCD for 4–8 wk followed by conventional diet	16	10.7	1 yr: 11.5 2 yr: 12.0
Sikand et al. (1988)	30 F (21; 15)	102.7	38.8	1. BT + VLCD for 16 wk	16	17.5	2 yr: 0.8
				2. BT + exercise + VLCD for 16 wk	16	21.8	2 yr: 9.1
Wadden et al. (1989)	89 F (76; 68; 55)	106.0	42.1	1. PSMF for 8 wk; 1000–1200 kcal/day for 8 wk	16	13.1_a	1 yr: 4.7_a 5 yr: +1.0
				2. BT + 1200 kcal/day	26	13.0_a	1 yr: 6.6_{ab} 5 yr: +2.7
				3. BT + PSMF for 8 wk; 1000–1200 kcal/day for 18 wk	26	16.8_b	1 yr: 10.6_b 5 yr: +2.9
Wing et al. (1991)	26 F, 10 M (33; 33)	103.8	51.0	1. BT + 1000–1500 kcal/day	20	10.1_a	1 yr: 6.8
				2. BT + PSMF/VLCD for 8 wk; 1000–1500 kcal/day for 12 wk	20	18.6_b	1 yr: 8.6

Note. Numbers in parentheses indicate the number of persons remaining at the end of treatment and at successive follow-up evaluations. VLCD, very low calorie diet; BT, behavior therapy; PSMF, protein-sparing modified fast. Dissimilar lowercase subscripts indicate statistically significant differences between conditions.

loss of 10.7 kg) to the 1-year (11.5 kg) and 2-year (12.0 kg) follow-up evaluations.

Reasons for Miura et al.'s (1989) superior results are not clear, but may include cultural differences between American and Japanese dieters. In addition, the Japanese patients were significantly less obese than their American counterparts, were treated by VLCD for a briefer period, and lost one-third to one-half less weight than patients in the American studies. It is possible that briefer treatment and smaller weight losses do not create as many biological pressures to regain weight (Brownell, 1982). Positive results, similar to those of Miura et al. (1989), were reported by Pavlou, Krey, and Steffee (1989) in a study of police officers who averaged only 22% overweight before treatment. Subjects who received a 420-kcal/day diet in combination with an intensive program of exercise appeared to achieve excellent results at a 3-year follow-up evaluation. The long-term results were reported in graphic form only, however, and must be regarded with caution, given an attrition rate of 31% during treatment and the limited number of persons who participated in the follow-up.

Conclusion

The majority of the evidence from randomized trials indicates that patients treated by VLCDs are likely to regain substantial amounts of weight in the first 2 years following treatment—a finding that is consistent with the results of several uncontrolled investigations (Genuth, Vertes, & Hazelton, 1978; Hovell et al., 1988; Kanders et al., 1991; Wadden, Foster, Letizia, & Stunkard, in press). Combining the VLCD with a program of intensive lifestyle modification is likely to improve weight losses 1 year after treatment but not 5 years.

We note that none of the studies reviewed above included a formal program of weight loss maintenance. Such programs have been shown to improve the maintenance of weight loss following treatment by a conventional 1200-kcal/day diet (Perri, Chapter 19, this volume) and may improve the long-term outcome of VLCD therapy, as discussed in a later section.

Health Benefits

Recent findings have shown that obese patients are likely to maintain some of the health benefits of weight loss even with partial weight regain. Kanders and Blackburn (Chapter 9, this volume) have provided a thorough review of the literature on cardiovascular risk factors, and Wing (Chapter 10, this volume) has done the same for findings in Type II diabetics. In the Wing et al. (1991) study described above, patients treated by VLCD demonstrated significantly better glycemic control at 1-year follow-up than did persons who consumed a 1200-kcal/day conventional reducing diet. The superiority of the VLCD was observed despite the fact that patients treated by this method regained significantly more weight than those who received the conventional diet, and the fact that weight losses of the two conditions did not differ significantly at follow-up. Thus, VLCDs may be of particular benefit to persons with Type II diabetes (Wing, Chapter 10, this volume; Wing et al., 1991).

Relative Efficacy of Very Low Calorie Diets

Any meaningful assessment of the efficacy of VLCDs must include an evaluation of the results of other weight control approaches, as well as comparison with the results of no treatment. In addition, the cost of different therapies must be considered.

There are few published studies of the efficacy of proprietary weight loss programs that treat patients by diets of 1000–1500 kcal/day, composed of either conventional or prepackaged foods. As with VLCDs, this is an alarming omission, given the millions of persons treated by these programs each year at a cost of billions of dollars (Subcommittee on Regulation, Business Opportunities, and Energy, 1990). These programs appear to suffer from high attrition, which may reach as great as 70% within 12 weeks (Feuerstein et al., 1989; Volkmar et al., 1981). This attrition limits the size of average weight losses, and a majority of persons are probably unlikely to achieve clinically significant reductions of 10% or more of initial body weight.

Behavior Therapy with a Conventional Reducing Diet

In the absence of findings from proprietary programs, we will review the results of research studies that have assessed the efficacy of behavior therapy combined with a conventional diet of 1000–1500 kcal/day. As used here, "behavior therapy" refers to group treatment, often provided by a psychologist and/or dietitian, which is designed to modify eating, exercise, dietary, and thinking habits (Wadden & Foster, Chapter 13, this volume). Behavior therapy is probably the most thoroughly researched approach to weight control (Brownell & Wadden, 1986).

Table 3.4 provides a summary of behavioral studies that were published between 1974 and 1990 in the following journals: *Addictive Behaviors*, *Behavior Therapy*, *Behaviour Research and Therapy*, and *Journal of Consulting and Clinical Psychology*. The reader will note that the 13 studies published in 1974 showed an average weight loss of only 3.8 kg, the size of the modest losses reported by Stunkard (1958) in his classic review. By contrast, current behavioral treatment (i.e., studies from 1988–1990) produces an average loss of 8.5 kg. The increased weight loss appears attributable to the longer duration of treatment, which increased from 8.4 to 21.3 weeks from 1974 to 1990. The rate of weight loss in earlier and later studies has remained constant over time at about 0.4–0.5 kg per week. Attrition more than doubled from 1974 to 1990 with the increased duration of treatment, but remains a very modest 13.5% today.

TABLE 3.4. Summary Analysis of Selected Studies from 1974 to 1990 Providing Treatment by Behavior Therapy and Conventional Reducing Diet

	1974	1978	1984	1985–1987	1988–1990
Number of studies included	15	17	15	13	5
Sample size	53.1	54.0	71.3	71.6	21.2
Initial weight (kg)	73.4	87.3	88.7	87.2	91.9
Initial % overweight	49.4	48.6	48.1	56.2	59.8
Length of treatment (wk)	8.4	10.5	13.2	15.6	21.3
Weight loss (kg)	3.8	4.2	6.9	8.4	8.5
Loss per week (kg)	0.5	0.4	0.5	0.5	0.4
Attrition (%)	11.4	12.9	10.6	13.8	21.8
Length of follow-up (wk)	15.5	30.3	58.4	48.3	53.0
Loss at follow-up	4.0	4.1	4.4	5.3	5.6

Note. The data, adapted and updated, are from Brownell and Wadden (1986).

There is a common perception that a slow but steady weight loss, such as that produced by behavioral treatment, is associated with better maintenance of weight loss than that produced by more aggressive approaches. This belief is confirmed by the results of studies from 1974, as it is by more recent studies in which patients lost approximately 5 kg or less (Lavery et al., 1989). Examination, however, of the studies in Table 3.4 published between 1984 and 1990 shows that, on average, patients regained approximately one-third of their weight loss in the year following treatment. Patients gain increasing amounts of weight with longer follow-up (Brownell & Jeffery, 1987; Kramer, Jeffery, Forster, & Snell, 1989). Thus, the larger weight losses produced by current behavioral treatment are associated with substantially greater weight regain than was observed in earlier studies.

Table 3.5 presents in greater detail the results of the five studies from 1988 to 1990 that are summarized in Table 3.4. We note that in none of the treatment conditions shown in Table 3.5 did patients participate in a formal program of weight loss maintenance (which has been shown to improve long-term outcome). We wish to present the results of behavior therapy as practiced in the vast majority of university- and hospital-based clinics.

Randomized Comparison of Very Low Calorie Diets and Conventional Diets

Our review of these studies suggests that patients treated by conventional reducing diets typically lose only about half as much weight (i.e., 8.5 kg) in

TABLE 3.5. Summary Analysis of Five Studies Providing Treatment by Behavior Therapy and Conventional Reducing Diet

	Craighead & Blum (1989)	Perri et al. (1988)	Perri et al. (1989)	Perri et al. (1989)	Rodin et al. (1988)	Wing et al. (1988)
Sample size	20	21	24	24	18	20
Initial weight (kg)	67.6	89.0	96.6	100.4	100.1	97.5
Initial percentage overweight	—	—	53.6	52.4	81.3	52.0
Length of treatment (wk)	12	20	20	40	20	16
Weight loss (kg)	3.8	10.8	8.9	13.6	7.6	6.0
Weight loss per week (kg)	0.3	0.5	0.4	0.3	0.4	0.4
Attrition (%)	30	24	33	33	11	0
Length of follow-up (wk)	52	78	52	32	52	52
Weight loss at follow-up (kg)	2.0	3.6	4.6	9.9	4.5	3.7

20 weeks as individuals treated by a VLCD for 12 weeks (i.e., 18–20 kg). This belief is generally supported by findings from three randomized trials in which patients received behavior therapy in combination with either a 1200-kcal/day diet or a VLCD (Miura et al., 1989; Wadden et al., 1989; Wing et al., 1991) (see Table 3.3).

VLCDs clearly increase short-term weight losses to a degree that is unlikely to be achieved by simply extending the length of traditional treatment. Patients in our randomized trial who received a 1200-kcal/day diet lost an average of 13.0 kg in 26 weeks (Wadden et al., 1989). This finding was replicated in a second study, which yielded a mean weight loss of 11.9 kg in 26 weeks (Wadden, Foster, & Letizia, 1990). Patients lost only 2.6 kg more, however, when this treatment program was extended to 52 weeks. Perri, Nezu, Patti, and McCann (1989) have reported similar findings for treatments of 20 and 40 weeks, as shown in Table 3.5. Thus, the standard behavioral approach is unlikely to produce average weight losses of 15 kg or more, even with very long-term, intensive therapy.

The possibility of more rapid regaining of weight following treatment by VLCD, as compared with conventional reducing diets, may offset the short-term advantages of the former approach. Thus, Wing et al. (1991) observed a difference of 8.5 kg in the end-of-treatment weight losses produced by these two approaches, which decreased to a mere 1.8 kg at 1-year follow-up. The VLCD was still associated with better glycemic control at 1 year than was the conventional diet. Comparable health benefits might not be observed with other medical conditions, however.

In the Miura et al. (1989) study, the difference of 6 kg observed at the end of treatment between the two approaches remained at both the 1-year and 2-year follow-up evaluations. Patients in both conditions showed excellent maintenance of weight loss. In the Wadden et al. (1989) study, the difference of 4 kg between a VLCD and a conventional diet was maintained 1 year later. However, patients in both conditions had regained weight, and the difference between groups was no longer statistically significant. Moreover, both conditions were associated with marked weight regain at the 3-year and 5-year follow-up evaluations.

Cost-Effectiveness

The high cost of VLCDs may further detract from the short-term benefits of this approach. Hospital-based programs typically charge $2500 to $3000 for therapy, which might include 12 weeks of a VLCD within a total program of 26 weeks. By contrast, weight loss by a 1200-kcal/day conventional diet may cost only a few dollars per week (e.g., Weight Watchers or a worksite program).

We will make the following assumptions in trying to assess the cost-effectiveness of treatment by VLCD as compared with a 1200-kcal/day diet combined with behavior therapy:

1. The cost of VLCD is estimated at $2750—the midpoint of the commonly heard estimates of $2500 to $3000 (Henderson, 1991). This $2750 is reduced to $2150 to account for the fact that the diet supplement costs about $600 for 12 weeks of modified fasting, plus 6 weeks of refeeding. Patients would ordinarily pay approximately $600 to eat conventional foods during this 18-week period of time.

2. The mean weight loss for patients who complete the VLCD is estimated at 20 kg (Wadden, Foster, Letizia, & Stunkard, in press). Mean weight loss 1 year after treatment is projected at 12 kg, equal to a weight regain of 40% (Wadden, Foster, Letizia, & Stunkard, in press).

3. The cost of 26 weeks of a 1200-kcal/day diet combined with behavior therapy, and delivered by a clinical psychologist as in research trials, is estimated at $1150. This includes $35 per week for attending group sessions (i.e., $910), plus $100 for an initial evaluation as described by Wadden and Foster (Chapter 13, this volume), and $140 for a medical evaluation as described by Atkinson (Chapter 12, this volume). We believe that all markedly obese individuals should receive a medical evaluation prior to weight reduction, regardless of the type of treatment that they select.

4. The mean weight loss for patients who complete 26 weeks of behavioral treatment is estimated, based on Table 3.4, at 11 kg (i.e., approximately 0.4 kg a week for 26 weeks). This estimate is substantially greater than that which would be anticipated with treatment in a self-help or worksite program (Stunkard, Chapter 2, this volume). That is why the estimated cost is substantially greater. Mean weight loss 1 year after treatment is estimated at 7.33 kg, equivalent to a regain of one-third of lost weight (see Table 3.4).

Short-Term Costs

Given these assumptions, the cost of weight loss by VLCD at the end of treatment is $107.50 per kilogram ($48.86 per pound). That for behavior therapy with a diet of 1200 kcal/day is $104.54 per kilogram ($47.52 per pound). Thus, the costs of these two approaches, per kilogram of lost weight, are roughly comparable at the end of treatment.

Long-Term Costs

With weight regain, however, the cost of the VLCD starts to exceed that for the 1200-kcal/day diet. Thus, assuming a 40% regain in 1 year for the VLCD patients, the cost of weight loss increases to $179.17 per kilogram ($81.43 per pound). That for the 1200-kcal/day diet, after patients regain one-third of lost weight, is only $156.89 per kilogram ($71.31 per pound). The cost for each kilogram of weight loss by VLCD will increase substantially, relative to the cost for the 1200-kcal/day diet, as patients regain increasing amounts of weight.

Cost-Benefit Ratio

We note, however, that by virtue of their larger initial weight losses, patients treated by VLCD will maintain a weight loss of 10 kg or more for a longer period than will persons treated by a 1200-kcal/day diet. Weight loss of this magnitude is likely to confer important health benefits, even with weight regain, as discussed by Kanders and Blackburn (Chapter 9, this volume). In our randomized trial, 90.3% and 63.6% of the patients who received the VLCD and the 1200-kcal/day diet, respectively, lost 10 kg or more at the end of treatment (Wadden et al., 1989). At the 1-year follow-up, the percentages of patients maintaining a loss of this size were 52.0% and 22.7%, respectively. Thus, studies are required that examine not only the cost of weight loss per kilogram, but also the health benefits associated with the weight loss. VLCDs may deliver significantly greater benefits in some cases, which would justify their increased costs. The treatment of Type II diabetes is a case in point, as discussed by Wing (Chapter 10, this volume).

Comparison with No Treatment

It is impossible to assess fully the costs and benefits of different weight reduction therapies without considering the potential costs and liabilities of not treating obesity. For example, should we count as a success or a failure an 80-kg woman who loses 20 kg in 6 months, but regains 7 kg (i.e., one-third) 1 year after treatment, and 14 kg (i.e., two-thirds) 3 years later? The answer depends, in part, upon whether she still experiences significant medical benefits of weight loss (e.g., improved blood pressure or glycemic control) and continues to feel more positive about her appearance and increased mobility.

The answer also depends upon what would have happened to her weight and health had she not reduced. Epidemiological data suggest that, without treatment, she would have gained 2 to 3 kg from baseline to the 3-year follow-up (Hartz & Rimm, 1980; National Center for Health Statistics, 1981). Thus, instead of weighing 74 kg 3 years after therapy, if left untreated she probably would have weighed 83 kg. Weight gain during this time might have been even more precipitous. Women who enrolled in the proprietary program of VLCD and behavior therapy reviewed earlier reported that they gained an average of 16 kg in the 5 years prior to treatment (Wadden, Foster, Letizia, & Stunkard, in press).

Brownell and Jeffery (1987) have called for the evaluation of obese persons who do not enter weight reduction programs, so that long-term changes in their weight, physical health, and psychological well-being can be compared with those of persons who receive treatment. The option of "no treatment" may, in fact, prove preferable to cycles of weight loss and regain, which may increase the risk of cardiovascular morbidity and mortality (Lissner et al., 1991) and may be associated with adverse psychological effects (Wadden, Stunkard, & Liebschutz, 1988). However, careful studies of this issue are required before obese individuals can be encouraged to abandon weight control efforts, in view of the clear adverse health effects associated with this disorder (Manson et al., 1990).

The Future of Very Low Calorie Diets: Critical Issues

Several key research and clinical issues must be resolved if VLCDs are to continue to play a significant role in the treatment of obesity. These include determining the optimal caloric and macronutrient content and the most suitable method of patients' consuming the diets. Moreover, new efforts must be devoted to the problem of weight loss maintenance, which remains the Achilles' heel of all obesity therapies.

Caloric Content

How few calories must a VLCD contain to produce a satisfactory weight loss? By definition, it must provide fewer than 800 kcal/day to qualify as a VLCD (by the American criteria). Clearly, however, the weight loss resulting from a 900-kcal/day liquid diet would not differ substantially (i.e., perhaps 0.167 kg/week) from that of a 750-kcal/day diet.

In explaining the effectiveness of VLCDs, investigators have focused almost exclusively upon caloric content and have overlooked the form and manner in which these diets are consumed. We increasingly believe that the form of the diets is more important than their caloric content. Liquid diets, in particular, provide patients a fixed energy intake and allow them to avoid all contact with conventional foods; thus, they facilitate excellent adherence, particularly when patients are warned that they may become ill if they "go off the diet."

We suspect that patients would lose significantly more weight in consuming a 1000-kcal/day liquid diet than they would on a 1000-kcal/day diet of conventional foods. This is because adherence to conventional diets is not satisfactory, as Stunkard (1958) discussed more than 30 years ago. Recent studies using doubly labeled water have shown that obese individuals may underestimate their caloric intake by as much as 40%, even when they know that their diet diaries are going to be evaluated (Bandini, Schoeller, Cyr, & Deitz, 1990). Thus, many persons who believe that they are adhering to a conventional reducing diet of 1000 kcal/day may, in actuality, be consuming 1400 kcal or more. Liquid diets—and, to a lesser degree, diets of lean meat, fish, and fowl—take the guess-work out of calorie counting.

Our belief that the caloric content of VLCDs is not critical to their success is based upon findings from a recent study in which we compared liquid diets providing 420, 660, and 800 kcal daily (Foster et al., in press). Patients who were randomized to these three conditions lost 18.2, 18.5, and 16.6 kg, respectively, after 12 weeks. Weight losses after the full 26-week program were 19.5, 22.6, and 19.9 kg, respectively. Thus, despite a difference of 380 kcal/day between the lowest and highest diets, patients in all three conditions achieved large weight losses, which did not differ significantly from each other. Similar findings have been reported by several other research teams (Blondheim, Horne, Kaufmann, & Rozen, 1981; Kanders, Blackburn, Lavin, & Norton, 1989; Ohno, Miura, Arai, Tsukahara, & Ikeda, 1989; Vertes, 1985). Treatment by a 1000-kcal/day liquid diet might produce weight losses roughly comparable to those of the other three diets described above.

These findings raise the possibility that a majority of markedly obese patients might be treated satisfactorily with a liquid diet providing 1000 kcal/day. Moreover, increasing the caloric content should reduce the intensity of the medical supervision required, and thus, the cost of treatment. Traditional VLCDs (providing fewer than 800 kcal/day) would be reserved for short individuals and possibly those with abnormally low energy requirements.

Form of the Diet

Most persons treated by a VLCD consume one of the commercially manufactured liquid diets. Research is needed, however, to assess the merits of this approach as compared with a diet of lean meat, fish, and fowl (i.e., a protein-sparing modified fast). We are aware of only one such comparison, and it was limited to 1 month (Wadden et al., 1985). It showed, however, that patients treated by the two approaches lost comparable amounts of weight. In addition, the protein-sparing modified fast was rated as more convenient and was associated with greater reductions in hunger than was the equivalent-calorie liquid diet.

Use of diets comprised of conventional foods (i.e., lean meat, fish, and fowl) might reduce the severe dietary deprivation that patients frequently report. In particular, the protein-sparing modified fast could possibly facilitate the transition from severe caloric deprivation to the resumption of a conventional diet, as a result of patients' consuming small quantities of conventional foods throughout treatment. This is only a hypothesis, but it deserves to be tested.

To take this concept a step further, studies are needed that assess short- and long-term weight changes resulting from a traditional VLCD as compared with the results of treatment in which patients consume a liquid diet for two meals daily but eat a third meal of conventional foods. This approach is similar to a popular over-the-counter weight loss plan. The approach holds promise of producing large weight losses by the use of a portion-controlled diet, but without subjecting patients to the possible adverse behavioral effects of severe dietary deprivation.

Maintenance of Weight Loss

Improving the maintenance of weight loss following treatment by conventional reducing diets, VLCDs, and surgery remains the foremost challenge facing researchers and clinicians. Practice is advancing, although at times it must seem painfully slow to both patients and their health care providers. The discovery of effective methods of maintaining weight loss following VLCD therapy would justify the added expense and risks associated with this approach. We review briefly the most promising leads in this area.

Exercise

Exercise is perhaps the single best predictor (or correlate) of weight maintenance following treatment by a conventional reducing diet (Fox, Chapter 15, this volume). It also improves treatment by VLCD. Pavlou et al. (1989) found that persons who received exercise training in combination with a diet of either 420 or 800 kcal/day maintained almost their entire weight loss 3 years after treatment. Persons who did not exercise had a poor outcome. Caution is required in interpreting these findings, as noted earlier, because they were obtained with mildly obese police officers (who are likely to have differed significantly from usual clinic patients). Nevertheless, the findings are encouraging and suggest that current programs should intensify their exercise instruction, including on-site supervision.

Maintenance Therapy

Behavior modification provided during a VLCD improves the maintenance of weight loss 1 year after therapy, as compared with treatment by diet alone (Wadden & Stunkard, 1986). Despite this improvement, patients are still likely to regain one-third of their weight loss during the year. Perri has shown with a 1200-kcal/day diet that patients will maintain their full end-of-treatment weight loss at 1-year follow-up if they participate in a biweekly program of weight loss maintenance during this time (Perri, Chapter 19, this volume; Perri et al., 1988). Such a program might improve the maintenance of weight loss following a VLCD, although our research team's preliminary results were disappointing (Wadden, Foster, & Letizia, 1990).

Long-Term Meal Replacement

Investigators should also explore whether patients benefit from continuing to use a diet supplement as a replacement for one meal daily, or two meals daily in response to weight gain. Current practice is to discontinue fully the use of the supplement once refeeding is completed. The supplement, however, might be used on a long-term basis if it were found to facilitate weight control.

Pharmacotherapy

Finer, Finer, and Naoumova (1989) found that maintenance of weight loss following a VLCD was enhanced by pharmacotherapy. After a mean loss of 13.9 kg achieved in 8 weeks on a 330-kcal/day diet, patients were refed to approximately 70% of their energy needs and randomly assigned to dexfenfluramine (a serotonin agonist) or placebo. Those who received the drug lost an additional 5.9 kg in the ensuing 18 weeks, whereas those on placebo regained 3.0 kg. These are promising findings that await replication. We are currently participating in a large multicenter trial (i.e., 500 patients) to assess the efficacy of sertraline (a serotonin reuptake inhibitor) in the maintenance of weight loss following a VLCD.

Summary and Conclusions

This chapter has shown that current VLCDs are safe when used under medical supervision by persons 30% or more over ideal body weight and produce average weight losses of 18 to 20 kg in 12 weeks. These end-of-treatment losses are more than double those produced by conventional 1200-kcal/day reducing diets in an equivalent period of time. Weight regain, however, of 30–40% is likely with both dietary approaches in the year following treatment. This regain decreases the long-term attractiveness of VLCDs, as compared with the more economical 1200-kcal/day diets.

Despite the safety of current VLCDs, we question whether a majority of markedly obese patients need to be subjected to diets providing fewer than 800 kcal daily. We suspect that the vast majority of patients would achieve very satisfactory weight losses by consuming diets that resemble current VLCDs in form, but provide approximately 1000 kcal daily. Increasing the caloric content of the diets should reduce the need for such intensive medical supervision, and thus decrease the cost of therapy.

The findings reviewed in this chapter clearly show that researchers and clinicians have significantly improved the treatment of obesity during the last 30 years. The field has advanced dramatically from the state of affairs described by Stunkard in 1958. Practitioners are now able to induce large, clinically significant weight losses by a number of means. The next and admittedly more challenging task is to improve the maintenance of these losses. Several approaches hold significant promise.

References

Apfelbaum, M. (1967). Traitement de l'obésité par la diète protodique. *Entriens de Bichat, 1,* 62.

Amatruda, J. M., Richeson, F., Welle, S. L., Brodows, R. G., & Lockwood, D. H. (1988). The safety and efficiency of a controlled low energy diet in the treatment of non-insulin dependent diabetes and obesity. *Archives of Internal Medicine, 148,* 873–877.

Andersen, T., Backer, O. G., Stokholm, K. H., & Quaade, F. (1984). Randomized trial of diet and gastroplasty compared with diet alone in morbid obesity. *New England Journal of Medicine, 310,* 352–356.

Ashwell, M. (1978). Commercial weight loss programs. In G. Bray (Ed.), *Recent advances in obesity research: II. Proceedings of the Second International Congress on Obesity* (pp. 266–276). London: Newman.

Atkinson, R. L., & Kaiser, D. L. (1981). Nonphysician supervision of a very-low-calorie diet: Results in over 200 cases. *International Journal of Obesity, 5,* 237–241.

Ballor, D. L., Katch, V. L., Becque, M. D., & Marks, C. R. (1988). Resistance weight training during caloric restriction enhances lean body weight maintenance. *American Journal of Clinical Nutrition, 47,* 19–25.

Ballor, D. L., McCarthy, J. P., & Wilterdink, E. J. (1990). Exercise intensity does not affect the composition of diet- and exercise-induced body mass loss. *American Journal of Clinical Nutrition, 51,* 142–146.

Bandini, L. G., Schoeller, D. A., Cyr, H. N., & Dietz, W. H. (1990). Validity of reported energy intake in obese and non-obese adolescents. *American Journal of Clinical Nutrition, 52,* 421–425.

Barrows, K., & Snook, J. T. (1987). Effect of a high-protein, very-low-calorie diet on body composition and anthropometric parameters of obese middle-aged women. *American Journal of Clinical Nutrition, 45,* 381–390.

Bistrian, B. R. (1978). Clinical use of a protein sparing modified fast. *Journal of the American Medical Association, 240,* 2299–2302.

Bistrian, B. R., Blackburn, G. L., & Stanbury, J. B. (1977). Metabolic aspects of protein sparing modified fast in the dietary management of Prader-Willi obesity. *New England Journal of Medicine, 296,* 774–779.

Bistrian, B. R., & Hoffer, L. J. (1982). Obesity. In H. Conn (Ed.), *Current therapy* (pp. 444–447). Philadelphia: W. B. Saunders.

Blackburn, G. L., Bistrian, B. R., & Flatt, J. P. (1975). Role of a protein sparing modified fast in a comprehensive weight reduction program. In A. N. Howard (Ed.), *Recent advances in* obesity research: Proceedings of the First International Congress on Obesity (pp. 279-281). London: Newman.

Blackburn, G. L., Flatt, J. P., Clowes, G. H., Jr., O'Donnell, T. F., & Hensle, T. E. (1973). Protein sparing therapy during periods of starvation with sepsis or trauma. *Annals of Surgery, 177,* 588-594.

Blackburn, G. L., Lynch, M. E., & Wong, S. L. (1986). The very-low-calorie diet: A weight-reduction technique. In K. D. Brownell & J. P. Foreyt (Eds.), *Handbook of eating disorders: Physiology, psychology, and treatment of obesity, anorexia, and bulimia* (pp. 198-212). New York: Basic Books.

Blondhein, S. H., Horne, T., Kaufmann, N. A., & Rozen, P. (1981). Comparison of weight loss on low calorie (800-1200) and very-low-calorie (300-600) diets. *International Journal of Obesity, 5,* 313-317.

Bloom, W. L. (1959). Fasting as an introduction to the treatment of obesity. *Metabolism, 8,* 214-220.

Bollinger, R. E., Lukert, B. D., Brown, R. V., Guevara R. W., & Steinberg, R. (1966). Metabolic balance of obese subjects during fasting. *Archives of Internal Medicine, 118,* 3-8.

Broomfield, P. H., Chopra, R., Sheinbaum, R. C., Bonorris, G. G., Silverman, A., M. Schoenfield, L. J., & Marks, J. W. (1988). Effects of ursodeoxycholic acid and aspirin on the formation of lithogenic bile and gallstones during loss of weight. *New England Journal of Medicine, 319,* 1567-1572.

Brownell, K. D. (1982). Obesity: Understanding and treating a serious, prevalent, and refractory disorder. *Journal of Consulting and Clinical Psychology, 50,* 820-840.

Brownell, K. D. (1988). The yo-yo trap. *American Health Magazine,* pp. 78-84.

Brownell, K. D., Greenwood, M. R. C., Stellar, E., & Shrager, E. E. (1986). The effects of repeated cycles of weight loss and regain in rats. *Physiology and Behavior, 38,* 459-464.

Brownell, K. D., & Jeffery, R. W. (1987). Improving long-term weight loss: Pushing the limits of treatment. *Behavior Therapy, 18,* 353-374.

Brownell, K. D., & Wadden, T. A. (1986). Behavior therapy for obesity: Modern approaches and better results. In K. D. Brownell & J. P. Foreyt (Eds.), *Handbook of eating disorders: Physiology, psychology, and treatment of obesity, anorexia, and bulimia* (pp. 180-197). New York: Basic Books.

Craighead, L. W., & Blum, M. D. (1989). Supervised exercise in behavioral treatment for moderate obesity. *Behavior Therapy, 20,* 49-59.

Committee on Medical Aspects of Food Policy. (1987). *Report of the working group on very low calorie diets: The use of very low calorie diets in obesity.* London: Her Majesty's Stationery Office.

Doherty, J. U., Wadden, T. A., Zuk, L., Letizia, K. A., Foster, G. D., & Day, S. C. (1991). Long-term evaluation of cardiac function in obese patients treated with a very-low-calorie diet: A controlled clinical study of patients without underlying cardiac disease. *American Journal of Clinical Nutrition, 53,* 854-858.

Donnelly, J. E., Pronk, N. P., Jacobsen, D. J., Pronk, S. J., & Jakicic, J. M. (1991). Effects of a very-low-calorie diet and physical training regimens on body composition and resting metabolic rate in obese females. *American Journal of Clinical Nutrition, 54,* 56-61.

Drapkin, R. G., Wing, R. R., Shiffman, S., Buchoff, L., & Grillo, C. (1991, May 21). *Comparison of lapses occurring on a moderate versus a very low calorie diet.* Poster presented at the annual meeting of the Society of Behavioral Medicine, Washington, DC.

Drenick, E. J., & Smith, R. (1964). Weight reduction by prolonged starvation. *Postgraduate Medicine,* A95-A100.

Elliot, D. L., Goldberg, L., Kuehl, K. S., & Bennett, W. M. (1989). Sustained depression of the resting metabolic rate after massive weight loss. *American Journal of Clinical Nutrition, 49,* 93-96.

Feuerstein, M., Papciak, A., Shapiro, S., & Tannenbaum, S. (1989). The weight loss profile: A biopsychosocial approach. *International Journal of Psychiatric Medicine, 19,* 181-192.

Feurer, I. D., & Mullen, J. L. (1986). Measurement of energy expenditure. In J. Rombeau & M. Caldwell (Eds.), *Clinical nutrition* (pp. 224–236). Philadelphia: W. B. Saunders.

Finer, N., Finer, S., & Naoumova, R. P. (1989). Prolonged use of a very low calorie diet (Cambridge diet) in massively obese patients attending an obesity clinic: Safety, efficacy and additional benefit from dexfenfluramine. *International Journal of Obesity, 13*(Suppl. 2), 91–93.

Fisler, J. S., Drenick, E. J., Blumfield, D. E., & Swendseid, M. E. (1982). Nitrogen economy during very low calorie diets: Quality and quantity of dietary protein. *American Journal of Clinical Nutrition, 35*, 471–486.

Forbes, G. B. (1987). Lean body mass–body fat interrelationships in humans. *Nutrition Review, 45*, 225–231.

Forbes, G. B., & Drenick, E. J. (1979). Loss of body nitrogen on fasting. *American Journal of Clinical Nutrition, 32*, 1570–1574.

Foster, G. D., Wadden, T. A., Feurer, I. D., Jennings, A. S., Stunkard, A. J., Crosby, L. O., Ship, J., & Mullen, J. (1990). Controlled trial of the metabolic effects of a very low calorie diet: Short and long-term effects. *American Journal of Clinical Nutrition, 51*, 167–172.

Foster, G. D., Wadden, T. A., Mullen, J. L., Stunkard, A. J., Wang, J., Feurer, I. D., Pierson, R. N., Yang, M.-U., Presta, E., VanItallie, T. B., Lemberg, P. S., & Gold, J. (1988). Resting energy expenditure, body composition and excess weight in the obese. *Metabolism, 37*, 467–472.

Foster, G. D., Wadden, T. A., Peterson, F. J., Letizia, K. A., Bartlett, S. J., & Conill, A. M. (1992). A controlled comparison of three very-low-calorie diets: Effects on weight, body composition, and symptoms. *American Journal of Clinical Nutrition, 55*, 802–810.

Garrow, J. S. (1981). *Treat obesity seriously: A clinical manual.* New York: Churchill Livingstone.

Genuth, S. (1979). Supplemented fasting in the treatment of obesity and diabetes. *American Journal of Clinical Nutrition, 32*, 2579–2586.

Genuth, S. M., Castro, J. H., & Vertes, V. (1974). Weight reduction in obesity by outpatient semi-starvation. *Journal of the American Medical Association, 230*, 987–991.

Genuth, S. M., Vertes, V., & Hazelton, J. (1978). Supplemented fasting in the treatment of obesity. In G. Bray (Ed.), *Recent advances in obesity research: II. Proceedings of the Second International Congress on Obesity* (pp. 370–378). London: Newman.

Hartz, A. J., & Rimm, A. A. (1980). Natural history of obesity in 6946 women between 50 and 59 years of age. *American Journal of Public Health, 70*, 385–388.

Henderson, N. (1991, October). Choose a weight-loss plan that keeps the weight off. *Kiplinger's Personal Finance Magazine*, pp. 104–106.

Hoffer, L. J., Bistrian, B. R., Young, V. R., Blackburn, G. L., & Matthews, D. E. (1984). Metabolic effects of very low calorie weight reduction diets. *Journal of Clinical Investigations, 73*, 750–758.

Honig, J. F., & Blackburn, G. L. (1991). *Practice guidelines for preventing symptomatic gallstones during obesity treatment.* Manuscript submitted for publication.

Hovell, M. F., Loch, A., Hofstetter, C. R., Sipan, C., Faucher, P., Dellinger, A., Borok, G., Forsythe, A., & Felitti, V. J. (1988). Long-term weight loss maintenance: Assessment of a behavioral and supplemented fasting regimen. *American Journal of Public Health, 78*, 663–666.

Howard, A. N. (1989). The historical development of very-low-calorie diets. *International Journal of Obesity, 13*, 1–9.

Howard, A. N., Grant, A., Edwards, O., Littlewood, E. R., & McLean Baird, I. (1978). The treatment of obesity with a very-low-calorie liquid-formula diet: An inpatient/outpatient comparison using skimmed milk as the chief protein source. *International Journal of Obesity, 2*, 321–332.

Howard, A. N., & McLean Baird, I. (1977). A long-term evaluation of very low calorie semi-synthetic diets: An inpatient/outpatient study with egg albumin as the protein source. *International Journal of Obesity, 1*, 63–78.

Isner, J. M., Sours, H. E., Paris, A. L., Farrans, V. J., & Roberts, W. C. (1979). Sudden unexpected death in avid dieters using the liquid protein modified fast diet: Observations in 17 patients and the role of the prolonged QT interval. *Circulation, 60,* 1401–1412.

Kanders, B. S., Blackburn, G. L., Lavin, P. T., & Norton, D. (1989). Weight-loss outcome and health benefits associated with the Optifast Program in the treatment of obesity. *International Journal of Obesity, 13*(Suppl. 2), 131–134.

Kanders, B. S., Blackburn, G. L., Lavin, P. T., Norton, D. E., Peterson, F. J., & Istfan, N. (1991). *Long-term health effects of obesity treatment with a multidisciplinary very low calorie diet program.* Manuscript submitted for publication.

Keefe, P. H., Wyshogrod, D., Weinberger, E., & Agras, W. S. (1984). Binge eating and outcome of behavioural treatment of obesity: A preliminary report. *Behaviour Research and Therapy, 22,* 319–321.

Kirschner, M. A., Schneider, G., Ertel, N. H., & Gorman, J. (1988). An eight-year experience with a very-low-calorie formula diet for control of major obesity. *International Journal of Obesity, 12,* 69–80.

Kramer, F. M., Jeffery, R. W., Forster, J. L., & Snell, M. K. (1989). Long-term follow-up of behavioral treatment for obesity: Patterns of weight regain in men and women. *International Journal of Obesity, 13,* 123–136.

LaPorte, D. J., & Stunkard, A. J. (1990). Predicting attrition and adherence to a very-low-calorie diet: A prospective investigation of the Eating Inventory. *International Journal of Obesity, 14,* 197–206.

Lavery, M. A., Loewy, J. W., Kapadia, A. S., Nichaman, M. Z., Foreyt, J. P., & Gee, M. (1989). Long-term follow-up of weight status of subjects in a behavioral weight control program. *Journal of the American Dietetic Association, 89,* 1259–1264.

Liddle, R. A., Goldstein, R. B., & Saxton, J. (1989). Gallstone formation during weight-reduction dieting. *Archives of Internal Medicine, 149,* 1750–1753.

Life Sciences Research Office. (1979). *Research needs in management of obesity by severe caloric restriction* (Contract No. FDA 223-75-2090). Washington, DC: Federation of American Societies for Experimental Biology.

Lindner, P. G., & Blackburn, G. L. (1976). Multidisciplinary approach to obesity utilizing fasting modified by protein-sparing therapy. *Obesity/Bariatric Medicine, 5,* 198–216.

Linn, R., & Stuart, S. L. (1976). *The last chance diet.* Secaucus, NJ: Lyle Stuart.

Lissner, L., Odell, P. M., D'Agostino, R. B., Stokes, J., Kreger, B. E., Belanger, A. J., & Brownell, K. D. (1991). Variability of body weight and health outcomes in the Framingham population. *New England Journal of Medicine, 324,* 1839–1844.

Marcus, M. D., Wing, R. R., & Lamparski, D. M. (1985). Binge eating and dietary restraint in obese patients. *Addictive Behaviors, 10,* 163–168.

Manson, J. E., Colditz, G. A., Stampfer, M. J., Willett, W., Rosner, B., Monson, R. R., Speizer, F. E., & Hennekens, C. H. (1990). A prospective study of obesity and risk of coronary heart disease in women. *New England Journal of Medicine, 322,* 882–889.

McLean Baird, I., & Howard, A. N. (1977). A double-blind trial of mazindol using a very low calorie formula diet. *International Journal of Obesity, 1,* 271–278.

Miura, J., Arai, K., Tsukahara, S., Ohno, M., & Kideda, Y. (1989). The long term effectiveness of combined therapy by behavior modification and very low calorie diet: 2 year follow up. *International Journal of Obesity, 13*(Suppl. 2), 73–77.

Munro, J. F., & Stolarek, I. (1989). Very-low-calorie diets: Future perspectives. *International Journal of Obesity, 13,* 11–15.

National Center for Health Statistics. (1981). Height and weight of adults ages 18–74 years by socioeconomic status and geographic variables: United States. *Vital Statistics, 224.*

Nettleton, J. A., & Hegsted, D. M. (1975). Protein–energy interrelationships during dietary restriction: Effects on tissue nitrogen and protein turnover. *Nutrition Metabolism, 18,* 31–40.

Ohno, M., Miura, J., Arai, K., Tsukahara, S., & Ikeda, Y. (1989). The efficacy and metabolic effects of two different regimens of very-low-calorie diet. *International Journal of Obesity, 13,* 79–85.

O'Neill, M. (1990, April 1). Dieters, craving balance, are battling fears of food. *The New York Times*, p. 1.

Palgi, A., Read, J. L., Greenberg, I., Hoffer, M. A., Bistrian, B. R., & Blackburn, G. L. (1985). Multidisciplinary treatment of obesity with a protein-sparing modified fast: Results in 688 outpatients. *American Journal of Public Health, 75*, 1190-1194.

Pavlou, K. N., Krey, S., & Steffee, W. P. (1989). Exercise as an adjunct to weight loss and maintenance in moderately obese subjects. *American Journal of Clinical Nutrition, 49*, 1115-1123.

Perri, M. G., McAllister, D. A., Gange, J. J., Jordan, R. C., McAdoo, W. G., & Nezu, A. M. (1988). Effects of four maintenance programs on the long-term management of obesity. *Journal of Consulting and Clinical Psychology, 56*, 529-534.

Perri, M. G., Nezu, A. M., Patti, E. T., & McCann, K. L. (1989). Effect of length of treatment on weight loss. *Journal of Consulting and Clinical Psychology, 57*, 450-454.

Phinney, S. D., Bistrian, B. R., Kosinski, E., Chan, D. P., Hoffer, L. J., Rolla, A., Schachtel, B., & Blackburn, G. L. (1983). Normal cardiac rhythm during hypocaloric diets varying carbohydrate content. *Archives of Internal Medicine, 143*, 2258-2261.

Polivy, J., & Herman, C. P. (1985). Dieting and bingeing: A causal analysis. *American Psychologist, 40*, 193-201.

Rodin, J., Elias, M. Silberstein, L. R., & Wagner, A. (1988). Combined behavioral and pharmacologic treatment for obesity: Predictors of successful weight maintenance. *Journal of Consulting and Clinical Psychology, 56*, 399-404.

Rosen, J. C., Gross, J., Loew, D., & Sims, E. A. H. (1985). Mood and appetite during minimal carbohydrate and carbohydrate-supplemented hypocaloric diet. *American Journal of Clinical Nutrition, 42*, 371-379.

Sikand, G., Kondo, A., Foreyt, J. P., Jones, P. H., & Gotto, A. M. (1988). Two year follow-up of patients treated with very low calorie dieting and exercise testing. *Journal of the American Dietetic Association, 88*, 487-488.

Sours, H. E., Frattali, V. P., Brand, C. D., Feldman, R. A., Forbes, A. L., Swanson, R. C., & Paris, A. L. (1981). Sudden death associated with very low calorie weight reduction regimens. *American Journal of Clinical Nutrition, 34*, 453-461.

Spencer, I. O. B. (1968). Death during therapeutic starvation for obesity. *Lancet, i*, 1288-1290.

Spitzer, R. L., Devlin, M., Walsh, B. T., Hasin, D., Wing, R., Marcus, M., Stunkard, A. J., Wadden, T., Yanovski, S., Agras, W. S., Mitchell, J., & Nonas, C. (in press). Binge eating disorder: A multisite field trial of the diagnostic criteria. *International Journal of Eating Disorders*.

Stunkard, A. J. (1958). The management of obesity. *New York State Journal of Medicine, 58*, 79-87.

Stunkard, A. J., & McLaren-Hume, M. (1959). The results of treatment for obesity. *Archives of Internal Medicine, 103*, 79-85.

Stunkard, A. J., & Rush, J. (1974). Dieting and depression reexamined: A critical review of reports of untoward responses during weight reduction for obesity. *Annals of Internal Medicine, 81*, 526-533.

Subcommittee on Regulation, Business Opportunities, and Energy, Committee on Small Business, U.S. House of Representatives. (1990). *Deception and fraud in the diet industry: Part I. Testimony of Ray Johnson, Assistant Attorney General, State of Iowa* (Series No. 101-50, pp. 47-51). Washington, DC: U.S. Government Printing Office.

Telch, C. F., Agras, W. S., Rossiter, E., Wilfley, D., & Kenardy, J. (1990). Group cognitive-behavioral treatment for the non-purging bulimic: An initial evaluation. *Journal of Consulting and Clinical Psychology, 58*, 629-635.

Thomson, T. J., Runcie, J., & Miller, V. (1966). Treatment of obesity by total fasting for up to 249 days. *Lancet, ii*, 992-996.

Tuck, M. L., Sowers, J., Dornfeld, L., Kledzik, G., & Maxwell, M. (1981). The effect of weight reduction on blood pressure, plasma renin activity, and plasma aldosterone levels in obese patients. *New England Journal of Medicine, 304*, 930-933.

VanItallie, T. B. (1978). Liquid protein mayhem. *Journal of the American Medical Association, 240*, 140-141.
VanItallie, T. B. (1988). Obesity. In K. M. Jeejeebhoy (Ed.), *Current therapy and nutrition* (pp. 314-324). Toronto: Decker.
VanItallie, T. B., & Yang, M. U. (1977). Current concepts in nutrition: Diet and weight loss. *New England Journal of Medicine, 297*, 1158-1161.
VanItallie, T. B., & Yang, M.-U. (1984). Cardiac dysfunction in obese dieters: A potentially lethal complication of rapid massive weight loss. *American Journal of Clinical Nutrition, 39*, 695-702.
Vertes, V. (1985). Clinical experience with a very low calorie diet. In G. L. Blackburn & G. A. Bray (Eds.), *Management of obesity by severe caloric restriction* (pp. 349-358). Littleton, MA: PSG.
Vertes, V., Genuth, S. M., & Hazelton, I. M. (1977). Supplemented fasting as a large scale outpatient program. *Journal of the American Medical Association, 238*, 1251-1253.
Volkmar, F. R., Stunkard, A. J., Woolston, J., & Bailey, R. A. (1981). High attrition rates in commercial weight reduction programs. *Archives of Internal Medicine, 141*, 426-428.
Wadden, T. A., Foster, G. D., & Letizia, K. A. (1990). *Long-term treatment of obesity with and without very-low-calorie diet*. Unpublished manuscript.
Wadden, T. A., Foster, G. D., & Letizia, K. A. (in press). Response of obese binge eaters to treatment by behavior therapy combined with very low calorie diet. *Journal of Consulting and Clinical Psychology*.
Wadden, T. A., Foster, G. D., Letizia, K. A., & Mullen, J. L. (1990). Long-term effects of dieting on resting metabolic rate in obese outpatients. *Journal of the American Medical Association, 264*, 707-711.
Wadden T. A., Foster, G. D., Letizia, K. A., & Stunkard, A. J. (in press). A multi-center evaluation of a proprietary weight reduction program for the treatment of marked obesity. *Archives of Internal Medicine*.
Wadden, T. A., Sternberg, J. A., Letizia, K. A., Stunkard, A. J., & Foster, G. D. (1989). Treatment of obesity by very low calorie diet, behavior therapy, and their combination: A five-year perspective. *International Journal of Obesity, 13*(Suppl. 2), 39-46.
Wadden, T. A., & Stunkard, A. J. (1986). Controlled trial of very low calorie diet, behavior therapy, and their combination in the treatment of obesity. *Journal of Consulting and Clinical Psychology, 54*, 482-488.
Wadden, T. A., Stunkard, A. J., & Brownell, K. D. (1983). Very low calorie diets: Their efficacy, safety, and future. *Annals of Internal Medicine, 99*, 675-684.
Wadden, T. A., Stunkard, A. J., Brownell, K. D., & Day, S. C. (1985). A comparison of two very-low-calorie diets: Protein-sparing-modified fast versus protein liquid formula diet. *American Journal of Clinical Nutrition, 41*, 533-539.
Wadden T. A., Stunkard, A. J., Day, S. C., Gould, R. A., & Rubin, C. J. (1987). Less food, less hunger: Reports of appetite and symptoms in a controlled study of a protein sparing modified fast. *International Journal of Obesity, 11*, 239-249.
Wadden, T. A., Stunkard, A. J., & Liebschutz, J. (1988). Three year follow-up of the treatment of obesity by very-low-calorie diet, behavior therapy, and their combination. *Journal of Consulting and Clinical Psychology, 56*, 925-928.
Wadden, T. A., Stunkard, A. J., & Smoller, J. W. (1986). Dieting and depression: A methodological study. *Journal of Consulting and Clinical Psychology, 54*, 869-871.
Wadden, T. A., VanItallie, T. B., & Blackburn, G. L. (1990). Responsible and irresponsible use of very-low-calorie diets in the treatment of obesity. *Journal of the American Medical Association, 263*, 83-85.
Weltman, A., Matter, S., & Stamford, B. A. (1980). Caloric restriction and/or mild exercise: Effects on serum lipids and body composition. *American Journal of Clinical Nutrition, 33*, 1002-1009.
Webster, J. D., Hesp, R., & Garrow, J. S. (1984). The composition of excess weight in obese

women estimated by body density, total body water and total body potassium. *Human Nutrition: Clinical Nutrition, 38C*, 299-306.

Wing, R. R. (in press). Weight cycling in humans: A review of the literature. *Annals of Behavioral Medicine*.

Wing, R. R., Marcus, M. D., Epstein, L. H., & Kupfer, D. (1983). Mood and weight loss in a behavioral treatment program. *Journal of Consulting and Clinical Psychology, 51*, 153-155.

Wing, R. R., Marcus, M. D., Salata, R., Epstein, L. H, Miaskiewicz, S., & Blair, E. H. (1991). Effects of a very-low-calorie diet on long-term glycemic control in obese Type II diabetics. *Archives of Internal Medicine, 151*, 1334-1340.

Yang, M. U. (1988). Body composition and resting metabolic rate in obesity. In R. T. Frankle & M.-U. Yang (Eds.), *Obesity and weight control* (pp. 71-96). Rockville, MD: Aspen.

Yang, M. U., Barbosa-Saldivar, J. L., Pi-Sunyer, F. X., & VanItallie, T. B. (1981). Metabolic effects of substituting carbohydrate for protein in a low-calorie diet: A prolonged study in obese patients. *International Journal of Obesity, 5*, 231-236.

PART TWO

BIOLOGICAL RESPONSE TO CALORIC RESTRICTION

4

Effect of Energy Restriction on Body Composition and Nitrogen Balance in Obese Individuals

MEI-UIH YANG

THEODORE B. VANITALLIE

Excessive loss of fat-free mass (FFM) by obese patients during prolonged, severe caloric restriction can result in iatrogenic illness of varying severity and, rarely, in sudden death. For this reason alone, the effect of therapeutic caloric restriction on body composition should be a matter of great concern to physicians who treat obesity.

In a metabolic ward setting, it is possible to determine with considerable accuracy the effects of various diets on FFM, particularly the protein moiety of the FFM, by measuring nitrogen (N) balance. The determination of N balance entails meticulous measurement of the amount of N consumed and that lost from the body in the urine and feces. The small quantity of N represented by the shedding of skin, hair, and nail fragments, and the loss of various bodily secretions, has to be estimated from the data obtained by investigators who have carefully quantified these losses (Calloway, Odell, & Margen, 1971).

Because it is usually impossible to conduct N balance studies on patients, physicians have to rely on more feasible approaches to the problem of monitoring composition of weight lost during prolonged caloric restriction. These approaches include (1) use of any of a variety of methods to measure body composition and its changes during weight loss (VanItallie & Segal, 1989; Yang, Wang, Pierson, & VanItallie, 1977); and (2) determinations of various serum indicators of protein nutriture—notably, albumin and the protein moieties that turn over more rapidly, such as prealbumin, transferrin, and retinol-binding protein (RBP) (Shetty, Watrasiewicz, Jung, & James, 1979). In view of the fast-changing nature of body composition measurement technology, a brief discussion of some of the methods currently in use may be helpful.

Measurement of Body Composition and Its Changes: Methods and Interpretation

In Vivo Methods of Measurement of Body Constituents

During therapeutic weight loss, it is helpful to be able to measure both the initial composition of the body and the changes that occur as a result of caloric restriction. Such measurements help investigators and clinicians assess the effect of various diets on the composition of weight lost, and, accordingly, the safety and appropriateness of such diets. In the past, the body constituents of greatest interest have been FFM, body fat mass (BFM), total body potassium (TBK), and total body water (TBW), as well as extracellular and intracellular water (ECW and ICW). More recently, *in vivo* neutron activation (IVNA) analysis has made it possible to estimate with considerable precision additional body constituents, such as total body nitrogen (TBN), calcium, phosphorus, chloride, carbon, and hydrogen (Heymsfield et al., 1989; Kehayias, Heymsfield, LoMonte, Wang, & Pierson, 1991).

Intracellular versus Extracellular Protein

The measurement of TBN by IVNA analysis now permits *in vivo* estimation of total body protein; however, it needs to be stressed that the protein component of greatest interest to those concerned with monitoring the composition of weight lost is intracellular protein. Total body protein can be divided into two broad categories: (1) intracellular protein and (2) extracellular protein. Extracellular protein includes (a) "structural proteins" (notably collagen and the protein components of bone, tendons, ligaments, etc.); and (b) the proteins that circulate in blood (albumin and other carrier proteins, such as RBP, transferrin, prealbumin, and the protein moieties of lipoproteins). Although erythrocytes are cells, their principal protein component (the globin portion of hemoglobin) is less labile than many of the proteins in muscle or viscera.

When one is concerned about the protein depletion that can occur during chronic energy deficit, the component of greatest interest is intracellular protein (i.e., the protein within the cells of the heart, liver, kidneys, skeletal muscle, etc.). It is this protein source that constitutes the major part of the body's "labile" protein reserve. Unfortunately, there is no convenient way to measure intracellular protein directly; however, the change that occurs in TBN during chronic energy deficit (and in other catabolic conditions) is most likely attributable to loss of intracellular protein, inasmuch as extracellular protein is not depleted rapidly during subsistence on diets deficient in calories and/or protein.

In healthy individuals, intracellular protein is about 53% of total body protein (International Commission on Radiological Protection, 1984); hence, when total body protein is determined to be decreasing at some given rate, the extent of the decrease taking place in intracellular protein can be seriously underestimated unless the difference in lability between the extra- and intracellular protein components is kept in mind. (See Figure 4.1.)

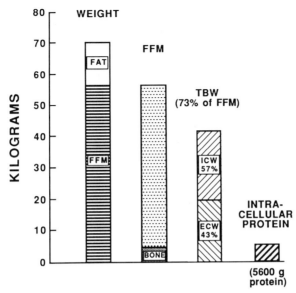

FIGURE 4.1. Body composition of a 70-kg reference man. (Values are from International Commission on Radiological Protection, 1984.)

Traditional Body Composition Methods

Historically, body composition has been determined by means of underwater weighing (hydrodensitometry) and by anthropometry (measurement of skinfold thicknesses at various sites as indices of subcutaneous fat content, and of various limb and trunk circumferences as indicators of muscle mass, as well as fatness).

Use of anthropometry has permitted investigators in the field to obtain reasonably accurate data for surveys of the nutritional status of various population groups; however, measurement of skinfold thickness is subject to a variety of errors, both methodological and biological. For example, it is difficult to obtain satisfactory and reproducible skinfold measurements in severely obese individuals; moreover, visceral fat, which may vary rather widely among obese persons (Sjöström & Kvist, 1988), can only be guessed at when adiposity is estimated from anthropometric data.

Hydrodensitometry is a more satisfactory method for estimating BFM and FFM; however, its accuracy is impaired by biological variations in bone mass and density and in the degree of hydration of the FFM. In addition, there are technical errors associated with measuring residual lung volume and obtaining accurate underwater weights, particularly in massively obese individuals.

FFM can be estimated from TBK (obtained by measurement of naturally occurring ^{40}K in a whole-body gamma ray counter). Unfortunately, this method for determining FFM and BFM is not always satisfactory, owing to errors in individual measurements that range from approximately 4% in phantoms to as much as 10% in human subjects (Pierson, Wang, Thornton, VanItallie, & Colt, 1984). Moreover, during weight reduction, rate of K loss from the body (particularly during the glycogen depletion phase) may be far more rapid than the concurrent rate of N loss. It also has to be kept in mind that the efficiency of ^{40}K counting in a whole-body counter increases as obese patients lose subcutaneous fat and thereby reduce self-absorption of ^{40}K-generated gamma emissions during successful treatment.

Measurement of energy–nitrogen (E-N) balance is a useful method against which the accuracy of serial body composition determinations performed by other techniques can be judged (Yang et al., 1977). In addition to providing information about N (protein) balance data, the E-N balance method permits estimation of fat balance from the measurement of energy balance corrected for N-derived energy (Passmore, Strong, & Richie, 1958). Change in TBW is then inferred from careful measurement of changes in body weight, after allowance has been made for the putative effects on body weight of changes in body protein (extrapolated from N balance data) and body fat content. This method is most accurate when applied after the occurrence of the early phase of rapid weight loss, which is normally associated with a water diuresis and glycogen depletion.

Newer Body Composition Methods

Recent advances in body composition technology include the development of IVNA techniques, dual photon absorptiometry, computerized tomography, and magnetic resonance imaging. These techniques are still in the investigative stage and, for the time being, have their greatest value in clinical investigation and as independent reference methods to help validate such recently developed rapid and clinically convenient procedures as those that estimate FFM by total body electrical conductivity (TOBEC) or biological impedance analysis (BIA).

The two latter methods (TOBEC and BIA) are based on the fact that the FFM, because of its content of water and electrolytes, is electrically conductive, whereas body fat is virtually nonconductive. Since the conductivity or impedance of the FFM varies systematically with its size, instruments designed to measure conductivity (or some related electrical property) can provide reasonably accurate estimations of the size of the FFM, assuming that the proper regression equations are available and are used to translate conductivity data into a quantitative estimate of FFM in kilograms. If FFM and body weight are known, body fat mass can be calculated by subtracting FFM from total body weight.

Interpretation

Advantages and Limitations of Various Methods

For the most part, the technologies for estimating body composition described above are not accessible to the practitioner. Because of the convenience and the rapidity with which they provide reasonably accurate results, the newer "electrical" methods such as BIA and TOBEC will probably be used increasingly to monitor composition of weight lost during therapeutic caloric restriction. However, both methods have certain limitations that need to be taken into consideration when the body composition data they generate are interpreted.

In the first place, as mentioned earlier, both bioelectrical methods measure such parameters as conductivity, resistivity, or impedance—indices that must be translated into metric units of volume (liters) or mass (kilograms) before they can be used by the practitioner. The equations to carry out this translation have to be derived from studies on appropriate, comparable populations in which the results obtained with the electrical method under consideration have been systematically compared with results obtained in the same subjects by an established reference method, such as hydrodensitometry or TBW by tracer dilution. Thus, if the equations used to derive kilograms of FFM or liters of water from conductivity/impedance units were based on studies of inappropriate population groups (because of differences in age, race, muscularity, stature, etc.), then significant errors could well result.

Another potential problem with the electrical methods is that they are quite responsive to changes in TBW. Hence, if the ECW volume changes disproportionately to a concurrent change in TBW (as often occurs during treatment of obesity), it may become very difficult to interpret the resulting changes measured in kilograms of FFM. For example, a recent study of the use of TOBEC to monitor changes in body composition in obese patients during caloric restriction reported that the water diuresis occurring early in weight loss significantly confounded interpretation of the long-term results (Vaswani, Gamble, & VanItallie, in press). Accordingly, the authors recommended that during TOBEC monitoring, body composition measurements obtained 2 to 3 weeks after initiation of caloric restriction be used as a more reliable benchmark against which to compare later measurements.

The problem of interpreting changes in FFM when the distribution of ICW and ECW is not known also arises when measurements such as hydrodensitometry are performed. There is, however, some hope that refinements in the TOBEC and BIA methods will ultimately permit a rapid estimation of ICW and ECW as well as of TBW. Currently, the methods that attempt to distinguish the proportions of ECW and ICW in TBW are under study in research settings.

Relation of Rate of Weight Loss to Composition of Weight Loss

It is important that practitioners who treat obese patients distinguish between quantity of weight loss and its quality. What is weight loss of "acceptable quality"? One way of answering this question is to examine the composition of the excess weight present in obese persons. Webster, Hesp, and Garrow (1984) studied this problem by analyzing body composition measurements made on 104 women whose ages ranged from 14 to 61 and whose BFM varied from 6%

to 60% of body weight. They discovered that differences in weight between obese and nonobese women of similar height are attributable to a mixture of constituents that is 70–78% fat and 22–30% FFM. In a later study conducted on 24 men, these investigators obtained similar results for the composition of "excess weight." The conclusion arrived at by the authors was that during therapeutic caloric restriction, it is prudent to ensure that no more than 25% of the weight loss be FFM.

Subsequent studies performed by Vaswani and colleagues have tended to confirm the findings of Webster and colleagues (Vaswani et al., in press; Webster et al., 1984). Accordingly, we believe that an acceptable composition of weight lost over time would be one that is at least 75% fat and does not exceed 25% FFM. If this criterion is taken as one standard by which to evaluate the long-term safety of low calorie regimens, then it is possible to derive tentative guidelines for the design of calorie-restricted diets that will induce weight loss of acceptable composition.

To this end, the first step is to consider the calorie value of 1 pound (0.45 kg) of "lost weight" of acceptable composition. The appropriate calculations are shown in Figure 4.2, which indicates that 1 pound of acceptable composition corresponds to an energy deficit of approximately 3200 kilocalories (kcal). Thus, at an energy deficit of 1000 kcal/day, it will take 3.2 days to lose 1 pound of weight of acceptable composition. This means that at a daily energy deficit

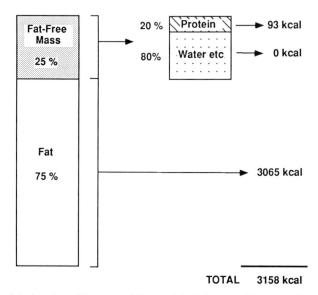

FIGURE 4.2. Caloric value of 1 pound of "lost weight" of acceptable composition (25% fat-free mass and 75% fat). At a 1000-kcal/day deficit, it will take 3.2 days to lose 1 pound. Thus, to maintain a weight loss of acceptable composition, the rate of loss should not exceed (on the average) 0.3 pound/day.

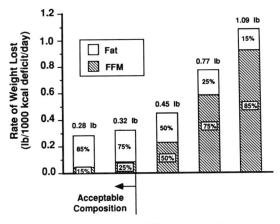

FIGURE 4.3. Composition of weight loss at different rates of weight reduction (assuming water equilibrium). Values are normalized to pounds per 1000-kcal/day deficit.

of 1000 kcal and assuming water equilibrium, the rate of weight loss per day should not exceed 0.3 pound (1 pound/3.2 days = 0.31).

If the rate of weight loss on a diet that creates a daily deficit of 1000 kcal is consistently more rapid than 0.3 pound/day, then the quality of the loss becomes increasingly unsatisfactory as the rate increases, as shown in Figure 4.3. Thus, at an energy deficit of 1000 kcal/day and a rate of weight loss of 0.45 pound/day, an obese person on a low calorie diet is actually losing equal amounts of FFM and fat. If this state of affairs is allowed to continue for a prolonged period, the body will become increasingly depleted of protein, with the attendant adverse consequences of such depletion.

On the basis of the calculations outlined above, one can reason that if the size of the patient's energy deficit is known with reasonable accuracy, the practitioner can then estimate whether or not the associated daily rate of weight reduction is compatible with an acceptable composition of loss of body constituents. By restraining rate of weight reduction to that associated with a loss of acceptable composition, the practitioner can increase the likelihood that the rate of weight loss exhibited by the patient is within a safe range as far as conservation of FFM is concerned. If the practitioner deems it important to obtain a more accurate representation of the size of the daily energy deficit, then it would be prudent to obtain the consultative assistance of a registered dietitian or a suitably qualified nutritionist.

Body Composition Terminology: Problems in Interpretation

As suggested earlier, the principal body constituents that are measured by various *in vivo* methods include FFM (lean body mass), BFM, and the total body content of water (TBW), potassium (TBK), sodium, chloride, calcium, and certain other minerals. As implied, values for the FFM are particularly subject to misinterpretation because FFM includes ECW, a fairly variable component, and body cell mass (BCM), a somewhat less variable component. The latter component includes ICW as well as various cell solids. Bone, except for the fat in its marrow, is part of the FFM, but much of bone cannot be considered to be part of the BCM. Because FFM embodies fluid components that can vary and, indeed, may change in opposite directions (i.e., ECW may increase while ICW is decreasing), changes in FFM must be interpreted with great caution, particularly in the absence of independent information about ECW, ICW, and TBN.

In a two-compartment analysis of body composition in which only FFM and BFM are estimated, it is most useful in individual patients to express changes in these two compartments in absolute terms—that is, in kilograms. As we have pointed out recently (VanItallie, Yang, Heymsfield, Funk, & Boileau, 1990), expressing BFM and/or FFM as percentages of body weight can be misleading. Since body weight in this context is composed of two components, FFM and BFM, one of which may be changing more rapidly than the other, it is obvious that the more slowly decreasing component paradoxically would appear to increase as a percentage of body weight, while the extent of the decrease of the more rapidly decreasing component would be underestimated because of the confounding effect of the more slowly decreasing component. It makes sense to use absolute values rather than percentages, which are often misleading and difficult to interpret. For example, an individual who embarks on a muscle-building project may greatly increase muscle mass. In this person, if BFM remains unchanged, it will nevertheless decrease as a percentage of total body weight. If BFM decreases while muscle mass remains constant, then FFM, expressed as a percentage of body weight, artifactually increases. The confusion often generated by the use of percentages can be avoided if individuals with a changing body composition are looked at in terms of the absolute changes that are occurring or have occurred in FFM and BFM.

Using Height-Normalized Indices of Fat-Free Mass and Body Fat Mass

In view of the fact that in population samples, variance in FFM and to a lesser extent in BFM is significantly affected by height, it seems logical to attempt to normalize values for FFM and BFM for height to facilitate comparison of individuals of differing heights. In this regard, we (VanItallie et al., 1990) have proposed the use of height-normalized indices for FFM and BFM. These indices have been termed the fat-free mass index (FFMI) and the body fat mass index (BFMI). The body mass index (BMI) is used as the model:

$$BMI = \frac{\text{weight (kg)}}{\text{height}^2 \text{ (m)}}$$

FFMI is then

$$FFMI = \frac{FFM \text{ (kg)}}{\text{height}^2 \text{ (m)}}$$

BFMI is

$$BFMI = \frac{BFM \text{ (kg)}}{\text{height}^2 \text{ (m)}}$$

Thus, FFMI + BFMI = BMI.

We (VanItallie et al., 1990) have suggested that FFMI and BFMI values be determined in a representative sample of the U.S. population (similar to the BMIs calculated for such a population by the National Center for Health Statistics during the second National Health and Nutrition Examination Survey [NHANES II] conducted during 1976–1980). Once compiled, such values could be used to develop reference standards by which to assess the status of FFMI and BFMI in a given individual.

Changes in Body Composition during Caloric Restriction

Regrettably, the scientific literature on changes in body composition associated with caloric restriction is sparse. Although many N balance studies have been reported in individuals who were losing weight, such experiments, at best, tell us only about "protein balance" and fail to throw much light on concurrent changes in fat and water. In addition, many N balance studies have been carried out under conditions that render the findings unreliable. For example, there has often been failure to control for the many factors that influence N balance (see below). Moreover, many studies have been performed on outpatients or patients in regular hospital facilities, where adequacy of control of intake and output cannot be guaranteed. Some studies have been flawed for reasons such as the following: (1) Only urinary N was measured; (2) the study failed to take into account "noncollectible" losses of N; (3) N excretion was estimated from urinary urea N; (4) the accuracy of laboratory measurements of dietary, urinary, and fecal N was questionable; and (5) the investigators failed to carry out concurrent measurements of daily creatinine excretion to validate the completeness of collection of 24-hour urines.

Only a few E-N balance studies conducted under metabolic ward conditions have been reported in patients or volunteer subjects. Nor have there been many published reports on the composition of weight lost during energy restriction that were based on serial estimations of body composition. Of the sequential body composition studies that have been reported, several have been difficult to interpret because the putative changes in body composition (i.e., TBK, TBW, body density) that were determined often fell within the range of measurement error.

In 1977, we (VanItallie & Yang, 1977, 1978) reviewed the literature on changes in body composition during weight loss. The harvest was disappointingly small; however, the few studies that provided sufficient data for analysis all demonstrated clearly that obese and nonobese individuals differ markedly in their metabolic response to caloric restriction, particularly if such restriction is prolonged. This effect is shown in Figure 4.4 and will be discussed in some detail in the next section of this chapter.

Factors That Influence Nitrogen Balance and Body Composition during Caloric Restriction

Obviously, a number of variables influence N balance and body composition during energy deficit. We consider such variables under three broad headings: (1) dietary factors; (2) physical exercise; and (3) host factors.

Dietary Factors

Calorie (Energy) Content of the Diet

The diet's energy content (or, better, the amount of energy actually consumed per day) is one of the major factors affecting N balance and body composition. If energy intake is low, the body must not only draw on its energy reserves (principally fat) for sustenance, but may also have to catabolize both endogenous and dietary protein for gluconeogenesis. As a consequence of energy deficiency, body protein synthesis rate decreases (Millward, Garlick, Stewart, Nnanyelugo, & Waterlow, 1975; Swick & Benevenga, 1977) and muscle protein synthesis, which is particularly sensitive to a reduced intake of energy and/or protein, can exhibit a substantial decrease. Yet, because of the body's continuing need for amino acids for synthesis of other critically needed proteins (for gluconeogenesis or simply as a fuel), body protein catabolism is not correspondingly inhibited. When the protein synthesis rate decreases to a point below the rate of protein breakdown, the result is N deficit and, ultimately, body protein depletion.

When energy intake is sufficiently low (i.e., 25% or less of the requirement for maintenance of normal body composition), dietary protein is increasingly catabolized to meet the body's overriding need for glucogenic amino acids and fuel. There is a systematic (albeit rough) inverse relationship between calorie intake on the one hand, and nitrogen deficit on the other hand. This relation-

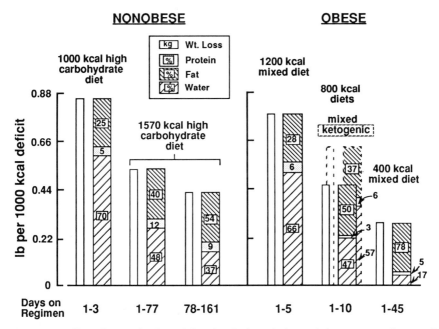

FIGURE 4.4. Effect of energy intake and duration during caloric restriction on rate and composition of weight loss in nonobese and obese subjects. All values have been normalized to pounds per 1000-kcal deficit. Adapted from "Current Concepts in Nutrition: Diets and Weight Loss" (p. 1159) by T. B. VanItallie and M.-U. Yang, 1977, *New England Journal of Medicine, 297,* 1158–1161. Copyright 1977 by *New England Journal of Medicine.* Adapted by permission.

ship (also observed in obese individuals; see Figure 4.5) is to some degree independent of the protein content of the diet.

Many studies of N balance in normal-weight adults at or near energy equilibrium have disclosed that, in such individuals, a selective reduction in energy intake is associated with a negative N balance. Several studies have shown that energy intake affects requirements for protein (Garza, Scrimshaw, & Young, 1976; Goranzon & Forsum, 1985; Kishi, Miyatani, & Inoue, 1978; Rao, Naidu, & Rao, 1975; Torun, Scrimshaw, & Young, 1977). For example, if a 20% energy deficit is induced in a subject (whether by decreasing food intake or increasing level of physical activity), a deficit in N will ensue. Collectively, these observations indicate that there is at least a transient linear relationship between energy intake and N balance at various levels of protein intake (see Figure 4.6).

Effect of Energy Deficit on Protein Requirement

Rao et al. (1975) found that at an energy intake of 2066 kcal, 60 g of protein per day was necessary to maintain N equilibrium in five "normal healthy young men" (p. 1116). In contrast, those consuming less protein (40 g/day)

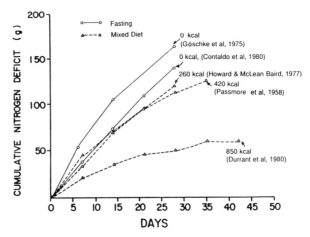

FIGURE 4.5. Cumulative nitrogen deficits in obese subjects on daily energy intakes ranging from 0 to 850 kcal.

required more dietary energy (2245 kcal/day) to achieve N equilibrium. Based on their studies, Rao and colleagues concluded that at a protein intake of 60 g/day, a change in energy intake of 100 kcal/day results in a change in N balance of 0.16 g/day. Kishi and colleagues observed that at a level of 40 kcal/kg/day, 15 nonobese young men gradually lost 1–2 pound over a 2-week test period (Kishi et al., 1978). At this submaintenance level of energy intake, the amount of protein required to sustain N equilibrium was about 0.775 g of egg protein per kilogram of body weight per day—about 105% of the U.S. recommended daily allowance for protein. This finding is consonant with other

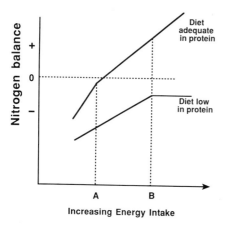

FIGURE 4.6. Relationship among protein, energy intake, and nitrogen balance. Adapted from "General Aspects of the Regulation of Protein Metabolism by Diet and by Hormones" (p. 420) by H. N. Munro, 1964, in H. N. Munro and J. B. Allison (Eds.), *Mammalian Protein Metabolism* (Vol. 1, pp. 381–481). New York: Academic Press. Copyright 1964 by Academic Press. Adapted by permission.

studies suggesting that even at moderate levels of energy deficit, the requirement for protein increases. Yet, despite the important effect of the energy intake on the body's protein requirement, it appears that changes in protein intake may be more effective than changes in energy intake in causing an alteration in N balance to take place (Garza et al., 1976).

Calorie–N relationships have been the subject of a number of reviews published in the 1950s and 1960s (Allison, 1951, 1958; Calloway & Spector, 1954; Munro, 1964). These reviews tended to focus on the results of relatively short-term experiments conducted on nonobese subjects or animals. Nevertheless, more recent evidence compiled by VanItallie and Abraham (1985) suggests that the N-sparing effect of increasing levels of energy intake occurs in obese as well as nonobese persons (see Figure 4.5). However, the dynamics of the calorie–N relationship can be influenced by the size of the fat depot as well as the state of the protein reserves, as will be discussed below under "Host Factors."

Flaws in the Design of Experiments Concerned with Calorie–Nitrogen Relationships

It is often difficult to interpret findings of experiments in which the "experimental" condition involves the alteration of more than one independent variable at one time. Davies et al. (1989) compared the metabolic responses of 16 obese women to a low calorie diet (780 kcal/day) versus a very low calorie diet (VLCD) (330 kcal/day). After consuming a 2000-kcal diet for 1 week, the obese women were randomly assigned to either a 330-kcal diet (providing 34 g of high quality protein, 44 g of carbohydrate, and 3 g of fat per day) or a 780-kcal diet (providing 63 g of high quality protein, 85 g of carbohydrate, and 17 g of fat per day). Over an 8-week period, average N balance was -1.46 ± 0.57 ($\pm$ SD) g of N per day in the 330-kcal group and $+1.39 \pm 0.73$ g of N per day in the 780-kcal group ($p < .05$). Thus, mean N balance in the 330-kcal group remained negative throughout the study.

One problem in interpreting these results lies in the fact that in the experimental (780-kcal diet) group, energy intake was increased over that of the control (VLCD) group by a factor of 2.36, while protein intake was simultaneously increased by a factor of 1.85. Clearly, it is difficult in such a study to separate the effect on N balance of increasing nonprotein calories from that of simultaneously increasing protein intake.

A more pervasive problem in the design of nutritional experiments involving caloric restriction lies in the failure of many investigators to be concerned with the size of the energy deficits induced by various low calorie diets. "Energy deficit" is a term that describes the difference between the energy level provided by a calorie-reduced diet and the energy level required to maintain one's current body weight and composition ("maintenance energy requirement" [MER]). Thus, as shown in Figure 4.7, the MER of individuals of similar age and stature will differ materially, depending on such factors as BMI and

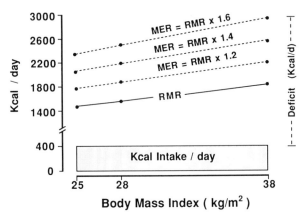

FIGURE 4.7. A 400-kcal/day diet will induce diverse energy deficits depending on factors such as sex, age, body size, physical activity level, and so on. The values shown are for three females 40 years old and 67 inches in height with different body mass indices. Energy deficit is determined by subtracting the appropriate maintenance energy requirement (MER) from the daily calorie intake, and MER is estimated from resting metabolic rate (RMR).

habitual physical activity (including its nature, duration, and intensity). Other attributes such as sex, age, and body composition also influence the MER.

In effect, MER is often estimated from an individual's resting metabolic rate (RMR), either calculated or measured, together with a careful appraisal of the amount of energy expended in physical activity. (This is often calculated by multiplying the RMR by a factor [e.g, 1.2–1.6] that attempts to allow for the contribution of daily physical activity to the MER.) As shown in Figure 4.7, a 400-kcal/day diet fed to subjects with different MERs can induce diverse energy deficits, whether expressed in absolute kilocalories or more appropriately, as percentages of MER. Thus, a 400-kcal/day diet will induce a 2515-kcal deficit (86%) in a physically active woman, age 40, height 67 inches (BMI = 38) whose MER is 2915 kcal/day, and a 1351-kcal deficit (77%) in a very sedentary and thinner woman of the same age and height (BMI = 25) whose MER is 1751 kcal/day.

Absolute Energy Deficit versus Percentage Energy Deficit

Countless nutritional experiments have demonstrated that the size of the energy deficit induced by a calorically restricted diet is a key consideration in determining metabolic response, rather than simply the energy content of the diet. For this reason, it makes little sense to study the effects of calorically restricted diets on N balance and other dependent variables unless the percentage energy deficit induced in each experimental subject is known and, if possible, controlled. Therefore, in conducting experiments on the metabolic effects of caloric restriction, investigators may have to compare individuals or groups whose MERs are inherently similar, or, alternatively, adjust the experimental diet so as to create a comparable degree of deficit, calculated as percentage of MER ([Energy intake − MER] × 100/MER). Unfortunately, most reports of experiments that examined the effect of various low calorie diets on N balance, body composition, and other dependent variables have failed to specify the percentage energy deficit induced in the subjects under study.

By the nature of the mathematics used to calculate percentage energy deficit, the percentage value is always less striking than the absolute value for calorie deficit. For example, as shown in Figure 4.7, if a 40-year-old female with a BMI of 38 and an MER of 2915 kcal/day is maintained on a 400-kcal diet, the energy deficit will be 2515 kcal/day. If the same woman on the same diet reduces her physical activity and thereby decreases her MER to 2551 kcal/day, the energy deficit will be 2151 kcal/day, 364 fewer kcal/day (and over a 10-day period 3641 kcal, equivalent to approximately 1 pound of lost weight). This substantial difference in negative energy balance (expressed as kilocalories) between the two levels of MER represents only a 2% difference when expressed as percentage energy deficit.

Although it is obviously difficult to obtain an accurate estimate of the daily MER (except by measuring energy expenditure in a room calorimeter), the principle of calculating the percentage energy deficit is an important one and, in our judgment, should be adhered to by investigators who are conducting studies of the metabolic effects of calorie-restricted diets.

Dietary Protein Intake: Quantity and Quality

The relationship between levels of dietary protein intake and N balance has been extensively studied in nonobese individuals, but far less is known about the effect in obese persons of varying protein consumption at different fixed levels of energy intake. The general relationship seems to be that at any given level of energy intake, there may be an improvement in N balance as the protein content of the diet is increased (see Figure 4.6). However, the ability of any particular level of protein intake to reduce N deficit may be influenced by the number and type of nonprotein calories consumed at the same time, as well as by the size of the N "reserve" present in the subject. Thus, there may be an initial rise in the quantity of N stored in the body (or a reduction in the N deficit) as protein intake increases, but this could quickly be replaced by an equilibrium or even a deficit condition, depending on a variety of factors, only one of which is the energy intake level (Nettleton & Hegsted, 1975).

There is evidence suggesting that the level of protein intake per se can have an important influence on N balance. Thus, Oi et al. (1987) have reported that normal-weight subjects fed diets providing 1100 kcal/day and at least 70 g of protein per day were able to remain in N equilibrium. In contrast, subjects receiving the same number of calories but only 50 g of protein per day exhibited a negative N balance. In another experiment, Durrant et al. (1980) studied obese subjects who remained on diets providing 850 kcal and 43 g of protein per day for 6 weeks. All of the subjects on this regimen exhibited N deficits during the first 5 weeks, and only some achieved N equilibrium or a positive N balance by the 6th week.

If the protein consumed is of poor quality (i.e., having a low protein efficiency ratio [PER]), then one would expect the fraction of the absorbed N retained in the body for anabolism to be suboptimal. This is the same as saying that the protein in question also has a reduced biological value. In other words, if two low calorie diets equal in energy and protein content are fed, one of which provides a protein of reduced biological value, then the N balance is likely to be more negative in the subjects consuming the poor quality protein diet. Increasing intake of the poor quality protein may or may not reduce the nitrogen deficit, depending on the nutritional circumstances. (A protein source's quality can be estimated from its content of essential and nonessential amino acids. Thus, the potential nutritive value of a protein can be predicted by comparing its essential amino acid composition with the amino acid compositions of reference proteins [i.e., egg albumin or lactalbumin] known to be of high quality.)

Optimizing the Protein Content of Low Calorie Diets

It is also not at all clear what the optimal level of protein intake is for obese individuals who continue to adhere faithfully to a low calorie diet. There appears to be a limit to how much protein one can add to a low calorie diet and still obtain an increasingly beneficial effect on N balance. In this regard, we (Yang & VanItallie, 1984) studied a series of obese individuals maintained for 64 days on either of two low calorie diets (600–800 kcal/day as determined by bomb calorimetry), consisting of protein alone at 1.5 g per kilogram of desirable weight per day or an equal mixture of protein and carbohydrate (each at 0.75 g/kg/day). On the average, the diet that consisted almost entirely of protein did not spare body protein better or induce a greater rate of weight loss than did the mixture of protein and carbohydrate.

Although a case could therefore be made for limiting the protein content of a low energy diet to a point where it provides no more than half of the calories (i.e., 75 g in a 600-kcal diet), no one seems to know how far the protein content of an energy-restricted diet can be reduced without having undesirable metabolic and clinical effects. In one study of obese patients who lost weight following therapeutic gastroplasty, Rasmussen and Andersen (1985) found that the patients who consistently consumed less than 34 g of protein per day exhibited adverse changes in rapidly turning over plasma proteins (prealbumin and RBP), and were at considerable risk of developing QTc interval prolongation and ventricular arrhythmia. Accordingly, when a weight reduction diet is prescribed, it seems prudent to provide more protein (perhaps an excessive amount) rather than to risk inducing protein depletion with a hypocaloric diet that is too low in protein content.

Role of Nonprotein Calories: Carbohydrate versus Fat

There is considerable evidence that during caloric restriction, dietary carbohydrate is better than fat at sparing body protein. In a study of the effect of dietary fat, carbohydrate, and protein on branched-chain amino acid catabolism during caloric restriction, Vazquez, Morse, and Adibi (1985) found a sharp contrast between the effect of carbohydrate and that of fat and protein on branched-chain amino acid oxidation. In this experiment, after 1 week of consumption of a 500-kcal diet, body protein was spared more effectively by dietary carbohydrate than by an equicaloric quantity of fat. Also, we (Yang & VanItallie, 1976) found that over a 10-day period, the N deficit associated with an 800-kcal diet providing 45% of calories from carbohydrate was somewhat less than the deficit associated with an equicaloric diet providing the same amount of protein but only 5% of calories from carbohydrate.

Richardson, Wayler, Scrimshaw, and Young (1979) examined the effect on N balance of an isocaloric exchange of carbohydrate for fat (and vice versa) in subjects consuming 0.57 g/kg/day of milk protein at energy intakes ranging from excessive to submaintenance. These investigators found that when the fat in the diets was replaced by carbohydrate, N retention was enhanced. Indeed, improvement in protein utilization even occurred in those subjects who were losing weight on a restricted calorie intake. Richardson and colleagues concluded that "a diet supplying twice as much energy from carbohydrate as from fat . . . when compared to one providing equal proportions of energy from [those] nonprotein sources . . . significantly improved overall N balance" (1979, p. 2223).

Exercise

The effect of increased muscular exertion on N balance and on body protein content can be quite variable, depending, *inter alia*, on the type of the exercise (e.g., jogging vs. weight lifting), the intensity and duration of the exercise, and the individual's nutritional status and degree of physical fitness.

The studies of Todd, Butterfield, and Calloway (1984) and Walberg et al. (1988) suggest that to remain in N equilibrium, dieters who also exercise require protein in excess of the U.S. recommended daily allowance. Not surprisingly, the energy deficit that can be created by increased physical activity may bring about a negative N balance. In studies conducted by Goranzon and Forsum (1985), subjects (nonobese young men and women) were fed 0.57 g/kg/day of protein and energy to maintain body weight under normal conditions. When they increased their expenditures by 20% by exercising on a stationary bicycle, they lost weight and exhibited significantly negative N balances. In a review of the pertinent literature, Lemon (1987) concluded that exercise increases protein need when energy intake is inadequate. According to Lemon, "there are several groups that are at higher risk [of experiencing an exercise-induced need for protein] . . . including individuals who may not consume a diet with sufficient total energy" (1987, p. S187).

Exercise can be a healthy way to induce an energy deficit sufficient to bring about weight loss; however, certain kinds of exercise may also enlarge muscle mass, which could increase the need for dietary protein as well as energy. For this reason, in overweight dieters who are being subjected to therapeutic caloric restriction, it is important to assess carefully the effect of a concurrent increase in physical exercise on the energy deficit and on protein need. In his review, Lemon has called attention to studies in which exercise increased N loss and has warned that "if allowed to continue . . . [the] negative nitrogen balance could decrease muscle mass and strength and adversely affect performance" (1987, p. S186).

Host Factors

Concurrent Nutritional Status

The metabolic response of an individual to any given diet depends not only on the nature of the diet, but on the nutritional status of the individual *at the time*. In this context, the expression "at the time" is very important, because it reflects the fact that a change in nutritional status over time will alter the metabolic response to a constant diet.

There are many examples of this phenomenon in the nutrition literature. Nitrogen retention is more likely to occur on a VLCD as protein stores continue to diminish. The effect of body protein depletion on the efficiency of the utilization of dietary N was well illustrated by Allison and Fitzpatrick in 1960 (see Figure 4.8). Accordingly, it is not surprising that during adherence to a VLCD, patients frequently exhibit a gradual improvement in N balance and, after a time, may approach or even achieve N equilibrium. It should be kept in mind, however, that in some instances at least, achievement of N equilibrium on a VLCD may be transient, being followed by a subsequent return to N deficit (Yang, Barbosa-Saldivar, Pi-Sunyer, & VanItallie, 1981). Also, the attainment of N equilibrium on a VLCD may be illusory, resulting from the fact that noncollectible N losses (and, in some cases, fecal N losses) have been disregarded. Also, N intake may have been calculated from food tables or simply not measured properly.

Thus, a part of the improved retention of N exhibited by obese patients as they continue to adhere to a VLCD is attributable to the concurrent depletion of body protein. What is not clear is just how much protein depletion must occur before the N excretion rate tends to stabilize at a new, lower level. Moreover, there is no assurance that if a diet is sufficiently low in protein and/or energy content, the patient will not continue to remain in protein deficit until severe illness or death supervenes.

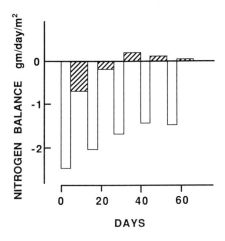

FIGURE 4.8. Nitrogen balances in dogs fed a protein-free diet (white bars) alternating with wheat gluten protein (hatched bars). Note that once protein depletion has occurred, there may be transient retention of dietary nitrogen on a relatively low intake of wheat protein. From *Dietary Proteins in Health and Disease* (p. 45) by J. B. Allison and W. H. Fitzpatrick, 1960, Springfield, IL: Charles C Thomas. Copyright 1960 by Charles C Thomas. Reprinted by permission.

Body Fat Content and Body Protein Conservation during Caloric Restriction

The evidence is convincing that during severe caloric restriction, body protein is more efficiently conserved by obese than by lean individuals. As an example, in one study (Passmore et al., 1958) obese subjects on a 400-kcal/day diet for 6 weeks lost far less nitrogen per day than nonobese individuals did while adhering to a 1570-kcal/day diet for 6 months (Keys, Brozek, Henschel, Mickelsen, & Taylor, 1950) (see Figure 4.4).

Because MERs in obese individuals are often higher than those in nonobese persons, some sort of normalization of the daily N excretion rate is needed if an appropriate comparison of people in these two categories is to be made. Thus, N excretion rate can be normalized to grams of N per kilogram of weight loss, grams of N per square meter of body surface, or grams of N per 1000-kcal deficit. Several studies have shown that during weight loss induced by therapeutic caloric restriction, an inverse relationship is obtained between the N deficit–weight loss ratio and degree of fatness (Durrant et al., 1980; Forbes & Drenick, 1979; VanItallie & Yang, 1977). Thus, at any given energy deficit, the N deficit–weight loss ratio is likely to be lower in severely obese (i.e., BMI of 32 to 42) than in moderately obese (i.e., BMI of 27 to 30) patients. In other words, in severely obese patients who lose weight on a hypocaloric diet, it is likely that a smaller proportion of the loss will be protein than would be the case if a nonobese or less obese person were subjected to a similar percentage energy deficit. The protective function of body fat stores during severe caloric restriction was evidenced in 17 dieters who died suddenly during or shortly after prolonged adherence (2–8 months) to a VLCD consisting entirely of collagen hydrolysates (liquid protein diet). We (VanItallie & Yang, 1984) reported that the duration of survival among these victims was positively correlated with their prediet body fat content as inferred from BMI. Thus, in this small subset, the fattest dieters lived the longest.

Weight control programs often lose sight of the fact that when patients are successful at losing large quantities of excess fat, they become more and more like nonobese individuals. This means that the same percentage energy deficit that was associated with reasonable conservation of body protein early in treatment could induce an excessive body protein loss in a patient whose fat stores have substantially diminished. Accordingly, it seems prudent to reduce in a systematic way the severity of the percentage energy deficit imposed on a patient as that patient's obesity increasingly lessens during treatment.

Does an Increased Fat-Free Mass Protect against Protein Depletion during Severe Caloric Restriction?

Obese people are not simply fatter than nonobese people; they also possess a larger FFM. This fact has been demonstrated by a number of anthropometric and body composition studies (Forbes, 1987; Forbes & Welle, 1983; James, Bailes, & Davies, 1981; Webster et al., 1984). Although some reports indicate that the composition of the excess weight of obese individuals is approximately 25% FFM and 75% fat, it is likely that proportions of these two constituents can vary appreciably, depending on such factors as severity of the obesity, age, sex, physical fitness, age of onset of the obesity, and so on.

If excess weight includes a substantial proportion of FFM, then it can be argued that during diet-induced weight reduction, some loss of body protein is obligatory. This argument is based on the unproven premise that during caloric restriction, components of excess weight will be lost in the same proportions in which they were present in the body. While such an assumption is at present unwarranted, further research into this matter is needed. In theory, an N deficit of as much as 3.6 g of N per pound of weight loss could be considered obligatory, assuming that the composition of the excess weight is 75% fat and 25% FFM and that the composition of the loss is 25% FFM of "normal" composition and 75% fat.

It is conceivable that obese individuals are somehow protected by their "extra" protein stores against the harmful effects of drastic caloric restriction. If this were true, a severely restricted diet should be tolerated better by people with a large musculature (e.g., body builders) than by normal-weight individuals with an average-sized musculature. To our knowledge, experiments designed to test this hypothesis have not been reported. Indeed, the physiological significance of the protein moiety of excess weight during weight reduction remains obscure.

Serum Triiodothyronine Changes and Nitrogen Conservation

There is inconclusive evidence suggesting that one of the mechanisms that help the body adapt to caloric deprivation is the ability to lower triiodothyronine

(T_3) during energy deficit. In a study of six subjects maintained on diets providing 600 to 800 kcal/day for 64 days, we (Yang & VanItallie, 1984) observed an inverse correlation between the magnitude of the T_3 drop by the end of the weight loss period and the magnitude of the cumulative N deficit exhibited by the subjects. Subsequently, Kaptein, Fisler, Duda, Nicoloff, and Drenick (1985) reported that in 10 obese men consuming 400 kcal/day for 40 days, there was a good inverse correlation between N deficit during this period and the degree of concurrent fall in T_3. A similar inverse correlation was also observed when the hypocaloric study period was shorter (2 weeks) in obese subjects on a 200-kcal/day regimen (Koppeschaar, Meinders, & Scharz, 1985).

However, other investigators who studied T_3 changes in subjects losing weight over a 21-day period of dieting were unable to find any correlation between thyroid hormones, energy deficit, or body cell mass (estimated from urinary creatinine) with N losses (Hendler & Bonde, 1990). There is also some controversy as to whether the decrease that occurs in T_3 during caloric restriction can be correlated with a proportionate decrease in resting metabolic rate. In our study, we (Yang & VanItallie, 1984) were unable to find such a correlation. On the other hand, Rozen, Abraham, Falcou, and Apfelbaum (1986) reported that when obese women were given 40 μg of T_3 per day for 2 weeks, their T_3 levels had increased by 20%; at the same time, the RMR failed to decrease, as would have been expected. In contrast, a control group of dieting women who did not receive T_3 exhibited a 22% decrease in T_3 levels and showed an appreciable drop in RMR.

In view of the conflicting results reported by research groups using markedly different experimental designs, the issue of whether the ability to lower T_3 during caloric restriction affects one's ability to conserve body protein must be considered unresolved.

Potential Nitrogen-Sparing Effects during Therapeutic Caloric Restriction for Human Growth Hormone and Insulin-Like Growth Factor I

It has been reported that injections of human growth hormone (HGH) (0.1 mg/kg ideal body weight) every 48 hours for 3 weeks improved N balance in seven of eight obese subjects maintained on diets providing 24 kcal and 1 g of protein per day (per kilogram of ideal body weight) (Clemmons, Snyder, Williams, & Underwood, 1987). The mean daily N deficit was -0.35 ± 2.14 (SD) g/day during 3 weeks of HGH administration and -2.21 ± 1.45 g/day during vehicle administration. (All of the subjects had been maintained on the same hypocaloric diet for 2 weeks before HGH or vehicle administration was begun.)

It has also been observed that HGH has N-retaining effects in malnourished surgical patients receiving hypocaloric parenteral nutrition (Ziegler, Young, & Manson, 1988) and in elderly adults with recent weight loss (Binnerts, Wilson, & Lamberts, 1988; Marcus et al., 1990). Collectively, these observations suggest that HGH, as well as insulin-like growth factor I (through which HGH presumably exerts its N-retaining action), may someday prove to be useful in reducing N deficits in severely obese patients while they are adhering to VLCDs. However, any conclusion concerning the utility of these hormones in the treatment of obesity will have to be deferred, pending the receipt of more definitive experimental evidence.

References

Allison, J. B. (1951). Interpretation of nitrogen data. *Federation Proceedings, 10*, 676–683.
Allison, J. B. (1958). Calories and protein nutrition. *Annals of the New York Academy of Sciences, 69*, 1009–1018.
Allison, J. B., & Fitzpatrick, W. H. (1960). *Dietary proteins in health and disease*. Springfield, IL: Charles C Thomas.
Binnerts, A., Wilson, J. H. P., & Lamberts, S. W. J. (1988). The effects of human growth hormone administration in elderly adults with recent weight loss. *Journal of Clinical Endocrinology and Metabolism, 67*, 1312–1384.
Calloway, D. H., Odell, A. C. F., & Margen, S. (1971). Sweat and miscellaneous nitrogen losses in human balance studies. *Journal of Nutrition, 101*, 775–786.
Calloway, D. H., & Spector, H. (1954). Nitrogen balance as related to caloric and protein intake in active young men. *American Journal of Clinical Nutrition, 2*, 405–412.
Clemmons, D. R., Snyder, D. K., Williams, R., & Underwood, L. E. (1987). Growth hormone administration conserves lean body mass during dietary restriction in obese subjects. *Journal of Clinical Endocrinology and Metabolism, 64*, 878–883.
Contaldo, F., DiBiase, G., Scalfi, L., Presta, E., & Mancini, M. (1980). Protein-sparing modified fast in the treatment of severe obesity: Weight loss and nitrogen balance. *International Journal of Obesity, 4*, 189–196.
Davies, H. J., McLean Baird, I., Fowler, J., Mills, I. H., Baillie, J. E., Rattan, S., & Howard, A. N. (1989). Metabolic response to low- and very-low-calorie diets. *American Journal of Clinical Nutrition, 49*, 745–751.
Durrant, M., Garrow, J. S., Royston, P., Stalley, S. F., Sunkin, S., & Warwick, P. M. (1980). Factors influencing the composition of the weight loss by obese patients on a reducing diet. *British Journal of Nutrition, 44*, 275–285.
Forbes, G. B. (1987). Lean body mass–body fat interrelationship in humans. *Nutrition Reviews, 45*, 225–231.
Forbes, G. B., & Drenick, E. J. (1979). Loss of body nitrogen on fasting. *American Journal of Clinical Nutrition, 32*, 1570–1574.
Forbes, G. B., & Welle, S. L. (1983). Lean body mass in obesity. *International Journal of Obesity, 7*, 99–107.
Garza, C., Scrimshaw, N. S., & Young, V. R. (1976). Human protein requirements: The effect of variations in energy intake within the maintenance range. *American Journal of Clinical Nutrition, 29*, 280–287.
Goranzon, H., & Forsum, E. (1985). Effect of reduced energy intake versus increased physical activity on the outcome of nitrogen balance experiments in man. *American Journal of Clinical Nutrition, 41*, 919–928.
Göschke, H., Stahl, M., & Tholen, H. (1975). Nitrogen loss in normal and obese subjects during total fasting. *Klinische Wochenshrift, 53*, 605–610.
Hendler, R., & Bonde, A. A. (1990). Effects of sucrose on resting metabolic rates, nitrogen balance, leucine turnover, and oxidation during weight loss with low calorie diets. *International Journal of Obesity, 14*, 927–938.
Heymsfield, S. B., Wang, J., Kehayias, J., Heshka, S., Lichman, S., & Pierson, R. N., Jr. (1989).

Chemical determination of human body density in vivo: Relevance to hydrodensitometry. *American Journal of Clinical Nutrition, 50,* 1282-1289.

Howard, A. N., & McLean Baird, I. (1977). A long-term evaluation of very low calorie semi-synthetic diets: An inpatient/outpatient study with egg albumin as the protein source. *International Journal of Obesity, 1,* 63-78.

International Commission on Radiological Protection. (1984). *Report of the Task Group on Reference Man.* Elmsford, NY: Pergamon Press.

James, W. P. T., Bailes, J., & Davies, H. L. (1981). Elevated metabolic rates in obesity. *Lancet, i,* 1122-1125.

Kaptein, E. M., Fisler, J., Duda, M. J., Nicoloff, J. T., & Drenick, E. J. (1985). Relationship between the changes in serum thyroid hormone levels and protein status during prolonged protein supplemented caloric deprivation. *Clinical Endocrinology, 22,* 1-15.

Kehayias, J., Heymsfield, S. B., LoMonte, A., Wang, J., & Pierson, R. N., Jr. (1991). In vivo determination of body fat by measuring total body carbon. *American Journal of Clinical Nutrition, 53,* 1339-1344.

Keys, A., Brozek, J., Henschel, A., Mickelsen, F., & Taylor, H. L. (1950). *The biology of human starvation.* Minneapolis: University of Minnesota Press.

Kishi, K., Miyatani, S., & Inoue, G. (1978). Requirement and utilization of egg protein by Japanese young men with marginal intakes of energy. *Journal of Nutrition, 108,* 658-669.

Koppeschaar, H. P., Meinders, A. E., & Scharz, F. (1985). Metabolic responses during modified fasting and refeeding: The role of sympathetic nervous system activity and thyroid hormones. *Human Nutrition: Clinical Nutrition, 39C,* 17-28.

Lemon, P. W. R. (1987). Protein and exercise: Update 1987. *Medicine and Science in Sports and Exercise, 19*(5), S179-S190.

Marcus, R., Butterfield, G., Holloway, L., Gilliand, L., Baylink, D. J., Hintz, R. L., & Sherman, B. M. (1990). Effects of short term administration of recombinant human growth hormone to elderly people. *Journal of Clinical Endocrinology and Metabolism, 70,* 519-527.

Millward, D. J., Garlick, P. J., Stewart, R. J. C., Nnanyelugo, D. O., & Waterlow, J. C. (1975). Skeletal muscle growth and protein turnover. *Biochemistry Journal, 150,* 235-243.

Munro, H. N. (1964). General aspects of the regulation of protein metabolism by diet and by hormones. In H. N. Munro & J. B. Allison (Eds.), *Mammalian protein metabolism* (Vol. 1, pp. 381-481). New York: Academic Press.

Nettleton, J. A., & Hegsted, D. M. (1975). Protein-energy interrelationships during dietary restriction: Effects on tissue nitrogen and protein turnover. *Nutrition Metabolism, 18,* 31-40.

Oi, Y., Okuda, T., Koishi, H., Koh, H., Waki, M., Kurata, M., & Nambu, S. (1987). Relationship between protein intake and nitrogen balance in obese patients on low energy diet. *Journal of Nutrition, Science, and Vitaminology, 33,* 219-226.

Passmore, R., Strong, J. A., & Ritchie, F. J. (1958). The chemical composition of the tissue lost by obese patients on a reducing regimen. *British Journal of Nutrition, 12,* 113-122.

Pierson, R. N., Jr., Wang, J., Thornton, C., VanItallie, T. B., & Colt, E. W. D. (1984). Body potassium by four-pi ^{40}K counting: An anthropometric correction. *Journal of Applied Physiology, 246,* F234-F239.

Rao, C. N., Naidu, A. N., & Rao, B. S. N. (1975). Influence of varying energy intake on nitrogen balance in men on two levels of protein intake. *American Journal of Clinical Nutrition, 28,* 1116-1121.

Rasmussen, L. H., & Andersen, T. (1985). The relationship between QTc changes and nutrition during weight loss after gastroplasty. *Acta Medica Scandinavica, 217,* 271-275.

Richardson, D. Q., Wayler, A. H., Scrimshaw, N. S., & Young, V. R. (1979). Quantitative effect of an isoenergetic exchange of fat for carbohydrate on dietary protein utilization in healthy young men. *American Journal of Clinical Nutrition, 32,* 2217-2226.

Rozen, R., Abraham, G., Falcou, R., & Apfelbaum, M. (1986). Effects of a "physiological" dose of triiodothyronine on obese subjects during a protein-sparing diet. *International Journal of Obesity, 10,* 303-312.

Shetty, P. S., Watrasiewicz, K. E., Jung, R. T., & James, W. P. T. (1979). Rapid-turnover transport proteins: An index of subclinical protein malnutrition. *Lancet, ii*, 2310–2320.

Sjöström, L., & Kvist, H. (1988). Regional body fat measurements with CT-scan and evaluation of anthropometric predictions. *Acta Medica Scandinavica*, Suppl. 723, 169–177.

Swick, R. W., & Benevenga, N. J. (1977). Labile protein reserves and protein turnover. *Journal of Dairy Science, 604*, 505–515.

Todd, K. S., Butterfield, G. E., & Calloway, D. H. (1984). Nitrogen balance in men with adequate and deficient energy intake at three levels of work. *Journal of Nutrition, 114*, 2107–2118.

Torun, B., Scrimshaw, N. S., & Young, V. R. (1977). Effect of isometric exercise on body potassium and dietary protein requirements on young men. *American Journal of Clinical Nutrition, 30*, 1983–1993.

VanItallie, T. B., & Abraham, S. (1985). Some hazards of obesity and its treatment. In J. Hirsch & T. B. VanItallie (Eds.), *Recent advances in obesity research: IV* (pp. 1–19). London: John Libbey.

VanItallie, T. B., & Segal, K. R. (1989). Nutritional assessment of hospital patients: New methods and new opportunities. *American Journal of Human Biology, 1*, 205–208.

VanItallie, T. B., & Yang, M.-U. (1977). Current concepts in nutrition: Diets and weight loss. *New England Journal of Medicine, 297*, 1158–1161.

VanItallie, T. B., & Yang, M.-U. (1978). Nitrogen balance during weight reduction: Effect of body stores of protein and fat. In G. A. Bray (Ed.), *Recent advances in obesity research: II* (pp. 379–384). London: Newman.

VanItallie, T. B., & Yang, M.-U. (1984). Cardiac dysfunction in obese dieters: A potentially lethal complication of rapid, massive weight loss. *American Journal of Clinical Nutrition, 39*, 695–702.

VanItallie, T. B., Yang, M.-U., Heymsfield, S. B., Funk, R. C., & Boileau, R. A. (1990). Height normalized indices of the body's fat-free mass and fat mass: Potentially useful indicators of nutritional status. *American Journal of Clinical Nutrition, 52*, 953–959.

Vaswani, A., Gamble, M. V., & VanItallie, T. B. (in press). Use of electromagnetic scanning in the determination of body composition in obese subjects undergoing weight reduction. In J. Kral & T. B. VanItallie (Eds.), *Human body composition: Technology and clinical applications.* London: Smith-Gordon.

Vazquez, J. A., Morse, E. L., & Adibi, S. A. (1985). Effect of dietary fat, carbohydrate, and protein on branched-chain amino acid catabolism during caloric restriction. *Journal of Clinical Investigation, 76*, 734–743.

Walberg, J. L., Leidy, M. K., Sturgill, D. J., Kinkle, D. E., Ritchey, S. J., & Sebolt, D. R. (1988). Macronutrient content of a hypoenergy diet affects nitrogen retention and muscle function in weight lifters. *International Journal of Sports Medicine, 9*, 261–266.

Webster, J. D., Hesp, R., & Garrow, J. S. (1984). The composition of excess weight in obese women estimated by body density, total body water, and total body potassium. *Human Nutrition: Clinical Nutrition, 38C*, 299–306.

Yang, M.-U., Barbosa-Saldivar, J. L., Pi-Sunyer, F. X., & VanItallie, T. B. (1981). Metabolic effects of substituting carbohydrate for protein in a low-calorie diet: A prolonged study in obese patients. *International Journal of Obesity, 5*, 231–236.

Yang, M.-U., & VanItallie, T. B. (1976). Composition of weight loss during short-term weight reduction. Metabolic responses of obese subjects to starvation and low calorie ketogenic and non-ketogenic diets. *Journal of Clinical Investigation, 58*, 722–730.

Yang, M.-U., & VanItallie, T. B. (1984). Variability in body protein loss during protracted severe caloric restriction: Role of triiodothyronine and other possible determinants. *American Journal of Clinical Nutrition, 40*, 611–622.

Yang, M.-U., Wang, J., Pierson, R. N. Jr., & VanItallie, T. B. (1977). Estimation of composition of weight loss in man: A comparison of methods. *Journal of Applied Physiology, 43*(2), 331–338.

Ziegler, T. R., Young, L. S., & Manson, J. M. (1988). Metabolic effects of recombinant human growth hormone in patients receiving parenteral nutrition. *Annals of Surgery, 208*, 6–16.

5

Marked Caloric Restriction and Organ Response in Normal-Weight and Obese Experimental Animals

ELEANOR A. YOUNG

Although scientific evidence supports the association of obesity with serious health hazards (Committee on Diet and Health, 1989; National Institutes of Health, 1985; U.S. Department of Health and Human Services, 1988; VanItallie, 1985), the traditional dietary approaches to weight control have been notoriously ineffective (Council on Scientific Affairs, 1988; Bray, 1970; Drenick & Johnson, 1978). This has led to more aggressive approaches to the treatment of obese patients. Very low calorie diets (VLCDs) currently lead the long list of treatment modalities (Gelfand & Hendler, 1989; Lockwood & Amatruda, 1984; Wadden, Stunkard, & Brownell, 1983). Their use has been heightened by aggressive marketing strategies and consumer demand for a quick and easy solution to the complex and serious problems of obesity (Beck, Springen, Beachy, Hager, & Buckley, 1990; Goode, 1990; Wyden, 1990).

The nutritional composition of VLCDs currently on the market is designed to provide 45 to 100 g/day of protein of high biological value, 400 to 800 kilocalories (kcal)/day, and all essential nutrients. These factors contribute to the apparently safe use of VLCDs (Amatruda, Richeson, Welle, Brodows, & Lockwood, 1988; Gelfand & Hendler, 1989; Hoffer, Bistrian, Young, Blackburn, & Matthews, 1984; Wadden et al., 1983), in contrast to the documentation of morbidity and mortality associated with very low calorie, liquid protein diets used in the mid-1970s (Felig, 1978; Sours et al., 1981; VanItallie, 1978). Nevertheless, there are still many unanswered questions regarding the use and abuse of VLCDs (Gelfand & Hendler, 1989; Wadden, VanItallie, & Blackburn, 1990), and debate continues regarding whether these diets should (Stordy, 1989) or should not (Garrow, 1989) be used.

The use of animal models can provide insights into the metabolic, physiological, and biochemical alterations that occur in response to severe caloric restriction. This chapter will focus on the advantages and disadvantages of the use of animal models in probing the effects of restricted caloric intake, and on animals' responses to low calorie diets that are designed to mimic the currently marketed commercial VLCDs.

Animal Models of Obesity

Despite numerous scientific investigations of human obesity, the genetic, physiological, and biochemical factors that underlie this disorder are often difficult or impossible to study directly in human subjects. These limitations have spurred many investigators to search for appropriate animal models of obesity. Since many laboratory animals become obese, they provide opportunities for fundamental research that may either complement or give direction to investigations of human obesity.

Species Variation

An excellent review by McCarthy (1979) and several experimental studies illustrate the normal variations of body fat and its inheritance in animal models (Fowler, 1962; Hayes & McCarthy, 1976; Kownacki, Keller, & Gebler, 1975; Lang & Legates, 1969; Larsson, 1967). Variations in body fat are attributable primarily to genetic and environmental factors, with approximately 40% to 50% of the total variance of body fatness due to genetic differences among animals (McCarthy, 1979). Examples of variations are given in Table 5.1. Body fat tends to increase with age, with variations occurring in relation to the site of fat deposition and the rate of adipose tissue synthesis. The food composition, the rate of food consumption, and the total time spent in feeding are some of the variables observed in animal models of obesity. Meal size has been suggested as one of the more important correlates in overall energy intake. Variations in the relative rates of energy expenditure (per unit weight of food–energy consumption) and the rates at which energy deposition is partitioned between adipose tissues influence an animal's overall adiposity.

Of particular interest are the variations that occur in the digestion and absorption of nutrients among different animal models. The gastrointestinal

TABLE 5.1. Factors Contributing to Variation in Body Fat in Animal Models of Obesity

1. Genetic inheritance
2. Age
3. Specific adipose depots
4. Fast versus slow rate of growth
5. Patterns of food consumption, palatability, meal size, time spent feeding
6. Rate of development of adipose tissue
7. Distribution of fat among fat depots with age
8. Utilization of energy efficiency in converting food energy to weight/fat gain
9. Physical activity level
10. Relative metabolic rate/energy expenditure per unit weight

tract acts as the interface between the multitude of complex biological molecules in foods and the nutrients that are ultimately absorbed to provide nourishment. The gastrointestinal tracts of animal models differ widely, thus limiting the number of animals available as possible models of human obesity (Buffington, 1984). An example of such a disqualifying characteristic is the extensive fermentation that occurs in ruminant pregastric chambers and in the horse hindgut. Among domestic animals, the dog and pig have a gastrointestinal anatomy and physiology that most closely resemble those in humans. Rabbits, guinea pigs, hamsters, mice, and rats all have been extensively used as animal models (Neil & Kesel, 1984). Among these models, the rat gastrointestinal system most closely approximates the form and function of the human gastrointestinal system. Rats and mice have been the animal models selected for most studies of obesity.

Values and Limitations

Numerous diseases appear to be similar in humans and some common laboratory animals. These include inborn errors of metabolism, congenital abnormalities, hormonal deficiencies or insensitivities, various types of cancer, diabetes, and obesity. Although these models may be useful in the investigation of the etiology, pathogenesis, and treatment of diseases in humans, both the value and limitations of such models must be clearly appreciated.

Animal models can be investigated under rigidly controlled conditions, maintained on defined nutrient intake, and held under pathogen-free or germfree environmental conditions. Breeding, inbreeding, and propagation of mutant types can be controlled. Animal models are usually small and economical to maintain. While animals are maintained under strict regulations (Committee on Care and Use of Laboratory Animals, 1985), they may be used for experiments that could not be conducted on humans.

On the other hand, there are a number of limitations in the use of animal models of obesity. As previously mentioned, there is no assurance that a selected animal model is indeed fundamentally similar to the human model. Some models may be useful for one investigation and unrealistic or unreliable for others. Animal size or scale can significantly influence energy balance via energy expenditure, thereby making comparisons difficult, even though the animal model may behave in a manner biochemically similar to the human counterpart. Careful considerations must be given to the interpretation of research findings generated by studies utilizing animal models.

Nongenetic Models of Obesity

A number of nongenetic models of obesity have been described (Miller, 1979; Stock & Rothwell, 1979). Table 5.2 lists the most widely used models. The

TABLE 5.2. Nongenetic Animal Models of Obesity

1. Dietary models	2. Chemical models	3. Surgical models
Early overfeeding in limited litter number	Gold thioglucose	Hypothalamic lesions
Force feeding via tube or gavage	Monosodium glutamate	Castration
Palatable "cafeteria" diets	Bipiperidyl mustard	
Energy-dense or high fat diets	Insulin	
	Steroid hormones	
	Antimetabolite	

animals in which obesity is induced by diet, as well as those in which it is chemically induced, exhibit a body fat content significantly greater than that of their controls; however, they do not get as fat as genetically obese animal models. Underlying mechanisms of obesity in these different models may be quite different. This point needs to be kept in mind when these animal models are used to investigate the metabolic responses to a restricted energy intake and/or refeeding after semistarvation. As pointed out by Stock and Rothwell (1979), obesity that results from intragastric tube feeding is associated with increased metabolic efficiency without an increase in energy intake. When tube-fed obese rats are returned to the control stock diet, weight loss occurs, associated with marked hypophagia. At the same time, energy expenditure remains normal. In contrast, "cafeteria" diet models become obese as a result of hyperphagia without exhibiting any changes in resting oxygen consumption. When these now obese animals are switched to a stock diet, they return close to the body weight of control animals, as a result of decreased energy intake.

Genetic Models of Obesity

Genetic obesity in animal models has been classified and described by several investigators (Bray, Ricquier, & Spiegelman, 1990; Bray & York, 1971; Festing, 1979; Greenwood & Turkenkopf, 1983; Stauffacher, Orci, Cameron, Burr, & Rendd, 1971). The obese ob/ob mouse and the Zucker fa/fa rat have been the most widely used models in the study of obesity. When such genetic models are used in studies involving energy restriction, one has to consider the profound influence on metabolism of genetically determined biochemical characteristics. For example, hyperglycemia accompanies the obesity seen in the ob/ob mouse; therefore, this model is not the most appropriate one for typical early-onset hypercellular–hypertrophic human obesity—a disorder that is not necessarily associated with diabetes. In contrast, while the Zucker fa/fa rat is normoglycemic during most of its lifespan, it does exhibit both hyperinsulinemia and hyperlipemia—conditions that are commonly observed in human early onset obesity.

Although single-gene Mendelian animal models of obesity are known, the underlying biochemical lesions have been difficult to detect. A number of metabolic abnormalities can arise as a consequence of the underlying lesion. In animal models whose obesity is thought to be polygenetically determined, multiple genetic lesions may be present. Indeed, these models probably have an array of genes that act by influencing growth rate, metabolic rate, fatness, appetite, and activity. Such animal models may be more realistic counterparts of human obesity. As Falconer (1960) proposed, the polygenic threshold model of inheritance will depend on the genes controlling fatness, which act through a variety of underlying factors (including the response to the composition, form, and palatability of the diet; the cage size; and ambient temperatures) and by influencing metabolic rate, growth rate, and activity level.

Factors Modifying the Effects of Restricted Energy Intake

The term "homeostasis" was coined by Cannon (1929) to describe the propensity of living organisms to preserve constancy in their internal environment. Since that time, numerous investigators have observed that when energy restriction is imposed, growth is retarded. When the restriction is removed, a compensatory growth rate is frequently observed. This rate may exceed the normal growth rate. This compensatory response may be modified by a number of factors, as shown in Table 5.3. Thus, each of these factors needs to be taken into account in the interpretation of studies of marked caloric restriction in animal models. Any one (or a combination) of these factors may have a profound influence on the whole body's and/or a specific organ's response to marked caloric restriction and/or refeeding.

Effects of Restricted Caloric Intake in Selected Animal Models

During the early 1960s and 1970s, numerous studies were designed to utilize fasted–refed animal models in an effort to determine the effects of total fasting on a variety of physiological, metabolic, and biochemical mechanisms. Many of these studies provided substantial evidence of undesirable effects of total fasting and corroborated similar adverse effects of fasting that were reported in

TABLE 5.3. Factors Modifying the Effects of Restricted Energy Intake

1. Characteristics of calorie restriction
2. Severity of undernutrition imposed
3. Duration of the energy restricted period
4. Stage of development–nutritional status as initiation of the energy restriction
5. Relative rate of maturity of the species
6. Pattern of refeeding
7. Species variations

human studies (Drenick, 1973; Duncan, Duncan, Schless, & Cristofori, 1965; Lawlor & Wells, 1969; Saudek & Felig, 1976). These observations helped spur the use of semistarvation or VLCDs for weight reduction in obese humans. Such intervention was thought to be a more reasonable and safer approach to the dietary therapy of obesity. As a consequence, a number of scientific studies were undertaken to explore the effects of restricted caloric and/or protein intake on the metabolism of adipose and muscle tissue and the body's nitrogen economy. Particular consideration was given to factors influencing the synthesis and catabolism of skeletal muscle and gastrointestinal organ systems, including the liver. This section provides a summary of selected examples of restricted caloric intake in animal models. Although these studies were not designed to assess caloric–protein restriction as a method of weight loss, they have provided useful scientific data regarding some of the underlying physiological, biochemical, and metabolic mechanisms that may be responsible for the development of obesity.

Intestinal Morphology and Absorption

Following a 15-day semistarvation period in Sprague–Dawley rats weighing 150–175 g, Esposito (1967) studied the rate of disappearance of glucose and 3-*O*-methyl-glucose from the jejunum. Utilizing an *in vivo* jejunal loop perfusion, he found that the active disappearance of glucose, but not 3-*O*-methyl-glucose, was significantly faster in semistarved than in control animals when these sugars were delivered at low concentrations. It was speculated that this effect was due to altered metabolism in the epithelial cells when metabolizable glucose was present, but not when nonmetabolizable glucose was the substrate. The faster rate of glucose disappearance was thought to be related to an atrophied, thinner gut wall in the semistarved animals. This concept was supported by Kershaw, Neame, and Wiseman (1960), who reported that active intestinal transport of glucose and L-histidine *in vitro* increased rapidly in semistarved rats as a result of a thinner, narrower, and shorter gut, as compared with the gut of control animals. However, the *in vivo* intestinal transport of these nutrients also increased significantly. This was thought to be more closely related to a higher concentration of the infused nutrients into a limited space within the gut of semistarved animals, as compared with the normal (but larger) gut space in the control animals.

Utilizing everted duodenal sacs, Adams, Hill, Wain, and Taylor (1974) studied the effects of undernutrition on intestinal transport of calcium in a Wistar rat model. Animals were made to grow slowly or rapidly by adjusting litter size. Some of the undernourished animals were rehabilitated with unlimited amounts of a full pellet diet. Calcium transport studies in well-fed, undernourished, and rehabilitated animals clearly showed that calcium transport was uniformly reduced in undernourished animals, and was inappropriately low (relative to age) when compared to that of the well-fed animals. Calcium transport in the undernourished animals was also inappropriately low (as indicated by the length and mineral concentration of the femur). The bones were always too short and contained too little mineral for the age of these undernourished animals when compared to those of the well-fed animals. Calcium transport improved in the rehabilitated animals, but these animals continued to manifest distorted growth patterns (as shown by the reduced size and composition of the femur), as compared with controls. Reduced calcium transport by everted sacs of rat duodenum, as a result of semistarvation, has also been reported by Kessner and Epstein (1965).

The effects of semistarvation on the transport of calcium in the large intestine were studied by Petith and Schedl (1979). Charles River CD male rats were fed commercial rat chow *ad libitum* (controls) or 50% of the amount fed to control animals (semistarved). After 11 to 14 days, an *in vivo* perfusion technique demonstrated that semistarvation decreased the dry weight of cecum and colon to one-half that of the controls. Specific colonic lumen-to-plasma flux remained unchanged; however, since the total weight of the colon decreased, the total calcium flux out of the lumen decreased. Because the flux of calcium from plasma to lumen was also depressed, the effect on total net movement was not significantly different, as compared with control animals. Decreased plasma-to-lumen flux was thought to be a reflection of atrophy of the colon as a result of semistarvation. This study suggests that the excretion of endogenous calcium may be decreased in semistarved rats, and definitely confirms atrophy of the colonic mucosa in the semistarved animals.

Using Lewis rats, Lipscomb and Sharp (1982) examined the effects on kinetic and morphometric parameters of the small intestine of reducing the food intake to 60% of that provided to *ad libitum*-fed controls. After 20 days of semistarvation, the weight of jejunum and ileum, the thickness of muscularis externa of the duodenum, the crypt depth throughout the intestine, and the intestinal uptake of tritiated thymidine in the ileum were decreased in the experimental group, as compared with the controls. Reducing food intake to 60% of the amount fed to paired untreated controls confirmed the development of distinct adverse effects of semistarvation on small intestine morphology.

Utilizing a gastric stapling model of restricted feeding in Zucker (fa/fa) rats, my colleagues and I (Young et al., 1984) studied the adaptive response of the gastrointestinal tract to semistarvation over a 14-day period. Female animals weighing 225 to 275 g were randomly assigned to the following study groups: Group I, Roux-en-Y, stapled, fed *ad libitum*; Group IIA, Roux-en-Y, nonstapled, pair-fed to Group I; Group IIB, Roux-en-Y, nonstapled, fed *ad libitum*; Group IIIA, intact, laparotomy, pair-fed to Group I; and Group IIIB, intact, laparotomy, fed *ad libitum*. Group I animals showed significant decreases in body weight gain, calorie intake, gastric mucosal weight, serum gastrin, and pancreatic amylase activity, as compared with Group IIIB animals. Intestinal segment weight, mucosal weight, and protein content reflected the atrophy observed in the duodenum and the hypertrophy seen in the jejunal segment of animals in Group I. A number of factors may influence intestinal adaptation to undernutrition, including the presence or absence of luminal nutrients, and changes in the volume of pancreaticobiliary secretions and of gastrointestinal hormones. All of these factors were altered by the gastric stapling procedure, since the stapled animals had no luminal nutrient exposure in the duodenum, thus effectively lessening proteolytic activity in the proximal intestine. On the other hand, the jejunal segment received a much greater nutrient load than would have been received under normal physiological conditions. All of these factors affected the gastrointestinal response to gastric stapling as a model of restricted caloric intake to effect weight loss.

Lipid Metabolism in Adipose Tissue

Considerable research has been published concerning the metabolism of adipose tissue in a variety of animal models. Recent reviews (Greenwood, 1985a, 1985b) describe the numerous factors that control normal as well as abnormal growth, development, and metabolism of adipose tissue. The metabolism of fatty acids in adipose tissue has been reviewed by Arner (1990); in addition, a description of recent developments in human fat cell adrenoreceptor characterization, with consideration of animal and cellular models for regulation of adipose tissue metabolism, has been provided by Lafontan et al. (1990).

Utilizing the Zucker "fatty" rat model, York and Bray (1973) examined the effects of food restriction on adipose tissue metabolism. Fatty rats were (1) fed *ad libitum*; (2) pair-fed to the food intake of lean rats; or (3) given only two-thirds of the food intake of the lean rats (restricted) from 8 weeks to 15–18 weeks of age. Food-restricted animals exhibited decreased serum insulin levels, smaller parametrial and subcutaneous fat cells, decreased glycerol release from adipose tissue, and a decreased conversion of glucose to adipocytes, as compared with *ad libitum*-fed fatty rats. However, controlling the serum insulin concentration and reducing adipose cell size to that of lean rats did not restore either lipogenesis or lipolysis to normal in the food-restricted animals.

When Zucker (fa/fa) rat models are pair-fed from birth at the same caloric intake as lean litter mates, the fa/fa animals still become obese (Cleary, Vasselli, & Greenwood, 1980). Animals reared in such experiments weigh the same as their lean litter mates at 15 weeks of age, but by 33 weeks of age they have outgained their lean litter mates by 100 g. Despite caloric restriction, the fa/fa animals have a body composition that is 50% fat. Moreover, adipose tissue, lipoprotein lipase (LPL) activity (Cleary et al., 1980), and triglyceride removal rate (Maggio & Greenwood, 1982) are increased.

Quig, Layman, Bechtel, and Hackler (1983) compared the effects of ad libitum feeding and restricted feeding on LPL activity in obese Zucker (fa/fa) rats and their lean litter mates. Pairs of lean and obese rats were randomly assigned to one of three feeding groups. During restricted caloric intake, LPL was reduced by 52% in adipose tissue. On refeeding, adipose tissue LPL was dramatically increased by 300% in both the lean and obese Zucker rats. The LPL activities of the heart and skeletal muscles returned to control levels on refeeding; however, the perirenal fat pad LPL activity was increased by 300% in both the lean and obese animals. The investigators suggest that the lower skeletal muscle mass and reduced muscle LPL activity found in the obese rats may have brought about an increase in the availability of plasma triglycerides to adipose tissue. The threefold increase in adipose LPL activity indicates the tremendous potential ability of adipose tissue to deposit lipid upon refeeding after caloric restriction. The rebound of rat adipose tissue (i.e., hyperlipogenesis after partial caloric restriction and after fasting) has been noted by a number of investigators (Björntorp et al., 1980; Björntorp & Yang, 1982; Cleary et al., 1980; Fried, Hill, Nickel, & Digirolamo, 1983; Greenwood, 1985b; Maggio & Greenwood, 1982; Timmers & Knittle, 1980). This phenomenon is considered to be of potential significance in human obesity, in view of the evidence of rapid regain of body weight in approximately 60% of patients who have undergone substantial weight reduction by caloric restriction.

Protein Catabolism–Anabolism in Muscle

Since the early 1960s, numerous studies have sought to gain knowledge of the numerous factors that control the synthetic and catabolic processes in muscle tissue. Because muscle constitutes the largest protein reservoir of the body, this tissue plays a dominant role in the overall protein economy of the body, in addition to its mechanical functions. Studies designed to uncover the impact of the diet on muscle metabolism in animal models have focused largely on restricted dietary protein and/or calories. Early studies confirmed that protein was lost from different tissues disproportionately during semistarvation (Addis, Poo, & Lew, 1936; Allison, 1964; Waterlow & Stephen, 1968). Dietary experiments designed to quantify the effect of dietary factors on the synthesis or breakdown of tissue protein were limited by the available technology (Millward, 1970; Waterlow & Stephen, 1968); however, the availability of a variety of labeled compounds for use in turnover studies has significantly improved the methodology of studying muscle metabolism in animal models, both *in vivo* and *in vitro*.

Using male Wistar rats, Millward, Garlick, Nnanyelugo, and Waterlow (1976) studied changes in muscle protein synthesis and breakdown in hypophysectomized animals fed *ad libitum*, as compared with an unoperated group of controls fed a similar amount of the stock diet. Since the food intake of the pair-fed, unoperated group was less than the normal intake for such animals, this group was designated a "low energy group." The rates of protein synthesis and catabolism were measured *in vivo* on combined quadriceps and gastrocnemius muscles by a constant intravenous infusion of [^{14}C]tyrosine. With restricted caloric intake in the low energy group, the protein fractional synthesis rate was significantly decreased to only 55% of that for the *ad libitum*-fed group. Protein fractional breakdown rate was decreased to 85% of that for the *ad libitum* group, and the RNA activity was also decreased, with a consequent growth-suppressing effect. A variety of growth-suppressing and muscle-wasting treatments (hypophysectomy, low caloric intake, diabetes, glucocorticoids) depress protein synthesis, and some also depress protein catabolism. Measurements of protein turnover indicate that the regulation of protein content in skeletal muscle is achieved primarily by modulation of the synthesis rates, with catabolism being more variable. Refeeding brings about a rapid return to normal growth rate, with an increase in synthesis rates and a decrease in muscle breakdown. The effect of refeeding is modulated by degree and duration of the earlier caloric and/or protein restriction, as well as the overall nutritional status of the animal (Millward et al., 1976; Millward & Waterlow, 1978; Young, Stothers, & Vilaire, 1971).

Using a male mouse model from the Q strain, Hooper, Thacker, Newby, Sykes, and Digirolamo (1984) conducted a study to determine the effect of caloric restriction on muscle fiber length. Animal groups included *ad libitum*-fed controls and food-restricted animals, which received 60% by weight of the intake of the controls, given in a single daily feeding for 21 days. One-half of the food-restricted mice, as well as the controls, were sacrificed on day 42. The remaining restricted mice were allowed *ad libitum* feeding until they achieved the mean body weight of their control litter mates, and were then sacrificed. After excision and preparation, the left biceps brachii and tibialis were studied to determine the effect of caloric restriction on mean muscle fiber length and mean sarcomere length for 15 randomly selected fibers per muscle. The results showed that caloric restriction produced a reduction in body weight and in the weight and length of the two muscles studied. Unrestricted refeeding abolished these differences. Shorter fiber length was due to reduced numbers of sarcomeres along the fibers and not to changes in the sarcomere length. The authors speculated that the decreased fiber length may have resulted from the reduced formation of new sarcomeres and not the loss of established ones. This study provides a possible new index that should be considered in studies designed to determine the effects of restricted caloric intake on muscle mass.

Carefully controlled studies of the functional and metabolic characteristics of rat gastrocnemius muscle after total fasting and caloric restriction provide valuable new information (Russell et al., 1984). Male Wistar rats weighing 250 g were used; controls were fed Purina Laboratory Chow *ad libitum*, while other groups of rats (experimental) were totally fasted for 2 to 5 days, or were fed 25% of the intake of pair-fed controls. Functional studies were conducted under anesthesia; at sacrifice, biopsies were taken for subsequent analyses. Caloric restriction resulted in loss of force during high frequency stimulation but in preservation of contraction–relaxation characteristics during low frequency stimulation. In addition, the energy-restricted animals showed a slower muscle relaxation rate and increased muscle fatigue on high frequency stimulation, reduction in glycolytic and oxidative enzymes, and increased intracellular calcium and adenosine diphosphate levels. The investigators have suggested that disturbances in the intracellular energy status of the myocytes with altered calcium flux may help explain the muscle dysfunction caused by caloric restriction.

Structure and Function of the Diaphragm

Using a Syrian hamster model, Kelsen, Ference, and Kapoor (1985) examined the effects of restricted caloric intake on the gross and microscopic anatomy of the diaphragm and its ability to generate force. The behavior of three fiber types in the diaphragm—slow oxidative, fast oxidative, and fast glycolytic fibers—was assessed. Diaphragm function was determined by measurements of the isometric force generated during electrically stimulated contractions and at a given length, and from the force generated in response to a range of stimulus frequencies. A total of 118 hamsters were randomly assigned either to a control group fed *ad libitum*, or to a calorie-restricted group. The intake of the latter group was approximately 33% of the controls. The low caloric intake was maintained over a 4-week period, at the end of which the total weight loss was between 25% and 33% of starting weight. Compared to the controls, the calorie-restricted hamsters showed decreases in diaphragm wet and dry weights, in muscle thickness, and in the cross-sectional area of fast glycolytic and fast oxidative fibers. Reduced maximum isometric tension and muscle force were also observed. This well-designed study clearly demonstrated that the respiratory muscles are not spared the wasting associated with caloric restriction. Similar findings have been reported in rats subjected to total caloric restriction for 4 days (Dureuil et al., 1989). These animals showed impaired diaphragmatic contractility and transdiaphragmatic pressures.

Animal model studies designed to determine the effect of caloric restriction on diaphragm morphology and function suggest that a severely restricted caloric intake could adversely affect patients with chronic obstructive pulmonary disease because of diet-induced impairment of respiratory muscle function, owing to atrophy of muscle fibers.

Alterations of Pulmonary Structure and Function

Emphysema-like changes in the structure and function of the lungs have been studied by Sahebjami and Wirman (1981), using hooded male rats of Long-Evans descent. *Ad libitum*-fed control animals were compared with calorie-restricted animals, which were allowed one-third of their usual daily food intake until they lost approximately 40% of their initial body weight. Mechanical and morphometric changes observed in the calorie-restricted rats included the following: fewer, shorter, and irregular elastic fibers; enlarged air spaces and alveolar wall destruction; reduced elastic recoil pressure over the entire range of volume pressure; reduced lung weight, wet and dry; reduced internal surface area; enlarged and irregular air spaces; alveolar wall rupture; and thin, irregular interalveolar septa. These investigators describe the scanning electron-microscopic features of the calorie-restricted lungs as similar to those observed in human emphysema. Refeeding after prolonged food deprivation in this animal model was associated with a return of surface forces to normal, while morphometric characteristics remained mostly unchanged (Sahebjami & Vassallo, 1979). In studies of pre-existing emphysematous process in rat lungs, starvation significantly aggravated this deleterious process (Sahebjami & Vassallo, 1980). It is speculated that similar processes may be responsible for the clinical deterioration that is frequently seen in underweight patients with emphysema.

Weight Cycling

Repeated cycles of restricted calorie intake following by overfeeding, popularly referred to as "yo-yo dieting," "elevator dieting," or "weight cycling," have been a focus of recent studies using animal models. Serious and concerned interest in this model comes largely from estimates that in the United States, the desire for slimness supported a lucrative $32 billion business in 1989, with expectations to exceed $50 billion by 1995. Some 90% of those who lose weight on a diet will regain it and possibly more (Beck et al., 1990). This concept is supported by human studies and has been recently reviewed (Blackburn et al., 1989). Several studies using animal models corroborate these findings from human studies (Archambault, Czyzewski, Cordua y Cruz, Foreyt, & Mariotto, 1989; Brownell, Greenwood, Stellar, & Shrager, 1986; Cleary, 1986; Contreras & Williams, 1989; Hill, 1990; Hill, Thacker, Newby, Sykes, & Digirolamo, 1988). Although these studies have utilized a variety of experimental designs, there is fairly consistent agreement on the basic premise that repeated periods of weight loss followed by weight gain lead to an increase in food efficiency that tends to inhibit future weight loss and promote weight gain. Possible mechanisms for increased food efficiency are currently being explored.

Brownell et al. (1986) examined the metabolic effects of weight cycling, using three groups of adult male Sprague-Dawley rats: (1) chow controls fed *ad libitum*; (2) obese controls fed a high fat diet; and (3) an obese cycling group fed a high-fat diet *ad libitum*, followed by periods of food restriction to 50% (18 g/day) of the average intake of the chow controls. After two cycles, the obese cycling animals were at the same body weight as the obese controls, but their food efficiency increased significantly. During the second cycle, the cycling animals required twice the amount of time to lose the same amount of weight as compared with the first cycle, and on refeeding they needed only one-third the time to regain weight as compared with the first cycle. Refeeding during the second cycle caused a 25% increase in food intake and a 52% increase in food efficiency. Overall, the cycling animals had a fourfold increase in food efficiency, as compared with the noncycling obese controls. Cycling did not prevent the increase in body fat produced by the high fat diet.

An experimental design similar to that of Brownell et al. (1986) was investigated by Archambault et al. (1989), using female Sprague–Dawley rats. Two factors were added to this study: *ad libitum* wheel running and maturity. Neither factor was influenced by weight cycling; however, during one cycle, the cycling rats showed marked increases in the rate of weight gain and efficiency of calorie utilization. This was not observed in the maturity control group that cycled only once, suggesting that the cycling results were not due to maturation. During the second cycle, cycling rats did not lose weight more slowly or show increased caloric efficiency as compared with the first cycle period. This failure to confirm the findings reported by Brownell et al. (1986) may be related to differences in gender, activity, or difficulty in feed acceptance after switching from the high fat diet to rodent chow.

Cleary (1986) selected female lean (FA/?) and obese (fa/fa) Zucker rats as models for determining the effects of four sequential periods of food restriction followed by refeeding. Both lean and obese animals were assigned to *ad libitum* and restricted feeding groups and were cycled over four 6-week periods. The restricted lean rats lost and then regained weight during each cycle to weigh the same as the *ad libitum*-fed lean animals. The restricted lean rats and *ad libitum*-fed lean rats were similar in body fat content and fat cell size. The restricted obese rats lost and regained weight with each cycle, but always weighed less than the *ad libitum* obese rats. At completion of the cycling periods, the following results were obtained for the restricted obese animals as compared with the *ad libitum* obese rats: lower fat pad weights and fat cell numbers; lower liver weight and lipogenic enzyme activity; similar fat cell size; significantly less heart weight and DNA; significantly less kidney weight and DNA; and little catch-up growth in adipose tissue. These observations in obese versus lean animals require further study to sort out the underlying differences.

The influence of food restriction coupled with weight cycling on carcass energy restoration during *ad libitum* feeding has been studied by Hill et al. (1988) and Hill (1990), using mature male Wistar rats. After four 10-day cycles, the calorie-restricted animals had elevated levels of LPL activity. Following the cycling periods, animals were allowed *ad libitum* access to a stock diet for 18 days. The cycling animals gained significantly more total carcass energy and total fat-free dry weight than noncycling animals, even though food intake during refeeding did not differ between the cycling and noncycling groups. Cycling in a food-restricted fashion tends to increase food efficiency. Hill (1990) speculates that sustained high fat feeding leads to obesity that is defended more by an increased gain in carcass energy during refeeding than by maintaining carcass energy during food restriction.

The use of different techniques of caloric restriction to produce weight cycling in animal models has caused serious problems of interpretation. Despite the fact that some similar results have been obtained, the differences in experimental design, animal models used, age and sex of the animals, duration of the cycling periods, and specific dietary manipulations raise new questions that call for further study.

Responses to Very Low Calorie Diets

This section focuses on the few studies of animal models that were designed specifically to use a VLCD in a manner that mimicked the treatment of obese humans. These studies should be interpreted in light of the limitations of animal models previously outlined.

Electrocardiographic Responses

In the study by Anderson, Ahn, and Hegarty (1981), obese and nonobese Osborne-Mendel rats were fed a high fat diet over an 11-week period. Rats reared on the high fat diet were then divided into the following groups: (1) controls, examined at the start of the weight loss period; (2) liquid protein (LP) diet only; (3) LP diet plus vitamin/mineral mix; and (4) high fat diet *ad libitum*. Rats reared on the low fat diet were divided into two groups: (1) controls, examined at the start of the weight loss period; and (2) those fed the LP diet only. All animals on the LP diet were allowed 5 ml/day (10 kcal), an amount said to be comparable to human consumption of approximately 300–600 kcal/day. Electrocardiograms were recorded weekly during the weight loss period. Rats reared on the high fat diet had higher body weights at the start of caloric restriction, and these animals had a longer survival time (28 days) as compared with animals reared on the low fat diet (21 days), which had lower weights entering into the weight restriction phase of the study. All animals on the LP diet had diarrhea; however, nitrogen loss was not reported. The weight of the heart, skeletal muscle, and liver decreased in all animals on the LP diet.

A normal electrocardiogram was recorded for all animals prior to the caloric restriction and for the control animals receiving the high fat diet for the entire experimental period. For all animals with decreasing weight, sinus bradycardia (sometimes less than 200 beats/minute), was a consistent finding. Abnormal cardiac findings in all of the obese rats placed on the LP diet were most frequently recorded after a 40% reduction in body weight. Arrhythmias observed in this group included atrial premature contractions in three animals; second-degree atrioventricular block in two; atrial beats in one animal; sinoatrial block in two animals; irregular sinus arrhythmias in two animals; and junctional escape beats in one rat. In contrast, the obese animals placed on the LP diet plus vitamins and minerals had normal electrocardiographic tracings at the time of death. All of the lean rats placed on the LP diet showed arrhythmias after only 17% to 30% loss of body weight.

Zinc and copper concentrations in hearts and skeletal muscles of animals receiving the LP diet were lower than levels observed in the controls, while the levels of potassium and magnesium were normal. Heart calcium concentrations were significantly decreased in the animals reared on the low fat diet and then placed on the LP diet. Serum potassium levels were significantly decreased in the lean rats that were placed on the LP diet.

These findings suggest that the low biological value of the protein in the LP diet (Centers for Disease Control, 1977), plus the lack of vitamins and minerals in the LP-diet-only group, probably contributed to the electrocardiographic abnormalities associated with this diet. Furthermore, these findings are similar to some of the findings observed in human subjects who adhered to the same or similar LP diets (Felig, 1978; Sours et al., 1981; VanItallie, 1978).

Metabolic Effects

In the study of Timmons, Slaten, and Svacha (1983), young Sprague–Dawley rats weighing 208 g were reared on an *ad libitum*-fed high calorie diet. Animals were then divided into three groups: (1) animals sacrificed at initiation of caloric restriction; (2) controls fed a nutritionally complete 10% casein diet *ad libitum*; and (3) animals fed an LP diet containing 44% protein and designed to approximate the Prolinn diet (Linn & Stuart, 1976), plus a vitamin/mineral mix. After 13 days on these respective diets, all animals were sacrificed. The LP rats lost 22% of initial weight, while the controls gained 8%. The liver weight, liver weight as a percentage of body weight, heart weight, and plasma calcium were significantly decreased in the LP animals as compared with control animals. Amino acid analysis of the LP diet was consistent with an amino acid imbalance, as were altered plasma amino acid patterns in animals on the LP diet. Methionine was the most limited amino acid. Fatty infiltration was seen in the liver, but no histological abnormalities of the myocardium were noted in the LP animals.

In this experiment, all essential vitamins and minerals were added to the commercial LP formula and may have contributed to the prevention of abnormalities. In preliminary studies, these investigators demonstrated that this LP diet without vitamin/mineral supplementation could not support growth in young rats, a finding similar to that observed by Anderson et al. (1981). Despite the addition of vitamins and minerals, total body weight decreased and the liver and heart atrophied as a result of restricted caloric intake.

Stock (1989) has reported the effects of low calorie diets (LCDs) and VLCDs on the metabolic rate and body composition of genetically obese (fa/fa) and lean (Fa/?) male Zucker rats. Two groups of weight-matched obese animals were fed either 3 g/day of the Cambridge diet (VLCD) or 11 g/day of a stock diet. A control group was fed the stock diet *ad libitum*. The LCD and VLCD groups were sacrificed when their body weight reached that of the lean control rats. The equivalent intake of energy for humans provided by these diets was calculated to be 330 kcal (VLCD) and 1400 kcal (LCD). The VLCD rats reached the control weight by day 16, while the LCD group required 30 days to reach the control weight.

Energy expenditure reductions were similar in the VLCD and LCD groups, and, based on metabolic size, were 54% and 57% of the control values, respectively. On day 8 of caloric restriction, the oxygen consumption ($\dot{V}O_2$ values (ml/kg$^{0.75}$/min) of the LCD and VLCD groups were similar and were significantly reduced ($p < .001$) to about 70% of control values. By day 14, the $\dot{V}O_2$ had further dropped to 60% of control values. Compared to the lean rats, the obese rats had a significantly greater percentage of the body weight as fat, and less as water and protein. The VLCD animals did not alter their proportions of body water or fat as compared with the initial proportions of these constituents; however, the proportion of protein increased in the carcass ($p < .01$). When the VLCD and LCD were compared, the contributions to weight loss were 38% and 41% from fat and 57% and 63% from water, respectively. The rate of weight loss in the VLCD was double that of the LCD, yet the effect of weight loss on metabolic rate and body composition was not significantly different from that observed in the LCD group. In this study, it appeared that beyond a certain level of caloric restriction, further restriction had no additional influence on metabolic rate. Stock (1989) suggested that the maximal capacity for compensatory increases in energetic efficiency may be reached at relatively modest levels of caloric restriction. At least in the Zucker rat model used in this study, gradual weight loss had no metabolic advantage over a rapid weight loss. In both the VLCD and LCD groups, metabolic rate was reduced significantly, the final body composition measurements were similar, and both groups were lighter but not leaner. Stock (1989) suggested that future studies should explore methods to prevent the compensatory reduction in metabolic rate (thus improving weight loss) and to discover how to promote the loss of excess body fat while preserving lean body mass.

These observations relate to a recent report by Wadden, Foster, Letizia, and Mullen (1990), who studied the long-term effects of dieting on resting metabolic rate in markedly obese outpatients. These investigators compared changes in weight and resting metabolic rate in obese women who consumed a balanced-deficit diet (1200 kcal/day) for 48 weeks with changes in women maintained on a VLCD (420 kcal/day) for 16 weeks and then kept on a conventional reducing diet for the remaining 32 weeks. At 48 weeks, the decreases in metabolic rate and weight loss were similar in both groups. The authors suggest that neither diet was associated with a long-term reduction in resting metabolic rate that exceeded decreases expected with the reduction of body weight. This finding reminds us again of the complexity of the weight cycling phenomenon and of the many questions still to be answered.

Nitrogen, Protein Losses, and Body Composition

Schemmel, Stone, Warren, and Stoddart (1983) used male Osborne-Mendel rats to determine nitrogen and protein losses during weight reduction induced by a high protein, low energy (HPLE) diet, as compared with fasting. Animals were reared on a high fat diet until mean body weight was 701 g and were then randomly divided into three groups: (1) controls fed a high fat diet; (2) animals fed a HPLE diet; and (3) fasted animals. Results of the 12-day weight reduction period disclosed that the HPLE and fasted animals weighed significantly less than the control animals. The HPLE animals voluntarily consumed only 30 g of the 56 g (53%) of the allotted diet available to them; thus, the weight loss in this group was not significantly different from that of the fasted animals. The cumulative 12-day nitrogen loss, calculated from composite urine and fecal nitrogen loss, was significantly greater in the fasted rats (-808 mg) than in the control and HPLE groups, with nitrogen gains of $+22$ and $+26$ mg, respectively. Liver weight, liver nitrogen, and liver protein were similar in the control and HPLE groups, but significantly lower in the fasted animals. Heart weight, heart protein, and heart RNA of HPLE and fasted rats were significantly lower than in the controls. This study indicated that the HPLE diet, as compared with fasting, tended to protect nitrogen balance and to preserve liver weight, liver protein, and kidney weight. On the other hand, the HPLE group was not protected against losses in body weight, heart weight, protein, or RNA. These findings are similar to results of human studies (Sours et al., 1981), which show that high protein calorie-restricted diets do not necessarily protect against losses of nitrogen from certain organ systems. This study also indicates that whole-body nitrogen balance studies cannot provide information about nitrogen losses from specific organs or tissues that may occur during caloric restriction and weight loss.

Gastrointestinal, Cardiac, and Renal Response

My colleagues and I have reported the effects of VLCD or semistarvation and refeeding on the gastrointestinal tract, the heart, and the kidneys (Young, Ramos, & Harris, 1988); and Young, Cantu, & Harris, 1989). The gastrointestinal tract, an organ system that is exquisitely sensitive to nutrient intake, serves as the interface between nutrient intake and subsequent nutrient uptake for metabolism. It is therefore surprising that the effects of VLCDs and refeeding on the gastrointestinal tract have not been studied with greater intensity. Over 40 years ago, Keys, Henschel, and Taylor (1947) demonstrated that in human subjects undergoing nutritional rehabilitation after semistarvation, the heart was closer to failure in the refeeding phase than in the semistarvation phase of the study. Following a 6-month period during which 32 young men were maintained on an LCD and lost 24% of their total body weight, some physiological indices still were not recovered fully 20 weeks after initiation of refeeding. It was noted that, although body weight was fully restored and total heart size was slightly greater than before starvation after 20 weeks of refeeding, cardiac work per minute was still 10% below control values, and only half of the lost margin of safety had been restored. Since the publication of the monumental study of human starvation conducted by Keys, Brozek, Henschel, Mickelsen, and Taylor (1950), little has been discovered to explain how refeeding after prolonged restriction of caloric intake may affect various body organs. Although it is understood that selected organ systems may be spared nitrogen loss at the expense of others during caloric restriction, much less is known about possible adaptive responses to refeeding.

In one experiment (Young et al., 1989), Sprague–Dawley rats weighing 440–445 g were randomly divided into three groups: (1) a control group receiving a nutritionally complete defined formula diet designed to meet the caloric and essential nutrient allowances of the laboratory rat; (2) a semistarved group that received 23% of the total caloric intake of the control group; and (3) a semistarved group that was subsequently refed. The level of semistarvation for the latter two groups was selected to mimic the percentage of caloric reduction of a popular commercial regimen that is designed and advertised as a safe, rapid weight loss supplement with protein, vitamins, and minerals. The diet for the semistarved animals contained the same quantity and quality of vitamins and minerals as the formula for the control animals, thus meeting the protein and other nutrient requirements of the rat.

Nitrogen balance findings during the semistarvation and semistarvation-refeeding cycles are shown in Table 5.4. Body and organ weights of the control, semistarved, and semistarved–refed groups are summarized in Table 5.5. Body weight and all organ weights decreased significantly in the semistarved animals as compared with the control animals. Not only was this trend reversed by refeeding, but the semistarved–refed group exhibited weight rebound to a significantly higher level, as compared with that observed in the control group.

Proximal-to-distal intestinal mucosal protein, DNA, and protein–DNA ratios are shown in Figure 5.1. The liver was the organ most severely affected by caloric restriction. This was not surprising as the liver weight of semistarved rats was less than one-half the liver weight of control animals (see Figure 5.2). Heart protein, DNA, and protein–DNA ratio for the control, semistarved, and semistarved–refed animals are shown in Figure 5.3.

The effects of caloric restriction and refeeding in this animal model reflected a somewhat similar pattern for the total small intestine, intestinal mucosa, heart, liver, pancreas and kidney, although the degree of weight loss and rebound varied for different organs. In the semistarved animals, intestinal mucosal protein concentration was 50%, total liver protein was 39%, total pancreatic protein was 62%, and total heart protein was 53%, as compared with the control animals. Tissues of the small intestinal mucosa, liver, pancreas, heart, and kidney in calorie-restricted animals were generally characterized by decreased tissue mass, decreased total protein per gram of tissue, a large number of cells per gram of tissue, and a decreased protein–DNA ratio.

Refeeding reversed these trends; however, the pattern of protein repletion on refeeding was somewhat variable. In the semistarved–refed animals, repleted protein was equal to or greater than that observed in the control group for intestinal segments, liver, pancreas, and heart. DNA concentrations in the intestinal segments, liver, and pancreas remained lower than those in the control group; however, DNA concentrations in the heart were equal to those of the control group. The protein–DNA ratio was consistently higher in the

TABLE 5.4. Nitrogen Balance during Semistarvation and Semistarvation-Refeeding

Group	Day 1	Day 5	Day 10	Day 15	Day 20	Day 23	Day 28	Day 33	Day 38	Day 43
Control ($n = 6$)	699 ± 87	632 ± 65	795 ± 67	858 ± 55	909 ± 145	—	—	—	—	—
Semistarved ($n = 6$)	605 ± 132	53 ± 18	64 ± 22	−37 ± 24	−82 ± 42	—	—	—	—	—
Semistarved–refed	639 ± 134	57 ± 21	−3 ± 21	−93 ± 41	−105 ± 25	384 ± 83	889 ± 55	994 ± 111	894 ± 88	1033 ± 116
p^*	n.s.	<.001	<.001	<.001	<.001	—	—	—	—	—

Note. Values expressed as mean ± *SEM*, urinary nitrogen retention (mg/day).
*Significance level of the two semistarvation groups versus the control group (one-way analysis of variance, Duncan's multiple-range test).

TABLE 5.5. Body and Organ Weights of Control Animals (C) and Animals after Semistarvation (SS) and Semistarvation–Refeeding (SS→RF)

Organ	Weights at sacrifice (g)[a]			p*		
	C	SS	SS→RF	SS vs. C	SS vs. SS→RF	SS→RF vs. C
Total body weight	456 ± 10	277 ± 11	438 ± 6	<.001	<.001	n.s.
Total small intestine	5.6826 ± 0.3706	4.0542 ± 0.4057	6.7193 ± 0.4166	<.05	<.01	n.s.
Total intestinal mucosa	3.4362 ± 0.2722	2.1868 ± 0.2569	4.0083 ± 0.3664	<.01	<.005	n.s.
Heart	1.3428 ± 0.0684	0.8665 ± 0.0379	1.2677 ± 0.0360	<.001	<.001	n.s.
Liver	14.8402 ± 0.6024	6.2028 ± 0.3893	17.3455 ± 0.4650	<.005	<.001	<.05
Pancreas	1.3929 ± 0.0650	1.0410 ± 0.0776	1.5752 ± 0.1995	<.05	<.01	n.s.

[a]Mean ± *SEM*.
*One-way analysis of variance and Duncan's multiple-range test.

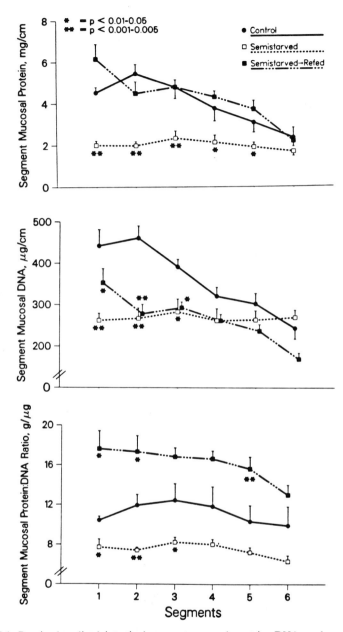

FIGURE 5.1. Proximal-to-distal intestinal segment mucosal protein, DNA, and protein–DNA ratio (by weight, $\times 10^6$) are plotted for control (filled circles), semistarved (open squares), and semistarved–refed (filled squares) animals. From "Gastrointestinal and Cardiac Response to Refeeding after Low-Calorie Semistarvation" (p. 925) by E. A. Young, T. L. Cantu, and M. M. Harris, 1989, *American Journal of Clinical Nutrition, 50*, 922–929. Copyright 1989 by American Society for Clinical Nutrition, Inc. Reprinted by permission.

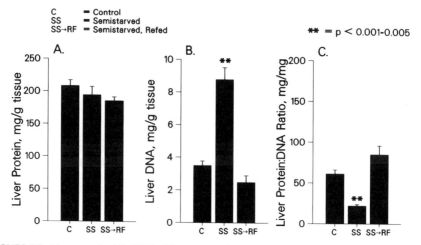

FIGURE 5.2. Liver protein (A), DNA (B), and protein–DNA ratio (C) are given for control (C), semistarved (SS), and semistarved–refed animals (SS → RF). From "Gastrointestinal and Cardiac Response to Refeeding after Low-Calorie Semistarvation" (p. 926) by E. A. Young, T. L. Cantu, and M. M. Harris, 1989, *American Journal of Clinical Nutrition*, 50, 922–929. Copyright 1989 by American Society for Clinical Nutrition, Inc. Reprinted by permission.

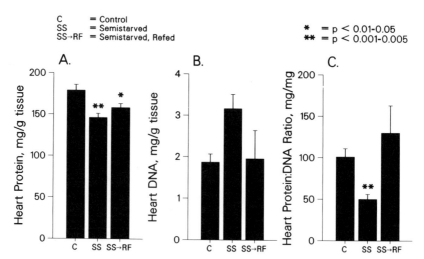

FIGURE 5.3. Heart protein (A), DNA (B), and protein–DNA ratio (C) are given for control (C), semistarved (SS), and semistarved–refed animals (SS → RF). From "Gastrointestinal and Cardiac Response to Refeeding after Low-Calorie Semistarvation" (p. 927) by E. A. Young, T. L. Cantu, and M. M. Harris, 1989, *American Journal of Clinical Nutrition*, 50, 922–929. Copyright 1989 by American Society for Clinical Nutrition, Inc. Reprinted by permission.

semistarved-refed group than in the control or semistarved animals for all indices studied. This finding suggests that existing cells in these tissues repleted their protein stores more rapidly than new cells were created. This probably reflects initial cellular hypertrophy with new cell synthesis lagging behind, thus characterizing this tissue as having fewer but larger cells, as compared with that of the control animals.

Histological examination of tissue disclosed significant atrophy of the liver tissues of semistarved rats, with cells devoid of glycogen and lipid. These characteristics were not seen in the liver cells of semistarved-refed animals; however, fatty infiltration was observed in two of six of these animals. Autolysis and blunting of intestinal epithelial villi were characteristic of all semistarved rats, but not in the control or semistarved-refed animals. Myocardial fiber size was decreased in four of six animals in the semistarved group.

Systematic studies are needed of the adaptive responses that occur after caloric restriction by VLCD is terminated. Studies of how caloric restriction and refeeding affect the function of organ systems also are needed. A number of as yet unknown factors may modulate adaptive responses to VLCDs in the obese animal model (Figure 5.4). It is probable that the adaptation that takes place during the refeeding period may influence the ability of the obese patient who has lost weight to remain at the lower weight achieved by conscientious dieting. Energy conservation and adaptation to semistarvation seem to persist during refeeding; however, adaptation to refeeding in a rat model may involve such mechanisms as increased glucose turnover rate, increased synthesis of

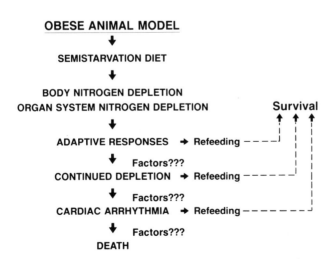

FIGURE 5.4. Possible adaptive response of the obese rat model to semistarvation and to semistarvation and refeeding. From "Gastrointestinal and Cardiac Response to Refeeding after Low-Calorie Semistarvation" (p. 928) by E. A. Young, T. L. Cantu, and M. M. Harris, 1989, *American Journal of Clinical Nutrition, 50*, 922-929. Copyright 1989 by American Society for Clinical Nutrition, Inc. Reprinted by permission.

glycogen and lipid in the liver and adipose tissue, increased substrate flux, enhanced ability of the peripheral tissues to capture circulating substrates, or increased efficiency in accumulating energy (Björntorp, Edstrom, & Kral, 1982); increased enzyme activity in various anabolic energy pathways (Björntorp et al., 1980); and moderate overeating (Björntorp & Yang, 1982). It is also possible that the adaptation of the gastrointestinal organ system to undernutrition takes the form of a more efficient absorptive process (Young et al., 1989).

Conclusion and Future Outlook

Although VLCDs currently lead the long list of treatment approaches to weight reduction, there are still many unanswered questions regarding the use of these diets. From the few studies utilizing animal models, several concepts have emerged that are relatively consistent and are supported by scientific evidence. Yet the need for creative, sophisticated approaches to solve the problem of obesity constitutes a high priority in health promotion and disease prevention.

An outlook for the future may include the following considerations:

1. The marketing strategists of VLCDs seemingly have been more successful in their sophisticated sales than scientists have been in sorting out the basic, fundamental aspects of restricting calories as a method of weight reduction for the obese.

2. The general public, as well as the scientific community, may not yet have come to an insightful realization of the complexity of obesity, including the many factors that may alter caloric restriction and weight maintenance.

3. Animal models have contributed a number of concepts that have broadened our knowledge of obesity and have stimulated new approaches of scientific inquiry.

4. The interpretation of data generated from studies using animal models must be tempered by serious considerations of species variations, genetic inheritance, diet composition and feeding modalities, age of the animal model used, a host of disease states that may modify the response to caloric restriction, and experimental design.

5. The findings of several studies utilizing animal models of restricted caloric intake have suggested that certain clinical problems may occur in patients as a by-product of consuming a VLCD. Examples include intestinal adaptation that may alter specific nutrient absorptive capabilities; the regulatory effect of LPL activity; altered calcium flux that adversely affects muscle function; possible impairment of respiratory muscle function, owing to atrophy of muscle fibers; and mechanical and morphometric changes in the lung similar to those seen in some human patients with emphysema.

6. Expansion of the duration and development of sophisticated animal models is needed to determine more definitively the metabolic effects of weight cycling, especially since weight maintenance is the ultimate goal of caloric restriction for the obese.

7. More studies of adaptation to refeeding after caloric restriction are needed. Examples are better measurements of fuel efficiency, glucose turnover rate, synthesis of glycogen and lipid in the liver and adipose tissue, diet-induced variations in the efficiency of the absorptive processes, and changes in the ability of peripheral tissues to capture energy substrate.

References

Adams, P. H., Hill, L. F., Wain, D., & Taylor, C. (1974). The effects of undernutrition and its relief on intestinal calcium transport in the rat. *Calcified Tissue Research, 16,* 293–304.

Addis, T., Poo, L. J., & Lew, W. (1936). The quantity of protein lost by various organs and tissues of the body during a fast. *Journal of Biological Chemistry, 115,* 111–118.

Allison, J. B. (1964). Nutritive value of dietary proteins. In H. N. Munro & J. B. Allison (Eds.), *Mammalian protein metabolism* (Vol. 2, pp. 41–68). New York: Academic Press.

Amatruda, J. M., Richeson, J. F., Welle, S. L., Brodows, R. G., & Lockwood, D. H. (1988). The safety and efficacy of a controlled low-energy (very-low-calorie) diet in the treatment of non-insulin-dependent diabetes and obesity. *Archives of Internal Medicine, 148,* 873–878.

Anderson, Y. A., Ahn, P. C., & Hegarty, P. V. J. (1981). Electrocardiograph abnormalities in obese rats fed a commercially available liquid protein diet. *Journal of Nutrition, 111,* 568–578.

Archambault, C. M., Czyzewski, D., Cordua y Cruz, G. D., Foreyt, J. P., & Mariotto, M. J. (1989). Effects of weight cycling in female rats. *Physiology and Behavior, 46,* 417–421.

Arner, P. (1990). Metabolism of fatty acids: An overview. In G. A. Bray, D. Ricquier, & B. M. Spiegelman (Eds.), *Obesity: Towards a molecular approach* (pp. 159–172). New York: Wiley.

Beck, M., Springen, K., Beachy, L., Hager, M., & Buckley, L. (1990, April 30). The losing formula. *Newsweek,* pp. 52–58.

Björntorp, P., Edstrom, S., & Kral, J. G. (1982). Refeeding after fasting in the rat: Energy substrate fluxes and replenishment of energy stores. *American Journal of Clinical Nutrition, 36,* 450–456.

Björntorp, P., Enzi, G., Karlsson, M., Kral, J., Larsson, B., Sjöström, L., & Smith, U. (1980). Effects of refeeding on adipocyte metabolism in the rat. *International Journal of Obesity, 4,* 11–19.

Björntorp, P., & Yang, M.-U. (1982). Refeeding after fasting in the rat: Effects on body composition and food efficiency. *American Journal of Clinical Nutrition, 36,* 444–449.

Blackburn, G. L., Wilson, G. T., Kanders, B. S., Stein, L. J., Lavin, P. T., Adler, J., & Brownell, K. D. (1989). Weight cycling: The experience of human dieters. *American Journal of Clinical Nutrition, 49,* 1105–1109.

Bray, G. A. (1970). The myth of diet in the management of obesity. *American Journal of Clinical Nutrition, 23,* 1141–1148.

Bray, G. A., Ricquier, D., & Spiegelman, B. M. (Eds.). (1990). *Obesity: Towards a molecular approach.* New York: Wiley.

Bray, G. A., & York, D. A. (1971). Genetically transmitted obesity in rodents. *Physiological Review, 51,* 598–646.

Brownell, K. D., Greenwood, M. R. C., Stellar, E., & Shrager, E. E. (1986). The effects of repeated cycles of weight loss and regain in rats. *Physiology and Behavior, 38,* 459–464.

Buffington, C. A. (1984). Comparative digestion and absorption in domestic animals. In R. W. Phillips (Ed.), *Animal models for nutrition research* (pp. 2–4). Columbus, OH: Ross Laboratories.

Cannon, W. B. (1929). Organization for physiological homeostasis. *Physiological Review, 9,* 399–431.

Centers for Disease Control. (1977). Deaths associated with liquid protein diets. *Morbidity and Mortality Weekly Reports, 26,* 383.

Cleary, M. P. (1986). Consequences of restricted feeding/refeeding cycles in lean and obese female Zucker rats. *Journal of Nutrition, 166,* 290-303.
Cleary, M. P., Vasselli, J. R., & Greenwood, M. R. C. (1980). Development of obesity in the Zucker obese (fa/fa) rat in the absence of hyperphagia. *American Journal of Physiology, 238,* E284-E292.
Committee on Care and Use of Laboratory Animals, Institute of Laboratory Animal Resources. (1985). *Guide for the care and use of laboratory animals.* Bethesda, MD: National Institutes of Health.
Committee on Diet and Health. (1989). *Diet and health: Implications for reducing chronic disease risk.* Washington, DC: National Academy Press.
Contreras, R. J., & Williams, V. L. (1989). Dietary obesity and weight cycling: Effects on blood pressure and heart rate in rats. *American Journal of Physiology, 256,* R1209-R1219.
Council on Scientific Affairs, American Medical Association. (1988). Treatment of obesity in adults. *Journal of the American Medical Association, 260,* 2547-2551.
Drenick, E. J. (1973). Weight reduction by prolonged fasting. In G. A. Bray (Ed.), *Obesity in perspective* (DHEW Publication No. NIH 75-708, pp. 341-360). Washington, DC: U.S. Government Printing Office.
Drenick, E. J., & Johnson, D. (1978). Weight reduction by fasting and semistarvation in morbid obesity: Long-term follow-up. *International Journal of Obesity, 2,* 25-34.
Duncan, G. G., Duncan, T. G., Schless, G. L., & Cristofori, F. C. (1965). Contraindications and therapeutic results of fasting in obese patients. *Annals of the New York Academy of Sciences, 131,* 632-636.
Dureuil, B., Viires, N., Veber, B., Pavlovic, D., Pariente, R., Desmonts, J., & Aubier, M. (1989). Acute diaphragmatic changes induced by starvation in rats. *American Journal of Clinical Nutrition, 49,* 738-744.
Esposito, G. (1967). Intestinal absorption of sugars in semistarved rats. *Proceedings of the Society for Experimental Biology and Medicine, 125,* 452-455.
Falconer, D. S. (1960). *Introduction to quantitative genetics.* Edinburgh: Oliver & Boyd.
Felig, P. (1978). Four questions about protein diets. *New England Journal of Medicine, 298,* 1025-1026.
Festing, M. F. W. (1979). The inheritance of obesity in animal models. In M. F. W. Festing (Ed)., *Animal models of obesity* (pp. 15-37). New York: Oxford University Press.
Fowler, R. E. (1962). The efficiency of food utilization, digestibility of foodstuffs, and energy expenditure of mice selected for large or small body size. *Genetic Research, 3,* 51-68.
Fried, S. K., Hill, J. O., Nickel, M., & Digirolamo, M. (1983). Prolonged effects of fasting-refeeding on rat adipose tissue lipoprotein lipase activity: Influence of calorie restriction during refeeding. *Journal of Nutrition, 113,* 1861-1869.
Garrow, J. S. (1989). Very low calorie diets should not be used. *International Journal of Obesity, 13*(Suppl. 2), 145-147.
Gelfand, R. A., & Hendler, R. (1989). Effect of nutrient composition on the metabolic response to very low calorie diets: Learning more and more about less and less. *Diabetes/Metabolism Review, 5,* 17-30.
Goode, E. E. (1990, May 14). Getting slim. *U.S. News and World Report,* pp. 56-57.
Greenwood, M. R. C. (1985a). Adipose tissue: Cellular morphology and development. *Annals of Internal Medicine, 103*(Suppl. 2), 996-999.
Greenwood, M. R. C. (1985b). Normal and abnormal growth and maintenance of adipose tissue. In J. Hirsch & T. B. VanItallie (Eds.), *Recent advances in obesity research: IV. Proceedings of the Fourth International Congress on Obesity* (pp. 20-32). London: John Libbey.
Greenwood, M. R. C., & Turkenkopf, I. J. (1983). Genetic and metabolic aspects. In M. R. C. Greenwood, (Ed.), *Obesity* (pp. 193-208). New York: Churchill Livingstone.
Hayes, J. F., & McCarthy, J. C. (1976). The effects of selection at different ages for high and low body weight on the pattern of fat deposition in mice. *Genetic Research, 27,* 389-403.

Hill, J. O. (1990). Body weight regulation in obese and obese-reduced rats. *International Journal of Obesity, 14*(Suppl. 1), 31–37.
Hill, J. O., Thacker, S., Newby, D., Sykes, M. N., & Digirolamo, M. (1988). Influence of food restriction couples with weight cycling on carcass energy restoration during ad-lib refeeding. *International Journal of Obesity, 12,* 547–555.
Hoffer, L. J., Bistrian, B. R., Young, G. L., Blackburn, G. L., & Matthews, D. E. (1984). Metabolic effects of very low calorie weight reduction diets. *Journal of Clinical Investigation, 73,* 750–758.
Hooper, A. C. B., Thacker, S., Newby, D., Sykes, M. N., & Digirolamo, M. (1984). The effect of dietary restriction on muscle fibre length in mice. *British Journal of Nutrition, 51,* 479–483.
Kelsen, S. G., Ference, M., & Kapoor, S. (1985). Effects of prolonged undernutrition on structure and function of the diaphragm. *Journal of Applied Physiology, 58,* 1354–1359.
Kershaw, T. G., Neame, K. D., & Wiseman, G. (1960). The effect of semistarvation on absorption by the rat small intestine in vitro and in vivo. *Journal of Physiology, 152,* 182–190.
Kessner, D. N., & Epstein, F. H. (1965). Effect of renal insufficiency on gastrointestinal transport of calcium. *American Journal of Physiology, 209,* 141–145.
Keys, A., Henschel, A., & Taylor, H. L. (1947). The size and function of the human heart at rest in semistarvation and in subsequent rehabilitation. *American Journal of Physiology, 50,* 153–169.
Keys, A., Brozek, J., Henschel, A., Mickelsen, F., & Taylor, H. L. (1950). *The biology of human starvation* (2 vols.). Minneapolis, MN: University of Minnesota Press.
Kownacki, M., Keller, J., & Gebler, E. (1975). Selection of mice for high weight gains: Its effect on the basal metabolic rate. *Genetica Polonica, 16,* 359–363.
Lafontan, M., Galitzky, J., Saulnier-Blache, J. S., Mauriege, P., Taouis, M., Langin, D., Carpene, C., Valet, P., & Berlan, M. (1990). Recent developments in human fat cell adrenergic-receptor characterization: Interests and limits of animal and cellular models for regulation studies. In G. A. Bray, D. Ricquier, & B. M. Spiegelman (Eds.), *Obesity: Towards a molecular approach* (pp. 173–188). New York: Wiley.
Lang, B. J., & Legates, J. E. (1969). Rate, composition and efficiency of growth in mice selected for large and small body weight. *Theoretical and Applied Genetics, 39,* 306–314.
Larsson, S. (1967). Factors of importance for the etiology of obesity in mice. *Acta Physiologica Scandinavica, 71* (Suppl. 294), 1–80.
Lawlor, T., & Wells, D. G. (1969). Metabolic hazards of fasting. *American Journal of Clinical Nutrition, 22,* 1142–1149.
Linn, R., & Stuart, S. L. (1976). *The last chance diet.* Secaucus, NJ: Lyle & Stuart.
Lipscomb, H. L., & Sharp, J. G. (1982). Effects of reduced food intake on morphometry and cell production in the small intestine of the rat. *Virchows Archives [Cell Pathology], 41,* 285–292.
Lockwood, D. H., & Amatruda, J. M. (1984). Very low calorie diets in the management of obesity. *Annual Review of Medicine, 35,* 373–381.
Maggio, C., & Greenwood, M. R. C. (1982). Triglyceride clearance and adipose tissue lipoprotein lipase activity and triglyceride uptake in Zucker rats. *Physiology and Behavior, 29,* 1147–1152.
McCarthy, J. C. (1979). Normal variation in body fat and its inheritance. In M. F. W. Festing (Ed.), *Animal models of obesity* (pp. 1–14). New York: Oxford University Press.
Miller, D. S. (1979). Non-genetic models of obesity. In M. F. W. Festing (Ed.), *Animal models of obesity* (pp. 131–140). New York: Oxford University Press.
Millward, D. J. (1970). Protein turnover in skeletal muscle: II. The effect of starvation and a protein-free diet on the synthesis and catabolism of skeletal muscle proteins in comparison to liver. *Clinical Science, 39,* 591–603.
Millward, D. J., Garlick, P. J., Nnanyelugo, D. O., & Waterlow, J. C. (1976). The relative importance of muscle protein synthesis and breakdown in the regulation of muscle mass. *Biochemical Journal, 156,* 185–188.

Millward, D. J., & Waterlow, J. C. (1978). Effect of nutrition on protein turnover in skeletal muscle. *Federation Proceedings, 37*, 2283-2289.

National Institutes of Health. (1985). Consensus Development Conference: Health implications of obesity. *Annals of Internal Medicine, 103*(Suppl. Pt. 2), 979-1077.

Neil, D. H., & Kesel, M. L. (1984). Some features of the digestive systems and absorption in rabbits and rodents. In R. W. Phillips (Ed.), *Animal models for nutrition research* (pp. 5-9). Columbus, OH: Ross Laboratories.

Petith, M. M., & Schedl, H. P. (1979). Effects of semistarvation on large intestinal calcium transport: In vivo studies in the rat. *American Journal of Clinical Nutrition, 32*, 1006-1010.

Quig, D. W., Layman, D. K., Bechtel, P. J., & Hackler, L. R. (1983). The influence of starvation and refeeding on the lipoprotein lipase activity of skeletal muscle and adipose tissue of lean and obese Zucker rats. *Journal of Nutrition, 113*, 1150-1156.

Russell, D. M., Atwood, H. L., Whittaker, J. C., Itakura, T., Walker, P. M., Mickle, D. A. G., & JeeJeebhoy, K. N. (1984). The effect of fasting and hypocaloric diets on the functional and metabolic characteristics of rat gastrocnemius muscle. *Clinical Science, 67*, 185-194.

Sahebjami, H., & Vassallo, C. L. (1979). Effects of starvation and refeeding on lung mechanics and morphometry. *American Review of Respiratory Diseases, 119*, 443-451.

Sahebjami, H., & Vassallo, C. L. (1980). Influence of starvation on enzyme-induced emphysema. *Journal of Applied Physiology, 48*, 284-288.

Sahebjami, H., & Wirman, J. A. (1981). Emphysema-like changes in the lungs of starved rats. *American Review of Respiratory Diseases, 124*, 619-624.

Saudek, C. D., & Felig, P. (1976). The metabolic events of starvation. *American Journal of Medicine, 60*, 117-126.

Schemmel, R. A., Stone, M., Warren, M. J., & Stoddart, K. A. (1983). Nitrogen and protein losses in rats during weight reduction with a high protein, low energy diet or fasting. *Journal of Nutrition, 113*, 727-734.

Sours, H. E., Frattali, V. P., Brand, C. D., Feldman, R. A., Forbes, A. L., Swanson, R. C., & Paris, A. L. (1981). Sudden death associated with very low calorie weight reduction regimens. *American Journal of Clinical Nutrition, 34*, 453-461.

Stauffacher, W., Orci, L., Cameron, D. P., Burr, I. M., & Rendd, A. E. (1971). Spontaneous hyperglycemia and/or obesity in laboratory rodents: An example of the possible usefulness of animal disease models with both genetic and environmental components. *Recent Progress in Hormone Research, 27*, 41-91.

Stock, M. J. (1989). Effects of low (LCD) and very low (VLCD) energy diets on metabolic rate and body composition in obese (fa/fa) Zucker rats. *International Journal of Obesity, 13*(Suppl. 2), 61-65.

Stock, M. J., & Rothwell, N. J. (1979). Energy balance in reversible obesity. In M. F. W. Festing (Ed.), *Animal models of obesity* (pp. 141-151). New York: Oxford University Press.

Stordy, B. J. (1989). Very low calorie diets should be used. *International Journal of Obesity, 13*(Suppl. 2), 141-143.

Timmers, K., & Knittle, J. L. (1980). Effects of undernutrition and refeeding on enzyme activities and rate of glucose catabolism in rat epididymal adipose tissue. *Journal of Nutrition, 110*, 1176-1184.

Timmons, K. H., Slaten, B. L., & Svacha, A. J. (1983). Metabolic effects of liquid protein. *Journal of the American Dietetic Association, 82*, 53-57.

U.S. Department of Health and Human Services. (1988). *The Surgeon General's report on nutrition and health* (DHHS Publication No. PHS 88-50210). Washington, DC: U.S. Government Printing Office.

VanItallie, T. B. (1978). Liquid protein mayhem. *Journal of the American Medical Association, 240*, 140-141.

VanItallie, T. B. (1985). Health implications of overweight and obesity in the United States. *Annals of Internal Medicine, 103*, 983-988.

Wadden, T. A., Foster, G. D., Letizia, K. A., & Mullen, J. L. (1990). Long-term effects of dieting on resting metabolic rate in obese outpatients. *Journal of the American Medical Association, 264,* 707–711.

Wadden, T. A., Stunkard, A. J., & Brownell, K. D. (1983). Very low calorie diets: their efficacy, safety, and future. *Annals of Internal Medicine, 99,* 675–684.

Wadden, T. A., VanItallie, T. B., & Blackburn, G. L. (1990). Responsible and irresponsible use of very-low-calorie diets in the treatment of obesity. *Journal of the American Medical Association, 263,* 83–85.

Waterlow, J. C., & Stephen, J. M. L. (1968). The effect of low protein diets on the turnover rate of serum, liver and muscle protein in the rat, measured by continuous infusion of L-[^{14}C]-lysine. *Clinical Science, 35,* 287–305.

Wyden, R. (1990, May 7). *Opening statement: Deception and fraud in the diet industry, Part II.* Hearings before the Subcommittee on Regulation, Business Opportunities and Energy, Committee on Small Business, U.S. House of Representatives (Serial No. 101-57, pp. 1–4). Washington, DC: U.S. Government Printing Office.

York, E. A., & Bray, G. A. (1973). Genetic obesity in rats: II. The effect of food restriction on the metabolism of adipose tissue. *Metabolism, 22,* 443–454.

Young, E. A., Cantu, T. L., & Harris, M. M. (1989). Gastrointestinal and cardiac response to refeeding after low-calorie semistarvation. *American Journal of Clinical Nutrition, 50,* 922–929.

Young, E. A., Ramos, R. G., & Harris, M. M. (1988). Gastrointestinal and cardiac response to low-calorie semistarvation diets. *American Journal of Clinical Nutrition, 47,* 981–988.

Young, E. A., Taylor, M. M., Taylor, M. K., McFee, A. S., LaWayne Miller, O., & Gleiser, C. A. (1984). Gastric stapling for morbid obesity: Gastrointestinal response in a rat model. *American Journal of Clinical Nutrition, 40,* 293–302.

Young, V. R., Stothers, S. C., & Vilaire, G. (1971). Synthesis and degradation of mixed proteins, and composition changes in skeletal muscle of malnourished and refed rats. *Journal of Nutrition, 101,* 1379–1390.

6

Cardiac Structure and Function in Markedly Obese Patients before and after Weight Loss

STEVEN B. HEYMSFIELD
PRASOON JAIN
OSCAR ORTIZ
MASAKO WAKI

Excess adipose tissue, which is the hallmark of obesity, has both direct and indirect effects on cardiac structure and function. These physiological and pathological interrelations are summarized in Figure 6.1. The aim of this chapter is twofold: to provide an overview of obesity–heart interactions; and to explore in detail the effects of obesity and weight loss on cardiac structure, myocardial performance, and electrophysiological function.

Obesity and the Heart

Cardiomegaly

"Fatty heart" was a nonspecific diagnosis of Victorian times that included many pathologies unrelated to obesity (Messerli & Engel, 1986). A clarification of the relation between obesity and the heart was first advanced by Smith and Willius at the Mayo Clinic (1933). A total of 136 autopsies were completed in obese patients who had no major pathology of the heart valves or coronary arteries. The investigators divided subjects into two groups, those with and without a history of high blood pressure. Their results for total heart weight as a function of body mass index (BMI) in females are presented in Figure 6.2. The conclusion is clear: Obesity by itself is associated with cardiomegaly, and obesity combined with high blood pressure is accompanied by a marked enlargement of the heart.

Echocardiography has now confirmed that many otherwise healthy obese patients develop eccentric left ventricular hypertrophy and that obesity combined with high blood pressure is associated with a combination of eccentric

Cardiac Structure and Function

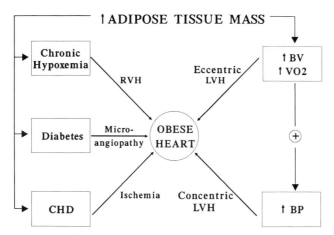

FIGURE 6.1. Interrelations between the excess adipose tissue mass of obesity and the heart. BP, blood pressure; BV, blood volume; CHD, coronary heart disease; LVH, left ventricular hypertrophy; RVH, right ventricular hypertrophy; $\dot{V}O_2$, oxygen consumption.

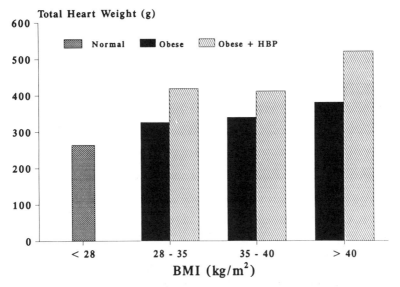

FIGURE 6.2. Total heart weight at autopsy as a function of body mass index (BMI) in normal and obese normotensive and hypertensive (HBP) females. The data are from the study of Smith and Willius (1933). All of the groups were of similar height.

and concentric left ventricular hypertrophy (see Figure 6.1) (Messerli et al., 1983a, 1983b).

Chronic Hypoxemia

A further clarification of obesity–heart interactions was provided by Burwell, Robin, Whaley, and Bickelmann (1956). These investigators first described the "Pickwickian syndrome," which is characterized by severe obesity, somnolence, polycythemia, hypoxemia, hypercapnia, pulmonary hypertension, right ventricular hypertrophy, and right-sided congestive heart failure. The cause of alveolar hypoventilation and hypoxemia appears to be multifactorial and to include obese patients with obstructive sleep apnea, idiopathic hypoventilation syndrome, and restrictive lung disease (Prakash, 1989). Hypoxemia at rest is observed in over 40% of obese patients who are 45 kg or more overweight (Prakash, 1989).

Coronary Artery Disease

Obesity is often associated with coronary risk factors such as hyperlipidemia, hypertension, and glucose intolerance. Obesity, independent of other risk factors, is also a determinant of coronary artery disease. Results from the Framingham Heart Study demonstrate that weight gain in adults conveys an increased risk of cardiovascular disease in both men and women that is independent of age, serum cholesterol, blood pressure, glucose tolerance, and smoking history (Hubert, Feinleib, McNamara, & Castelli, 1983).

Upper body fat distribution associated with obesity is a component of the recently described "deadly quartet" that includes glucose intolerance, hypertriglyceridemia, and high blood pressure (Kaplan, 1989). Patients who have this combination of findings are at high risk of developing atherosclerotic cardiovascular disease. The mechanisms linking upper body obesity and high blood pressure with abnormalities in insulin, glucose, and lipid metabolism are unknown.

Microangiopathy

Although Smith and Willius (1933) excluded diabetics from their autopsy series, direct and indirect effects of glucose intolerance are now known to influence the patency of cardiac blood vessels. Myocardial ischemia can develop in diabetic patients, secondary to a microangiopathy that is characterized by glycoprotein deposition in the vascular endothelium (Shafrir, Bergman, & Felig, 1987). Atherosclerotic lesions of the larger coronary arteries are also more common in obese patients with diabetes (Shafrir et al., 1987).

Ventricular Arrhythmias and Weight Loss

The influence of obesity on cardiac structure and function became of practical relevance to practitioners involved in weight reduction therapy with the report of Garnett, Barnard, Ford, Goodbody, and Woodehouse (1969). During the 1950s and 1960s, total starvation was gaining popularity as a means of treating severe obesity (Bloom, 1959). Garnett and his colleagues described the history of an otherwise healthy 20-year-old girl who weighed 118 kg at the time of hospital admission. The subject successfully completed a 30-week fast as an inpatient and achieved her ideal body weight of 60 kg with only a brief episode of mild hypokalemia and slightly prolonged QT interval (0.38 seconds, with normal for heart rate <0.37 seconds). The patient was then cautiously refed, but on the seventh day she developed a series of refractory ventricular arrhythmias, low QRS voltage in the precordial leads, prolonged QT interval (0.56 seconds), and hypotension. She subsequently died, despite normal serum electrolytes and intensive resuscitative measures.

Although the exact cause of death in this patient was unknown, Garnett and his colleagues made a series of key observations that were later confirmed by other investigators (Isner, Sours, Paris, Ferrans, & Roberts, 1979; Michiel, Sneider, Dickstein, Hayman, & Eich, 1978; Sours et al., 1981). During the total fast, the patient lost 1969 mmol of potassium, 784 mmol of sodium, and 670 g of nitrogen. These results, converted to body composition estimates (Forbes, 1984), are presented in Figure 6.3. Over 50% of the patient's weight loss consisted of fat-free body mass. Compared to a nonobese matched control, Garnett et al.'s patient demonstrated the classic body composition changes of protein–energy malnutrition following weight loss, depletion of body cell mass (−58% from baseline and −46% vs. the control), and a relative increase in extracellular fluid. The investigators linked these changes with a 36% reduction in myofiber diameter and gross myofibrillar fragmentation observed in the postmortem histological inspection of the sectioned myocardium. All other aspects of the patient's heart, including coronary arteries, valves, and myocardium, were normal at autopsy.

The fatality reported by Garnett et al. (1969) and those reported by others (Cubberly, Polster, & Schulman, 1965; Spencer, 1968), during this period led to a decline in total fasting as a means of weight control. However, similar arrhythmias or deaths during weight reduction therapy have appeared either as isolated cases (Sandhofer, Dienstl, Bolzano, & Schwingshackl, 1973) or in clusters related to specific weight loss programs (Isner et al., 1979; Sours et al., 1981).

The remainder of this chapter describes the hemodynamic and cardiac functional, structural, and electrophysiological effects of obesity and weight reduction therapy. A concluding section provides recommendations for the evaluation and monitoring of obese patients prior to and during weight reduction therapy.

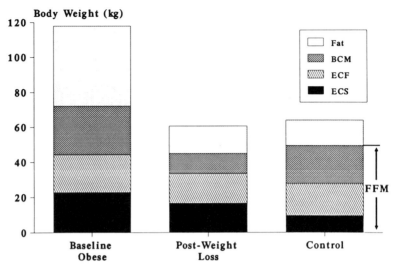

FIGURE 6.3. Body composition before and after 30 weeks of a total fast in the patient of Garnett, Barnard, Ford, Goodbody, and Woodehouse (1969). The data for the matched control patient (sex, age, weight, and height) are from the archives of the Obesity Research Center, St. Luke's–Roosevelt Hospital Center. BCM, body cell mass; ECF, extracellular fluid; ECS, extracellular solids; FFM, fat-free body mass.

Cardiac Structure and Function in Relation to Physiological Demands

Cardiac Output

Cardiac output in the healthy adult is determined by tissue oxygen requirements and circulating blood volume (Schlant & Sonnenblick, 1982; Schlant, Sonnenblick, & Gorlin, 1982). Circulatory demands in the obese patient are increased due to both an elevated total body tissue oxygen requirement and an expanded blood volume.

Tissue oxygen requirements are increased in the obese patient due to an increase in metabolically active cell mass (Bernstein, Redmond, & VanItallie, 1981). As body weight increases in the presence of positive nutrient balance, the tissue formed consists of both adipocytes and non-fat-containing cell mass (e.g., the myofibers of skeletal muscle). The result is that body cell mass is larger in the obese individual than in a lean counterpart. Whole-body resting oxygen consumption is proportionately increased (Ravussin & Bogardus, 1989). The increase in body weight associated with obesity also causes an augmentation in the absolute oxygen cost of exercise. Long-term (14-day) studies of ambulatory obese patients demonstrate an increase in whole-body

24-hour oxygen consumption in relation to their enlarged body cell mass and greater body weight (Schoeller, 1990).

As adipose and other tissues increase in mass with the development of obesity, there is a parallel expansion of blood volume, extracellular fluid, and plasma volume (Feldschuh & Enson, 1977). Obese patients have a relative expansion of extracellular fluid even in the absence of clinical symptoms of congestive heart failure (Waki et al., 1991). This is because adipose tissue fluid is almost entirely extracellular, and adipose tissue represents about 75% of excess body weight (Webster, Hesp, & Garrow, 1984). Adipose tissue perfusion at rest is about 2–3 ml/min/100 g, which contributes to the increased requirement for cardiac output (DiGirolamo & Esposito, 1975).

The relation between BMI, total blood volume, and 24-hour energy expenditure is presented in Figure 6.4. The increase in cardiac output is accomplished via an augmentation in stroke volume, and resting heart rate is unchanged. A high resting cardiac output and increased stroke volume are characteristic of obesity (Lavie, Ventura, & Messerli, 1988). In the absence of high blood pressure, the increase in cardiac output of obesity is associated with a reciprocal lowering of total peripheral vascular resistance (i.e., resistance = mean blood pressure/cardiac output) (Licata et al., 1990; Reisin & Frohlich, 1981). The relation between BMI, heart rate, stroke volume, cardiac output, and total peripheral vascular resistance is presented in Figure 6.5.

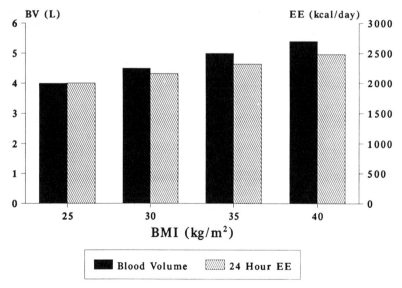

FIGURE 6.4. The relation between BMI, total blood volume, and 24-hour energy expenditure (EE) in a metabolic chamber. The data are from Feldschuh and Enson (1977) and Ravussin, Lillioja, Anderson, Christin, and Bogardus (1986).

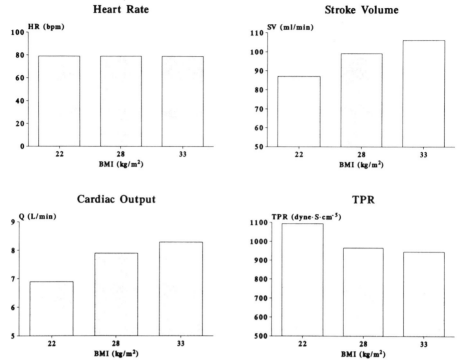

FIGURE 6.5. The relation between BMI, heart rate (HR), stroke volume (SV), cardiac output (Q), and total peripheral vascular resistance (TPR) in normotensive subjects evaluated using first-pass radionuclide angiography. Adapted from "Effect of Obesity on Left Ventricular Function Studied by Radionuclide Angiocardiography" by G. Licata, R. Scaglione, M. Barbagallo, G. Parrinello, G. Capuana, R. Lipari, G. Merlino, and A. Ganguzza, 1990, *International Journal of Obesity, 15,* 295-302. Copyright 1990 by Macmillan Press Ltd. Adapted by permission.

Cardiac Structure

The high cardiac output observed in obese patients is accompanied by an expansion of atrial and ventricular chamber volumes (de Divitiis et al., 1981; Nakajima et al., 1985; Messerli et al., 1983a, 1983b). For example, both the end-diastolic and end-systolic volumes of the left ventricle are increased in obese patients compared to lean controls.

The expanded left ventricular end-diastolic volume (preload) of obesity contributes to an elevation in the afterload—the force required to eject blood into the systemic circulation during contraction of the myocardium. An additional increase in afterload occurs in the obese patient who has high blood pressure and elevated peripheral vascular resistance. The higher preload and afterload in obese patients increase ventricular wall stress and myofiber tension, which then stimulate cardiac muscle protein synthesis and promote hypertrophy (Alpert, 1986; Ford, 1976; Grossman, Jones, & McLaurin, 1975; Kao, Rannels, Whitman, & Morgan, 1978).

The enlargement in cardiac muscle proceeds with the development of obesity in relation to the relative increase in preload and afterload. In the absence of high blood pressure, the increase in blood volume and venous return to the heart elevate mainly preload. The result is "magnification" or "eccentric" cardiac enlargement, consisting of a proportional increase in both heart muscle mass and chamber volumes (Alexander, 1982; Messerli et al., 1983a). When high blood pressure and an elevation in peripheral vascular resistance are also present, afterload is further increased, which stimulates additional thickening of the left ventricular wall. The resulting change in cardiac anatomy is referred to as "concentric hypertrophy" (see Figure 6.6) (Messerli et al., 1983a). Obese patients with high blood pressure can have a combination of eccentric and concentric hypertrophy (Figure 6.6).

In an important recent study, Lauer, Anderson, Kannel, and Levy (1991) examined changes in left ventricular mass and geometry in the Framingham Heart Study. A total of 3922 healthy nonhypertensive subjects ranging widely

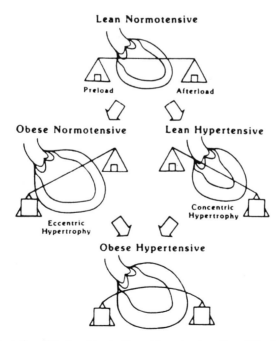

FIGURE 6.6. .Adaptation of the heart to obesity and hypertension. From "Cardiopathy of Obesity" (p. 64) by C. J. Lavie, H. O. Ventura, and F. H. Messerli, 1988, *Internal Medicine, 9,* 57–71. Copyright 1988 by Lancet, Ltd. Reprinted by permission.

in BMI were evaluated using M-mode echocardiography. After adjusting for the effects of age and blood pressure, left ventricular mass normalized for stature increased 10.2 g/m and 9.3 g/m for men and women, respectively, for each 4 kg/m² increment in BMI. The investigators also observed an increase in left ventricular wall thickness as a function of BMI which exceeded the increase observed in left ventricular end-distolic dimension. This finding differs from previous studies and suggests that the increase in left ventricular mass associated with obesity in the absence of high blood pressure is not due solely to eccentric hypertrophy but is also accompanied by a change in relative left ventricular wall thickness.

Mechanical Function

The presence of glucose intolerance, coronary artery disease, high blood pressure, and chronic hypoxemia all contribute to the abnormalities in cardiac mechanical function observed in obese patients. Uncomplicated mild or moderate obesity is accompanied by normal systolic left ventricular function, as estimated by preload-dependent indices such as ejection fraction and circumferential fiber shortening (Lavie et al., 1988; Nakajima et al., 1985; Messerli et al., 1983a). A recent study by Lavie et al. (1988) suggests that diastolic ventricular dysfunction is an early finding in obesity. Using the M-mode echocardiographic left atrial emptying index as a measure of early diastolic ventricular filling, these investigators observed a 25% and 35% reduction in obesity alone and obesity combined with high blood pressure, respectively.

Cardiac catheterization studies of severely obese patients demonstrate the hemodynamic characteristics of a congestive circulatory state, including high cardiac output, increased circulating blood volume, elevated left ventricular filling pressures at rest or following the increased venous return stimulated by leg raising or exercise, and pulmonary hypertension without a transpulmonary diastolic pressure gradient (Alexander, 1982; de Divitiis et al., 1981). Left ventricular pressure–volume studies also demonstrate a reduction in diastolic compliance (de Divitiis et al., 1981).

The presence of cardiac dysfunction may be related to the severity and duration of obesity. Using first-pass radionuclide angiography, Licata et al. (1990) observed an inverse correlation between BMI, resting left ventricular ejection fraction, and duration of obesity. Nakajima et al. (1985) observed a larger relative end-diastolic volume and ratio of left ventricular end-diastolic radius to posterior wall thickness in patients who were overweight for more than 15 years than in those who were obese for less than that time.

The systolic and diastolic abnormalities in cardiac function may predispose obese patients to congestive heart failure. The Framingham Study indicated that high blood pressure, obesity, and glucose intolerance are major, related risk factors for the development of congestive heart failure and sudden death (Kannel & Schatzkin, 1985; Kannel, Plehn, & Cupples, 1988).

Electrophysiological Function

The electrocardiogram of the obese patient reflects multiple cardiac pathologies, including coronary artery disease, high blood pressure (e.g., increased QRS voltage due to left ventricular hypertrophy), and severe chronic hypoxia (e.g., P-pulmonale and right axis deviation secondary to pulmonary hypertension). More rarely occurring are arrhythmias related to fatty infiltration of the myocardium, sinus node, and bundle of His (Balsaver, Morales, & Whitehouse, 1967). A number of studies have reviewed the electrocardiographic findings in obese patients, and the results of these investigations can be summarized as follows.

Heart Rate and Rhythm

The resting heart rate (i.e., the R-R interval) is normal in over 97% of patients (Eisenstein, Edelstein, Sarma, Sanmarco, & Selvester, 1982; Frank, Colliver, & Frank, 1986). Rare conduction disturbances are observed, including junctional rhythms and atrial fibrillation. The frequency of these abnormalities is the same as in the nonobese population.

The 24-hour ambulatory electrocardiogram is a more sensitive method of detecting extrasystoles and arrhythmias than the conventional 12-lead electrocardiogram. Uncomplicated obesity does not appear to be accompanied by abnormalities in the ambulatory electrocardiogram. An example is the study of Zwiauer, Schmidinger, Klipsera, Mayr, and Widhalm (1989), who investigated 36 grossly obese children and adolescents and found no increase in ventricular ectopic beats or arrhythmias.

In contrast, the presence of high blood pressure combined with eccentric left ventricular hypertrophy in the obese patient is associated with abnormalities in the 24-hour ambulatory electrocardiogram. Messerli, Nunez, Ventura, and Snyder (1987) evaluated three groups of hypertensive patients. One group had a normal body weight and the other two were obese, one with and the other without eccentric left ventricular hypertrophy. A 10-fold increase in premature ventricular contractions was observed in the obese hypertensive patients with normal cardiac anatomy as compared to the normal weight hypertensive group. In the obese hypertensives with cardiac enlargement, a 30-fold increase in premature ventricular contractions was observed compared to the normal-weight group, and 2 of the 14 patients had short runs of ventricular tachycardia.

The observations of Messerli et al. (1987) complement those from other studies of left ventricular hypertrophy in nonobese populations. Patients with longstanding high blood pressure and left ventricular hypertrophy have more premature ventricular contractions and high grade arrhythmias than do patients without cardiac enlargement or subjects who are normotensive (Koren, Devereux, Cassale, Savage, & Laragh, 1991; McLenachan, Henderson, Morris, & Dargie, 1987). Left ventricular hypertrophy was also a risk factor for sudden death in the Framingham Study, independent of blood pressure (Kannel, Gordon, & Affutt, 1969; Kannel, Doyle, McNamara, Quickenton, & Gordon, 1975).

Echocardiography combined with ambulatory monitoring thus demonstrates frequent ventricular ectopy and abnormalities in heart rhythm in obese hypertensive patients with eccentric left ventricular hypertrophy. Although it has not been proven, the suggestion is that these patients are at increased risk of sudden death due to cardiac arrhythmias.

P Wave and P-R Interval

The P-R interval is normal in obese patients (Eisenstein et al., 1982; Frank et al., 1986). P wave amplitude and axis may be abnormal in patients with right atrial enlargement secondary to severe chronic hypoxia.

QRS Complex

Obese patients often have a horizontal axis (Frank et al., 1986), although a QRS axis of $>-30°$ is unusual in the otherwise healthy patient. Frank et al. (1986) observed a small linear increase in precordial QRS voltage as a function of percentage overweight in 1029 obese adults.

QT Interval

The QT interval, measured from the beginning of the QRS complex to the end of the T wave, represents ventricular repolarization during diastole. Several intervals are usually measured in the leads showing the highest amplitude T waves, and the results are averaged (Lepeschkin & Surawicz, 1952). Because the QT interval is dependent on heart rate, a correction (QTc) is made by using Bazett's equation (QTc = $[QT/\sqrt{R-R}]$) or other published formulas (Ashman, 1942; Surawicz & Knoebel, 1984). The upper limit of normal for the QTc interval found in most reference sources is 0.44 seconds, although not all publications provide the same upper limit. For example, Myerburg (1991) gives the upper limit of normal for the QTc interval as 0.40 seconds for males and 0.45 seconds for females in *Harrison's Principles of Internal Medicine*.

Most published clinical studies of the QT interval in obese patients use these measurement techniques, the Bazett equation, and the upper limit of 0.44 seconds for the QTc interval. However, each one of these areas is controversial, and the interested reader should consult in-depth reviews for a thorough discussion of the QT interval (Ashman, 1942; Kremers, 1988; Surawicz & Knoebel, 1984).

Obese patients showed a linear increase in QTc interval duration as a function of percentage overweight in the study of Frank et al. (1986). For each 10% increment in excess body weight, the QTc duration was prolonged by 1.0 milliseconds. Frank and his colleagues observed a QTc interval of >0.44 seconds in 4% of obese subjects. A prolonged QTc interval (>0.44 seconds) was found in 14 out of 30 morbidly obese patients studied by Shalom, Santora, Iseri, and Henry (1981). Rasmussen and Andersen (1985), on the other hand, found a normal QTc interval in all 22 of the morbidly obese patients whom they evaluated prior to gastroplasty.

A prolonged QT interval increases the susceptibility to ventricular tachyarrhythmias and sudden death. There are two main concerns related to the QT interval in evaluating the obese patient prior to or during weight reduction therapy. The first is pre-existence of a prolonged QT interval in the patient. In such patients, the practitioner should search for the heritable and acquired causes of a prolonged QT interval that increase the vulnerability of individuals to ventricular arrhythmias (Bhandari & Scheinman, 1985; Moss, 1986) (see Table 6.1).

While the conditions listed in Table 6.1 are clearly associated with an increased risk of arrhythmias and sudden death, the relevance of a prolonged QT interval (>0.44 seconds) detected on routine electrocardiography is uncer-

TABLE 6.1. Prolonged QT Interval Syndromes

Congenital long QT syndrome
  Hereditary form
    Jervell–Lange–Nielsen syndrome
    Romano–Ward syndrome
  Sporadic type

Acquired long QT syndrome (drug-induced)
  Antiarrhythmic agents
  Phenothiazines
  Tricyclic antidepressants
  Lithium carbonate

Metabolic/electrolyte abnormalities

Total starvation or nutritionally incomplete very low calorie diets
  Central nervous system disorders
    Subarachnoid hemorrhage
    Acute cerebral thrombosis
    Head trauma
  Miscellaneous
    Coronary heart disease
    Mitral valve prolapse

Note. Adapted from "Prolonged QT-Interval Syndromes" by A. J. Moss, 1986, *Journal of the American Medical Association, 256,* 2985–2987. Copyright 1986 by American Medical Association. Adapted by permission.

tain. A 30-year follow-up of subjects enrolled in the Framingham Study with a prolonged QTc interval showed no increased risk of total mortality or sudden death due to coronary artery disease (Goldberg et al., 1991). Of the 5125 subjects followed, 279 (5.4%) had an initial QTc of >0.44 seconds. The ideal body weight for the group as a whole was 102%, with no influence of relative weight on the QTc interval.

The second concern is that the QT interval, or more precisely the QU interval, is prolonged by potassium deficiency, a problem that can arise during caloric restriction (Commerford & Lloyd, 1984; Singh et al., 1978; Surawicz, 1967). A prominent U wave usually accompanies severe hypokalemia. Untreated severe potassium deficiency can result in ventricular tachycardia and fibrillation. Hypokalemia alone, or particularly during antiarrhythmic drug therapy, can precipitate the rhythm disturbance referred to as *Torsade de Pointes*. This distinctive form of ventricular tachycardia, characterized by a gradual oscillation around the baseline by the peaks of successive QRS complexes, tends to be rapid, occurs in clusters, and leads to ventricular fibrillation and sudden death (Jackman et al., 1984).

S-T Segment

Nonspecific ST and T wave changes were detected in 11% and 50% of the patients studied by Eisenstein et al. (1982) and Frank et al. (1986). T wave flattening in the precordial leads is a common electrocardiographic finding in morbidly obese patients.

Weight Loss and the Heart

The general description presented in this section refers to weight loss during ingestion of a low or very low calorie diet with a high quality protein source and adequate amounts of electrolytes and micronutrients. A later section describes the sudden death syndrome associated with total starvation or intake of nutritionally incomplete very low calorie diets. It should be emphasized, however, that this is an arbitrary separation of modern very low calorie diet treatments and sudden death during starvation. Under certain circumstances, very low calorie dieting may be physiologically indistinct from total starvation as, for example, in the case of a noncompliant patient who ingests less than the prescribed amount of formula and loses weight rapidly.

Composition of Body Weight Loss

Early weight loss (weeks 1 and 2) is rapid and consists of a high proportion of protein, glycogen, and water (Heymsfield, Casper, Hearn, & Guy, 1989).

Weight loss beyond the second week slows, with activation of adaptive mechanisms and diminution in the rate of nitrogen depletion. With total starvation, the composition of weight loss during this later phase is about half fat and half fat-free body mass. Very low calorie diets reduce the proportion of fat-free mass loss to about one-quarter of weight loss, which is similar to the composition of excess body weight (75:25, fat:fat-free body mass). Fat and fat-free body mass have caloric densities of 9 kilocalories (kcal)/g and about 1 kcal/g, respectively. Accordingly, 1 kg of weight loss during very low calorie diet treatment optimally has a caloric content of about 7000 kcal. As the average moderate or severely obese adult achieves a negative energy balance of between 1000 and 2000 kcal/day during very low calorie diet treatment, weight loss should range between 1 and 2 kg per week.

The usual recommendation is that patients maintain a rate of weight loss in this range during very low calorie diet treatment. Higher rates of weight loss suggest excessive losses of fat-free body mass, resulting in a depletion of visceral tissue proteins such as the actomyosin in cardiac myofibers. It should be emphasized that all of these aforementioned associations—the composition of excess weight, composition of weight loss on very low calorie diet, and relation between loss in fat-free body mass and catabolism of myofibrils—are approximations or hypotheses, but form a reasonable framework for recommending safe weight loss guidelines.

Cardiac Changes in Relation to Reduced Physiological Demands

A combination of hormonal mechanisms (Landsberg & Young, 1978; Osburne et al., 1983; Yang & VanItallie, 1984), reductions in body cell mass, and negative fluid balance reduce whole-body oxygen consumption (Montgomery, 1962), heart rate, and cardiac output (Keys, Brozek, Henschel, Mickelsen, & Taylor, 1950). Although refeeding reverses some of the hormonal and adaptive mechanisms of semistarvation, the reduced-obese patient has an appropriately lower body cell mass, whole-body oxygen consumption (Ravussin, Burnand, Schutz, & Jéquier, 1985), and blood volume (Alexander, 1982; Alexander & Peterson, 1971; Henschel, Mickelsen, Taylor, & Keys, 1947). Many studies have now demonstrated that with weight loss, obese individuals also have an appropriate reduction in left ventricular end-diastolic volume, stroke volume, and cardiac output compared to baseline levels (Alexander & Peterson, 1971; Alpert, Terry, & Kelly, 1985; Ramhamadany et al., 1989; Reisin et al., 1983).

As preload, afterload, and ventricular wall tension decrease with weight loss, a predictable effect of dieting would be negative myocardial protein balance, as ventricular wall tension is the major determinant of cardiac protein synthesis. There is now good evidence that a lowering of ventricular wall tension is the major determinant of cardiac protein balance during underfeeding. For example, increasing afterload by banding the aorta in rats reduces the loss in myocardial mass that occurs with starvation (Heymsfield, Hoff, Gray, Galloway, & Casper, 1987). A related experiment is that increasing the mechanical load on the rat soleus muscle reduces the degree of atrophy produced by total starvation that appears in a contralateral soleus muscle not subjected to an increased workload (Goldberg, 1971). Regression of cardiac hypertrophy promptly occurs following the reduced physiological demands associated with antihypertensive therapy in patients with high blood pressure, with relief of ventricular outflow obstruction in patients with cardiac valvular disease, and with completion of training in athletes (Hickson, Foster, Pollock, Galassi, & Rich, 1985).

Both human and animal studies clearly demonstrate a loss in myocardial mass with weight loss (Alpert et al., 1985; Heymsfield & Nutter, 1979; Ramhamadany et al., 1989; Nutter, Heymsfield, Murray, & Fuller, 1979). Studies by Crandall, Lizzo, and Cervoni (1985) in the spontaneously obese rat revealed that the reduction in total heart weight with underfeeding consisted of lipid, water, and protein. The pre- and post-obese heart contained equal proportions of water and protein, and, as expected, there was a relative reduction in lipid due to a loss of myocardial adipose tissue.

In addition to a decrease in ventricular wall tension, the multiple metabolic changes that accompany the negative energy balance of dieting create a pattern of hormonal alterations that favor net cardiac protein catabolism (Heymsfield et al., 1987) (see Figure 6.7). Mechanical and hormonal mechanisms thus appear to regulate the reduction in heart mass that accompanies weight loss in a manner that closely balances organ size and physical needs (Beznak, 1964; Beznak, Korecky, & Thomas, 1969).

Electrocardiogram

As the patient continues to lose weight during treatment, the electrocardiogram often demonstrates a reduction in heart rate, secondary to the overall hypometabolic state that develops during semistarvation. Several studies of obese children, adolescents, and adults who used diets that ranged widely in their caloric, protein, and carbohydrate content, revealed no major increase in ventricular premature beats or cardiac arrhythmias (Amatruda, Biddle, Patton, & Lockwood, 1983; Baird, 1981; Brown, Klish, Hollander, Campbell, & Forbes, 1983; Doherty et al., 1991; Linet, Butler, Caswell, Metzler, & Reele, 1983; Narasimhan & Bennett, 1985; Phinney et al., 1983; Wilson, Lamberts, & Swart, 1983; Zwiauer et al., 1989). The P-R interval is unchanged with weight loss, the QRS voltage remains unchanged or decreases slightly, and the flattened T waves associated with morbid obesity often revert to normal.

In general, studies of the QT interval during weight loss demonstrate either no change or a normalization of a pre-existing prolonged QTc interval. One of the clearest studies of the QTc interval during weight loss was the Minnesota experiment in which male volunteers with a mean BMI of 21.7 kg/

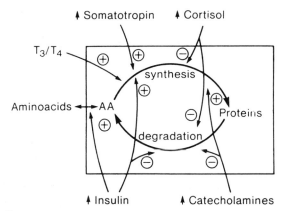

FIGURE 6.7. Metabolic signals that can influence the rate of protein synthesis or degradation in the heart. The exact role of these factors *in vivo* is unknown. T_3/T_4, thyroid hormones; AA, intracellular amino acids. From "Nutrition and the Heart: Fundamental Relations and Therapeutic Principles" (p. 495) by S. B. Heymsfield, R. D. Hoff, T. F. Gray, J. Galloway, and K. Casper, 1987, in J. M. Kinney (Ed.), *Nutrition and Metabolism in Patient Care* (pp. 477–509). Philadelphia: W. B. Saunders. Copyright 1987 by W. B. Saunders Co. Reprinted by permission.

m² ingested a semistarvation diet for 24 weeks (Keys et al., 1950; Simonson, Henschel, & Keys, 1948). A relative reduction in body weight of 24% was associated with no change in the QTc interval. A small increase in the QTc interval was observed with refeeding. A similar lack of change in the QTc interval during weight loss was observed by Doherty et al. (1991) in obese patients who ingested a 420-kcal/day liquid diet for 16 weeks. Studies at our center also support these observations, as we have found no change in the mean QTc interval during 8 weeks of weight loss in 47 obese patients ingesting an 800 kcal/day liquid diet. One of the largest follow-up studies of the QTc interval was completed on 22 markedly obese subjects (50% to 90% above ideal body weight) maintained on a supplemented fasting program (300–450 kcal/day) for an average of 8.5 months (Narasimhan & Bennett, 1985). There was no significant change in the QTc interval during the fast (initial 0.41 ± 0.05 seconds and final 0.39 ± 0.03 seconds) and all QTc intervals fell within the normal range of 0.34–0.43 seconds.

Weight Loss in Obese Patients with Medical Complications

Obese patients with noninsulin-dependent diabetes are also safely treated using a very low calorie diet, to judge by the limited number of subjects evaluated by Amatruda, Richeson, Welle, Brodows, and Lockwood (1988). No 12-lead or 24-hour electrocardiographic abnormalities were detected in six obese diabetic women studied on a metabolic ward for 48 days.

The lowering of blood pressure in weight loss patients with hypertension has a beneficial effect in reversing left ventricular hypertrophy. Obese patients with high blood pressure were randomized by MacMahon, Wilcken, and Macdonald (1986) to placebo, metoprolol, or weight reduction treatment. Subjects in the weight loss condition lost 8.3 kg and had greater reductions in left ventricular wall thickness and left ventricular mass than did both the placebo and metoprolol groups.

Angina pectoris in response to exercise was not found by Sharma, Thadani, and Taylor (1974) to improve over 1 year in six moderately obese patients who lost 16.3 kg on a weight reduction diet. No adverse effects of weight loss were reported by the investigators.

A recent study (Sweeney et al., 1991) examined the safety and efficacy of severe caloric restriction (785 kcal/day food diet) combined with exercise in 18 obese patients (149 ± 4% of ideal body weight) with documented coronary artery disease. Subjects were randomized to a 13-week protocol that consisted of diet plus either aerobic exercise or aerobic exercise plus circuit weight training. Blood pressure, heart rate, and electrocardiographic telemetry were measured during selected exercise sessions. The group as a whole lost weight (14.3 ± 1.0 kg) and weight loss was similar for both types of exercise. No significant arrhythmias or electrocardiographic changes were observed in any patient at rest or with exercise during the study.

Patients who are on cardiac medications at the time of initial evaluation should have a careful review of all pharmacological agents. Diuretics must often be discontinued or dosages reduced and potassium supplements given. Antihypertensive drugs can usually be reduced in dose or discontinued during very low calorie diet therapy. The reduced calorie intake of dieting potentiates the absorption of oral anticoagulants and digoxin. Clinical status, the prothrombin time, and serum digoxin levels should therefore be monitored in patients who take these medications during treatment by very low calorie diet.

Sudden Death Syndrome

Although by the early 1970s the deaths associated with therapeutic total starvation were well documented, it was the "Last Chance Diet" described by Linn and Stuart (1976) that focused national attention on the relation between weight loss and cardiac arrhythmias. According to the Centers for Disease Control, 100,000 persons used the 320-kcal/day collagen or gelatin hydrolysate "liquid protein" as their sole source of nutrition for at least 1 month during 1977 (Gregg, 1977; Schucker & Gunn, 1978). By January 1978, 60 deaths related to the consumption of a liquid protein modified fast had been reported to the Food and Drug Administration. Of these 60 fatalities, investigators ultimately selected for further study 17 of the deceased subjects who (1) were previously healthy; (2) were free of any risk factors associated with QTc prolongation; (3) were not taking any cardiotoxic medications; (4) had died suddenly during or immediately following the diet; and (5) had complete clinical records or necropsy information available (Isner et al., 1979; Sours et al., 1981).

Of the 17 deaths, 16 occurred in obese women between the ages of 23 and 51 years (median of 35 years) who consumed liquid protein for between 2 and 8 months (median of 5 months). There was one 43-year-old male subject who was on the diet for 7 months. The weight loss of the group as a whole was very large, ranging between 9 and 82 kg, with a median for females of 39 kg. The median rate of weight loss for the females was 2.1 kg per week. Ten of the patients were continuing the diet at the time of death, and seven were refeeding.

Six of the patients died outside of the hospital, and 11 were hospitalized at the time of death. The presenting symptoms of those who were hospitalized included weakness, dizziness, palpitations, transient chest pain, and recurrent syncope. All 11 had ventricular tachycardia and fibrillation that were refractory to antiarrhythmic therapy. *Torsade de Pointes*, the atypical form of ventricular tachycardia, was present in 4 of the 11 hospitalized patients. Electrolyte abnormalities on admission included clinically insignificant hypokalemia (6/11) and hypocalcemia (1/11). Ten electrocardiograms were available for detailed review, nine of which were taken on the final hospitalization. Low QRS voltage and prolonged QTc interval (>0.44 seconds) were present in 9 and 10 of the patients, respectively. Of the 10 patients with prolonged QTc intervals at the time of admission, 4 had prediet electrocardiograms. The QTc interval was prolonged in one of these patients and was normal in the remaining three.

Autopsy disclosed normal coronary arteries and valves in 14 of the patients on whom examinations were completed. Histological examination of the myocardium showed attenuated myofibers ($n = 12$), increased lipofuscin pigment ($n = 11$), and mononuclear cell myocarditis ($n = 1$). Similar histologic findings were observed in cachectic control subjects, although none of these individuals had a prolonged QTc interval.

Studies indicated that the commercial liquid protein products were deficient in selected vitamins and trace elements, had inadequate electrolyte content, and provided protein of a low biological value (Frank, Graham, & Frank, 1981; Klevay, 1979; Lowy, Fisler, Drenick, Hunt, & Swendseid, 1986).

Severe arrhythmias or sudden death were subsequently reported during total starvation or treatment with other nutritionally incomplete very low calorie diets (Lantigua, Amatruda, Biddle, Forbes, & Lockwood, 1980; Michiel et al., 1978; Pringle, Scobie, Murray, Kesson, & Maccuish, 1982; Rose & Greene, 1979; Siegel, Cabeen, & Roberts, 1981; Singh et al., 1978), as well as with the large weight losses resulting from obesity surgery (Drenick & Fisler, 1988). In a study of morbidly obese patients subjected to total starvation for a mean of 97 days, Pringle et al. (1982) observed a progressive decrease in QRS voltage, and there was no change in the QRS axis. QTc prolongation (>0.44 seconds) was present in seven patients by the end of the fast, mainly those who had fasted longer and had lost a greater percentage of their initial body weight.

One patient developed atrial fibrillation, and another had syncope with frequent premature ventricular contractions and ventricular tachycardia. The nutritionally incomplete formula evaluated in obese patients by Lantigua et al. (1980) showed similar results. The investigators studied six obese patients for 40 days during ingestion of 300 kcal/day of hydrolyzed collagen (liquid protein) supplemented with tryptophan. Electrocardiograms were normal at baseline and during the treatment period. In contrast, 24-hour ambulatory electrocardiograms showed serious arrhythmias in three subjects, including second-degree heart block and ventricular premature beats, bigeminy, and tachycardia. One-third of the morbidly obese patients studied by Rasmussen and Andersen (1985) following gastroplasty had prolongation of the QTc interval. These individuals appeared to ingest inadequate amounts of protein and showed other signs of protein deficiency.

It is clear that in some cases of death during dieting, an underlying cause such as acute myocardial infarction or pulmonary embolus is evident at postmortem. The more complex question is the cause of death in patients such as the one described by Garnett et al. (1969) or those who consumed the liquid protein products. These unexplained fatalities have several factors in common: (1) total starvation or near total starvation on nutritionally incomplete diets; (2) relatively large amounts or rapid rates of weight loss; (3) preterminal electrocardiographic abnormalities and cardiac rhythm disturbances; and (4) postmortem evidence of reduced cardiac myofiber diameter. It is not clear whether or how a connection exists between these observations. Proposed mechanisms of the sudden death syndrome associated with dieting and weight loss are summarized in Table 6.2.

Although these are not the subject of our review, electrocardiographic abnormalities, arrhythmias, and sudden death are well documented in nonobese subjects. Severe weight loss in famine victims (Ellis, 1946; Keys, 1948; Wharton, Balmer, Somers, & Templeton, 1969), anorexia nervosa and depletion of body cell mass (Gottdiener, Gross, Henry, Borer, & Ebert, 1978;

TABLE 6.2. Proposed Mechanisms of Sudden Death during Weight Reduction Treatment

Prolonged QTc syndromes (Moss, 1986)
Electrolyte abnormalities (Frank et al., 1981; Singh et al., 1978)
Myofiber atrophy with membrane alterations in potassium flux and delayed repolarization (de Silva, 1985; Moss, 1985; VanItallie & Yang, 1984)
Autonomic imbalance (de Silva, 1985; Landsberg & Young, 1978; Moss, 1985) and sudden physical stress (Thompson & Mitchell, 1984) or emotional stress (Brodsky, Sato, Iseri, Wolff, & Allen, 1987)
Micronutrient deficiencies (Drenick, Blumfield, Fisler, & Lowy, 1985; Klevay, 1979; Lowy et al., 1986)
Sinus node ganglionitis and neuritis (Siegel, Cabeen, & Roberts, 1981)
Congenital cardiac abnormalities and thromboembolus (Brown, Yetter, Spicer, & Jones, 1978)
Lactic acidosis (Cubberly, Polster, & Schulman, 1965)
Arrhythmias secondary to increased free fatty acids (de Silva, 1985)

Schocken, Holloway, & Powers, 1989; St. John-Sutton et al., 1985; Thurston & Mark, 1974), and wasting illnesses associated with cachexia (Heymsfield & Nutter, 1979) are all associated with prolongation of the QTc interval, ventricular tachyarrhythmias, loss of left ventricular mass, and sudden death. Thus, a link may exist between sudden death during dieting in obese patients and other states that are characterized by negative nitrogen balance and depletion of myocardial tissue mass. Further support for this hypothesis is provided by the observations of VanItallie and Yang (1984) that survival time on liquid protein diet for the 17 victims of sudden death was correlated with initial BMI. Not only would more obese subjects have a larger energy store as fat, but a protein-sparing effect of adipose tissue is well recognized. The greater the body weight, the better the retention of nitrogen during severe caloric restriction (VanItallie & Yang, 1984).

Summary

Several conclusions are clear from our review of cardiac structure and function in obese patients before weight loss and during treatment with very low calorie diets. Cardiomegaly, with elevations in both preload and afterload, is a characteristic feature of obesity. The specific anatomic adaptation of the heart to obesity appears to depend on blood pressure level, degree of excess adipose tissue accumulation, and duration of obesity. The electrocardiogram of the obese patient tends to have a horizontal QRS axis, a normal QTc interval, and nonspecific T wave abnormalities; the QTc interval may be prolonged in the morbidly obese patient. Obese hypertensive patients with eccentric or concentric left ventricular hypertrophy have increased ventricular ectopy. Cardiac mechanical dysfunction, although asymptomatic, can be detected early in obesity. Severe obesity is often associated with a congestive state, and obese patients are at increased risk of developing congestive heart failure. Although in-depth studies are lacking, most research indicates that the cardiac changes associated with obesity are improved with weight loss.

During weight loss on a low or very low calorie diet with a high quality protein source and adequate amounts of electrolytes and minerals, the average QTc interval for groups of patients under medical supervision remains relatively unchanged. Ambulatory electrocardiographic monitoring demonstrates no increased risk of ventricular ectopy or tachyarrhythmias. A rare patient may demonstrate self-limiting arrhythmias during ambulatory monitoring.

Severe protein wasting may be associated with rapid weight loss in patients treated by total starvation or nutritionally incomplete very low calorie diets, as well as with weight loss in the morbidly obese patient following gastroplasty. Such protein wasting may occur in response to famine or disease. Proposed mechanisms of sudden death during weight reduction treatment are presented in Table 6.2.

Recommendations

A number of published reviews provide guidelines for the safe and effective use of very low calorie diets in the management of obesity (Bistrian, 1978; Wadden, Stunkard, & Brownell, 1983; Wadden, VanItallie, & Blackburn, 1990). These earlier guidelines are summarized and modified in this section to focus specifically on the cardiac aspects of dieting.

Baseline

1. Enroll and treat only patients who are moderately or severely obese. Other weight loss methods (e.g., behavior modification combined with meal replacement plan, etc.) are appropriate in less overweight patients.
2. Patients should have a medical evaluation prior to treatment.
3. Patients with a history of or newly detected cardiac abnormalities should have an in-depth medical evaluation prior to treatment. Consider an examination by a cardiologist. Review medications that might require dosage adjustments or discontinuation during weight loss therapy. Patients with severe or unstable angina, a recent myocardial infarction, severe arrhythmias, or prolonged QTc interval syndromes are usually not candidates for very low calorie diet therapy.

Weight Loss Phase

4. Always use a very low calorie diet that has appropriate amounts of a high quality protein source and sufficient amounts of electrolytes and micronutrients.
5. After the early phase of weight loss, rapid rates ($>$1-2 kg per week) or large amounts of weight loss should be discouraged.
6. Monitor vital signs and serum electrolytes as indicated for specific diet and patient. Promptly treat electrolyte abnormalities that develop during dieting.
7. If a prolonged QTc interval develops during weight loss, search for a cause (e.g., electrolyte abnormality). If no cause can be found and QTc prolongation persists, consider starting the patient on a refeeding program.
8. Patients with cardiac-related symptoms (e.g., syncope, palpitations, or chest pain) during treatment should have a thorough medical evaluation.
9. Reintroduce foods gradually, avoiding excessive salt and carbohydrate intake, which promote fluid retention and occasionally dependent edema.

References

Alexander, J. K. (1982). The heart and obesity. In J. W. Hurst (Ed.), *The heart* (5th ed., pp. 1584–1590). New York: McGraw-Hill.

Alexander, J. K., & Peterson, K. L. (1971). Cardiovascular effects of weight reduction. *Circulation, 45*, 310-318.

Alpert, M. A., Terry, B. E., & Kelly, D. L. (1985). Effect of weight loss on cardiac chamber size, wall thickness and left ventricular function in morbid obesity. *American Journal of Cardiology, 55*, 783-786.

Alpert, N. R. (1986). Cellular and subcellular basis of myocardial hypertrophy. *Federation Proceedings, 45*, 2561-2562.

Amatruda, J. M., Biddle, T. L., Patton, M. L., & Lockwood, D. H. (1983). Vigorous supplementation of a hypocaloric diet prevents cardiac arrhythmias and mineral depletion. *American Journal of Medicine, 74*, 1016-1022.

Amatruda, J. M., Richeson, F., Welle, S. L., Brodows, R. G., & Lockwood, D. H. (1988). The safety and efficiency of a controlled low energy diet in the treatment of non-insulin dependent diabetes and obesity. *Archives of Internal Medicine, 148*, 873-877.

Ashman, R. (1942). The normal duration of the QT interval. *American Heart Journal, 23*, 522-534.

Baird, I. M. (1981). Low-calorie-formula diets—are they safe? *International Journal of Obesity, 5*, 249-256.

Balsaver, A. M., Morales, A. R., & Whitehouse, F. W. (1967). Fat infiltration of myocardium as a cause of cardiac conduction defect. *American Journal of Cardiology, 19*, 261-265.

Bernstein, R. S., Redmond, A., & VanItallie, T. B. (1981). Prevalence and interrelationship of metabolic abnormalities in obese patients. In A. Howard & I. M. Baird (Eds.), *Recent advances in clinical nutrition* (pp. 191-201). London: John Libbey.

Beznak, M. (1964). Hormonal influences in regulation of cardiac performance. *Circulation, 14-15*(Suppl. 2), 141-149.

Beznak, M., Korecky, B., & Thomas, G. (1969). Regression of cardiac hypertrophies of various origin. *Canadian Journal of Physiology and Pharmacy, 47*, 579-585.

Bhandari, A. K., & Scheinman, M. (1985). The long QT syndrome. *Modern Concepts of Cardiovascular Disease, 54*, 45-50.

Bistrian, B. R. (1978). Clinical use of a protein sparing modified fast. *Journal of the American Medical Association, 240*, 2299-2302.

Bloom, W. L. (1959). Fasting as introduction to treatment of obesity. *Metabolism, 8*, 214-220.

Brodsky, M. A., Sato, D. A., Iseri, L. T., Wolff, L. J., & Allen, B. J. (1987). Ventricular tachyarrhythmia associated with physical stress: The role of the sympathetic nervous system. *Journal of the American Medical Association, 257*, 2064-2067.

Brown, C. J., Yetter, M. J. F., Spicer, L. C. M. J., & Jones, C. J. D. (1978). Cardiac complications in protein-sparing modified fasting. *Journal of the American Medical Association, 240*, 120-122.

Brown, W. J., Klish, W. J., Hollander, J., Campbell, M. A., & Forbes, G. B. (1983). A high protein, low calorie liquid diet in the treatment of very obese adolescents: Long-term effect on lean body mass. *American Journal of Clinical Nutrition, 38*, 20-31.

Burwell, C. S., Robin, E. D., Whaley, R. D., & Bickelmann, A. G. (1956). Extreme obesity associated with alveolar hypoventilation—a Pickwickian syndrome. *American Journal of Medicine, 21*, 811-818.

Commerford, P. J., & Lloyd, E. A. (1984). Arrhythmias in patients with drug toxicity, electrolyte, and endocrine disturbances. *Medical Clinics of North America, 68*, 1051-1079.

Crandall, D. L., Lizzo, F. H., & Cervoni, P. (1985). Alteration in cardiac composition with weight reduction in obese rats. *Metabolism, 34*, 405-407.

Cubberley, P. T., Polster, S. A., & Schulman, C. L. (1965). Lactic acidosis and death after the treatment of obesity by fasting. *New England Journal of Medicine, 272*, 628-630.

de Divitiis, O., Fazio, S., Petitto, M., Maddadena, G., Contaldo, F., & Mancini, M. (1981). Obesity and cardiac function. *Circulation, 64*, 477-482.

DiGirolamo, M., & Esposito, J. (1975). Adipose tissue, blood flow, and cellularity in the growing rabbit. *American Journal of Physiology, 229*, 107-112.

de Silva, R. A. (1985). Ionic, catecholamine, and dietary effects on cardiac rhythm. In G. L.

Blackburn & G. A. Bray (Eds.), *Management of obesity by severe caloric restriction* (pp. 183-204). Littleton, MA: PSG.

Doherty, J. U., Wadden, T. A., Zuk, L., Letizia, K. A., Foster, G. D., & Day, S. C. (1991). Long term evaluation of cardiac function in obese patients treated with a very low calorie diet: A controlled clinical study of patients without underlying cardiac disease. *American Journal of Clinical Nutrition, 53,* 1-5.

Drenick, E. J., Blumfield, D. E., Fisler, J. S., & Lowy, S. (1985). Cardiac function during very low calorie diets with dietary protein of good and poor nutritional quality. In G. L. Blackburn & G. A. Bray (Eds.), *Management of obesity by severe caloric restriction* (pp. 223-234). Littleton, MA: PSG.

Drenick, E. J., & Fisler, J. S. (1988). Sudden cardiac arrest in morbidly obese surgical patients unexplained after autopsy. *American Journal of Surgery, 115,* 720-726.

Eisenstein, I., Edelstein, J., Sarma, R., Sanmarco, M., & Selvester, R. H. (1982). The electrocardiogram in obesity. *Journal of Electrocardiology, 15,* 115-118.

Ellis, L. B. (1946). Electrocardiographic abnormalities in severe malnutrition. *British Heart Journal, 8,* 53-61.

Feldschuh, J., & Enson, Y. (1977). Prediction of the normal blood volume: Relation of blood volume to body habitus. *Circulation, 56,* 605-611.

Forbes, G. B. (1984). *Human body composition: Growth, aging, nutrition, and activity.* New York: Springer-Verlag.

Ford, L. E. (1976). Heart size. *Circulation Research, 39,* 297-303.

Frank, A., Graham, C., & Frank, S. (1981). Fatalities on the liquid protein diet: An analysis of possible causes. *International Journal of Obesity, 5,* 234-248.

Frank, S., Colliver, J. A., & Frank, A. (1986). The electrocardiogram in obesity: Statistical analysis of 1,029 patients. *Journal of the American College of Cardiology, 7,* 295-299.

Garnett, E. S., Barnard, D. L., Ford, J., Goodbody, R. A., & Woodehouse, J. A. (1969). Gross fragmentation of cardiac myofibrils after therapeutic starvation for obesity. *Lancet, i,* 914-916.

Goldberg, A. (1971). Relationship between hormones and muscular work in determining muscle size. In N. J. Alpert (Ed.), *Cardiac hypertrophy* (pp. 39-54). New York: Academic Press.

Goldberg, R. J., Bengtson, J., Chen, Z., Anderson, K. M., Locati, E., & Levy, D. (1991). Duration of the QT interval and total and cardiovascular mortality in healthy persons (the Framingham Heart Study experience). *American Journal of Cardiology, 67,* 55-58.

Gottdiener, J. S., Gross, H. A., Henry, W. L., Borer, J. S., & Ebert, M. H. (1978). Effects of self-induced starvation on cardiac size and function in anorexia nervosa. *Circulation, 58,* 425-433.

Gregg, M. B. (1977). Deaths associated with liquid protein diets. *Morbidity and Mortality Weekly Report, 26,* 383.

Grossman, W., Jones, C., & McLaurin, L. P. (1975). Wall stress and patterns of hypertrophy in the human left ventricle. *Journal of Clinical Investigation, 56,* 56-64.

Henschel, A., Mickelsen, O., Taylor, H. L., & Keys, A. (1947). Plasma volume and thiocynate space in famine edema and recovery. *American Journal of Physiology, 50,* 170.

Heymsfield, S. B., Casper, K., Hearn, J., & Guy, D. (1989). Rate of weight loss during underfeeding: Relation to level of physical activity. *Metabolism, 38,* 215-233.

Heymsfield, S. B., Hoff, R. D., Gray, T. F., Galloway, J., & Casper, K. (1987). Nutrition and the heart: Fundamental relations and therapeutic principles. In J. M. Kinney (Ed.), *Nutrition and metabolism in patient care* (pp. 477-509). Philadelphia: W. B. Saunders.

Heymsfield, S. B., & Nutter, D. O. (1979). The heart in protein-caloric undernutrition. In J. W. Hurst (Ed.), *Update I: The heart* (pp. 191-209). New York: McGraw-Hill.

Hickson, R. C., Foster, C., Pollock, M. L., Galassi, T. M., & Rich, S. (1985). Reduced training intensities and loss of aerobic power, endurance, and caloric growth. *Journal of Applied Physiology, 58,* 492-499.

Hubert, H. B., Feinleib, M., McNamara, P. M., & Castelli, W. P. (1983). Obesity as an independent risk factor for cardiovascular disease: A 26-year follow-up of participants in the Framingham study. *Circulation, 67*, 968–977.

Isner, J. M., Sours, H. E., Paris, A. L., Ferrans, V. J., & Roberts, W. C. (1979). Sudden, unexpected death in avid dieters using the liquid-protein-modified-fast diet: Observations in 17 patients and the role of the prolonged QT interval. *Circulation, 60*, 1401–1412.

Jackman, W. M., Clark, M., Friday, K. J., Aliot, E. M., Anderson, J., & Lazzara, R. (1984). Ventricular tachyarrhythmias in the long QT symdomes. *Medical Clinics of North America, 68*, 1079–1109.

Kannel, W. B., Doyle, J. T., McNamara, P. M., Quickenton, M., & Gordon, T. (1975). Precursors of sudden coronary death: Factors related to the incidence of sudden death. *Circulation, 51*, 606–613.

Kannel, W. B., Gordon, T., & Affutt, D. (1969). Left ventricular hypertrophy by electrocardiogram: Prevalence, incidence, and mortality in the Framingham Study. *Annals of Internal Medicine, 71*, 89–105.

Kannel, W. B., Plehn, J. F., & Cupples, L. A. (1988). Cardiac failure and sudden death in the Framingham Study. *American Heart Journal, 115*, 869–875.

Kannel, W. B., & Schatzkin, A. (1985). Sudden death: Lessons from subjects in population studies. *Journal of the American College of Cardiology, 5*, 141B–149B.

Kao, R. L., Rannels, D. E., Whitman, V., & Morgan, H. E. (1978). Factors accounting for growth and atrophy of the heart. In T. Kobayashi, Y. Ito, & G. Rona (Eds.), *Cardiac adaptation* (pp. 105–113). Baltimore: University Park Press.

Kaplan, N. M. (1989). The deadly quartet: Upper body obesity, glucose intolerance, hypertriglyceridemia, and hypertension. *Archives of Internal Medicine, 149*, 1514–1520.

Keys, A. (1948). Cardiovascular effects of undernutrition and starvation. *Modern Concepts of Cardiovascular Disease, 17*, 21–22,

Keys, A., Brozek, J., Henschel, A., Mickelsen, O., & Taylor, H. L. (1950). *The biology of human starvation* (2 vols.). Minneapolis: University of Minnesota Press.

Klevay, L. H. (1979). Copper deficiency with liquid protien diet [Letter to the editor]. *New England Journal of Medicine, 300*, 48.

Koren, M. J., Devereux, R. B., Cassale, P. N., Savage, D. D., & Laragh, J. H. (1991). Relation of left ventricular mass and geometry to morbidity and mortality in uncomplicated essential hypertension. *Annals of Internal Medicine, 114*, 345–352.

Kremers, M. S. (1988). Southwestern Internal Medicine Conference: The premise, promise, and perils of the prevention of lethal ventricular tachyarrhythmias. *American Journal of Medical Science, 296*, 202–220.

Landsberg, L., & Young, J. B. (1978). Fasting feeding and regulation of the sympathetic nervous system. *New England Journal of Medicine, 298*, 1295–1301.

Lantigua, R. A., Amatruda, J. M., Biddle, T. L., Forbes, G. B., & Lockwood, D. H. (1980). Cardiac arrhythmias associated with a liquid protein diet for the treatment of obesity. *New England Journal of Medicine, 303*, 735–738.

Lauer, M. S., Anderson, K. M., Kannel, W. B., & Levy, D. (1991). The impact of obesity on left ventricular mass and geometry. *Journal of the American Medical Association, 266*, 231–236.

Lavie, C. J., Ventura, H. O., & Messerli, F. H. (1988). Cardiopathy of obesity. *Internal Medicine, 9*, 57–71.

Lepeschkin, E., & Surawicz, B. (1952). The measurement of the QT interval of the electrocardiogram. *Circulation, 6*, 378–388.

Licata, G., Scaglione, R., Barbagallo, M., Parrinello, G., Capuana, G., Lipari, R., Merlino, G., & Ganguzza, A. (1990). Effect of obesity on left ventricular function studied by radionuclide angiocardiography. *International Journal of Obesity, 15*, 295–302.

Linet, O. I., Butler, D., Caswell, K., Metzler, C., & Reele, S. B. (1983). Absence of cardiac arrhythmias during a very low calorie diet with high biological quality protein. *International Journal of Obesity, 7*, 313–320.

Linn, R., & Stuart, S. L. (1976). *The last chance diet*. Secaucus, NJ: Lyle & Stuart.

Lowy, S. L., Fisler, J. S., Drenick, E. J., Hunt, I. F., & Swendseid, M. E. (1986). Zinc and copper nutriture in obese men receiving very low calorie diets of soy or collagen protein. *American Journal of Clinical Nutrition, 43*, 272-287.

MacMahon, S. W., Wilcken, D. E., & Macdonald, G. J. (1986). The effect of weight reduction on left ventricular mass: A randomized controlled trial in young, overweight hypertensive patients. *New England Journal of Medicine, 314*, 334-339.

McLenachan, J. M., Henderson, E., Morris, K. I., & Dargie, H. J. (1987). Ventricular arrythmias in patients with hypertensive left ventricular hypertrophy. *New England Journal of Medicine, 317*, 787-792.

Messerli, F. H., & Engel, N. (1986). Cardiology of obesity: A not so Victorian disease. *New England Journal of Medicine, 314*, 378-380.

Messerli, F. H., Nunez, B. D., Ventura, H. O., & Snyder, D. W. (1987). Weight and sudden death: Increased ventricular ectopy in cardiopathy of obesity. *Archives of Internal Medicine, 147*, 1725-1728.

Messerli, F. H., Sundgaard-Riise, K., Reisin, E. D., Dreslinski, E., Dunn, F. G., & Frohlich, E. D. (1983a). Dimorphic cardiac adaptation to obesity and arterial hypertension. *Annals of Internal Medicine, 99*, 757-761.

Messerli, F. H., Sundgaard-Riise, K., Reisin, E. D., Dreslinski, E., Dunn, F. G., & Frohlich, E. D. (1983b). Disparate cardiovascular effects of obesity and arterial hypertension. *American Journal of Medicine, 74*, 808-812.

Michiel, R. R., Sneider, J. S., Dickstein, R. A., Hayman, H., & Eich, R. H. (1978). Sudden death in a patient on a liquid protein diet. *New England Journal of Medicine, 298*, 1005-1007.

Montgomery, R. D. (1962). Changes in the basal metabolic rate of the malnourished infant and their relation to body composition. *Journal of Clinical Investigation, 41*, 1653.

Moss, A. J. (1985). Caution: Very-low-calorie diets can be deadly. *Annals of Internal Medicine, 102*, 121-123.

Moss, A. J. (1986). Prolonged QT-interval syndromes. *Journal of the American Medical Association, 256*, 2985-2987.

Myerburg, R. J. (1991). Electrocardiography. In R. G. Petersdorf, R. D. Adams, E. Braumwald, T. J. Isselbacher, J. B. Martin, J. E. Wilson, A. S. Fauci, & R. K. Root (Eds.), *Harrison's principles of internal medicine* (pp. 850-860). New York: McGraw-Hill.

Nakajima, T., Fujioka, S., Tokunaga, K., Hirobe, K., Matsuzawa, Y., & Tarui, S. (1985). Noninvasive study of left ventricular performance in obese patients: Influence of duration of obesity. *Circulation, 71*, 481-486.

Narasimhan, N., & Bennett, W. M. (1985). Very low calorie diets and electrocardiographic changes. *Annals of Internal Medicine, 102*, 716.

Nutter, D. O., Heymsfield, S. B., Murray, T. M., & Fuller, E. O. (1979). The effect of chronic protein-calorie undernutrition in the rat on myocardial function and cardiac function. *Circulation Research, 45*, 144-152.

Osburne, R. C., Myers, E. A., Rodbard, D., Burman, K. D., Georges, L. P., & O'Brian, J. T. (1983). Adaption to hypocaloric feeding: Physiologic significance of the fall in serum T_3 as measured by the pulse wave arrival time (QKd). *Metabolism, 32*, 9-13.

Phinney, S. D., Bistrian, B. R., Kosinski, E., Chan, D. P., Hoffer, L. J., Rolla, A., Schachtel, B., & Blackburn, G. L. (1983). Normal cardiac rhythm during hypocaloric diets varying carbohydrate content. *Archives of Internal Medicine, 143*, 2258-2261.

Prakash, L. B. S. (1989). Endocrine and metabolic diseases. In G. L. Baum & E. Wolinsky (Eds.), *Textbook of pulmonary diseases* (4th ed., Vol. 7, pp. 1351-1369). Boston: Little, Brown.

Pringle, T. H., Scobie, I. N., Murray, R. G., Kesson, C. M., & Maccuish, A. C. (1982). Prolongation of the QT interval during therapeutic starvation: A substrate for malignant arrhythmias. *International Journal of Obesity, 7*, 253-261.

Ramhamadany, E., Dasgupta, P., Brigden, G., Lahiri, A., Raftery, E. B., & Baird, I. M. (1989). Cardiovascular changes in obese subjects on very-low-calorie diet. *International Journal of Obesity, 13*(Suppl. 2), 95-99.

Rasmussen, L. H., & Andersen, T. (1985). The relationship between QTc changes and nutrition during weight loss after gastroplasty. *Acta Medica Scandinavica, 217*, 271–275.

Ravussin, E., Burnand, B., Schutz, Y., & Jécquier, E. (1985). Energy expenditure before and during energy restriction in obese patients. *American Journal of Clinical Nutrition, 41*, 753–759.

Ravussin, E., & Bogardus, C. (1989). Relationship of genetics, age, and physical fitness to daily energy expenditure and fuel utilization. *American Journal of Clinical Nutrition, 49*, 968–975.

Ravussin, E., Lillioja, S., Anderson, T. E., Christin, L., & Bogardus, C. (1986). Determinants of 24-hour energy expenditiure in man: Methods and results using a respiratory chamber. *Journal of Clinical Investigation, 78*, 1568–1578.

Reisin, E., & Frohlich, E. D. (1981). Obesity: Cardiovascular and respiratory pathophysiological alterations. *Archives of Internal Medicine, 141*, 431–434.

Reisin, E., Frohlich, E. D., Messerli, F. H., Dreslinski, G. R., Dunn, F. G., Jones, M. M., & Boston, H. M. (1983). Cardiovascular changes after weight reduction in obesity hypertension. *Annals of Internal Medicine, 98*, 315–319.

Rose, M., & Greene, R. M. (1979). Cardiovascular complications during prolonged starvation. *Western Journal of Medicine, 130*, 170–177.

St. John-Sutton, M. G., Plappert, T., Crosby, L., Douglas, P., Mullen, J., & Reichek, N. (1985). Effects of reduced left ventricular mass on chamber architecture, load, and function: A study of anorexia nervosa. *Circulation, 72*, 991–1000.

Sandhofer, F., Dienstl, F., Bolzano, K., & Schwingshackl, H. (1973). Severe cardiovascular complication associated with prolonged starvation. *British Medical Journal, i*, 462–463.

Schlant, R. C., & Sonnenblick, E. H. (1982). Pathophysiology of heart failure. In J. W. Hurst (Ed.), *The heart* (5th ed., pp. 382–407). New York: McGraw-Hill.

Schlant, R. C., Sonnenblick, E. H., & Gorlin, R. (1982). Normal physiology of the cardiovascular system. In J. W. Hurst (Ed.), *The heart* (5th ed., pp. 75–114). New York: McGraw-Hill.

Schocken, D. D., Holloway, J. D., & Powers, P. S. (1989). Weight loss and the heart: Effects of anorexia nervosa and starvation. *Archives of Internal Medicine, 149*, 877–881.

Schoeller, D. A. (1990). How accurate is self-reported dietary energy intake? *Nutrition Review, 48*, 373–379.

Schucker, R. E., & Gunn, W. J. (1978). *A national survey of the use of protein products in conjugation with weight reduction diets among American women*. Atlanta: Centers for Disease Control.

Shafrir, E., Bergman, M., & Felig, P. (1987). The endocrine process: Diabetes mellitus. In P. Felig, J. D. Bacter, A. E. Broadus, & L. A. Frohman (Eds.), *Endocrinology and metabolism* (2nd ed., pp. 1043–1178). New York: McGraw-Hill.

Shalom, F. M., Santora, L. J., Iseri, L. T., & Henry, W. L. (1981). Electrocardiogram observations before, during and after rapid weight loss in morbidly obese subjects. *Circulation, 64*, 81. (Abstract)

Sharma, B., Thadani, U., & Taylor, S. H. (1974). Cardiovascular effects of weight reduction in obese patients with angina pectoris. *British Heart Journal, 36*, 854–858.

Siegel, R. J., Cabeen, W. R., Jr., & Roberts, W. C. (1981). Prolonged QT interval–ventricular tachycardia syndrome from massive rapid weight loss utilizing the liquid-protein-modified-fast diet: Sudden death with sinus node ganglionitis and neuritis. *American Heart Journal, 102*, 121–122.

Simonson, E., Henschel, A. J., & Keys, A. (1948). The electrocardiogram of man in semi-starvation and subsequent rehabilitation. *American Heart Journal, 35*, 584–602.

Singh, B. N., Gaardner, T. D., Kanegae, T., Goldstein, M., Montgomerie, J. Z., & Mills, H. (1978). Liquid protein diets and *Torsade de Pointes*. *Journal of the American Medical Association, 240*, 115–119.

Smith, N. I., & Willius, F. A. (1933). Adiposity of the heart: A clinical and pathological study of one hundred and thirty-six obese patients. *Archives of Internal Medicine, 52*, 911–931.

Sours, H. E., Fratalli, V. P., Brand, C. D., Feldman, R. A., Forbes, A. L., Swanson, R. C., & Paris, A. L. (1981). Sudden death associated with very low calorie weight reduction regimens. *American Journal of Clinical Nutrition, 34*, 453–461.

Spencer, I. O. B. (1968). Death during therapeutic starvation for obesity. *Lancet, i*, 1288.

Surawicz, B. (1967). Relationship between electrocardiogram and electrolytes. *American Heart Journal, 73*, 814–834.

Surawicz, B., & Knoebel, S. B. (1984). Long QT: Good, bad, or indifferent? *Journal of the American College of Cardiology, 4*, 398–413.

Sweeney, M. E., Almon, L., Jensen, B., Lloyd-Ceisner, A., Sabatelle, M., & Fletcher, G. F. (1991). Safety and efficacy of severe caloric restriction in obese patients with coronary artery disease. *International Journal of Obesity, 15*(Suppl. 3), 57. (Abstract)

Thompson, P. D., & Mitchell, J. H. (1984). Exercise and sudden cardiac death. *New England Journal of Medicine, 344*, 914–915.

Thurston, J., & Mark, P. (1974). Electrocardiographic abnormalities in patients with anorexia nervosa. *British Heart Journal, 36*, 719–723.

VanItallie, T. B., & Yang, M.-U. (1984). Cardiac dysfunction in obese dieters: A potentially lethal complication of rapid massive weight loss. *American Journal of Clinical Nutrition, 39*, 695–702.

Wadden, T. A., Stunkard, A. J., & Brownell, K. D. (1983). Very low calorie diets: Their efficacy, safety, and future. *Annals of Internal Medicine, 99*, 675–684.

Wadden, T. A., VanItallie, T. B., & Blackburn, G. L. (1990). Responsible and irresponsible use of very low calorie diets in the treatment of obesity. *Journal of the American Medical Association, 263*, 83–85.

Waki, M., Kral, J. G., Mazariegos, M., Wang, J., Pierson, R. N., Jr., & Heymsfield, S. B. (1991). Relative expansion of extracellular fluid in obese versus non-obese women. *American Journal of Physiology: Endocrinology and Metabolism, 261*, E199–E203.

Webster, J. D., Hesp, R., & Garrow, J. S. (1984). The composition of excess weight in obese women estimated by body density, total body water, and total body potassium. *Human Nutrition: Clinical Nutrition, 38*, 299–306.

Wharton, B. A., Balmer, S. E., Somers, K., & Templeton, A. C. (1969). The myocardium in kwashiorkor. *Quarterly Journal of Medicine, 38*, 107–116.

Wilson, J. H. P., Lamberts, S. W. J., & Swart, G. R. (1983). A metabolic study of a high protein very low energy diet. *International Journal of Obesity, 7*, 345–352.

Yang, M.-U., & VanItallie, T. B. (1984). Variability in body protein loss during protracted, severe caloric restriction: Role of triiodothyronine and other possible determinants. *American Journal of Clinical Nutrition, 40*, 611–622.

Zwiauer, K., Schmidinger, H., Klipsera, M., Mayr, H., & Widhalm, K. (1989). 24-hour electrocardiographic monitoring in obese children during a three weeks low calorie diet (500Kcal). *International Journal of Obesity, 13*(Suppl. 2), 101–105.

7

Effect of Caloric Restriction and Weight Loss on Energy Expenditure

ERIC RAVUSSIN
BOYD A. SWINBURN

The prevalence of obesity is increasing dramatically throughout the world in parallel with the industrialization of countries. In the United States, obesity affects approximately 34 million adults aged 20–74 (National Center for Health Statistics, 1986), a slightly higher prevalence than that observed in England, Canada, or Australia (Bray, 1985; Millar & Stephens, 1987). Obesity represents one of the most important public health problems of the latter half of this century. As pointed out in the Surgeon General's Report on Nutrition and Health (U.S. Department of Health and Human Services, 1988), obesity is clearly a risk factor for the development of non-insulin-dependent diabetes mellitus, hypertension, hyperlipidemia, coronary heart disease and stroke, gallbladder disease, and certain types of cancer. Therefore, in the quest to reduce these "modern" diseases, much attention has been focused on the potentially reversible condition of obesity. However, the causes of obesity are not fully understood; not surprisingly, this makes its long-term treatment or prevention very difficult.

Despite the frustration related to the poor outcome of the treatment of obesity, the consistent observation that human obesity is a familial disorder that seems to be inherited has shed new light on its possible causes (Mueller, 1983). This familial occurrence could result from similarities among siblings in either an excessive caloric intake, a deficit in energy expenditure, or both. Since family members share not only genes but also cultural background and environmental conditions, it is often difficult to separate the genetic from the environmental conditions. Studies of twins (Bouchard et al., 1989, 1990) and adoptees (Stunkard et al., 1986; Stunkard, Harris, Pedersen, & McClearn, 1990) have given evidence of an important genetic basis for obesity. Using families and twins, Bouchard and colleagues could attribute approximately 25% of the variance in body fat to genetic factors and 30% to culturally transmissible factors (Bouchard, Savard, Després, Tremblay, & Leblanc, 1985).

Since obesity results from an imbalance between intake and expenditure, it is indisputable that the obvious treatment for the obese patient is a diet restricted in calories and/or increased physical activity. Very low calorie diets have therefore been designed to produce rapid weight loss while preserving the lean body mass (Wadden, Stunkard, & Brownell, 1983). Indeed, most regimens induce acceptable short-term weight loss, but the success of long-term weight loss is very limited. The features common to all hypocaloric diets is a rapid initial weight loss during the first few weeks of the diet, followed by a diminished and eventually flattened rate of weight loss. In most cases the subjects eventually regain some or most of the weight they lost (Johnson & Drenick, 1977). The decrease in the rate of weight loss, as well as the subsequent weight gain often observed after slimming, may be caused by relaxation of efforts to control weight (accompanied by increased food intake), but also has been attributed to changes in the metabolic rate in response to caloric restriction (Miller & Parsonage, 1975).

This chapter will outline the energy balance equation, the components of energy expenditure and their possible roles in the genesis of obesity. It will then review the studies that have addressed the question of the "metabolic adaptation" in response to caloric restriction, weight loss and weight cycling. Finally, it will examine other possible metabolic factors involved in the maintenance of body weight.

Energy Balance Equation

The principle of energy conservation is the underlying basis of energy balance in humans. This simple concept has led most scientists in this field to view the energy balance equation as a static equation:

$$\text{Change in energy stores} = \text{Energy intake} - \text{Energy expenditure}$$

Authors in many studies have estimated energy excess or deficit and predicted body weight gain or loss. However, in most studies, weight gain or weight loss has been far below these predicted values. The reason is that a static model cannot account for the dynamics of energy balance, and thus leads to exaggerated predictions for weight gain or weight loss. Since energy expenditure at rest as well as during exercise is mostly proportional to body weight, any body weight change in response to energy imbalances (overfeeding or caloric restriction) will cause a change in energy expenditure. Therefore, Alpert has proposed a very elegant model of energy balance under conditions of semistarvation (Alpert, 1988) and hyperphagia (Alpert, 1990), using a two-reservoir energy model (Alpert, 1979). Under these specific conditions of growth and tissue losses, not only the composition of the tissue deposited or lost plays a critical role in the prediction of weight gain or loss, but also small changes in body weight can offset the imbalance very easily. The example Alpert (1990) has used to highlight the inadequacy of the static model of energy balance is that of a 75-kg man who is initially in energy balance, but who then adds to this equilibrium a single piece of lightly buttered toast every morning for 40 years. If the toast equals 100 kilocalories (kcal) and the energy density of the weight gained is 7720 kcal/kg, this man would gain 189 kg over the 40 years, according to the static equation. The fact that this magnitude of weight gain does not happen in reality has led to the deduction that the body's metabolism has adapted to counter the weight gain. Although adaptation may have occurred, "it cannot be justified by a syllogism based on faulty premises" (Alpert, personal communication, 1989). Alpert used a dynamic, two-reservoir energy model to calculate that 40 years of eating the extra fatal piece of toast would result in a weight gain of 2.7 kg (93% fat and 7% fat-free mass), which is much more realistic. In parallel with this example, the failure of a hypocaloric diet to achieve the weight loss predicted from a static equation cannot be used as evidence for adaptation, because the use of a static model in this situation is inappropriate. Another energy balance equation has to be considered:

Rate of change in energy stores =
Rate of energy intake − Rate of energy expenditure

This new equation indicates explicitly the fundamental importance of the time variable over which both the rate of change in energy stores and the rate of energy expenditure vary, despite a constant rate of energy intake.

The body weight of most people remains remarkably stable over periods of years during adulthood, despite large fluctuations in food intake and exercise (Garrow, 1974). This has led to the idea that body weight is strongly regulated. The best evidence supporting the regulation of body weight comes from intervention studies in which a subject's "usual weight" is intentionally disturbed. Most of the millions of overweight individuals who successfully lose weight eventually regain most or all of their lost weight (Johnson & Drenick, 1977). Those few who maintain their weight loss do so, in most cases, at the cost of becoming "restrained eaters" (Herman & Polivy, 1980). Keys and colleagues' study of conscientious objectors, who lost 25% of their initial body weight on severe calorie restriction, showed that they quickly returned to their usual starting weight after returning to their normal diet (Keys, Brozek, Henschel, Mickelsen, & Taylor, 1950).

The stability of body weight suggests the presence of a mechanism that balances energy intake (which is intermittent and variable) and energy expenditure (which is continuous and variable) without conscious effort. Does energy intake vary in response to energy expenditure, or vice versa? Experiments in animals suggest that the body weight is maintained by variations in metabolic rate in response to food intake (Keesey, 1986). Keesey (1980) pointed out that apparent regulation of body weight still occurs in animals with lesions of the lateral hypothalamus or in obese Zucker rats; they simply defend a body weight that is greater than that of the lean animals. Their energy expenditure increases or decreases, depending upon whether weight is forced above or below habitual weight; however, intake and expenditure are appropriate for the "metabolic body size," which is equal to body weight raised to the 0.75

power (Kleiber, 1975). Keesey suggested that humans also appear to regulate weight around values that differ as much between individuals as between animal species. However, the controlling mechanisms of a putative "set point" for body weight have not yet been demonstrated in humans.

Other recent studies in animals (Flatt, 1988) and humans (Tremblay, Plourde, Després, & Bouchard, 1989) suggest that the majority of the energy balance on a day-to-day basis is maintained by variations in food intake in response to energy expenditure. However, larger increases or decreases in energy intake than are needed to match energy expenditure will lead to weight change, and consequently to an increased or decreased metabolic rate. Therefore, depending on the circumstances, it seems that energy intake can balance expenditure to maintain an equilibrium, or vice versa.

Components of Daily Energy Expenditure

In assessing the impact of caloric restriction on energy expenditure, it is imperative to consider separately the different components of energy expenditure. Daily energy expenditure has three major components (Figure 7.1): the resting metabolic rate (RMR), the thermic effect of food, and the energy cost of physical activity. In most sedentary adults, RMR accounts for about 60–

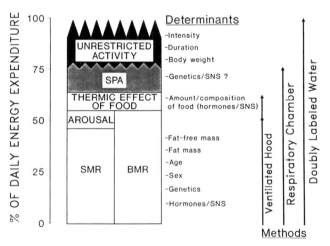

FIGURE 7.1. Components of daily energy expenditure in humans. Daily energy expenditure can be divided into three major components: (1) the basal metabolic rate (BMR; sum of the sleeping metabolic rate [SMR] and the energy cost of arousal), which represents 50–70% of daily energy expenditure; (2) the thermic effect of food, which represents ~10% of daily energy expenditure; and (3) the energy cost of physical activity (sum of spontaneous physical activity [SPA] and voluntary physical activity), which represents 20–40% of daily energy expenditure. The major determinants of the different components of daily energy expenditure components, as well as the methods to measure them, are presented in the figure. SNS, sympathetic nervous system.

70% of daily energy expenditure (Jéquier, 1984; Ravussin, Lillioja, Anderson, Christin, & Bogardus, 1986). The thermic effect of food accounts for about another 10%, and the contribution of physical activity is much more variable.

Resting Metabolic Rate

The tight relationship between the RMR and body size has been known for many years. Although earlier investigators observed some variance in RMR within the normal range (Boothby & Sandiford, 1922), they were more concerned with defining the limits of the normal range to identify such disease states as hypo- or hyperthyroidism. The RMR was considered essentially constant for a given body size, and this led to the development of equations now widely used to predict RMR based on height and weight (Harris & Benedict, 1919; Roza & Shizgal, 1984). More recent studies showed that at any given body size and composition, RMR can be quite different between individuals. In a study of 130 siblings from 54 families, Bogardus et al. (1986) showed that RMR correlated best with fat-free body mass. In addition, repeated measurements in individuals revealed that RMR varied over and above that which could be accounted for by differences in fat-free body mass, age, and sex; by daily fluctuations in RMR; and by methodological variability. Fat-free mass, fat mass, age, and sex are the major determinants of RMR, explaining approximately 80% of its variance (Ravussin, Zurlo, Ferraro, & Bogardus, 1991). In their study comparing the RMR among siblings, Bogardus et al. (1986) showed that some of the unexplained variance in RMR was explained by family membership, suggesting that RMR is at least partially genetically determined (Figure 7.2). Further support for a genetic determinant of RMR comes from studies of twins by Bouchard et al. (1989). These authors showed convincingly that RMRs of monozygotic twins were more alike than RMRs of dizygotic twins, even after adjustment for individual differences in body size and body composition. Recent data suggest that the sympathetic nervous system may be a regulator of the RMR under eucaloric conditions, perhaps explaining its familial aggregation (Saad et al., 1991). Also, resting skeletal muscle metabolism seems to be a major determinant of whole-body metabolism (Zurlo, Larson, Bogardus, & Ravussin, 1990).

Thermic Effect of Food

Since Pittet and colleagues' study showing a decreased thermic effect of glucose in obese individuals compared to controls (Pittet, Chappuis, Acheson, de Techtermann, & Jéquier, 1976), studies of energy expenditure in lean and obese persons have focused predominantly on the thermic effect of food. This seems to have occurred for two reasons. First, it was assumed that RMR was constant for a given body size and therefore an unlikely cause of variations in

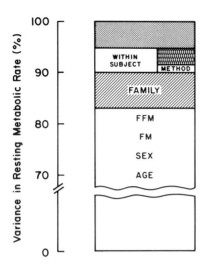

FIGURE 7.2. Proportion of the variance in resting metabolic rate explained by different determinants. Fat-free mass (FFM), fat mass (FM), age, and sex explain 83% of the variance in resting metabolic rate, whereas family membership (sum of genetic and shared environmental influences) explains a further 7%.

daily caloric expenditure among individuals. Second, studies using crude methods to assess physical activity have failed to demonstrate that obese subjects are consistently less active than lean persons. Thus, the thermic effect of food appeared to be the only component of daily energy expenditure that could cause variations in predisposition to obesity among individuals. However, it has also been shown that the thermic effect of food is the most difficult and the least reproducible component to measure (Ravussin et al., 1986). One of the major reasons for the poor reproducibility of the measurement is that many factors influence the thermic effect of food: the test meal size and composition; the time and duration of the measurement; the technique used for measurement; the palatability of the food; and the subjects' genetic background, age, physical fitness, and sensitivity to insulin. All of these factors might explain the inconsistency and the variability of the published data regarding the thermic effect of food in humans (Sims, 1986).

Stoichiometric calculations of the energy cost of nutrient absorption, transport, and storage provide numbers that are lower than the measured thermic effect of food (Flatt, 1978). This has led to the view that the thermic effect of food can be divided into two parts: (1) an "obligatory" component related to the metabolic processing of the nutrients; and (2) a "facultative" component, which seems to have a "cephalic phase" and a "postprandial phase" (Acheson, Ravussin, Wahren, & Jéquier, 1984; LeBlanc & Cabanac, 1989). Whereas the relevance of the cephalic facultative phase of the thermic effect of food has been questioned in humans (Hill, DiGirolamo, & Heymsfield, 1985), the postprandial facultative phase is believed to be mediated through activation of the sympathetic nervous system (Acheson et al., 1984; Schwartz, Jaeger, & Veith, 1988). In their review of the literature, D'Alessio et al. (1988) pointed out that half of the studies showed a blunted thermic effect of food in the obese, whereas the other half did not. D'Alessio et al. (1988) elegantly demonstrated that in any given subject, the thermic effect of food increases linearly with caloric intake, but is independent of leanness and obesity. Although this study does not totally refute the possibility that a low thermic effect of food might play a role in the pathogenesis of obesity, it does suggest the need for prospective studies comparing subjects with low and high thermic effect of food. It should be emphasized, however, that since the facultative component of the thermic effect of food comprises only a small percentage of the total daily energy expenditure, even large changes in this component are unlikely to explain either significant weight gain or significant adaptation to a hypocaloric diet.

Physical Activity

Reduced physical activity as a cause of obesity is an obvious and attractive hypothesis. The energy expended in physical activity is very variable, and the secular increase in obesity parallels the increase in sedentary lifestyles. However, until the very recent introduction of the doubly labeled water method to measure energy expenditure in free-living conditions (Schoeller & van Santen, 1982; Schoeller et al., 1986), there has been no satisfactory method by which to assess the impact of physical activity on daily energy expenditure. Under the conditions of a respiratory chamber, large differences in energy expenditure between individuals (100 to 800 kcal/day) could be attributed to differences in spontaneous physical activity (Ravussin et al., 1986). Clearly, these differences may be much larger in free-living conditions, in which voluntary physical activity varies widely among individuals. Also, since physical activity is mostly associated with weight-bearing exercise, the energy cost of this activity is closely related to body weight. Studies are needed to assess physical activity and its impact on the development of obesity in a large number of subjects.

Whether physical activity and physical fitness interact with the RMR and/or the thermic effect of food is still controversial. Some studies have shown increased RMR in well-trained individuals (Poehlman, Melby, Bradylak, & Calles, 1989; Tremblay et al., 1986), independent of body composition, while others have not (Hill, Sparling, Shields, & Heller, 1987; Schulz, Nyomba, Alger, Anderson, & Ravussin, 1991). Similarly, the possible increased thermic effect of food during or immediately after exercise is still very debatable (Miller, Mumford, & Stock, 1967; Segal, Gutin, Nyman, & Pi-Sunyer, 1985). Investigations of the role of exercise as an adjunct to diet therapy for weight loss have also led to inconclusive data: Some investigators have shown a beneficial impact of exercise on the rate of weight loss (Kenrick, Ball, & Canary, 1972; Pavlou et al., 1989), while others have not (Hill et al., 1987; Phinney, LaGrange, O'Connell, & Danforth, 1988). Similarly, some studies have shown a protective effect of exercise on the fat-free body mass reduction, thereby reducing the fall in RMR that commonly occurs with weight loss

(Donahoe, Lin, Kirschenbaum, & Keesey, 1984; Lennon, Nagle, Stratman, Shrago, & Dennis, 1985; Mole, Stern, Schultz, Bernauer, & Holcomb, 1989), whereas some have not (Bogardus et al., 1984; Warwick & Garrow, 1981). One of the major benefits of the addition of an exercise program for weight loss seems to be a better maintenance of the reduced weight. Studies using a combination of respiratory gas exchange measurements and the doubly labeled water method are likely to provide new insight into accurate assessments of physical activity and its impact on the development of obesity.

Low Energy Expenditure as a Risk Factor for Obesity

Before assessing the effect of weight loss on energy expenditure, it is important to know whether or not a reduced energy expenditure plays a role in the development of obesity. Clearly, *absolute* energy expenditure is generally increased in the obese state, because of the increased fat-free mass associated with obesity (James, Bailes, Davies, & Dauncey, 1978). At issue, however, is whether a low energy expenditure *relative* to body size is a cause of weight gain.

Using prospective designs, three studies have now convincingly shown that a reduced metabolic rate (relative to body size) is a risk factor for future weight gain. One study found that total energy expenditure in 3-month-old infants was, on average, 20% lower in those who became overweight at 12 months of age than in infants who did not become overweight (Roberts, Savage, Coward, Chew, & Lucas, 1988). In another set of studies, Griffiths and Payne (1976) reported that 5-year-old children of obese parents had lower 24-hour metabolic rates per kilogram of body weight than children of nonobese parents. Twelve years later, the female children of obese parents were substantially taller and heavier than those of nonobese parents (Griffiths, Payne, Stunkard, Rivers, & Cox, 1990). From our own longitudinal studies in adult Pima Indians, we found that both a low RMR and a low 24-hour energy expenditure were risk factors for body weight gain (Ravussin et al., 1988). After 4 years of follow-up, the risk of gaining 10 kg was approximately seven times greater in those subjects with the lowest RMR (lower tertile) than in those with the highest RMR (higher tertile). In 95 subjects the rate of 24-hour energy expenditure, adjusted for fat-free body mass, fat mass, age, and sex, correlated negatively with the rate of weight change ($r = -.39, p < .001$). However, the slope of this relationship indicated that a maximum of 40% of the weight change could be attributed to 24-hour energy expenditure, as measured in a respiratory chamber. Although a low *relative* metabolic rate clearly predicts weight gain, the results also indicate that metabolic rate is not the only contributor to the pathogenesis of obesity. Excess caloric intake and decreased physical activity also contribute, but the relative contribution of each in populations or individuals remains to be determined.

These longitudinal data, showing that a low *relative* metabolic rate predicts weight gain, seem to contradict the cross-sectional data showing that obese individuals (who have a higher fat mass) have normal, if not higher, metabolic rates for their fat-free mass as compared to lean subjects (Ravussin et al., 1986). An interesting observation in our study was the fact that in response to body weight gain, the new metabolic rate increased to "normal" or even higher values for the new body weight and composition. This might explain why so many cross-sectional studies have failed to show any difference in energy metabolism between lean and obese subjects. From two such cross-sectional studies, Garrow concluded that there was no evidence of a "thrifty metabolism" that might predispose individuals to obesity (Garrow, Warwick, Blaza, & Ashwell, 1980; Garrow & Webster, 1985). In response to weight loss, those subjects who became obese because of a reduced metabolic rate are likely to present an unusually low metabolic rate when compared to lean subjects, or even possibly when compared to postobese subjects who did not have a low metabolic rate before their obesity.

The concept of a "thrifty genotype," originally proposed by Neel (1962), implies that some people have an efficient metabolism that enables them to store more calories in times of plenty and/or use fewer calories in times of food shortages. This would then confer a survival advantage, and natural selection would ensure a high prevalence of that genotype under conditions of intermittent food supplies. By the same token, however, a "gluttony genotype" could also be responsible for a high prevalence of obesity in a population. In either case, this survival advantage has become a liability in industrialized societies, where food is consistently available and the physical effort to obtain, process, and prepare the food is reduced. This kind of interaction between the genotype and the environment (Bouchard et al., 1990) may explain the rapid increase in the prevalence of obesity over the last century in populations such as the Pima Indians (Knowler et al., 1991).

Predictable Effects of Low Energy Intake and Weight Reduction on Energy Expenditure

In response to a hypocaloric diet, there is an abrupt change from an energy balance steady state to a new imbalance, which will tend to reach a new equilibrium over time. The caloric restriction and the consequent weight loss will both cause predictable reductions in energy expenditure.

In the obese state, excess body weight is maintained by high energy intakes in proportion mainly to fat-free mass, but also to fat mass. In response to caloric deficit (e.g., 1000 kcal/day), body weight loss will be exponential until a new energy equilibrium is reached in which energy expenditure will be equal to energy intake; both will be 1000 kcal/day lower than in the initial energy equilibrium. The energy balance equation for both the obese and the reduced-obese equilibrium must be the same:

Energy intake = RMR +
Thermic effect of food + Thermic effect of exercise

Therefore, some or all of these components of energy expenditure must decrease to match the new energy intake. The question is this: At what new body size will this new steady state occur? To relate the question to energy expenditure, at what energy expenditure will the new steady state occur? If it occurs at an energy expenditure that is about what would be expected for the body size, then the metabolic changes can be called predictable, and "metabolic adaptation" need not be invoked.

Predictable decreases in the three components of daily energy expenditure are expected (Figure 7.3): (1) In response to lower energy intake, the thermic effect of food will decrease by at least 10% of the deficit (i.e., 100 kcal/day in the example above); (2) in response to weight loss, the RMR will decrease in a predictable manner according to the respective losses of fat-free mass and fat mass; and (3) since the energy cost of physical activity is mainly proportional to body weight, this component of daily energy expenditure will decrease even in the absence of a decreased level in physical activity. The decrease can vary from

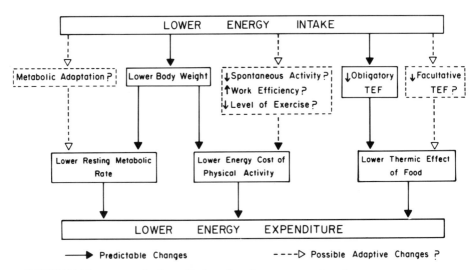

FIGURE 7.3. Factors contributing to the lowering of energy expenditure in response to a decreased food intake (negative energy balance). Solid lines indicate predictable effects, which include a lower energy cost of physical activity in relationship to lower body weight, lower resting metabolic rate in response to lower fat-free mass and fat mass, and lower thermic effect of food (TEF) related to lower food intake. Dashed lines represent more speculative adaptative mechanisms, mostly in relationship to metabolic adaptation and behavioral adaptation in response to caloric restriction. Adapted from *Energy Metabolism of Overweight Women before, during and after Weight Reduction, Assessed by Indirect Calorimetry* by C. P. G. de Groot, 1988, unpublished PhD thesis, University of Wageningen, The Netherlands. Adapted by permission of the author.

~16 kcal/kg body weight loss in very sedentary conditions to ~30 kcal/kg in more active conditions (Jéquier & Schutz, 1985; Flatt, 1983). Ideally, accurate assessments of energy intake and of the components of energy expenditure are feasible in the obese and the reduced-obese state, both while in energy balance.

The transition state during weight loss and energy deficit is considerably more complicated, since the dynamics of fat-free mass loss versus fat mass loss change over time and predictions based on cross-sectional relationships may not be valid. Alpert has proposed that the fat reserve provides energy to the fat-free reservoir at a rate proportional to the size of the fat store (Alpert, 1982). This assumption suggests a slow, exponential decay of the fat store, which was experimentally observed in the Minnesota semistarvation study (Keys et al., 1950). The different origins of the fuel to cover the energy deficit will cause not only marked differences in the rate of weight loss (Alpert, 1982, 1988), but also differences in energy expenditure. Because of these difficulties, the discussion on adaptation will place more emphasis on those studies in which measurements were performed under conditions of energy balance.

Adaptation to Hypocaloric Diet and Body Weight Loss

Flexibility of Metabolic Rate

More than 100 years ago, von Voit (1881) suggested that any excess energy intake was in some way wasted in the form of dissipated heat. Twenty years later, Neumann (1902) demonstrated that he was able to maintain his body weight constant over a 3-year period, despite considerable variability in caloric consumption during this time. He used the term *luxus-konsumption* to suggest that the maintenance of body weight was the result of burning off the excess calories. This finding was later confirmed by some classic overfeeding studies (Miller et al., 1967; Sims et al., 1973), but was also disputed by a re-examination of the data (Forbes, 1984) and a short-term (9-day) overfeeding study measuring 24-hour energy expenditure (Ravussin, Schutz, et al., 1985). This same concept of "flexibility" of the metabolic rate during overfeeding was proposed in situations of caloric restriction in lean subjects and called "adaptation" by Keys et al. (1950). Further support of this concept came from studies in obese subjects as reviewed by Apfelbaum, Fricker, and Igoin-Apfelbaum (1987), by Gelfand and Hendler (1989) and more recently by Shetty (1990).

In the pioneering studies on semistarvation by Keys et al. (1950), the basal oxygen consumption of 32 lean men declined promptly and steadily over 24 weeks of caloric restriction. At the end of the 24 weeks, the mean oxygen consumption per man had decreased by 39%. When expressed per unit of body size, the decrease in oxygen consumption was still very impressive: 31% per square meter of body surface area, 19% per kilogram of body weight, and 16% per kilogram of "active tissue." The data were later confirmed in another group of 25 normal young men studied for ~2 months by Grande, Anderson, and

Keys (1958). Interestingly enough, the RMR rose very rapidly during refeeding to reach baseline values after 4–6 days of refeeding (Grande et al., 1958). From the Minnesota experiment, Taylor and Keys (1950) concluded that 65% of the reduction in basal metabolism could be attributed to the "shrinkage of the metabolizing mass of the body cells" and only 35% to an actual decrease of the cellular metabolic rate. The Minnesota study provided the first quantitative description of metabolic adaptation to caloric restriction in humans—clearly an appropriate survival mechanism in the face of dangerously low energy intake and energy reserves. Forty years later, the debate continues on whether a low energy intake evokes such adaptive changes in those with adequate energy reserves (the obese).

Definition of Metabolic Adaptation

In their work on the biology of semistarvation, Keys et al. (1950) stated: "It might seem entirely reasonable that the energetic processes of the body diminish in intensity as the exogenous food supply is reduced. It is reasonable in the sense that a wise man reduces his expenditure when his income is cut." They defined adaptation as "a useful adjustment to altered circumstances." A more recent definition of adaptation has been proposed in a 1985 report as "a process by which a new or different steady state is reached in response to a change or difference in the intake of food and nutrients" (Food and Agriculture Organization/World Health Organization/United Nations University, 1985). In this context, the adaptation can be genetic, metabolic, and sociobehavioral. In nutritional balance studies, only relatively short-term adaptations can be studied, up to a period of 2–6 months.

Under conditions of a large deficit of energy intake, does the body adapt its metabolic rate (over and above the predictable effects just described) to minimize the impact of energy imbalance on body weight? This concept of "metabolic adaptation" implies a lowering of metabolic rate (incorrectly called "increased efficiency"), which is dependent upon the recent history of negative energy balance and leads to less of a reduction in body weight than would be predicted from the reduction in energy intake. Therefore, an operational definition of "adaptation" to a low calorie diet would be any significant decrease in energy expenditure that is *more than would be expected*, given its known determinants from cross-sectional data (Figure 7.4). For RMR, for example, this would mean a larger fall than could be explained by the decrease in fat-free mass and fat mass (Ravussin et al., 1991).

As noted by Alpert (1988), the static energy balance equation is an inappropriate method of determining the "expected" metabolic rate at the new body weight, or the "expected" body weight at the new energy intake. Another potential pitfall in determining an "expected" metabolic rate is using a denominator to normalize the data. The relationship between RMR and fat-free body mass has a positive y intercept, which means that heavier subjects have a lower

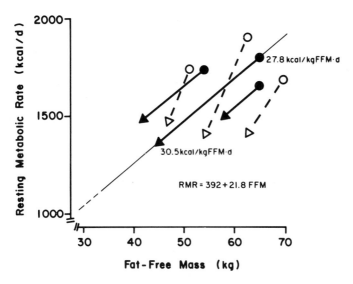

FIGURE 7.4. Relationship between resting metabolic rate (RMR; in kilocalories per day) and fat-free body mass (FFM; in kilograms). This figure illustrates the error introduced when RMR is expressed in kilocalories per kilogram of FFM. Because of the significant y intercept, larger subjects tend to have lower RMRs if FFM is the denominator. A subject who loses 20 kg of FFM, yet does not deviate from the predicted resting metabolic rate, would increase his RMR by 10% if it was expressed per kilogram of FFM. This figure also shows that metabolic adaptation is present only when the longitudinal relationship between the decrease in RMR and the decrease in FFM is steeper (dashed lines) than the slope of the cross-sectional relationship obtained from that population (solid lines).

RMR per kilogram of fat-free mass than lighter subjects do (Ravussin & Bogardus, 1989). As shown in Figure 7.4, a subject with a fat-free mass of 65 kg who lies on the regression line for the population has a RMR of 27.8 kcal/kg fat-free mass. For that person to lose 20 kg of fat-free mass and maintain a normal RMR, the RMR per kilogram of fat-free mass must *rise* to 30.5 kcal/kg. The expected RMR after the weight loss, as calculated from the normal population data (1373 kcal/day), is about 120 kcal/day more than that calculated from the original RMR per kilogram of fat-free mass (1251 kcal/day). While this difference may be trivial in an individual, it may be important when statistical tests are applied to groups looking for significant falls in RMR below expected values. Therefore, the best evidence that adaptation has occurred requires that a relationship containing the major determinants be used as a baseline. If individuals in the reduced-obese steady state fall below that cross-sectional regression line, or if the slope of the longitudinal data (ΔRMR corrected for age, sex, and fat mass, vs. Δfat-free mass) is steeper than the cross-sectional data, then that would represent "adaptation" by our definition. In other words, the new RMR or the change in RMR cannot be explained by the cross-sectional determinants of RMR.

When these definitions are used, then, what is the evidence that adaptation of metabolic rate occurs? Interesting studies by Minghelli and colleagues (Minghelli, Schutz, Charbonnier, Whitehead, & Jéquier, 1990; Minghelli, Schutz, Whitehead, & Jéquier, 1991) suggest that adaptation may occur in Gambian men during the "hungry" season. They found lower 24-hour energy expenditure and RMR (both adjusted for fat-free mass), lower thermic effect of food, and greater efficiency in walking among the Gambians than among European men matched for body composition. While this difference may indeed represent an adaptation to chronic low energy intake in lean subjects (similar to the Minnesota study), it may also be caused by underlying racial differences, independent of energy intake. Similarly, low RMRs were measured in 14 undernourished Indian laborers in comparison to age-matched controls (Shetty, 1984).

Studies of 24-Hour Energy Expenditure

Three studies have indirectly assessed 24-hour energy expenditure using accurate energy intake measurements in weight-stable subjects. Leibel and Hirsch (1984) studied 26 subjects in their obese state and their reduced-obese state. In the obese state, the subjects needed 9% more energy intake per surface area for weight maintenance than controls, whereas in the reduced-obese state they required 24% fewer calories while still being 38 kg heavier than controls. Weigle and colleagues found that the data from the reduced-obese subjects fell below the regression line between 24-hour energy expenditure and fat-free mass that was established in their baseline, obese state (Weigle, 1988; Weigle, Sande, Iverius, Monsen, & Brunzel, 1988). This was related mostly to the predictable decreased energy cost of physical activity.

Other studies, which have used indirect calorimetry in the steady obese state and in the nonsteady, weight-losing state, have also found a fall in 24-hour energy expenditure (Apfelbaum, Bostsarron, & Lacatis, 1971; Bessard, Schutz, & Jéquier, 1983; de Groot, van Es, van Raaij, Vogt, & Hautvast, 1990; de Boer, van Es, Roovers, van Raaij, & Hautvast, 1986; Garby, Kurzer, Lammert, & Nielsen, 1988; Ravussin, Burnand, Schutz, & Jéquier, 1985; Webb & Abrams, 1983). While these studies do not all agree on the presence or the absence of adaptation to hypocaloric diets, it is important to examine the changes in the three components of energy expenditure and their determinants before a final judgment can be made.

Resting Metabolic Rate

Several studies have found a decrease in absolute RMR, but have not reported the RMR normalized to fat-free mass (Apfelbaum, Brigant, & Joliff, 1977; Apfelbaum et al., 1971; Bray, 1969; Garrow & Webster, 1989; Morgan, 1984;

Welle, Amatruda, Forbes, & Lockwood, 1984). Hendler and colleagues have also shown that the decrease in RMR is influenced by the composition of the diet (Hendler, Walesky, & Sherman, 1986; Hendler & Bonde, 1988, 1990). In both studies by Weigle and colleagues, in cases where the 24-hour energy expenditure fell, the relationship between RMR and fat-free mass was similar before and after weight reduction (Weigle, 1988; Weigle et al., 1988). In two other studies in which subjects were close to weight maintenance at the time of measurement, the RMR reduction was greater than the reduction in fat-free mass (Elliot, Goldberg, Kuehl, & Bennett, 1989; Heshka, Yang, Wang, Burt, & Pi-Sunyer, 1990). These results were not confirmed by Wadden, Foster, Letizia, and Mullen (1990), who showed that RMR was absolutely normal for the new body weight 31 weeks after the end of a 17-week very low calorie diet. Similarly, Foster et al. (1990) found no significant, long-lasting decrease in RMR normalized for fat-free mass after 12 weeks of realimentation following an 8-week low calorie diet. In five studies where the follow-up measurements were not made during weight maintenance, four of these (Belko, Van Loan, Barbieri, & Mayclin, 1987; Davies et al., 1989; de Boer et al., 1986; Ravussin, Burnand, et al., 1985) found no fall in RMR per kilogram of fat-free mass, while one did (Henson, Poole, Donahoe, & Heber, 1987). Although a positive result (a fall in RMR per kilogram of fat-free mass) may have been masked in some of these studies because of the intercept error (see above), the weight of the evidence indicates that adaptation of RMR to weight loss does not occur, or that if it does occur, then it is only under certain circumstances. Garrow and Webster (1989) have suggested that the fall in RMR with weight loss may be greater in the lean than the obese, and with a rapid weight loss rather than a gradual weight loss.

Thermic Effect of Food

Investigators who found evidence for adaptation in the response of the 24-hour energy expenditure to weight loss, but none in the response of RMR (de Boer et al., 1986; Weigle 1988; Weigle et al., 1988), concluded that the discrepancy was to be found in the nonresting metabolic rate. The thermic effect of food has been examined for evidence of adaptation by Schutz and colleagues (Schutz, Bessard, & Jéquier, 1987; Schutz, Golay, Felber, & Jéquier, 1984) and Davies et al. (1989). Both found that the thermic effect of food decreased by about 50% in obese, nondiabetic subjects after weight loss. As previously mentioned, the thermic effect of food is difficult to measure and poorly reproducible; indeed, in two of these studies, the energy expenditure had not returned to resting levels by the time the tests were terminated. However, even assuming that a reduction in the thermic effect of food as large as 50% occurs (presumably by suppression of its facultative component), the impact of this adaptation (equivalent to about 3–5% of energy intake and expenditure) is not likely to influence the final body weight very much. Therefore, although the available evidence points to adaptation of the thermic effect of food to low calorie diets, its significance is questionable.

Thermic Effect of Exercise

The determinants of the energy cost of physical activity in free-living individuals are poorly defined because, until the introduction of the doubly labeled water method (Schoeller & van Santen, 1982), the techniques for measuring it have been relatively crude. Nevertheless, some studies have addressed the question of how much a reduction in the thermic effect of exercise might contribute to the fall in overall energy expenditure seen in reduced-obese individuals. Two possible effects need to be examined: the level of activity and the cost of this activity (which in turn is influenced by body weight and by work efficiency). Weigle (1988) conducted an elegant weight loss study in 12 obese men, in which the weight lost by 6 of them was replaced by lead weights worn in a vest during the day. This had no effect on the RMR, but it did decrease the fall in nonresting energy expenditure to about one-fifth of the fall experienced by the control group. After this difference between the groups (about 500 kcal/day) and the lower RMR (proportional to the lower fat-free mass) were accounted for, only about 100–200 kcal of the fall in overall energy expenditure could be considered "adaptive." A further interesting finding from this study was the decrease in activity levels (measured by a pedometer) in both groups over the duration of the weight loss. This was attributed to the increasing fatigue and cold intolerance reported by virtually all subjects. This decrease in activity levels at the lower body weights is contrary to the cross-sectional data showing the obese to be less active than the lean (Ferraro, Boyce, Swinburn, De Gregorio, & Ravussin, 1991), and this may be an example of an adaptation to negative energy balance. A decrease in spontaneous physical activity during weight loss was also found by de Groot, van Es, van Raaij, Vogy, and Hautvast (1989), but not by Ravussin, Burnand, et al. (1985). Although Minghelli et al. (1990) showed that the Gambian men studied during the "hungry" season were more efficient at walking than were weight-matched European men, Schutz et al. (1987), as well as Poole and Henson (1988) could find no effect of weight loss on the efficiency of moderate exercise on a bicycle ergometer.

Summary

There is general agreement that weight loss in obese subjects on hypocaloric diets causes a fall in 24-hour energy expenditure corrected for fat-free mass, the main but not sole determinant. This fall is mainly related to the nonresting metabolic rate, and the major part seems to be explained by the decreased cost of activity at the lower body weight. Possible adaptive changes to the weight loss include a decrease in the thermic effect of food (beyond that expected from the reduction in calories); a decrease in activity levels (as opposed to the expected increase); and perhaps, under certain circumstances, a decrease in RMR (beyond that expected from the reduced body size). A quantitative estimate of the contribution of these adaptive changes to the overall lower metabolic rate is clearly not possible, but our review of the current data indicates that it is likely to be minor. On the other hand, low calorie diets in lean subjects seem to evoke significant adaptive changes in RMR and probably in the energy cost of physical activity. This more dramatic response is not surprising, since the threat that a hypocaloric diet poses to survival is greater in leaner subjects.

Possible Mechanisms for Adaptation

If adaptation does occur, what are the possible mediating mechanisms? A fall in thyroid hormones has received considerable attention in the literature, with most (Barrows & Snook, 1987; Davies et al., 1989; Hendler & Bonde, 1988; Welle et al., 1984), but not all (Ravussin, Burnand, et al., 1985) investigators observing a fall in free triiodothyronine (T_3) on a hypocaloric diet. Welle and Campbell (1986) found that replacement of T_3 largely reversed the fall in energy expenditure from a hypocaloric diet. The sympathetic nervous system has also been implicated by Davies et al. (1989), who found a decreased 24-hour urinary excretion of noradrenaline during weight loss, and by Shetty, James, and Jung (1979), who found that the catecholamine precursor levodopa prevents the fall in RMR in response to semistarvation. Many subjects on very low calorie diets become cold-intolerant, but it is not clear whether this happens because the body temperature is a mediator of adaptive changes or whether it is just an effect of decreasing fat-free mass (a smaller furnace) and decreasing fat mass (less insulation). Other possible mechanisms to explain the fall in RMR have been suggested by Waterlow (1985, 1986): (1) decreased work of the heart; (2) decreased rate of protein turnover (Nair, Woolf, Welle, & Matthews, 1987); (3) decreased sodium pump activity; (4) alteration in metabolic pathways; (5) increased yield of adenosine triphosphate per oxygen used; and (6) decreased substrate cycling (Newsholme, 1980).

Other Metabolic Responses to Body Weight Loss

A recent study in our laboratory has indicated that energy balance is not maintained as such but is rather the sum of the three macronutrient balances (i.e., protein, carbohydrate, and fat). Abbott et al. (1988) showed that protein and carbohydrate balances are maintained in most energy imbalance conditions, whereas fat tends to buffer the imbalance. Similarly, addition of fat to the diet is not compensated for by increased fat oxidation and will result in positive fat balance, whereas protein and carbohydrate stores are maintained

(Flatt 1987; Flatt, Ravussin, Acheson, & Jéquier, 1985; Schutz, Flatt, & Jéquier, 1989; Danforth, 1985). Thus it seems that the fat content of the diet, rather than the total caloric intake, may influence the level at which body weight will plateau. Total energy intake alone is not the critical factor. Flatt (1988) also pointed out that a state of equilibrium can be reached only when the rates of oxidation of carbohydrate and fat correspond to their proportion in the diet. Therefore, in parallel to the energy balance equation is the energy substrate balance equation:

Rate of change in carbohydrate/fat stores ≈
Rate of carbohydrate/fat intake (food quotient) −
Rate of carbohydrate/fat oxidation (respiratory quotient)

As with energy intake and energy expenditure, a difference between respiratory quotient and food quotient seems to be a necessary and sufficient condition for weight change. We examined the effect of 24-hour respiratory quotient on body weight in Pima Indians (Zurlo, Lillioja, et al., 1990) and found striking parallels between respiratory quotient and energy expenditure, as might be predicted from their similar roles in their respective equations. We found that obesity was associated with a low respiratory quotient (low carbohydrate/fat oxidation), but that a high respiratory quotient (corrected for body size) predicted future weight gain. These results confirm the higher 24-hour respiratory quotient in postobese subjects compared to controls matched for weight and body composition (Lean & James, 1988). Also, in those subjects who had repeat measurements, weight gain or weight loss resulted in a greater fall or rise in respiratory quotient than would be predicted from the cross-sectional relationship. This suggests, again in parallel with some of the studies on energy expenditure, that adaptation of respiratory quotient to weight change may occur.

In a similar study of insulin resistance and weight change in Pima Indians, we found that, cross-sectionally, insulin resistance was associated with obesity but that insulin sensitivity predicted future weight gain (Swinburn et al., 1991). Again, with weight gain or weight loss, the increase or decrease in insulin resistance was greater than would be expected from the cross-sectional data. Perhaps these studies indicate that metabolic factors other than the classic components of energy expenditure may well be related to the maintenance of body weight and may play a role in adaptation to large energy imbalances.

Weight Cycling and Energy Expenditure

Finally, in this review it seems appropriate to mention one of the currently fashionable concepts in obesity—that is, weight cycling. According to the National Center for Health Statistics (1986), dieting has become a way of life for many Americans, since it seems that at any given time 25% of men and 50%

of women are trying to lose weight. However, some warnings have been expressed through the media and by some health care providers that repeated cycles of weight loss and gain through on-and-off dieting may be deleterious.

Rats put through cycles of caloric restrictions followed by refeeding seem to undergo a significant increase in "food efficiency," characterized by increased weight gain after refeeding (Brownell, Greenwood, Stellar, & Shrager, 1986). However, other studies have not been able to reproduce the same effect of feeding cycles on "food efficiency" (Gray, Fisher, & Bray, 1988; Hill et al., 1987). Despite the widely publicized possible side effects of weight cycling or "yo-yo dieting," there are few data available on the influence of weight cycling on energy requirements and metabolic rate in humans. Blackburn et al. (1989) reported a decline in the rate of weight loss in dieters during the second cycle of a very low calorie diet (protein-sparing modified fast), compared to the first cycle of the diet. In this retrospective chart review study, as many as 9 years could have elapsed from the first to the second dieting period, and therefore results could have been confounded by age-related changes in metabolic rate or activity. Also, this observation was not confirmed in four subjects enrolled in two 8-week weight loss periods 18 months apart (Beeson, Ray, Coxon, & Kreitzman, 1989). In a more direct fashion, Steen, Oppliger, and Brownell (1988) examined adolescent wrestlers and found that those wrestlers who engaged in repeated cycles of weight loss to "make the weight" had lower RMR than wrestlers who did not report weight cycling. However, such a cross-sectional study does not allow one to determine whether weight cycling contributes to a low metabolic rate or whether a low metabolic rate leads to weight gain (Ravussin et al., 1988), and therefore to weight cycling. In a similar study of wrestlers, but with longitudinal measurements of RMR before, during, and after the 6-month wrestling season, Melby, Schmidt, and Corrigan (1990) did not show that repeated cycles of weight loss and regain caused a decreased RMR. Furthermore, RMRs of wrestlers with reported weight cycling were found to be higher than those of nonwrestlers matched for age, weight, and body composition, but with no history of weight cycling. In essence, therefore, these few human studies have been done in young athletes (who are not necessarily equivalent to the general dieting population) and produce no evidence that repeated cycles of weight loss and gain lower metabolic rate, thereby predisposing to a rapid and easy regain of weight. Some preliminary data in seven moderately obese women enrolled through three consecutive cycles of a very low calorie diet in an 18-week study do not support the theory that repeated short periods of dieting lead to a decrease in metabolic rate (Goldberg, Parkinson, Savage, Murgatroyd, & Prentice, 1990). With the knowledge of the numerous health benefits of even small weight losses, any overweight persons should be encouraged to enroll in a weight loss program, not dissuaded from it.

Finally, one concern has been brought up by the popular "rotation diet" (Kathan, 1986). This diet, which alternates periods of low calorie intake with periods of higher calorie intake, proposed that such an alteration of calories would blunt the usual decline in metabolic rate induced by dieting and weight loss. One well-designed study by de Groot et al. (1989) showed that alternating the calories did not prevent the decrease in 24-hour energy expenditure. Once again, this study did not provide any argument in favor of adaptive metabolic mechanisms.

Summary

The high prevalence of obesity, and the fact that obesity is clearly a risk factor for the development of many diseases, represent one of the most important public health problems of the second half of this century. However, since the causes of obesity are not fully understood, it is of no surprise that long-term treatment or prevention of the disease has been very difficult. Since the weight loss achieved with any hypocaloric diet will depend on the caloric deficit, very low calorie diets have been designed to attempt to maximize the deficit by minimizing the calorie intake in most cases. However, the weight loss has been far below that predicted on the basis of the energy balance equation.

The failure of these hypocaloric diets to achieve the predicted weight loss cannot be used as evidence for metabolic adaptation, because the use of a static energy balance model in this situation is inappropriate. Another dynamic equation explicitly indicates the fundamental importance of the time variable, over which both the rate of change in energy stores and the rate of change of energy expenditure vary, despite a constant rate of energy intake. In response to the weight loss induced by the energy deficit, the different components of daily energy expenditure decrease in a predictable manner, mostly in proportion to the weight lost (for RMR and the energy cost of physical activity) and to the decreased energy intake (for the thermic effect of food). Also, the composition of the weight loss varying over time will introduce a confounding factor when one tries to predict weight loss from the energy deficit. The dynamic model proposed by Alpert (1988) predicts an exponentially decaying body weight in response to caloric restriction.

Whether metabolic adaptation occurs in response to caloric restriction has been debated for a long time. There is general agreement that weight loss on hypocaloric diet causes a fall in 24-hour energy expenditure. During or immediately after caloric restriction, the fall in metabolic rate is larger than can be accounted for by the loss of fat-free mass and fat mass. This can be attributed to adaptive decreases in the thermic effect of food, the level of activity, and the RMR. However, after refeeding some or all of the adaptive changes disappear. The adaptive response is much greater in lean individuals than in obese individuals, where the contribution of adaptive changes to the overall lower metabolic rate seems minor. After a few weeks or months of maintenance, reduced-obese individuals often have a metabolic rate that is "normal" for their new body weight, body composition, and food intake. Also, there is no good evidence that weight cycling lowers the metabolic rate and predisposes to rapid weight regain.

In conclusion, a fall in the metabolic rate on a hypocaloric diet will inevitably occur until it matches the new energy intake. The majority of the fall in metabolic rate is predictable, given the known determinants of energy expenditure, but a variable contribution (significant in the lean, minor in the obese) may come from adaptive changes. The causes of the original obesity and the weight regain after weight loss are likely to be the same; until these are more fully elucidated, treatment of obesity will continue to be difficult. Nevertheless, in light of the many beneficial effects of weight loss, every encouragement should be given to overweight individuals who want to lose weight on hypocaloric diets, and every effort should be made to avoid relapse after weight loss (James, Lean, & McNeill, 1987).

References

Abbott, W. G. H., Howard, B. V., Christin, L., Freymond, D., Lillioja, S., Boyce, V. L., Anderson, T. E., Bogardus, C., & Ravussin, E. (1988). Short-term energy balance: relationship with protein, carbohydrate, and fat balances. *American Journal of Physiology, 255*, E332–E337.

Acheson, K. J., Ravussin, E., Wahren, J., & Jéquier, E. (1984). Obligatory and facultative thermogenesis. *Journal of Clinical Investigation, 70*, 1570–1580.

Alpert, S. S. (1979). A two-reservoir energy model of the human body. *American Journal of Clinical Nutrition, 32*, 1710–1718.

Alpert, S. S. (1982). Optimal time response of the human body to food shortage and the two-reservoir energy model. *Angewandte Systemanalyse, 3*(2), 79–84.

Alpert, S. S. (1988). The energy density of weight loss in semistarvation. *International Journal of Obesity, 12*, 533–542.

Alpert, S. S. (1990). Growth, thermogenesis, and hyperphagia. *American Journal of Clinical Nutrition, 52*, 784–792.

Apfelbaum, M., Bostsarron, J., & Lacatis, D. (1971). Effect of caloric restriction and excessive caloric intake on energy expenditure. *American Journal of Clinical Nutrition, 24*, 1404–1409.

Apfelbaum, M., Brigant, L., & Joliff, M. (1977). Effects of severe diet restriction on the oxygen consumption of obese women during exercise. *International Journal of Obesity, 1*, 387–393.

Apfelbaum, M., Fricker, J., & Igoin-Apfelbaum, L. (1987). Low- and very-low-calorie diets. *American Journal of Clinical Nutrition, 45*, 1126–1134.

Barrows, K., & Snook, J. T. (1987). Effect of a high-protein, very-low-calorie diet on resting metabolism, thyroid hormones, and energy expenditure of obese middle-aged women. *American Journal of Clinical Nutrition, 45*, 391–398.

Beeson, V., Ray, C., Coxon, A., & Kreitzman, S. (1989). The myth of the yo-yo: Consistent rate of weight loss with successive dieting by VLCD. *International Journal of Obesity, 13*(Suppl. 2), 135–139.

Belko, A. Z., Van Loan, M., Barbieri, T. F., & Mayclin, P. (1987). Diet, exercise, weight loss, and energy expenditure in moderately overweight women. *International Journal of Obesity, 11*, 93–104.

Bessard, T., Schutz, Y., & Jéquier, E. (1983). Energy expenditure and postprandial thermogenesis in obese women before and after weight loss. *American Journal of Clinical Nutrition, 38*, 680–693.

Blackburn, G. L., Wilson, G. T., Kanders, B. S., Stein, L. J., Lavin, P. T., Adler, J., & Brownell, K. D. (1989). Weight cycling: The experience of human dieters. *American Journal of Clinical Nutrition, 49*, 1105–1109.

Bogardus, C., Lillioja, S., Ravussin, E., Abbott, W., Zawadzki, J. K., Young, A., Knowler, W. C.,

Jacobowitz, R., & Moll, P. P. (1986). Familial dependence of the resting metabolic rate. *New England Journal of Medicine, 315*, 96-100.

Bogardus, C., Ravussin, E., Robbins, D. C., Wolfe, R. R., Horton, E. S., & Sims, E. A. H. (1984). Effects of physical training and diet therapy on carbohydrate metabolism in patients with glucose intolerance and non-insulin dependent diabetes mellitus. *Diabetes, 33*, 311-318.

Boothby, W. M., & Sandiford, I. (1922). Summary of the basal metabolism data on 8,614 subjects with special reference to the normal standards for the estimation of the basal metabolic rate. *Journal of Biological Chemistry, 54*, 783-803.

Bouchard, C., Savard, R., Després, J. P., Tremblay, A., & Leblanc, C. (1985). Body composition in adopted and biological siblings. *Human Biology, 57*, 61-75.

Bouchard, C., Tremblay, A., Després, J. P., Nadeau, A., Lupien, P. J., Thériault, G., Dussault, J., Moorjani, S., Pinault, S., & Fournier, G. (1990). The response to long-term overfeeding in identical twins. *New England Journal of Medicine, 322*, 1477-1482.

Bouchard, C., Tremblay, A., Nadeau, A., Després, J. P., Thériault, G., Boulay, M. R., Lortie, G., Leblanc, C., & Fournier, G. (1989). Genetic effect in resting and exercise metabolic rates. *Metabolism, 38*, 364-370.

Bray, G. A. (1969). Effect of caloric restriction on energy expenditure in obese patients. *Lancet, ii*, 397-398.

Bray, G. A. (1985). Obesity: Definition, diagnosis and disadvantages. *Medical Journal of Australia, 142*, S2-S8.

Brownell, K. D., Greenwood, M. R. C., Stellar, E., & Shrager, E. E. (1986). The effects of repeated cycles of weight loss and regain in rats. *Physiological Behavior, 38*, 459-464.

D'Alessio, D. A., Kavle, E. C., Mozzoli, M. A., Smalley, J., Polansky, M., Kendrick, Z. V., Owen, L. R., Bushman, M. C., Boden, G., & Owen, O. E. (1988). Thermic effect of food in lean and obese men. *Journal of Clinical Investigation, 81*, 1781-1789.

Danforth, E., Jr. (1985). Diet and obesity. *American Journal of Clinical Nutrition, 41*, 1132-1145.

Davies, A. H., Baird, I. M., Fowler, J., Mills, I. H., Baillie, J. E., Rattan, S., & Howard, A. N. (1989). Metabolic response to low- and very-low-calorie diets. *American Journal of Clinical Nutrition, 49*, 745-751.

de Boer, J. O., van Es, A. J. H., Roovers, L. C. A., van Raaij, J. M. A., & Hautvast, J. G. A. J. (1986). Adaptation of energy metabolism of overweight women to low-energy intake, studied with whole-body calorimeters. *American Journal of Clinical Nutrition, 44*, 585-595.

de Groot, C. P. G. M. (1988). *Energy metabolism of overweight women before, during and after weight reduction, assessed by indirect calorimetry.* Unpublished PhD thesis, University of Wageningen, The Netherlands.

de Groot, C. P. G. M., van Es, A. J. H., van Raaij, J. M. A., Vogt, J. E., & Hautvast, J. G. A. J. (1989). Adaptation of energy metabolism of overweight women to alternating and continuous low energy intake. *American Journal of Clinical Nutrition, 50*, 1314-1323.

de Groot, C. P. G. M., van Es, A. J. H., van Raaij, J. M. A., Vogt, J. E., & Hautvast, J. G. A. J. (1990). Energy metabolism of overweight women 1 mo and 1 y after an 8-wk slimming period. *American Journal of Clinical Nutrition, 51*, 578-583.

Donahoe, C. P., Lin, D. H., Kirschenbaum, D. S., & Keesey, R. E. (1984). Metabolic consequences of dieting and exercise in the treatment of obesity. *Journal of Consulting and Clinical Psychology, 52*, 827-836.

Elliot, D. L., Goldberg, L., Kuehl, K. S., & Bennett, W. M. (1989). Sustained depression of the resting metabolic rate after massive weight loss. *American Journal of Clinical Nutrition, 49*, 93-96.

Ferraro, R., Boyce, V. L., Swinburn, B., De Gregorio, M., & Ravussin, E. (1991). Energy cost of physical activity on a metabolic ward in relationship to obesity. *American Journal of Clinical Nutrition, 53*, 1368-1371.

Flatt, J. P. (1978). Biochemistry of energy expenditure. In G. Bray (Ed.), *Recent advances in obesity research: II. Proceedings of the Second International Congress on Obesity* (p. 211). London: Newman.

Flatt, J. P. (1983). Metabolic cost of nutrient storage. *Journal of Obesity & Weight Regulation, 2,* 5-18.

Flatt, J. P. (1987). Dietary fat, carbohydrate balance, and weight maintenance: Effects of exercise. *American Journal of Clinical Nutrition, 45,* 296-306.

Flatt, J. P. (1988). Importance of nutrient balance in body weight regulation. *Diabetes/Metabolism Reviews, 6,* 571-581.

Flatt, J. P., Ravussin, E., Acheson, K. J., & Jéquier, E. (1985). Effects of dietary fat on postprandial substrate oxidation and on carbohydrate and fat balances. *Journal of Clinical Investigation, 76,* 1019-1024.

Food and Agriculture Organization/World Health Organization (WHO)/United Nations University. (1985). *Energy and protein requirements* (WHO Technical Report Series No. 724). Geneva: WHO.

Forbes, G. B. (1984). Energy intake and body weight: A re-examination of two "classic" studies. *American Journal of Clinical Nutrition, 39,* 349-350.

Foster, G. D., Wadden, T. A., Feurer, I. D., Jennings, A. S., Stunkard, A. J., Crosby, L. O., Ship, J., & Mullen, J. L. (1990). Controlled trial of the metabolic effects of a very-low-calorie diet: Short- and long-term effects. *American Journal of Clinical Nutrition, 51,* 167-172.

Garby, L., Kurzer, M. S., Lammert, O., & Nielsen, E. (1988). Effect of 12 weeks' light-moderate underfeeding on 24-hour energy expenditure in normal male and female subjects. *European Journal of Clinical Nutrition, 42,* 295-300.

Garrow, J. S. (1974). *Energy balance and obesity in man.* New York: American Elsevier.

Garrow, J. S., Warwick, P. M., Blaza, S. E., & Ashwell, M. A. (1980). Predisposition to obesity. *Lancet, i,* 1103-1104.

Garrow, J. S., & Webster, J. (1985). Are pre-obese people energy thrifty? *Lancet, i,* 670-671.

Garrow, J. S., & Webster, J. D. (1989). Effects on weight and metabolic rate of obese women of a 3-4 mJ (800 kcal) diet. *Lancet, i,* 1429-1431.

Gelfand, R. A., & Hendler, R. (1989). Effect of nutrient composition on the metabolic response to very low calorie diets: Learning more and more about less and less. *Diabetes/Metabolism Reviews, 5,* 17-30.

Goldberg, G. R., Parkinson, S. A., Savage, J. M., Murgatroyd, P. R., & Prentice, A. M. (1990). Repeated periods of dieting by women using a very low energy diet: 1. Effect on metabolic rate. *Proceedings of the British Nutrition Society, 9,* 11A.

Grande, F., Anderson, J. T., & Keys, A. (1958). Changes of basal metabolic rate in man in semistarvation and refeeding. *Journal of Applied Physiology, 12,* 230-238.

Gray, D. S., Fisler, J. S., & Bray, G. A. (1988). Effects of repeated weight loss and regain on body composition in obese rats. *American Journal of Clinical Nutrition, 47,* 393-399.

Griffiths, M., & Payne, P. R. (1976). Energy expenditure in small children of obese and non-obese parents. *Nature, 260,* 698-700.

Griffiths, M., Payne, P. R., Stunkard, A. J., Rivers, J. P. W., & Cox, M. (1990). Metabolic rate and physical development in children at risk of obesity. *Lancet, ii,* 76-78.

Harris, J. A., & Benedict, F. G. (1919). *A biometric study of basal metabolism in man.* Washington, DC: The Carnegie Institute.

Hendler, R. G., & Bonde, A. A. (1988). Very-low-calorie diets with high and low protein content: Impact on triiodothyronine, energy expenditure, and nitrogen balance. *American Journal of Clinical Nutrition, 48,* 1239-1247.

Hendler, R. G., & Bonde, A. A. (1990). Effects of sucrose on resting metabolic rate, nitrogen balance, leucine turnover and oxidation during weight loss with low calorie diets. *International Journal of Obesity, 14,* 927-938.

Hendler, R. G., Walesky, M., & Sherwin, R. S. (1986). Sucrose substitution in prevention and reversal of the fall in metabolic rate accompanying hypocaloric diets. *American Journal of Medicine, 81,* 280-284.

Henson, L. C., Poole, D. C., Donahoe, C. P., & Heber, D. (1987). Effects of exercise training on resting energy expenditure during caloric restriction. *American Journal of Clinical Nutrition, 46*, 893–899.

Herman, C. P., & Polivy, J. (1980). Restrained eating. In A. J. Stunkard (Ed.), *Obesity* (pp. 208–225). Philadelphia: W. B. Saunders.

Heshka, S., Yang, M.-U., Wang, J., Burt, P., & Pi-Sunyer, F. X. (1990). Weight loss and change in resting metabolic rate. *American Journal of Clinical Nutrition, 52*, 981–986.

Hill, J. O., DiGirolamo, M., & Heymsfield, S. B. (1985). Thermic effect of food after ingested versus tube delivered meals. *American Journal of Physiology, 248*, E370–E374.

Hill, J. O., Sparling, P. B., Shields, T. W., & Heller, P. A. (1987). Effects of exercise and food restriction on body composition and metabolic rate in obese women. *American Journal of Clinical Nutrition, 46*, 622–630.

James, W. P. T., Bailes, J., Davies, H. L., & Dauncey, M. J. (1978). Elevated metabolic rates in obesity. *Lancet, i*, 1122–1125.

James, W. P. T., Lean, M. E. J., & McNeill, G. (1987). Dietary recommendations after weight loss: How to avoid relapse of obesity. *American Journal of Clinical Nutrition, 45*, 1135–1141.

Jéquier, E. (1984). Energy expenditure in obesity. In W. P. T. James (Ed.), *Clinics in endocrinology and metabolism* (Vol. 13, pp. 563–580). Philadelphia: W. B. Saunders.

Jéquier, E., & Schutz, Y. (1985). New evidence for a thermogenic defect in human obesity. *International Journal of Obesity, 9*(Suppl. 2), 1–7.

Johnson, D., & Drenick, E. J. (1977). Therapeutic fasting in morbid obesity: Long-term follow-up. *Archives of Internal Medicine, 137*, 1381–1382.

Kathan, M. (1986). *The rotation diet*. New York: Norton.

Keesey, B. (1980). A set-point analysis of the regulation of body weight. In A. J. Stunkard (Ed.), *Obesity* (pp. 144–181). Philadelphia: W. B. Saunders.

Keesey, R. E. (1986). A set point theory of obesity. In K. D. Brownell & J. P. Foreyt (Eds.), *Handbook of eating disorders: Physiology, psychology, and treatment of obesity, anorexia, and bulimia* (pp. 63–87). New York: Basic Books.

Kenrick, M. M., Ball, M. F., & Canary, J. J. (1972). Exercise and weight reduction in obesity. *Archives of Physical and Medical Rehabilitation, 53*, 323–327.

Keys, A., Brozek, J., Henschel, A., Mickelsen, O., & Taylor, H. L. (1950). *The biology of human starvation* (Vol. 1). Minneapolis: University of Minnesota Press.

Kleiber, M. (1975). *The fire of life: An introduction to animal energetics* (rev. ed.). Huntington, NY: Krieger.

Knowler, W. C., Pettitt, D. J., Saad, M. F., Charles, M. A., Nelson, R. G., Howard, B. V., Bogardus, C., & Bennett, P. H. (1991). Obesity in the Pima Indians: Its magnitude and relationship with diabetes. *American Journal of Clinical Nutrition, 53*, 1543S–1551S.

Lean, M. E. J., & James, W. P. T. (1988). Metabolic effects of isoenergetic nutrient exchange over 24 hours in relation to obesity in women. *International Journal of Obesity, 12*, 15–27.

LeBlanc, J., & Cabanac, M. (1989). Cephalic postprandial thermogenesis in human subjects. *Physiology and Behavior, 46*, 479–482.

Leibel, R. L., & Hirsch, J. (1984). Diminished energy requirements in reduced-obese patients. *Metabolism, 33*, 164–170.

Lennon, D., Nagle, F., Stratman, F., Shrago, E., & Dennis, S. (1985). Diet and exercise training effects on resting metabolic rate. *International Journal of Obesity, 9*, 39–47.

Melby, C. L., Schmidt, W. D., & Corrigan, D. (1990). Resting metabolic rate in weight-cycling collegiate wrestlers compared with physically active, noncycling control subjects. *American Journal of Clinical Nutrition, 52*, 409–414.

Millar, W. J., & Stephens, T. (1987). The prevalence of overweight and obesity in Britain, Canada, and the United States. *American Journal of Public Health, 77*, 38–41.

Miller, D. S., Mumford, P., & Stock, M. J. (1967). Gluttony: 2. Thermogenesis in overeating man. *American Journal of Clinical Nutrition, 20*, 1223–1229.

Miller, D. S., & Parsonage, S. (1975). Resistance to slimming: Adaptation or illusion? *Lancet, i*, 773–775.

Minghelli, G., Schutz, Y., Charbonnier, A., Whitehead, R., & Jéquier, E. (1990). Twenty-four-hour energy expenditure and basal metabolic rate measured in a whole-body indirect calorimeter in Gambian men. *American Journal of Clinical Nutrition, 51*, 563-570.

Minghelli, G., Schutz, Y., Whitehead, R., & Jéquier, E. (1991). Seasonal changes in 24-h and basal energy expenditures in rural Gambian men as measured in a respiration chamber. *American Journal of Clinical Nutrition, 53*, 14-20.

Mole, P. A., Stern, J. S., Schultz, C. L., Bernauer, E. M., & Holcomb, B. J. (1989). Excercise reverses depressed metabolic rate produced by severe caloric restriction. *Medicine and Science in Sports and Exercise, 21*, 29-33.

Morgan, J. B. (1984). Weight-reducing diets, the thermic effect of feeding and energy balance in young women. *International Journal of Obesity, 8*, 629-640.

Mueller, W. H. (1983). The genetics of human fatness. *Yearbook of Physical Anthropology, 26*, 215-230.

Nair, K. S., Woolf, P. D., Welle, S. L., & Matthews, D. E. (1987). Leucine, glucose, and energy metabolism after 3 days of fasting in healthy human subjects. *American Journal of Clinical Nutrition, 46*, 557-562.

National Center for Health Statistics. (1986). *Health, United States 1986* (DHHS Publication No. PHS 87-1232). Washington, DC: U.S. Government Printing Office.

Neel, J. V. (1962). Diabetes mellitus: A "thrifty" genotype rendered detrimental by progress? *American Journal of Human Genetics, 14*, 353-363.

Neumann, R. O. (1902). Experimentelle Beiträge zur Lehre von dem täglichen Nahrungsbedarf des Menschen unter besonderer Berucksichtigung der notwendigen Eiweissmenge. *Archives of Hygiene, 45*, 1-87.

Newsholme, E. (1980). A possible metabolic basis for the control of body weight. *New England Journal of Medicine, 302*, 400-405.

Pavlou, K. N., Whatley, J. E., Jannace, P. W., DiBartolomeo, J. J., Burrows, B. A., Duthie, E. A. M., & Lerman, R. H. (1989). Physical activity as a supplement to a weight-loss dietary regimen. *American Journal of Clinical Nutrition, 49*, 1110-1114.

Phinney, S. D., LaGrange, B. M., O'Connell, M., & Danforth, E., Jr. (1988). Effects of aerobic exercise on energy expenditure and nitrogen balance during very low calorie dieting. *Metabolism, 37*, 758-765.

Pittet, P., Chappuis, P., Acheson, K., de Techtermann, F., & Jéquier, E. (1976). Thermic effect of glucose in obese subjects studied by direct and indirect calorimetry. *British Journal of Nutrition, 35*, 281-292.

Poehlman, E. T., Melby, C. L., Bradylak, S. F., & Calles, J. (1989). Aerobic fitness and resting energy expenditure in young adult males. *Metabolism, 38*, 85-90.

Poole, D. C., & Henson, L. C. (1988). Effect of acute caloric restriction on work efficiency. *American Journal of Clinical Nutrition, 47*, 15-18.

Ravussin, E., & Bogardus, C. (1989). Relationship of genetics, age, and physical fitness to daily energy expenditure and fuel utilization. *American Journal of Clinical Nutrition, 49*, 968-975.

Ravussin, E., Burnand, B., Schutz, Y., & Jéquier, E. (1985). Energy expenditure before and during energy restriction in obese patients. *American Journal of Clinical Nutrition, 41*, 753-759.

Ravussin, E., Lillioja, S., Anderson, T. E., Christin, L., & Bogardus, C. (1986). Determinants of 24-hour energy expenditure in man: Methods and results using a respiratory chamber. *Journal of Clinical Investigation, 78*, 1568-1578.

Ravussin, E., Lillioja, S., Knowler, W. C., Christin, L., Freymond, D., Abbott, W. G. H., Boyce, V., Howard, B. V., & Bogardus, C. (1988). Reduced rate of energy expenditure as a risk factor for body-weight gain. *New England Journal of Medicine, 318*, 467-472.

Ravussin, E., Schutz, Y., Acheson, K. J., Dusmet, M., Bourquin, L., & Jéquier, E. (1985). Short-term, mixed-diet overfeeding in man: No evidence for "luxuskonsumption." *American Journal of Physiology, 249*, E470-E477.

Ravussin, E., Zurlo, F., Ferraro, R., & Bogardus, C. (1991). Energy expenditure in man: determinants and risk factors for body weight gain. In *Recent advances in obesity research: VI. Proceedings of the Sixth International Congress on Obesity* (pp. 175–182). London: John Libbey.

Roberts, S. B., Savage, J., Coward, W. A., Chew, B., & Lucas, A. (1988). Energy expenditure and intake in infants born to lean and overweight mothers. *New England Journal of Medicine, 318,* 461–466.

Roza, A. M., & Shizgal, H. M. (1984). The Harris–Benedict equation reevaluated: Resting energy requirements and the body cell mass. *American Journal of Clinical Nutrition, 40,* 168–182.

Saad, M. F., Alger, S. A., Zurlo, F., Young, J. B., Bogardus, C., & Ravussin, E. (1991). Contribution of the sympathetic nervous system to energy expenditure: Ethnic differences. *American Journal of Physiology, 261,* E789–E794.

Schoeller, D. A., Ravussin, E., Schutz, Y., Acheson, K. J., Baertschi, P., & Jéquier, E. (1986). Energy expenditure by doubly labeled water: Validation in humans and proposed calculation. *American Journal of Physiology, 250,* R1–R8.

Schoeller, D. A., & van Santen, E. (1982). Measurement of energy expenditure in humans by doubly labeled water method. *Journal of Applied Physiology, 53,* 955–959.

Schulz, L. O., Nyomba, B. L., Alger, S., Anderson, T. E., & Ravussin, E. (1991). Effect of endurance training on sedentary energy expenditure measured in a respiratory chamber. *American Journal of Physiology, 260,* E257–E261.

Schutz, Y., Bessard, T., & Jéquier, E. (1987). Exercise and postprandial thermogenesis in obese women before and after weight loss. *American Journal of Clinical Nutrition, 45,* 1424–1432.

Schutz, Y., Flatt, J. P., & Jéquier, E. (1989). Failure of dietary fat intake to promote fat oxidation: A factor favoring the development of obesity [comment]. *American Journal of Clinical Nutrition, 50,* 307–314.

Schutz, Y., Golay, A., Felber, J. P., & Jéquier, E. (1984). Decreased glucose-induced thermogenesis after weight loss in obese subjects: A predisposing factor for relapse of obesity? *American Journal of Clinical Nutrition, 39,* 380–387.

Schwartz, R. S., Jaeger, L. F., & Veith, R. C. (1988). Effect of clonidine on the thermic effect of feeding in humans. *American Journal of Physiology, 254,* R90–R94.

Segal, K. R., Gutin, B., Nyman, A. M., & Pi-Sunyer, X. P. (1985). Thermic effect of food at rest, during exercise, and post exercise in lean and obese men of similar body weight. *Journal of Clinical Investigation, 76,* 1107–1112.

Shetty, P. S. (1984). Adaptive changes in basal metabolic rate and lean body mass in chronic undernutrition. *Human Nutrition: Clinical Nutrition, 83C,* 443–451.

Shetty, P. S. (1990). Physiological mechanisms in the adaptive response of metabolic rates to energy restriction. *Nutrition Research Reviews, 3,* 49–74.

Shetty, P. S., James, W. P. T., & Jung, R. T. (1979). Effect of catecholamine replacement with levodopa on the metabolic response to semistarvation. *Lancet, i,* 77–79.

Sims, E. A. (1986). Energy balance in human beings: the problems of plenitude. *Vitamins and Hormones, 43,* 1–101.

Sims, E. A. H., Danforth, E., Jr., Horton, E. S., Bray, G. A., Glennon, J. A., & Salans, L. B. (1973). Endocrine and metabolic effects of experimental obesity in man. *Recent Progress in Hormone Research, 29,* 457–496.

Steen, S. N., Oppliger, R. A., & Brownell, K. D. (1988). Metabolic effects of repeated weight loss and regain in adolescent wrestlers. *Journal of the American Medical Association, 260,* 47–50.

Stunkard, A. J., Harris, J. R., Pedersen, N. L., & McClearn, G. E. (1990). The body-mass index of twins who have been reared apart. *New England Journal of Medicine, 322,* 1483–1487.

Stunkard, A. J., Sorensen, T. I. A., Hanis, C., Teasdale, T. W., Chakraborty, R., Schull, W. J., & Schulsinger, F. (1986). An adoption study of human obesity. *New England Journal of Medicine, 314,* 193–198.

Swinburn, B. A., Nyomba, B. L., Saad, M. F., Zurlo, F., Raz, I., Knowler, W. C., Lillioja, S., Bogardus, C., & Ravussin, E. (1991). Insulin resistance associated with lower rates of weight gain in Pima Indians. *Journal of Clinical Investigation, 88,* 168–173.

Taylor, H. L., & Keys, A. (1950). Adaptation to caloric restriction. *Science, 112*, 215-218.
Tremblay, A., Fontaine, E., Poehlman, E. T., Mitchell, D., Perron, L., & Bouchard, C. (1986). The effect of exercise-training on resting metabolic rate in lean and moderately obese individuals. *International Journal of Obesity, 10*, 511-517.
Tremblay, A., Plourde, G., Després, J. P., & Bouchard, C. (1989). Impact of dietary fat content and fat oxidation on energy intake in humans. *American Journal of Clinical Nutrition, 49*, 799-805.
U.S. Department of Health and Human Services. (1988). *The Surgeon General's report on nutrition and health* (DHHS Publication No. PHS 88-50210). Washington, DC: U.S. Government Printing Office.
von Voit, C. (1881). Physiology of general metabolism and nutrition. In L. Hermann (Ed.), *Handbook of physiology* (Vol. 6, Part 1, pp. 1-566). Leipzig: Vogel.
Wadden, T. A., Foster, G. D., Letizia, K. A., & Mullen, J. L. (1990). Long-term effects of dieting on resting metabolic rate in obese outpatients. *Journal of the American Medical Association, 264*, 707-711.
Wadden, T. A., Stunkard, A. J., & Brownell, K. D. (1983). Very low calorie diets: Their efficacy, safety, and future. *Annals of Internal Medicine, 99*, 675-684.
Warwick, P. M., & Garrow, J. S. (1981). The effect of addition of exercise to a regime of dietary restriction on weight loss, nitrogen balance, resting metabolic rate and spontaneous physical activity in three obese women in a metabolic ward. *International Journal of Obesity, 5*, 25-32.
Waterlow, J. C. (1985). What do we mean by adaptation. In K. Blaxter & J. C. Waterlow (Eds.), *Nutritional adaptation in man*. London: John Libbey.
Waterlow, J. C. (1986). Notes on the new international estimates of energy requirement. *Proceedings of the Nutrition Society, 45*, 351-360.
Webb, P., & Abrams, T. (1983). Loss of fat stores and reduction in sedentary energy expenditure from undereating. *Human Nutrition: Clinical Nutrition, 37*, 271-282.
Weigle, D. S. (1988). Contribution of decreased body mass to diminished thermic effect of exercise in reduced-obese men. *International Journal of Obesity, 12*, 567-578.
Weigle, D. S., Sande, K. J., Iverius, P. H., Monsen, E. R., & Brunzell, J. D. (1988). Weight loss leads to a marked decrease in nonresting energy expenditure in ambulatory human subjects. *Metabolism, 37*, 930-936.
Welle, S. L., Amatruda, J. M., Forbes, G. B., & Lockwood, D. H. (1984). Resting metabolic rates of obese women after rapid weight loss. *Journal of Clinical Endocrinology and Metabolism, 59*, 41-44.
Welle, S. L., & Campbell, R. G. (1986). Decrease in resting metabolic rate during rapid weight loss is reversed by low dose thyroid hormone treatment. *Metabolism, 35*, 289-291.
Zurlo, F., Larson, K., Bogardus, C., & Ravussin, E. (1990). Skeletal muscle metabolism is a major determinant of resting energy expenditure. *Journal of Clinical Investigation, 86*, 1423-1427.
Zurlo, F., Lillioja, S., Esposito-Del Puente, A., Nyomba, B. L., Ryaz, I., Saad, M. F., Swinburn, B. A., Knowler, W. C., Bogardus, C., & Ravussin, E. (1990). Low ratio of fat to carbohydrate oxidation as predictor of weight gain: Study of 24-h RQ. *American Journal of Physiology, 259*, E650-E657.

8

The Effects of Increased Physical Activity on Food Intake, Metabolic Rate, and Health Risks in Obese Individuals

F. XAVIER PI-SUNYER

Exercise is commonly prescribed as a major component in the treatment of obesity. This is generally done because exercise is thought to be beneficial for a number of reasons. First, exercise enhances energy expenditure; second, it is thought to decrease energy intake; third, exercise may help to remedy the health risks associated with obesity. This chapter will discuss each of these in turn.

Energy Expenditure

Americans are extraordinarily inactive. This inactivity is apparently the price of technologically advanced societies. Labor-saving devices are continually being introduced, so that, from automobiles to electric blenders, we engage in less and less thermogenic activity each year. The decrease in activity, although it cannot be quantified precisely, is no doubt great. An outgrowth of this is that in the 50 years between 1900 and 1950, obesity in the United States approximately doubled, even though caloric consumption dropped 10% (U.S. Department of Agriculture, 1962; VanItallie, 1977). Some years ago, a study that determined the body weights and caloric intake of 500 pairs of Irish brothers, one of each pair living in Boston and one in Ireland, reported that while the American brothers ate significantly less, they were more obese. This was attributed to the less active lifestyle in the technologically more advanced country (Brown, Bourke, & Gerarty, 1970).

Obesity and Energy Expenditure

While our whole society is sedentary, there may be individuals who are particularly so and thus incur an even greater risk of becoming obese. The issue of whether obese persons are more inactive than lean ones is the subject of some controversy. The issue is clouded in both children and adults. In a number of studies, obese children have been reported to be less active than lean ones. In some of these, the children's activities were actually observed by the investigators (Bullen, Reed, & Mayer, 1974; Rose & Mayer, 1968), while in others the data were simply gathered by questionnaire, a rather imperfect method (Johnson, Burke, & Mayer, 1956; Stephanik, Heald, & Mayer, 1959). Other investigators, however, have found no difference in activity between obese and lean children (Bradfield, Paulos, & Grossman, 1971; Maxfield & Konishi, 1966; Stunkard & Peska, 1962; Wilkinson, Parkin, Pearlson, Strong, & Sykes, 1977).

In adults, a number of investigators have reported that obese persons are less active than lean ones (Bloom & Eidex, 1967; Chirico & Stunkard, 1960; Mayer, Roy, & Mitra 1956). However, actual energy expenditure was not measured in these studies; it was assessed either by self-report or by very crude measures of activity. Thus, whether obese adults are actually less active than lean adults has not been resolved to date. In addition, even if the obese are less active, they may expend more energy because they carry more weight. The net energy expended in a free-living state has not been well studied, and a definitive answer on whether the obese expend more or less energy overall is unclear. A recent, very well-conducted study (Blair & Buskirk, 1987) required careful activity diaries and measured the cost of energy expenditure for different activities for each individual. Obese persons were found to expend more energy in the nonresting than in the resting component of their 24-hour energy expenditure, suggesting that even if the obese are less active, they expend more energy per unit of activity than do their lean peers. This makes good sense, since they carry a much greater weight.

Exercise and Energy Expenditure

Since body weight is determined by the balance between energy intake and energy expenditure, if energy expenditure can be increased without changing food intake, then weight will be lost. Thus, the expenditure side of the equation can help in the prevention or treatment of obesity. There is a common misconception that exercise is not helpful in weight control because the energy expended is rather small (Franklin & Rubenfire, 1980; Harris & Halbauer, 1973). However, the effect is cumulative over time; because, as mentioned above, overweight individuals expend more energy for a given weight-bearing activity than do lean individuals (Williams, 1984), they get more benefit for each minute of activity.

An example of the ability to expend calories is given in Table 8.1. It is clear that the greater the obesity, the greater the energy expended in weight-bearing exercise. Of course, the table lists only the gross energy expenditure. The net increase is determined by subtracting from that amount what the energy expenditure would have been if the individual simply were sitting. This

TABLE 8.1. Gross Caloric Requirements per Mile for Running, Walking, and Outdoor Bicycling

Body weight		Caloric requirements (kcal/mile)		
(lb)	(kg)	Running	Walking	Bicycling
110	50	85	58	30
132	60	102	69	36
154	70	119	81	42
176	80	136	92	48
198	90	153	104	54
220	100	170	115	60
242	110	187	127	66
264	120	204	138	72

Note. Adapted from "Losing Weight through Exercise" by B. A. Franklin and M. Rubentire, 1980, *Journal of the American Medical Association, 244,* 377-379. Copyright 1980 by American Medical Association. Adapted by permission.

sedentary energy expenditure is on the order of 1.5 to 2.0 kilocalories (kcal) per minute for an obese person, so that if a 220-pound man were to walk 2 miles in 30 minutes, he would expend 230 kcal minus about 60 kcal, for a net increased expenditure of 170 kcal.

Postexercise Energy Expenditure

Whether there is a sustained elevation of oxygen consumption after exercise is controversial. Elevated oxygen consumption has been estimated in the literature to last from 7 to 48 hours (de Vries & Gray, 1983; Edwards, Thorndike, & Dill, 1935; Margaria, Edwards, & Dill, 1973; Passmore & Johnson, 1960). Steinhaus (1983), and earlier Karpovich (1941), both reviewed the available data and concluded that no change in subsequent basal metabolism could be demonstrated in response to exercise. My colleagues and I could not document a sustained effect of either moderate or intense exercise on metabolic rate (Freedman-Akabas, Colt, Kissileff, & Pi-Sunyer, 1985). This was true for males and females in all fitness categories. An example of this is given in Figure 8.1, which shows that within 40 minutes of the termination of exercise, the energy expenditure has returned to baseline. Similar results have been found by others (Brehm & Gutin, 1986; Staten, 1991).

Three studies have found a sustained effect after exercise. A recent study showed that resting metabolic rate (RMR) was 4.7% higher on the morning after a 3-hour bout of intense exercise than on a morning after a day when no such bout was done (Bielinski, Schutz, & Jéquier, 1985). However, the metabolic rates of 10 of 11 subjects were not significantly different from the rest day, with only one the following morning being 0.07 kcal/minute higher. In two subsequent studies that we conducted, a 30-minute bout of moderate intensity exercise raised the caloric expenditure over the next 3 hours by only a total of 14 kcal (Segal, Gutin, Albu, & Pi-Sunyer, 1987; Segal, Gutin, Nyman, & Pi-Sunyer, 1985). Thus, even when an effect can be documented, it is very small and cannot be considered of thermogenic significance.

Thermogenic Interaction between Food Intake and Exercise

There is controversy in the literature as to whether the thermic effect of food—that is, the rise in energy expenditure after ingestion of nutrients—is blunted in obese persons. Although many studies have found such a phenomenon, many others have not (Blaza & Garrow, 1983; Garrow, 1978; Jéquier, Pittet, & Gygax, 1978; Jung, Shetty, & James, 1979; Ravussin et al., 1983; Segal & Gutin, 1983; Shetty, Jung, James, Barrand, & Callingham, 1981). Similarly, there is controversy as to the effect of exercise on the thermogenic effect of food, with some studies finding a potentiation of thermogenesis and others not finding any (Dalloso & James, 1984; Welle, 1984). The differences between studies may be partly related to differences in meal size, length of measurement

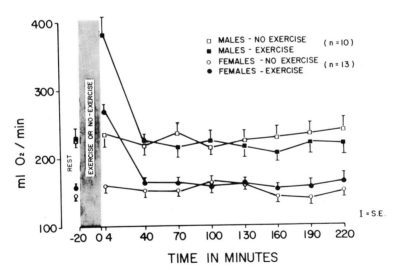

FIGURE 8.1. Summary of the oxygen consumption per minute by subjects before and after moderate exercise or rest. Subjects exercised for 20 minutes at the work rates associated with their anaerobic thresholds. From "Lack of Sustained Increase in VO_2 Following Exercise in Fit and Unfit Subjects" (p. 546) by S. Freedman-Akabas, E. Colt, H. R. Kissileff, and F. X. Pi-Sunyer, 1985, *American Journal of Clinical Nutrition*, 41, 545–549. Copyright 1985 by American Society for Clinical Nutrition. Reprinted by permission.

of thermogenesis, kind and intensity of exercise, and the time relation of the meal and the exercise.

In a study by Segal and Gutin (1983), the synergism of food and exercise was measured in lean and obese women. Every 30 minutes, cycle exercise was done for 5 minutes at a workload of 50 watts, with and without eating. Exercise was done 8 times for a total of 40 minutes over 4 hours. Exercise potentiated the thermic effect of food in the lean but not in the obese women. In the lean women, the caloric expenditure was about 11 kcal greater when exercise and food were combined than the simple sum of exercise alone and food alone. In the obese, the number of kilocalories expended did not exceed the simple sum. Thus, a potentiating effect of exercise on food could be found in the lean but not the obese women. Similar studies had been reported earlier by Zahorska-Markiewicz (1980).

While Bray, Whipp, and Koyal (1974) reported a greater thermic response to the combination of either a 1000- or 3000-kcal breakfast meal with cycle exercise in lean young men, Welle (1984) could not find such an effect when using low intensity exercise. Dalloso and James (1984) also could not find an effect, and neither could Swindells (1972) when the meal given was less than 1000 kcal. Segal, Presta, and Gutin (1984) measured the effect of the combination of food and exercise in lean and obese men. They exercised them at different levels of exertion, from very mild to the maximum, and determined the impact of a 910-kcal meal taken 60 minutes before on the thermogenic response. They found that the difference in the thermic response between the fed and the fasted day was greater in the lean than in the obese. This was true at all submaximal work intensities.

To summarize, a potentiation of exercise on the thermic effect of food has been found in the lean but not the obese by a number of investigators, although not all have been able to document this. Thus, obese persons may have a small defect in their ability to mount an enhanced thermogenic response when exercise is combined with food.

Effect of Prior Exercise on Thermic Response to Food

The effect of prior exercise on the subsequent thermic response to food has been investigated by a number of researchers. Bielinski et al. (1985) measured the effect of 3 hours of treadmill walking on the thermic effect of a meal and found that it was significantly enhanced. Because this was a rather heavy work load, unlikely to be approximated by a typical obese patient, my colleagues and I did a similar study in which we measured the effect of a 30-minute exercise bout on the thermic effect of a 750-kcal meal in lean and obese men (Segal et al., 1985). The postexercise effect, measured for 3 hours, was greater for lean than for obese men (44 kcal $\pm$ 7 vs. 16 $\pm$ 4; mean $\pm$ *SEM*). In a subsequent study, we compared the sequences of food and exercise (i.e., the meal given before or after exercise) in lean and obese men (Segal et al., 1987).

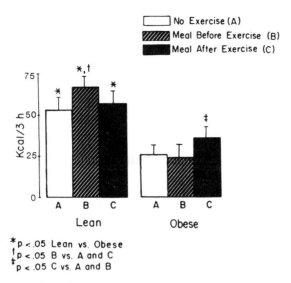

FIGURE 8.2. Thermic effect of food at rest and postexercise, with two sequences of meal and exercise in lean and obese men. From "Exercise and Obesity" (p. 227) by K. R. Segal and F. X. Pi-Sunyer, 1989, *Medical Clinics of North America, 73,* 217–236. Copyright 1989 by W. B. Saunders Co., Harcourt Brace Jovanovich, Inc. Reprinted by permission.

This is shown in Figure 8.2. The thermic response to food was greater in the lean than in the obese in all conditions. In addition, while no potentiating effect of the exercise could be found in the lean (either before or after the meal), there was an enhanced thermic response in the obese if the meal was taken after the exercise, though no such effect could be documented if the meal was taken before the exercise.

The blunted thermic response of the obese is probably at least partially due to their insulin resistance. During a euglycemic insulin clamp, a reduced thermic response to infused glucose has been related to a reduced glucose disposal (Ravussin et al., 1983; Ravussin, Acheson, Vernet, Danforth, & Jéquier, 1985). This has been associated with a reduced rate of glucose storage, which is costly in terms of energy (Acheson, Ravussin, Wahren, & Jéquier, 1984). Thus, the exercise taken before the meal may diminish insulin resistance, allowing greater glucose disposal and storage and enhancing thermogenesis.

Effects of Chronic Exercise on Energy Expenditure

The effects of chronic exercise on energy expenditure are complicated by the fact that exercise may affect aerobic capacity, body composition, and food intake, all of which may have an impact on expenditure. Since longitudinal studies are difficult to do, most studies in this area have been cross-sectional, taking a trained and an untrained group and comparing them. However, since there is a great deal of variability in energy expenditure between people, cross-sectional studies are not as good as longitudinal ones to determine the effect of long-term training.

Cross-sectional studies have been conducted by LeBlanc, Mercier, and Samson (1984) in women who chronically exercised at different levels, and by Tremblay, Coe, and LeBlanc (1983) in younger men. Neither study found a difference in RMR between the trained and untrained groups, but both found a decreased thermic effect of food in the more highly trained groups. Hammer, Barrier, Roundy, Bradford, and Fisher (1988) examined 16 weeks of exercise versus no exercise in women and found no effect on RMR. Poehlman and colleagues conducted two studies and found differing results. In the first, they found no effect of training on either RMR or TEF (Poehlman et al., 1986); in the second, they found an enhanced RMR in the most highly trained men, but a lower thermic effect of food (Poehlman, McCauliffe, Van Houten, & Danforth, 1990).

We have conducted longitudinal studies in which we asked lean women to exercise for 19-day periods so as to expend an extra 10% and 25% of their usual daily energy expenditure by walking on a treadmill (Woo & Pi-Sunyer, 1985). The exercise was a fast walk. The mean energy cost of the activities during the sedentary period and two exercise periods is shown in Figure 8.3. It can be seen that there was no difference among the periods; we could document no change in either the RMR or the cost of the various activities. We repeated the study in

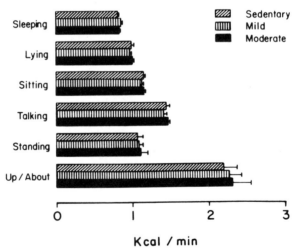

FIGURE 8.3. Mean energy cost of activities during a sedentary period and two exercise treatments for five women. The mild exercise treatment was walking on a treadmill to increase energy expenditure by 14% ± 4%, and the moderate treatment was walking to increase it by 29% ± 3%, of the sedentary 24-hour energy expenditure. From "Effect of Increased Physical Activity on Voluntary Intake in Lean Women" (p. 838) by R. Woo and F. X. Pi-Sunyer, 1985, *Metabolism, 34,* 836–841. Copyright 1985 by Grune & Stratton, Inc. Reprinted by permission.

obese women and obtained a similar result (Woo, Garrow, & Pi-Sunyer, 1982a). We then performed a study for a full 57-day period at the heavier exercise level, again with no change in RMR or the energy cost of various activities (Woo, Garrow, & Pi-Sunyer, 1982b).

Davis et al. (1983) also conducted a longitudinal study in a group of men and women whom they trained for 12 weeks. Neither body composition nor RMR changed. These studies suggest that there is little effect of exercise on thermogenesis in the obese beyond the energy cost of the exercise itself, except, as discussed above, in enhancing the thermic effect of a subsequent meal. The above-mentioned studies thus do not support the notion that training has any major effect on either resting or postprandial thermogenic response.

Effect of Exercise on Food Intake

Increased physical activity could have three possible effects on food intake: (1) increase it; (2) decrease it; or (3) have no effect. It is generally assumed that in a lean individual, as activity is increased, intake also rises proportionately to keep pace with the increased energy expenditure and thus to defend the body weight. Does this truly occur? And is the response different in obese persons?

In humans, there is little experimental evidence on the effect of exercise on food intake, because few studies have actually measured food intake. Generally, protocols either have estimated food intake or have simply followed body weight and interpreted weight loss (or weight stability) as reflecting a hypophagic response and weight gain as a hyperphagic response. The use of accurate body composition measures rather than body weight would have improved these studies, because exercise can increase muscle mass. Since muscle is denser than the fat that is lost, body weight changes may not appropriately reflect the changes in body composition. However, body composition has seldom been determined accurately in these exercise studies.

Normal-Weight Subjects

Studies of normal-weight persons have shown that they regulate food intake appropriately in response to exercise, so as to maintain weight. Lincoln (1972) studied caloric intake in 1836 individuals of both sexes who were 31 to 60 years of age. Subjects were divided by history into four quartiles of physical activity: hardly any, mild, moderate, and heavy. In these groups, caloric intake as measured by dietary recall increased to keep pace with increasing activity. Studies in which food intake was actually measured have been of relatively short duration. Passmore and colleagues studied five young men during hard walking for 1 week and found that weight did not significantly change, suggesting that food intake increased appropriately (Passmore, Meiklejohn, Dewar, & Thow, 1959; Passmore, Thomson, & Warnock, 1952). Warnold and Lenner

(1977) studied healthy normal-weight diabetic and normal subjects who underwent regimens of mild activity for 2 weeks. They also could not show a significant change in weight, suggesting an increase in food intake to compensate for the increased expenditure. A number of other studies also have inferred caloric compensation for maintenance of body weight, although food intake was not measured. Examples are the reports of Warnold and Lenner (1977), Boileau, Buskirk, Horstman, Mendez, and Nicholas (1971), and Wilmore et al. (1980). A minority, however, describe a loss of weight, implying incomplete caloric compensation (Carter & Phillips, 1969; Joseph, 1968).

Obese Subjects

If one then looks at obese persons and the effect of exercise on food intake, studies can be divided according to which showed weight loss and which did not. In about one-half of the studies, subjects did not show weight loss, implying a complete compensation for their increased exercise by decreased physical activity the rest of the day and/or increased food intake (Atomi & Miyashita, 1980; Björntorp et al., 1977; Krotkiewski et al., 1979). In the other studies, some weight loss occurred, implying incomplete compensation (Boileau et al., 1971; Dempsey, 1964; Dudleston & Benniou, 1970; Franklin et al., 1979; Gwinup, 1975; Leon, Conrad, Hunninghade, & Serfass, 1979; O'Hara, Allen, & Shepard, 1977; Oscai & Williams, 1968; Pollock et al., 1971). None of these studies addressed the issue of food intake directly, and thus they are not helpful in resolving the question as to whether activity regulates food intake. The best of these studies, however, are analyzed briefly below, although there is a disconcerting lack of consistency in the results.

Dempsey (1964) exercised seven obese men 1 hour daily, 5 days per week for 5 weeks, and found that they lost an average of 4.7 kg of weight. The subjects kept food records that demonstrated no change in intake, so it was assumed that the weight loss was attributable to the exercise. Dudleston and Benniou (1970), studying young obese women, also found a decrease in weight that could be accounted for by exercise alone, while food intake did not change. On the other hand, studies by Oscai and Williams (1968) of middle-aged obese men and by Boileau et al. (1971) of young obese men suggested a decreased intake, although actual food intake was not measured. Gwinup (1975) did a much more prolonged study of 1 year, with long exercise bouts of 70 to 190 minutes daily. Again, food intake was not measured. Less than a third of those who started the program finished it; those who did, however, lost an average of 10 kg. But again, since food intake was not measured, it is unclear whether it remained the same or increased or decreased slightly. If it changed downward, it could have been due to a motivation to lose weight. With such a radical change in behavior to increase physical activity, it is possible that subjects consciously changed their eating behavior, although the volunteers were told to continue eating as they wished. Two studies—one by

Dahlkoetter, Gallahan, and Linton (1979) and the other by Weltman, Matter, and Stamford (1980)—investigated the effect of exercise versus diet versus a combination of the two. Although the first study showed an effect of exercise in decreasing weight, the other did not. Since in both studies, however, subjects were enrolled in fitness and/or diet and weight control classes, it is difficult to know whether the exercise group took it upon themselves to diet, even though they were not told to do so. Thus, the studies are flawed.

Krotkiewski et al. (1979) found no change in weight after a 6-month exercise program in which food intake was not limited. Leon et al. (1979), on the other hand, observed significant weight losses in healthy obese graduate students at the University of Minnesota who were subjected to intense exercise. The students were told to continue eating as they wished. They exercised 5 days a week for 90 minutes daily, expending between 1000 and 1200 kcal a day. They lost 5.7 kg in 16 weeks. The loss was reported to consist entirely of fat with no loss of lean body mass. Using 3-day dietary records, the investigators documented that the volunteers initially ate more, but that by the 12th week they consumed fewer calories than at baseline (when they were sedentary). However, in calculations of the energy expenditure and the weight loss, the numbers do not add up, suggesting that the dietary records were probably very inaccurate. It is more likely that these subjects increased their intake somewhat, but not enough to keep up with expenditure, so that they lost some weight.

Studies Conducted on a Metabolic Unit

Because of the confusion in the literature (Pi-Sunyer & Woo, 1985) and the lack of studies that included adequate measurement of food intake, we conducted a series of studies to measure the effect of exercise on food intake in lean (Woo & Pi-Sunyer, 1985) and obese (Woo et al., 1982a, 1982b) women. Since the only way to measure food intake accurately was to weigh and analyze the food, we studied the volunteers in a metabolic unit. All women had maintained a stable body weight for at least 6 months. They were told that the purpose of the study was to measure the effect of exercise on protein metabolism and nitrogen balance, so as to prevent individuals from signing up because they wanted or expected to lose weight. Subjects initially came into the unit and underwent a short 5-day sedentary period, during which we measured their energy expenditure and food intake. Energy expenditure was determined by keeping very complete activity diaries and measuring the energy cost of each activity for the individual. Food was served "platter style," as previously perfected by our colleagues (Porikos, Booth, & VanItallie, 1977). Each item of food was served on a separate platter, with more on each platter than a person could eat. The volunteer then served herself as she wished. Unbeknownst to the volunteer, all food was weighed before and after eating, so that food intake was carefully monitored. Duplicate food was analyzed by bomb calorimetry. We calculated energy balance as the difference between intake and expenditure (Woo et al., 1982a).

The first group we studied consisted of six women who averaged 167% of ideal weight by the Metropolitan 1959 tables (Metropolitan Life Insurance Company, 1959). Each was studied for a total of 62 days on the unit. After the initial 5-day sedentary evaluation phase, there were 3 periods of 19 days each in which the volunteers either remained sedentary, exercised at a mild rate, or exercised at a more moderate rate. These periods were assigned randomly to the subjects. During the exercise periods, subjects exercised so as to expend either an extra 10% or 25% above their normal expenditure. Subjects walked on the treadmill at a 2.5% grade and chose a walking speed with which they were comfortable. They averaged a walking time of 39 minutes daily for the mild exercise period and 96 minutes daily for the moderate period. The results of this study are presented in Figure 8.4.

Mean expenditure rose significantly with increased activity, as had been expected. Mean food intake, however, did not change significantly between periods. That is, food intake did not keep pace with expenditure, so that energy balance was negative; as a result, over time, individuals lost weight (Woo et al., 1982a). We then conducted a longer study in which a similar group of women

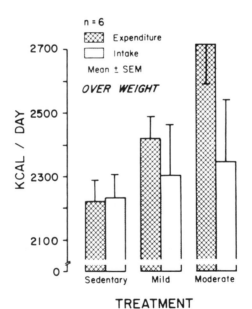

FIGURE 8.4. Mean energy expenditure and intake in six obese women over three 19-day periods in which they either were sedentary or exercised on a treadmill at a mild (+10% of sedentary daily activity) or moderate (+25% of sedentary activity) rate. From "Effect of Increased Physical Activity on Voluntary Intake in Lean Women" (p. 839) by R. Woo and F. X. Pi-Sunyer, 1985, *Metabolism, 34*, 836–841. Copyright 1985 by Grune & Stratton, Inc. Reprinted by permission.

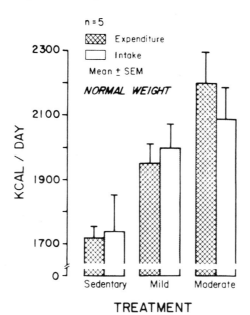

FIGURE 8.5. Mean energy expenditure and intake in five normal-weight women over three 19-day periods in which they either were sedentary or exercised on a treadmill at a mild (+14% ± 4%) of sedentary daily activity) or moderate (+29% ± 3%) rate. From "Effect of Increased Physical Activity on Voluntary Intake in Lean Women" (p. 837) by R. Woo and F. X. Pi-Sunyer, 1985, *Metabolism, 34*, 836–841. Copyright 1985 by Grune & Stratton, Inc. Reprinted by permission.

participated in a similar program of moderate exercise, but for a much longer period of 57 days (Woo et al., 1982b). They exhibited similar behavior, with their food intake not compensating for the increased activity. As a result, they also were in negative energy balance throughout the whole exercise period and lost weight at the rate of 0.12 kg/day.

Because of this lack of compensation in the two obese groups, we thought it important to determine the response to a similar protocol in a lean group. We therefore studied a group of women whose average weight was 97% of ideal and whose age was comparable to that of the obese group (Woo & Pi-Sunyer, 1985). The protocol was similar to the first described above, with three periods—one sedentary, one of mild exercise, and one of severe exercise. The results are shown in Figure 8.5. It can be seen that the lean women compensated for the increased activity by increasing their intake. As a result, weight and body composition remained the same over the period of the study.

Thus, in our studies, the obese and the lean women responded to increased activity very differently. While the lean increased their intake to meet the needs of their extra expenditure, this was not the case with the obese. The obese seemed to be eating in response to cues that did not relate to activity. It is possible that they did not discern these cues or were indifferent to them; more research is needed in order to clarify this further.

Palatability and Food Intake

Since it is possible that factors such as palatability, variety, and availability of foods are more important in determining food intake in obese than lean persons, we have conducted several studies to examine these issues (Pi-Sunyer, 1985). We fed obese young men a very palatable gourmet diet with a great deal of variety. This was again done by means of the platter method as described above. They exercised at basal activity level, at 110% of sedentary level, at 140% of sedentary level, and back to baseline. Once again, calorie intake did not vary with the different activity levels. But with such a palatable diet the intake was very high, on the order of 4000 kcal per day, so that the men only came into energy balance at their high level of activity. The fact that the food intake was again fixed in these subjects, despite major changes in energy expenditure, suggests that the regulation of food intake may depend more on sensory aspects of the diet than on activity cues in obese individuals. Such results are in accordance with studies by Rolls et al. (1981) and Rolls, Rowe, and Rolls (1982), which showed that variety and palatability of food enhances caloric intake.

Our studies summarized above show that obese individuals can use exercise to facilitate weight loss. This is so not because exercise inhibits food intake; rather, exercise seems to have little influence on food intake, which is seemingly regulated by other factors. Since expenditure is increased, negative energy balance supervenes and weight loss occurs.

Health Benefits of Exercise

Obesity is associated with an increased risk of diabetes mellitus, hypertension, cardiovascular disease, gallbladder disease, stroke, arthritis, and gout (Pi-Sunyer, 1991). In morbidly obese persons, there is also a greater incidence of thrombophlebitis, pulmonary embolus, pulmonary insufficiency, cardiac failure, and sleep apnea (VanItallie, 1985).

Diabetes

Obesity greatly increases the risk of diabetes. Close to 90% of diabetic patients in America have Type II (non-insulin-dependent) diabetes, and of these approximately 85% are obese (Pi-Sunyer, 1990). As a country's population becomes fatter, the incidence of diabetes increases. In situations where food becomes scarce and individuals lose weight, such as in Europe in World War II, the incidence of diabetes decreases. Exercise is important in diabetes in two ways. First, as weight loss ensues, insulin sensitivity is improved; second, exercise per se, independent of weight loss, increases insulin sensitivity (Björntorp, 1976; Björntorp et al., 1972; Schneider, Amorosa, Khachadurian, & Ruderman, 1984; Segal et al., 1989).

The insulin resistance of obesity induces a compensatory hyperinsulinemia. There is increasing evidence to suggest that hyperinsulinemia is associated with hypertension (Modan et al., 1985; Ferrannini et al., 1987). In addition, hyperinsulinemia has been implicated in atherogenesis, since a high correlation has been noted between hyperinsulinemia and coronary artery disease (Ducimetiere et al., 1980; Jarrett, 1988; Pyorala, 1979). Moreover, a strong correlation has also been noted between hyperinsulinemia and elevations in blood triglycerides (Garcia-Webb, Bosner, & Whitting, 1983; Zavonori et al., 1989) and cholesterol (Orchard, Becker, & Bates, 1983); hyperinsulinemia is also associated with low levels of high density lipoprotein (HDL) (Haffner, Fong, Hazuda, Pugh, & Patterson, 1988; Orchard et al., 1983; Stalder, Pometta, & Suenram, 1981). It is well known that exercise and physical training improve insulin sensitivity (DeFronzo, Sherwin, & Kraemer, 1987; Horton, 1986) and lower insulin levels. Thus, exercise is likely to be of benefit in preventing or slowing the health risks associated with hyperinsulinemia.

Hypertension and Lipid Disorders

Hypertension is strongly associated with obesity (Bjerkedal, 1957; Chiang, Perlman, & Epstein, 1969; Master & Lasser, 1958). The incidence of hypertension rises with increasing weight and improves with weight loss (Pi-Sunyer, 1991). Active men generally have blood pressures that are lower than those of sedentary men (Morris, 1960; Morris & Crawford, 1958). Exercise, by its ability to enhance weight loss, can have a beneficial effect on hypertension (Reisin et al., 1978). Also, as a consequence of its ability to improve insulin sensitivity in insulin-resistant patients, it can ameliorate hypertension. Finally, regular exercise, even in the absence of weight loss, seems to have a beneficial effect on blood pressure (Boyer & Kasch, 1970; Cogswell, Henderson, & Berryman, 1946; Rudd & Day, 1967). This seems to be particularly true in hypertensives (Choquette & Ferguson, 1973).

As weight increases, atherogenic lipid levels also increase (Ashley & Kannel, 1974; Kannel, Gordon, & Castelli, 1979) and HDL cholesterol decreases (Castelli, 1986). With exercise and physical training, the lipid profile improves. Triglycerides generally fall (Holloszy, Skinner, Toro, & Cureton, 1964; Lopez, Vial, Balart, & Arroyave, 1974; Oscai, Patterson, Bogard, Beck, & Rothermel, 1972). While HDL cholesterol levels have generally been reported to rise and low density lipoprotein (LDL) cholesterol levels to fall (Altekruse & Wilmore, 1973; Ballantyne et al., 1978; Lopez et al., 1974; Streja & Mymin, 1979), the former is much more common than the latter. Certainly, the ratio of HDL to LDL cholesterol improves with exercise in both obese (Lewis et al., 1976) and nonobese (Lopez et al., 1974) subjects.

Other Benefits of Exercise

Exercise is beneficial for the heart (Scheuer & Tipton, 1977). It can increase exercise tolerance (Clausen, 1976; Redwood, Rosing, & Epstein, 1972), enhance myocardial vascularity (Scheuer & Tipton, 1977), and improve cardiac efficiency (Clausen, 1976; Oberman & Kouchoukos, 1978; Redwood et al., 1972; Scheuer & Tipton, 1977). Thus, in patients with marked obesity who are at particular risk for cardiac failure and congestion, exercise is a good preventative strategy.

It is necessary to make clear that the beneficial effects of exercise are very short-lived; as a result, an exercise program must be continuously maintained to reduce health risks. Thus, obese individuals must commit themselves to permanent lifestyle change in order to ensure a positive effect on health.

In conclusion, it is clear that exercise can be beneficial to obese persons. It induces a negative energy balance, which leads to weight loss. It also increases insulin sensitivity and decreases existing insulin levels with beneficial effects on health risks. Finally, it may help enhance the thermic effect of food if the exercise is performed before eating.

It must be remembered, however, that the markedly obese patient is a special case. While all the benefits accruing to a less obese individual can also accrue to the markedly obese, their exercise tolerance is very limited (Pacy, Webster, & Garrow, 1986). These patients must be shown how to exercise, must be closely supervised, and must be given rather specific graded exercise programs. These issues are discussed in Chapter 15 by Fox.

References

Acheson, K. J., Ravussin, E., Wahren, J., & Jéquier, E. (1984). Thermic effect of glucose in man: Obligatory and facultative thermogenesis. *Journal of Clinical Investigation, 74*, 1572–1580.

Altekruse, E. B., & Wilmore, J. H. (1973). Changes in blood chemistries following a controlled exercise program. *Journal of Occupational Medicine, 15*, 110–113.

Ashley, F. W., & Kannel, W. B. (1974). Relation of weight change to changes in atherogenic traits: The Framingham Study. *Journal of Chronic Disease, 27*, 103–114.

Atomi, Y., & Miyashita, M. (1980). Effect of training intensity in adult females on aerobic power, related to lean body mass. *European Journal of Applied Physiology, 44*, 109–116.

Ballantyne, D., Clark, A., Dyker, G. S., Gillis, C. R., Hawthorne, V. M., Henry, D. A., Hole, D. S., Murdoch, R. M., Semple, T., & Stewart, G. M. (1978). Prescribing exercise for the healthy assessment of compliance and effects on plasma lipids and lipoproteins. *Health Bulletin, 36*(4), 169–176.

Bielinski, R., Schutz, Y., & Jéquier, E. (1985). Energy metabolism during postexercise recovery in man. *American Journal of Clinical Nutrition, 42*, 69–82.

Bjerkedal, T. (1957). Overweight and hypertension. *Acta Medica Scandinavica, 159,* 13–26.
Björntorp, P. (1976). Effect of exercise and physical training on carbohydrate and lipid metabolism in man. *Advances in Cardiology, 18,* 158–166.
Björntorp, P., Berchtold, P., Grimby, G., Lindholm, B., Sanne, H., Tibblin, G., & Willhelmsen, L. (1972). Effects of physical training on glucose tolerance, plasma insulin and lipids on body composition in men after myocardial infarction. *Acta Medica Scandinavica, 192,* 439–443.
Björntorp, P., Holm, G., Jacobsson, B., Schiller-deJounge, K., Lundberg, P., Sjöström, L., Smith, U., & Sullivan, L. (1977). Physical training in human hyperplastic obesity: IV. Effects of hormonal status. *Metabolism, 26,* 319–328.
Blair, D., & Buskirk, E. R. (1987). Habitual daily energy expenditure and activity levels of lean and adult-onset and child-onset obese women. *American Journal of Clinical Nutrition, 45,* 540–550.
Blaza, S., & Garrow, J. S. (1983). Thermogenic response to temperature, exercise, and food stimuli in lean and obese women, studied by 24-hour direct calorimetry. *British Journal of Nutrition, 49,* 171–180.
Bloom, W. L., & Eidex, M. F. (1967). Inactivity as a major factor in adult obesity. *Metabolism, 16,* 679–684.
Boileau, R. A., Buskirk, E. R., Horstman, D. H., Mendez, J., & Nicholas, W. C. (1971). Body compositional changes in obese and lean men during physical conditioning. *Medicine and Science in Sports, 3,* 183–189.
Boyer, J. L., & Kasch, F. W. (1970). Exercise therapy in hypertensive men. *Journal of the American Medical Association, 211,* 1668–1671.
Bradfield, R., Paulos, J., & Grossman, H. (1971). Energy expenditure and heart rate of obese high school girls. *American Journal of Clinical Nutrition, 24,* 1482–1486.
Bray, G. A., Whipp, B. J., & Koyal, S. N. (1974). The acute effects of food on energy expenditure during cycle ergometry. *American Journal of Clinical Nutrition, 27,* 254–259.
Brehm, B. A., & Gutin, B. (1986). Recovery energy expenditure for steady-state exercise in runners and nonexercisers. *Medicine and Science in Sports and Exercise, 18,* 205–210.
Brown, J., Bourke, G. J., & Gerarty, G. R. (1970). Nutritional and epidemiological factors related to heart disease. In G. H. Bourne (Ed.), *World reviews of nutrition and dietetics* (Vol. 12, pp. 1–12). Basel: Pitman Medical and Scientific.
Bullen, B. A., Reed, R. B., & Mayer, J. (1974). Physical activity of obese and non-obese adolescent girls appraised by motion picture sampling. *American Journal of Clinical Nutrition, 14,* 211–233.
Carter, J. E. L., & Phillips, W. H. (1969). Structural changes in exercising middle-aged males during a 2 year period. *Journal of Applied Physiology, 27,* 787–794.
Castelli, W. P. (1986). The triglyceride issue: A view from Framingham. *American Heart Journal, 112,* 432–440.
Chiang, B. N., Perlman, L. V., & Epstein, F. H. (1969). Overweight and hypertension: A review. *Circulation, 39,* 403–421.
Chirico, A., & Stunkard, A. J. (1960). Physical activity and human obesity. *New England Journal of Medicine, 263,* 935–940.
Choquette, G., & Ferguson, R. J. (1973). Blood pressure reduction in "borderline" hypertensives following physical training. *Canadian Medical Association Journal, 108,* 699–703.
Clausen, J. P. (1976). Circulatory adjustments to dynamic exercise and effect of physical training in normal subjects and in patients with coronary artery disease. *Progress in Cardiovascular Disease, 18,* 459–495.
Cogswell, R. C., Henderson, C. R., & Berryman, G. H. (1946). Some observations of effects of training on pulse rate, blood pressure and endurance, in humans using the step test (Harvard) treadmill and electrodynamic brake bicycle ergometer. *American Journal of Physiology, 146,* 422–430.
Dahlkoetter, J., Gallahan, E. J., & Linton, J. (1979). Obesity and the unbalanced energy equation: Exercise vs. eating habit change. *Journal of Consulting and Clinical Psychology, 47,* 898–905.

Dalloso, H. M., & James, W. P. T. (1984). Whole body calorimetry studies in adult men: The interaction of exercise and overfeeding on the thermic effect of a meal. *British Journal of Nutrition, 52*, 65-72.

Davis, J. R., Tagliaferro, A. R., Kertzer, R., Gerardo, T., Nichols, J., & Wheeler, J. (1983). Variations of dietary-induced thermogenesis and body fatness with aerobic capacity. *European Journal of Applied Physiology, 509*, 319-329.

DeFronzo, R. A., Sherwin, R. S., & Kraemer, N. (1987). Effect of physical training on insulin action in obesity. *Diabetes, 36*, 1379-1385.

Dempsey, J. A. (1964). Anthropometrical observations on obese and non-obese young men undergoing a program of vigorous physical exercise. *Research Quarterly, 35*, 275-287.

de Vries, H. A., & Gray, D. E. (1983). After effects of exercise upon resting metabolic rate. *Research Quarterly, 34*, 314-321.

Ducimetiere, P., Eschwege, R., Papoz, L., Richard, J. L., Claude, J. R., & Rosselin, G. (1980). Relationship of plasma insulin levels to the incidence of myocardial infarction and coronary heart disease mortality in a middle-aged population. *Diabetologia, 19*, 205-210.

Dudleston, A. K., & Benniou, M. (1970). Effect of diet and/or exercise on obese college women. *Journal of the American Dietetic Association, 56*, 126-129.

Edwards, H. T., Thorndike, A., & Dill, D. B. (1935). The energy requirement in strenuous muscular exercise. *New England Journal of Medicine, 213*, 532-535.

Ferrannini, E., Buzzigoli, G., Bonadonna, R., Giorico, M. A., Oleggini, M., Graziadei, L., Pedrinella, R., Brandi, L., & Bevilacqua, S. (1987). Insulin resistance in essential hypertension. *New England Journal of Medicine, 317*, 350-356.

Franklin, B. A., Buskirk, E., Hodgson, J., Gahagan, H., Kollias, J., & Mendez, J. (1979). Effects of physical conditioning on cardiorespiratory function, body composition and serum lipids in relatively normal weight and obese middle-aged women. *International Journal of Obesity, 3*, 97-109.

Franklin, B. A., & Rubenfire, M. (1980). Losing weight through exercise. *Journal of the American Medical Association, 244*, 377-379.

Freedman-Akabas, S., Colt, E., Kissileff, H. R., & Pi-Sunyer, F. X. (1985). Lack of sustained increase in VO_2 following exercise in fit and unfit subjects. *American Journal of Clinical Nutrition, 41*, 545-549.

Garcia-Webb, P., Bosner, A. M., & Whitting, D. (1983). Insulin resistance: A risk factor for coronary heart disease? *Scandinavian Journal of Clinical Laboratory Investigation, 43*, 677-685.

Garrow, J. S. (1978). The regulation of energy expenditure in man. In G. A. Bray (Ed.), *Recent advances in obesity research: II. Proceedings of the Second International Congress on Obesity* (pp. 200-210). London: Newman.

Gwinup, G. (1975). Effect of exercise alone on the weight of obese women. *Archives of Internal Medicine, 135*, 676-780.

Haffner, S. M., Fong, D., Hazuda, H. P., Pugh, J. A., & Patterson, J. K. (1988). Hyperinsulinemia, upper body adiposity, and cardiovascular risk factors in non-diabetics. *Metabolism, 37*, 338-345.

Hammer, R. L., Barrier, C. A., Roundy, E. S., Bradford, J. M., & Fisher, A. G. (1988). Calorie-restricted low-fat diet and exercise in obese women. *American Journal of Clinical Nutrition, 49*, 77-85.

Harris, M. B., & Halbauer, E. S. (1973). Self-directed weight control through eating and exercise. *Behaviour Research and Therapy, 11*, 523-529.

Holloszy, J. O., Skinner, J. S., Toro, G., & Cureton, T. K. (1964). Effects of a six month program of endurance exercise on the serum lipids of middle-aged men. *American Journal of Cardiology, 14*, 753-760.

Horton, E. S. (1986). Exercise and physical training: Effect on insulin sensitivity and glucose metabolism. *Diabetes and Metabolism Reviews, 2*, 1-17.

Jarrett, R. J. (1988). Is insulin atherogenic? *Diabetologia, 31*, 71-75.

Jéquier, E., Pittet, P., & Gygax, P. T. (1978). Thermic effect of glucose and thermal body insulation in lean and obese subjects: A calorimetric approach. *Proceedings of the Nutrition Society, 37*, 45–53.

Johnson, M. L., Burke, M. S., & Mayer, J. (1956). Relative importance of inactivity and overeating in the energy balance of obese high school girls. *American Journal of Clinical Nutrition, 4*, 37–44.

Joseph, J. J. (1968). Effects of exercise and sedentary living on middle-aged adults. *American Corrective Therapy Journal, 22*, 3–7.

Jung, R. T., Shetty, P. S., & James, W. P. T. (1979). Reduced thermogenesis in obesity. *Nature, 279*, 322–323.

Kannel, W. B., Gordon, T., & Castelli, W. P. (1979). Obesity, lipids and glucose intolerance: The Framingham Study. *American Journal of Clinical Nutrition, 32*, 1238–1245.

Karpovich, P. V. (1941). Metabolism and energy used in exercise. *Research Quarterly, 12*, 423–431.

Krotkiewski, M., Mandroukas, K., Sjöström, L., Sullivan, L., Wetterquist, H., & Björntorp, P. (1979). Effects of long-term physical training on body fat, metabolism and blood pressure in obesity. *Metabolism, 28*, 650–658.

LeBlanc, J., Mercier, P., & Samson, P. (1984). Diet-induced thermogenesis with relation to training state in female subjects. *Canadian Journal of Physiological Pharmacology, 62*, 334–337.

Leon, A. S., Conrad, J., Hunninghade, D. B., & Serfass, R. (1979). Effects of a vigorous walking program on body composition and lipid metabolism of obese young men. *American Journal of Clinical Nutrition, 33*, 1776–1787.

Lewis, S., Haskell, W. L., Wood, P. D., Manoogian, N., Bailey, J. E., & Pereira, M. B. (1976). Effects of physical activity on weight reduction in obese middle-aged women. *American Journal of Clinical Nutrition, 29*, 151–156.

Lincoln, J. E. (1972). Calorie intake, obesity, and physical activity. *American Journal of Clinical Nutrition, 25*, 390–394.

Lopez, A., Vial, R., Balart, L., & Arroyave, G. (1974). Effect of exercise and physical fitness on serum lipids and lipoproteins. *Atherosclerosis, 20*, 1–9.

Margaria, R., Edwards, H. T., & Dill, D. B. (1973). The possible mechanism of contracting and paying O_2 debt and the role of lactic acid in muscle contraction. *American Journal of Physiology, 106*, 689–715.

Master, A. M., & Lasser, R. P. (1958). Relationship of the blood pressure to weight, height and body build in apparently healthy subjects. *American Journal of Medical Science, 235*, 278–289.

Maxfield, E., & Konishi, F. (1966). Patterns of food intake and physical activity in obesity. *Journal of the American Dietetic Association, 49*, 406–408.

Mayer, J., Roy, P., & Mitra, K. P. (1956). Relation between caloric intake, body weight, and physical work: Studies in an industrial male population in West Bengal. *American Journal of Clinical Nutrition, 4*, 169–175.

Metropolitan Life Insurance Company. (1959). Metropolitan height and weight tables. *Statistical Bulletin of the Metropolitan Life Insurance Company, 40*, 1–4.

Modan, M., Halkin, H., Almog, S., Lusky, A., Eshkol, A., Shefi, M., Shitrit, A., & Fuchs, Z. (1985). Hyperinsulinemia: A link between hypertension, obesity and glucose intolerance. *Journal of Clinical Investigation, 75*, 809–817.

Morris, J. N. (1960). Epidemiology and cardiovascular disease of middle age. *Modern Concepts of Cardiovascular Disease, 29*, 625–632.

Morris, J. N., & Crawford, M. D. (1958). Coronary heart disease and physical activity of work. *British Medical Journal, ii*, 1485–1496.

Oberman, A., & Kouchoukos, N. T. (1978). Role of exercise after coronary artery bypass surgery. In N. K. Wenger (Ed.), *Exercise and the heart*. Philadelphia: F. A. Davis.

O'Hara, W. J., Allen, C., & Shepard, R. J. (1977). Treatment of obesity by exercise in the cold. *Canadian Medical Association Journal, 117*, 773–786.

Orchard, T. J., Becker, D. L., & Bates, M. (1983). Plasma insulin and lipoprotein cholesterol concentrations: An atherogenic association? *American Journal of Epidemiology, 118,* 326–337.

Oscai, L. B., Patterson, J. A., Bogard, D. L., Beck, R. J., & Rothermel, B. L. (1972). Normalization of serum triglycerides and lipoprotein electrophoretic patterns by exercise. *American Journal of Cardiology, 30,* 775–780.

Oscai, L. B., & Williams, B. T. (1968). Effect of exercise on overweight middle-aged males. *Journal of the American Geriatric Society, 16,* 794–797.

Pacy, P. J., Webster, J., & Garrow, J. S. (1986). Exercise and obesity. *Sports Medicine, 3,* 89–113.

Passmore, R., & Johnson, R. E. (1960). Some metabolic changes following prolonged moderate exercise. *Metabolism, 9,* 452–456.

Passmore, R., Meiklejohn, A. P., Dewar, A. D., & Thow, R. K. (1959). An analysis of the gain in weight of overfed thin young men. *British Journal of Nutrition, 13,* 27–37.

Passmore, R., Thomson, J. G., & Warnock, G. M. (1952). A balance sheet of the estimation of energy intake and energy expenditure as measured by indirect calorimetry using the Kofranyi–Michaelis calorimeter. *British Journal of Nutrition, 6,* 253–264.

Pi-Sunyer, F. X. (1985). Effect of exercise on food intake. In J. Hirsch & T. B. VanItallie (Eds.), *Recent advances in obesity research: IV. Proceedings of the Fourth International Congress on Obesity* (pp. 368–373). London: John Libbey.

Pi-Sunyer, F. X. (1990). Obesity and diabetes in blacks. *Diabetes Care, 13,* 1144–1149.

Pi-Sunyer, F. X. (1991). Health implications of obesity. *American Journal of Clinical Nutrition, 53,* 1595S–1603S.

Pi-Sunyer, F. X., & Woo, R. (1985). Effect of exercise on food intake in human subjects. *American Journal of Clinical Nutrition, 42,* 983–990.

Poehlman, E. T., McCauliffe, T. L., Van Houten, D. R., & Danforth, E., Jr. (1990). Influence of age and endurance training on metabolic rate and hormones in healthy men. *American Journal of Physiology, 259,* E66–E72.

Poehlman, E. T., Tremblay, A., Nadeau, A., Dussault, J., Theriault, G., & Bouchard, C. (1986). Heredity and changes in hormones and metabolic rates with short-term training. *American Journal of Physiology, 250,* E711–E717.

Pollock, M. L., Miller, D. S., Janeway, R., Linnerud, A. C., Robertson, B., & Valentino, R. (1971). Effects of walking on body composition and cardiovascular function of middle-aged men. *Journal of Applied Physiology, 30,* 126–130.

Porikos, K. P., Booth, G., & VanItallie, T. B. (1977). Effect of covert nutritive dilution on the spontaneous food intake of obese individuals: A pilot study. *American Journal of Clinical Nutrition, 30,* 1638–1644.

Pyorala, K. (1979). Relationship of glucose tolerance and plasma insulin to the incidence of coronary artery disease: Results from two population studies in Finland. *Diabetes Care, 2,* 131–141.

Ravussin, E., Acheson, K. J., Vernet, O., Danforth, E., & Jéquier, E. (1985). Evidence that insulin resistance is responsible for the decreased thermic effect of glucose in human obesity. *Journal of Clinical Investigation, 75,* 1268–1273.

Ravussin, E., Bogardus, C., Schwartz, R. S., Robbins, D. C., Wolfe, R. R., Horton, E. S., Danforth, E., Jr., & Sims, E. A. (1983). Thermic effect of infused glucose and insulin in man. Decreased response with increased insulin resistance in obesity and non insulin dependent diabetes mellitus. *Journal of Clinical Investigation, 72,* 893–902.

Redwood, D. R., Rosing, D. R., & Epstein, S. E. (1972). Circulatory and symptomatic effects of physical training in patients with coronary artery disease and angina pectoris. *New England Journal of Medicine, 286,* 959–965.

Reisin, E., Abel, R., Modan, M., Silverberg, D. S., Dliahon, H. E., & Modan, B. (1978). Effect of weight loss without salt restriction on the reduction of blood pressure in overweight hypertensive patients. *New England Journal of Medicine, 289,* 1–6.

Rolls, B. J., Rowe, E. A., & Rolls, E. T. (1982). How sensory properties of food affect human feeding behavior. *Physiology and Behavior, 26,* 409–417.
Rolls, B. J., Rowe, E. A., Rolls, E. T., Kingston, B., Megson, A., & Gunary, R. (1981). Variety in a meal enhances food intake in man. *Physiology and Behavior, 26,* 215–221.
Rose, H. E., & Mayer, J. (1968). Activity, caloric intake, and the energy balance of infants. *Pediatrics, 41,* 18–21.
Rudd, J. L., & Day, W. C. (1967). A physical fitness program for patients with hypertension. *Journal of the American Geriatric Society, 15,* 373–379.
Scheuer, J., & Tipton, C. M. (1977). Cardiovascular adaptations to physical training. *Annual Reviews of Physiology, 39,* 221–251.
Schneider, S. H., Amorosa, L. F., Khachadurian, A. K., & Ruderman, N. B. (1984). Studies on the mechanism of improved glucose control during regular exercise in type 2 (non-insulin dependent) diabetes. *Diabetologia, 26,* 355–360.
Segal, K. R., Abalos, A., Albu, J., Edano, E., Ginsberg-Fellner, F., & Pi-Sunyer, F. X. (1989). Effect of exercise training on insulin sensitivity and the thermic effect of glucose in lean, obese, and diabetic men. *Clinical Research, 39,* 334A.
Segal, K. R., & Gutin, B. (1983). Thermic effects of food and exercise in lean and obese women. *Metabolism, 32,* 581–589.
Segal, K. R., Gutin, B., Albu, J., & Pi-Sunyer, F. X. (1987). Thermic effect of food and exercise in lean and obese men of similar lean body mass. *American Journal of Physiology, 252,* E110–E117.
Segal, K. R., Gutin, B., Nyman, A. M., & Pi-Sunyer, F. X. (1985). Thermic effect of food at rest, during exercise, and after exercise in lean and obese men of similar body weight. *Journal of Clinical Investigation, 76,* 1107–1112.
Segal, K. R., & Pi-Sunyer, F. X. (1989). Exercise and obesity. *Medical Clinics of North America, 73,* 217–236.
Segal, K. R., Presta, E., & Gutin, B. (1984). Thermic effect of food during graded exercise in normal weight and obese men. *American Journal of Clinical Nutrition, 40,* 995–1000.
Shetty, P. S., Jung, R. T., James, W. P., Barrand, M. A., & Callingham, B. A. (1981). Postprandial thermogenesis in obesity. *Clinical Science, 60,* 519–525.
Stalder, M., Pometta, B., & Suenram, A. (1981). Relationship between plasma insulin levels and high density lipoprotein cholesterol levels in healthy men. *Diabetologia, 21,* 544–548.
Staten, M. A. (1991). The effect of exercise on food intake in men. *American Journal of Clinical Nutrition, 53,* 27–31.
Steinhaus, A. H. (1983). Chronic effects of exercise. *Physiological Review, 13,* 103–147.
Stephanik, P. A., Heald, F. L., & Mayer, J. (1959). Caloric intake in relation to energy output of obese and non obese adolescent boys. *American Journal of Clinical Nutrition, 7,* 55–62.
Streja, D., & Mymin, D. (1979). Moderate exercise and HDL cholesterol. *Journal of the American Medical Association, 242,* 2190–2192.
Stunkard, A. J., & Peska, J. (1962). The physical activity of obese girls. *American Journal of Diseases of Children, 103,* 812–817.
Swindells, Y. E. (1972). The influence of activity and size of meals on caloric response in women. *British Journal of Nutrition, 27,* 65–73.
Tremblay, A., Coe, J., & LeBlanc, J. (1983). Diminished dietary thermogenesis in exercise-trained human subjects. *European Journal of Applied Physiology, 52,* 1–4.
U.S. Department of Agriculture. (1962). *Consumption of food in the U.S. in 1909–1952* (Agricultural Handbook No. 2, Suppl. 1901). Washington, DC: U.S. Government Printing Office.
VanItallie, T. B. (1977). *Diets related to the killer diseases.* Testimony before the Senate Select Committee on Nutrition and Human Needs, Vol. II, Part 2: Obesity. Washington, DC: U.S. Government Printing Office.
VanItallie, T. B. (1985). Health implications of overweight and obesity in the United States. *Annals of Internal Medicine, 103,* 983–988.

Warnold, E., & Lenner, R. A. (1977). Evaluation of the heart rate method to determine the daily energy expenditure in disease. A study in juvenile diabetics. *American Journal of Clinical Nutrition, 30*, 304–315.

Welle, S. (1984). Metabolic responses to a meal during rest and low-intensity exercise. *American Journal of Clinical Nutrition, 40*, 990–994.

Weltman, A., Matter, S., & Stamford, B. A. (1980). Caloric restriction and/or mild exercise: Effects on serum lipids and body composition. *American Journal of Clinical Nutrition, 33*, 1002–1009.

Wilkinson, P. W., Parkin, J. M., Pearlson, G., Strong, H., & Sykes, P. (1977). Energy intake and physical activity in obese children. *British Medical Journal, i,* 756.

Williams, M. H. (1984). *Nutritional aspects of human physical and athletic performance* (2nd ed.). Springfield, IL: Charles C Thomas.

Wilmore, J. H., Davis, J. A., O'Brien, R., Vodak, P. A., Walder, G. R., & Amsterdam, E. A. (1980). Physiological alterations consequent to 20 week conditioning programs of bicycling, tennis and jogging. *Medicine and Science in Sports and Exercise, 12*, 1–8.

Woo, R., Garrow, J., & Pi-Sunyer, F. X. (1982a). Effect of exercise on spontaneous calorie intake in obesity. *American Journal of Clinical Nutrition, 36*, 470–477.

Woo, R., Garrow, J. S., & Pi-Sunyer, F. X. (1982b). Voluntary food intake during prolonged exercise in obese women. *American Journal of Clinical Nutrition, 36*, 478–484.

Woo, R., & Pi-Sunyer, F. X. (1985). Effect of increased physical activity on voluntary intake in lean women. *Metabolism, 34*, 836–841.

Zahorska-Markiewicz, B. (1980). Thermic effect of food and exercise in obesity. *European Journal of Applied Physiology, 44*, 231–235.

Zavanori, I., Bonora, E., Pagliara, M., Dall'Aglio, E., Luchetti, L., Buonann, G., Bonati, P. A., Bergonzani, M., Gnudi, L., Passeri, M., & Reaven, G. (1989). Risk factors for coronary artery disease in healthy persons with hyperinsulinemia and normal glucose tolerance. *New England Journal of Medicine, 320*, 703–706.

PART THREE

HEALTH CONSEQUENCES OF THERAPEUTIC WEIGHT LOSS

9

Reducing Primary Risk Factors by Therapeutic Weight Loss

BEATRICE S. KANDERS
GEORGE L. BLACKBURN

Obesity is an independent risk factor for cardiovascular disease, hypertension, and diabetes (Hubert, Feinleib, McNamara, & Castelli, 1983). Clearly, the most important reason to lose weight is to reduce the risk of disease and to improve health. However, long-term maintenance of weight loss is difficult; relapse has been reported to be as high as 95% past the second year (Leibel & Hirsch, 1984). Thus, most significantly obese persons treated in clinical settings are unlikely to achieve and maintain "ideal" body weight.

Increasing evidence indicates that a 10–20% weight loss can ameliorate most obesity-related diseases and should, in fact, serve as a goal of treatment. Most obese patients can achieve this weight loss in 12–16 weeks by consuming a balanced hypocaloric diet or a very low calorie diet (VLCD), and can maintain it for at least 18 months (Kanders, Blackburn, et al., 1991). Thus, therapeutic weight loss must be contrasted to the ideal weights proposed by life insurance actuary tables, which are based on a genetically, metabolically, and behaviorally diverse population.

This chapter will review the short- and long-term (more than 1-year) medical and health outcomes associated with a 10–20% reduction in initial weight. Although obesity is related to a number of chronic diseases, we will examine primarily diabetes, hypertension, and cardiovascular disease.

Non-Insulin-Dependent Diabetes Mellitus

Non-insulin-dependent diabetes mellitus (NIDDM) affects approximately 10 million middle-aged or older Americans. The prevalence of the disease increases steadily from the fourth decade. Approximately 90% of all diabetic individuals have Type II diabetes (NIDDM), and 80–90% of these are obese (National Institutes of Health [NIH], 1987). The association between obesity and NIDDM is well known. Individuals 20–30% overweight are clearly at increased risk for NIDDM, and the risk rises linearly with body weight.

Both obesity and NIDDM result in insulin resistance and subsequent hyperinsulinemia (Olefsky, Kolterman, & Scarlett, 1982; Reaven, 1988). In obese nondiabetic individuals, the principal target tissues for insulin (i.e., liver, skeletal muscle, adipose tissue) do not respond appropriately to those levels of the hormone found in nonobese individuals. Obese nondiabetic persons can compensate for the impairment in hormone action by secreting greater amounts of insulin, resulting in hyperinsulinemia. When obese persons become unable to compensate for the insulin resistance, hyperglycemia and NIDDM ensue.

Like obesity, the hyperglycemia that accompanies NIDDM results from a combination of metabolic defects, including peripheral insulin resistance and impaired insulin secretion (or beta cell dysfunction). Increased basal hepatic glucose output has also been cited as a key factor (Defronzo, Ferrannini, & Koivisto, 1983). However, the relative contribution of changes in each of these metabolic abnormalities to the onset and perpetuation of the diabetic state, as well as to improvements in hyperglycemia after weight loss, is not well defined.

Short-Term Effects of Weight Loss on Type II Diabetes

While much remains to be learned about the interactions between obesity and NIDDM, it is clear that weight loss confers beneficial changes in both disorders via glycemic control. Weight loss in obese patients with diabetes, as in obese nondiabetic patients, ameliorates insulin resistance, and there are usually accompanying improvements in carbohydrate tolerance. Weight loss reduces hyperglycemia and hyperinsulinemia, and, in patients with severe hyperglycemia, may lead to increased insulin secretion (Doar, Wilde, Thompson, & Sewell, 1975; Hadden et al., 1975). Weight loss has also been shown to increase high density lipoprotein (HDL) cholesterol levels in patients with Type II diabetes, who often have elevated total cholesterol levels and low HDL cholesterol levels (Gordon, Castelli, Hjortland, Kannel, & Dawber, 1977; Reckless, Betleridge, Wu, Payne, & Galton, 1978; Hughes, Gwynne, Switzer, Herbet, & White, 1984).

Hyperglycemia is frequently reduced when a low-calorie diet is employed, even before significant amounts of weight are lost; this suggests that caloric restriction has a beneficial effect, independent of weight loss (Greenfield, Kolterman, Olefsky, & Reaven, 1978). Furthermore, several studies have shown that a weight loss of 10–20% of initial weight greatly improves glycemic control in obese NIDDM subjects. Hughes et al. (1984) examined the effects of caloric restriction and weight loss on glycemic control in a sample of obese patients with Type II diabetes. Patients lost a mean of 25.5 kg (23% of initial body weight) over 6 months as a result of treatment by either protein-sparing modified fast (PSMF) or gastric bypass. Only three diet-treated patients and one surgically treated patient approached actuarial "ideal" body weight. Nonetheless, all patients showed significant improvements in fasting plasma glucose and total glycosylated hemoglobin (HbA$_{1C}$) values, irrespective of the final weight achieved.

Other studies have reported improvement in glycemic control and diabetes in response to a modest weight loss. Following a 23-kg weight loss (22% of initial body weight), Kirschner and colleagues reported that 100% of patients taking oral hypoglycemic agents were able to discontinue these medications, and that 87% of patients requiring exogenous insulin could be weaned entirely from their daily injections (Kirschner, Schneider, Ertel, & Gorman, 1988). The remaining patients decreased their daily insulin dosage as well. No long-term data were available on the health status of these individuals. These findings are similar to those of Fitz and colleagues, who observed improved glycemic control despite a mean weight loss of only 9.5 kg (Fitz, Sperling, & Fein, 1983). Seventy-two percent of patients had been taking insulin prior to treatment. At a mean 41-week follow-up, however, 77% of these patients remained off insulin. Studying nondiabetic and hyperlipoproteinemic subjects, Olefsky et al. (1982) found that weight losses of 10 kg were sufficient to produce short-term improvements in insulin sensitivity and in serum lipid levels. Finally, a modest weight loss of 16% in obese patients with Type II diabetes brought about significant improvements in glycemic control, which were sustained for 3 weeks after a VLCD with the resumption of a weight stabilization diet (Henry, Wallace, & Olefsky, 1986).

Long-Term Effects of Weight Loss on Type II Diabetes

Thus, even a modest weight loss of 10–20% of body weight will ameliorate NIDDM in obese individuals in the short term. Only a handful of studies have examined the long-term effects of such weight losses. Mancini et al. (1981) investigated the effects of weight loss with a VLCD (<400 kilocalories [kcal]/day) on medical outcome in morbidly obese patients at the 3-year follow-up visit. Glucose intolerance or overt diabetes was detected in more than 40% of women and about 50% of men at baseline; 162 of the original 390 patients attended the 3-year follow-up visit. Patients were divided into tertiles at this time, based upon whether they had lost ≤ 4% of initial body weight (mean of 2 kg); 5–9% of initial weight (mean of 8 kg); or ≥10% (mean 23 kg) of initial weight. Patients who maintained losses of 5–9% and ≥10% of initial body weight had lasting reductions from baseline in plasma glucose, whereas patients with losses of ≤4% of initial body weight had an increase in fasting plasma glucose levels with losses.

Wing et al. (1987) examined long-term effects of a modest 10% weight loss on glycemic control in patients with Type II diabetes. Through a combination of caloric restriction, exercise, and behavior modification, patients achieved a mean weight loss of 5.6 kg at the end of treatment and maintained a loss of 4.5 kg at 1 year. The long-term effects of specific amounts of weight loss on glycemic control were examined according to weight change from pretreatment to the 1-year follow-up. The categories of weight change were as follows: gained weight; lost 0–2.3 kg; lost 2.4–6.8 kg; lost 6.9–13.6 kg; or lost >13.6 kg.

Patients who lost more than 13.6 kg experienced significant improvements in HbA_{1C}, fasting blood sugar, and insulin at 1 year, and all subjects could be removed from oral hypoglycemic medication. However, patients with more modest weight losses of 6.9–13.6 kg also experienced significant improvements on these measures. These patients remained well above ideal body weight, having reduced only from 97.8 kg to 87.4 kg (10%). The authors concluded that a modest weight reduction of 10–20% was associated with significant decreases in HbA_{1C} that could be maintained for at least 1 year.

Finally, we (Kanders, Blackburn, et al., 1991) investigated the effect of weight loss on health outcome at an 18-month follow-up evaluation in a population of 1429 obese men and women who had undergone treatment by a VLCD. At baseline, men and women weighed a mean of 125.0 and 96.9 kg, respectively, and were 67.9% and 65.2% above ideal body weight, respectively. Eleven percent of patients had diabetes. Patients lost a mean of 20% of initial body weight during the active weight loss phase, during which time clinically and statistically significant health benefits were observed among patients with diabetes. Of the 154 patients with diabetes enrolled, the condition was resolved in 53 persons (34%) and improved in another 35 (23%). At study entry, 19% of patients with diabetes reported taking insulin or other diabetic agents; at the end of active weight loss, half of those on insulin and half of those on other diabetic agents discontinued use of the medications. During this same period, the number of patients requiring new medications also remained small, with only one patient starting insulin and only seven patients beginning other diabetic agents.

At an 18-month follow-up, weight and health outcome data were available for 821 patients. Men and women maintained losses of 13.7% and 11.8% of initial weight, respectively. Improvements in diabetes at 18 months corresponded directly to the degree of weight lost from baseline. Among patients losing ≥20% of body weight, 70% of those with diabetes had resolution or improvement of their disease condition. Among patients losing 10–19% of body weight, 55% of those with diabetes had resolution or improvement in their condition. Among patients who lost <10% of body weight, 30% of those with diabetes had improvement or resolution of their disease condition. Among the 34 patients with diabetes whose disease was completely resolved by the 18-month follow-up, 26 had been on baseline medications that were discontinued; among the 8 patients with diabetes whose disease status improved, 5 discontinued their baseline medications and 1 reduced baseline medications. For all patients with diabetes, the mean net percentages of weight loss from baseline through the 18-month follow-up as it related to change in disease status were as follows: 18% weight loss in patients in whom diabetes was resolved; 16% reduction for diabetes "improved"; 7% for no change in status; and 3% for worsening of condition. These results demonstrate that a modest weight loss of <20% is associated with the long-term amelioration of diabetes in a population of significantly obese patients.

Diet therapy, which includes weight loss, is considered the cornerstone of treatment for obese patients with NIDDM (NIH, 1987; Flood, Halford, Coopan, & Marble, 1985). While not all patients will respond equally to weight loss (Watts et al., 1990), these studies indicate that any reduction in body weight will bring about an improvement in glycemic control (Henry, Wiest-Kent, & Schaeffer, 1986; Wing, Epstein, Norwalk, Koeske, & Haag, 1985; Wing et al., 1987; D'Eramo, Wylie-Rosett, & Hagan, 1986; Henry, Wallace, & Olefsky, 1986). This includes modest reductions of 10–20% of initial body weight (Wing et al., 1987; D'Eramo et al., 1986). Among patients on diabetic agents, weight loss will also permit a reduction in the number and dosage of medications.

Hypertension

In the United States, hypertension now ranks as the leading cause both for physician office visits and for the use of prescription drugs (Koch & Knapp, 1987; McLemore & DeLozier, 1987). Hypertension affects more than 20% of adults aged 25–74 years (Lenfant & Roccella, 1984) and is a major risk factor for cardiovascular morbidity and mortality (U.S. Department of Health and Human Services [DHHS], 1988). Epidemiological studies of undeveloped as well as Westernized populations have confirmed the link between body weight and blood pressure (Dustan, 1983), and, specifically, the association of weight gain during adulthood with higher blood pressure levels. Individuals who are $\geq$20% above ideal body weight are twice as likely to have hypertension as are nonobese adults (Havlik, Hubert, Fabsitz, & Feinleib, 1983), and in the Framingham Study, the risk for normotensive subjects to develop hypertension was proportional to increases in body weight (Kannel, Brand, Skinner, Dawber, & McNamara, 1967).

It has been estimated that about 30% of cases of hypertension may be attributable to obesity, and in men less than 45 years of age, the figure may be as high as 60% (MacMahon, Blacket, MacDonald, & Hall, 1984). In the Framingham Offspring Study, adiposity, as measured by subscapular skinfold thickness, was the major controllable contributor to hypertension, with estimates of 78% of hypertension in men and 64% in women due to obesity (Garrison, Kannel, & Stokes, 1985). Given the high incidence of hypertension in this country and the strong correlation between obesity and elevated blood pressure, weight loss clearly remains one of the most potent nonpharmacological means of lowering blood pressure and is currently recommended for all overweight hypertensive individuals (U.S. DHHS, 1988).

Indeed, many studies have demonstrated that weight reduction in both normotensive and hypertensive obese individuals is associated with decreases in blood pressure, though the exact mechanism by which obesity elevates blood pressure and by which weight loss reduces it remains unknown. Some investigators have described hemodynamic changes and alterations in cardiac morphology and fluid volume distribution. Others have shown variations in adrenergic, metabolic, and endocrine factors. However, we have shown that obesity leads to worsening of insulin resistance, development of hyperinsulinemia (which increases the adrenergic activity), and reabsorption of sodium at the renal tubular levels (Istfan, Plaisted, Bistrian, & Blackburn, 1992). Clearly, more research is needed to clarify the complex role of obesity in the pathogenesis of hypertension.

Short-Term Effects of Weight Loss on Hypertension

Whatever the mechanism, it is well known that weight loss in overweight hypertensive individuals is associated with a fall in arterial pressure (MacMahon, Cutler, Brittain, & Higgins, 1987) (see Table 9.1). Indeed, over the last decade, few studies have reported that treatment of hypertension with weight loss did *not* result in lower blood pressure (Fagerberg, Anderson, Isaksson, & Björntorp, 1984; Haynes, Harper, & Costley, 1984). Although some investigators have attributed the change in blood pressure to a concomitant reduction in sodium, which typically occurs on a hypocaloric diet (Dahl, Silver, & Christie, 1958), the results of more recent studies show that weight loss has an independent antihypertensive effect in the absence of sodium restriction (Reisin et al., 1978; Maxwell, Kushiro, Dornfeld, Tuck, & Waks, 1984).

Significant reductions in blood pressure in obese subjects do not require attainment of ideal body weight. A reduction of only 10% of initial body weight is associated with significant effects. In a study by Tuck and colleagues, a 10–30% weight loss reduced diastolic blood pressure by 15 mm Hg (Tuck, Sowers, Dornfeld, Kledzik, & Maxwell, 1981). Reisin et al. (1978) also showed that blood pressure was significantly reduced in overweight hypertensive patients placed on a dietary program. Patients lost a mean of 10.5 kg and did not achieve goal weight; however, both systolic and diastolic blood pressure were reduced by about 20 mm Hg, and the arterial pressure levels of 75% of the obese hypertensive patients treated only by weight loss returned to normal. Ramsay and colleagues found that a mean weight loss of 5.1 kg in overweight patients who received individual counseling from a dietitian resulted in reductions in systolic and diastolic blood pressure of 12 mm Hg and 7 mm Hg, respectively (Ramsay, Ramsay, Hettiarachchi, Davies, & Wichester, 1978). There was a highly significant correlation between weight loss and the fall in blood pressure. Regression equations predicted a blood pressure fall of 2.5/1.5 mm Hg per kilogram of weight loss, or a decrease of 25/15 mm Hg for a 10-kg loss.

In a study by MacMahon and colleagues, a 7.7-kg weight loss over 5 months in middle-aged obese hypertensive women was associated with a greater reduction in blood pressure than was either a beta blocker or a placebo, with an average drop of 1 mm Hg in systolic and diastolic blood pressure per kilogram of weight loss as compared with placebo (MacMahon, MacDonald, Bernstein, Andrews, & Blacket, 1985a). Modest weight loss has also been effective in improving blood pressure control in individuals taking antihypertensive medication (Oberman et al., 1990), and in reducing the risk factors for cardiovascular disease exacerbated by medication use (MacMahon, Mac-

TABLE 9.1. Changes in Weight and Blood Pressure (BP) from Baseline to Follow-up in Treatment (Rx) and Control Groups of Five Randomized Controlled Trials

	n		Follow-up (mo)	Weight change (kg)		Systolic BP change		Diastolic BP change	
	Rx	Control		Rx	Control	Rx	Control	Rx	Control
Diet trials									
Reisin et al. (1978)	57	26	4	−14.9	−1.2	−37.4	−6.9	−23.3	−2.5
Heyden (1978)	63	64	12	−8.1	−1.9	−18.0	−12.0	−13.0	−8.0
Ramsay et al. (1978)	15	34	12	−5.1	−2.4	−11.9	−8.9	−6.9	−4.4
Haynes et al. (1984)	30	30	6	−4.1	−0.8	+4.8	−0.2	+1.4	−0.1
MacMahon et al. (1985b)	20	18	5	−7.4	+0.5	−13.3	−7.4	−9.8	−3.1
Pooled estimates[a] (Rx vs. controls)									
Diet trials	185	172		−9.2		−6.3		−3.1	
(95% confidence limits)				(−8.2, −10.2)		(−3.3, −9.4)		(−1.5, −4.7)	
Pooled estimates[a] (Rx vs. controls)									
All trials	336	254		−8.7		−5.3		−3.3	
(95% confidence limits)				(−7.9, −9.5)		(−3.4, −7.3)		(−1.8, −4.7)	

Note. Adapted from "Obesity and Hypertension: Epidemiological and Clinical Issues" by S. W. MacMahon, J. Cutler, E. Brittain, and M. Higgins, 1987, *European Heart Journal*, 8(Suppl. B), 57–70. Copyright 1987 by Academic Press, Ltd. Adapted by permission.

[a] See MacMahon et al. (1987) for methods.

Donald, Bernstein, Andrews, & Blacket, 1985b). Elihou and colleagues treated 212 hypertensive patients by diet and weight loss; 42% of patients complied with the diet and lost at least 5% of their initial body weight (Elihou, Iaina, Gaon, Schochat, & Modan, 1981). The authors observed that two-thirds of the compliant patients achieved a normal blood pressure, even though they lost only half of their excess weight.

Long-Term Effects of Weight Loss on Hypertension

Only a handful of studies have investigated the long-term effects of weight loss on the control of hypertension. In two such studies, weight loss was shown to be effective in slowing or preventing the return of hypertension after prolonged drug treatment had produced a normotensive level (Stamler et al., 1987; Langford et al., 1985). Both studies reported losses of approximately 4-5 kg, which were largely maintained by patients for the duration of the study. Stamler et al. (1987) followed participants for 4 years and found that 40% of patients were able to remain normotensive (as compared to 5% among the control group), as well as to maintain much of their weight loss. Langford et al. (1985) showed that a mean weight loss of 4.5 kg, which represented a 5% reduction in initial body weight by the end of 1 year of treatment, was effective in lowering blood pressure and keeping patients off antihypertensive medication. In both studies, weight loss was clearly beneficial, despite participants remaining well above ideal weight.

The Dietary Intervention Therapy for Obese Hypertensives (DITOH) was a randomized trial in which we investigated the effects of weight loss on blood pressure in a population of obese hypertensives (diastolic blood pressure = 90–105 mm Hg) over 30 months (Blackburn, Kanders, Lavin, Pontes, & Greenberg, 1989). Patients were randomly assigned to one of two multidisciplinary weight loss regimens: a balanced-deficit diet (BDD) providing 1200 ± 200 kcal/day, or a very low calorie PSMF providing 1.5 g of protein per kilogram of ideal body weight. Patients in the BDD and the PSMF groups lost a mean of 12% and 17% of initial body weight, respectively, which correlated with drops of 15/9 mm Hg and 20/13 mm Hg, respectively. During the 6 months of active maintenance, patients in the BDD group showed a 2% weight gain with good control of blood pressure, while patients in the PSMF group experienced a 5% increase in body weight. Eighteen months later, patients in the BDD group showed a net loss of 4% of initial body weight, maintaining 38% of their original loss; patients in the PSMF group showed a net loss of 7% of initial weight, maintaining 41% of their original weight loss. At the end of 2½ years of treatment, patients in the BDD and PSMF groups had maintained an average loss of 5.0 and 7.3 kg, respectively. There were no significant differences between the groups with regard to net weight change or blood pressure. At the conclusion of this 5-year study, only 41% of all DITOH patients had started or resumed single-dose medication to control their blood pressure, whereas 75% had a history of hypertension medication use at baseline.

Reducing Primary Risk Factors

Finally, in a study previously described, which investigated health outcome following weight loss on a VLCD, significant reductions in blood pressure and blood pressure medication use were observed in patients who began treatment for hypertension (Kanders, Blackburn, Lavin, & Norton, 1989; Kanders, Blackburn, et al., 1991). Patients lost a mean of 20% of body weight during active weight loss. Thirty-nine percent of hypertensive patients had complete resolution of their disease, and another 15% had improvement. Significant reductions in the incidence and severity of hypertension were still noted at 18 months, despite some weight regain.

In considering the primary prevention of hypertension in those at risk for the disease, Stamler et al. (1989) reported a significant difference in the incidence of hypertension between a lifestyle intervention group (8.8%), which included weight loss, and a control group (19.2%). The relative risk for developing hypertension was 2.4 times greater in the control group than in the intervention group, which achieved a mean loss of 2.7 kg. In another study directed at prevention, the Hypertension Prevention Trial (1990), dietary intervention strategies (including reduction in dietary sodium, weight loss, and increased consumption of potassium) were evaluated for their ability to effect changes in blood pressure. The mean net weight loss attributable to calorie restriction was 5.8 kg (7% of initial body weight) at 6 months and 3.4 kg (4% of initial body weight) at 3 years, with corresponding decreases in diastolic blood pressure of 2.8 mm Hg and 1.8 mm Hg, respectively. Not surprisingly, the largest changes were observed during the initial treatment phase, although evidence of change did persist over the 3-year follow-up period.

Risks Associated with Drug Therapy

Drug treatment that lowers or normalizes blood pressure can reduce morbidity and mortality (Joint National Committee [JNC], 1988). There are, however, documented side effects of antihypertensive drugs. Thiazide diuretics, for example, can induce short-term increases in serum cholesterol, low density lipoprotein (LDL), and triglyceride levels (Kaplan, 1985). In addition, recent evidence has demonstrated that there is a J-shaped relationship between treated diastolic blood pressure levels and cardiac diseases, such that low diastolic blood pressure levels (i.e., below 85 mm Hg) that are treated are associated with increased risk of cardiac events (Farnett, Mulrow, Linn, Lucey, & Tuley, 1991). Finally, antihypertensive therapy to date has not reduced the risk of coronary disease to normal.

Although the reasons for this J-shaped relationship remain unclear, coronary heart disease is multifactorial, and reduction of blood pressure by pharmacological measures does nothing to address other risk factors. Nonpharmacological treatment of hypertension clearly deserves increased attention. In particular, nonpharmacological treatment involving weight loss tends to ameliorate other risk factors (e.g., cholesterol levels improve, insulin resistance improves, and patients may quit smoking or start an exercise program). Weight loss also has been shown to reduce left ventricular hypertrophy (MacMahon, Wilkens, & MacDonald, 1986).

The use of weight loss and other nonpharmacological treatments as the initial therapy for most patients, at least for the first 3 to 6 months after the diagnosis of hypertension, is now widely advocated (JNC, 1988). It has been suggested that control of obesity would eliminate hypertension in 48% of whites and 28% of blacks (Tyroler, Heyden, & Hames, 1975). Even if blood pressure is not reduced to normal by diet therapy alone, nondrug therapy can aid in reducing blood pressure without risk, so that less drug therapy will be needed. The results from research to date clearly demonstrate that weight reduction can have a substantial and sustained antihypertensive effect, while simultaneously improving other risk factors as well.

Cardiovascular Disease

Cardiovascular disease (CVD) currently ranks as the leading cause of death in the United States. Among the many factors that contribute to the development of CVD, obesity clearly plays a significant (though indirect) role by affecting other risk factors. Obesity is associated with elevations in blood pressure, blood lipids, and blood glucose, as well as with insulin resistance and hyperinsulinemia (VanItallie, 1979; MacMahon et al., 1987; Reaven, 1988). Weight loss is known to reduce these risk factors. Whether obesity serves as an independent risk factor for CVD remains controversial, though recent evidence suggest that it does.

The relationship between body weight and morbidity and mortality from heart disease was first noted in data collected from insurance companies. The death rate from CVD among overweight men was 49% higher than among average-weight men (Marks, 1960). In a later study, the American Cancer Society showed a linear relationship between self-reported weight and subsequent coronary heart disease (Lew & Garfinkel, 1979), with the risk of CVD approximately doubling in persons more than 40% above average weight.

Despite this evidence, the relationship between CVD and obesity remains a complex one, surrounded by controversy. Data from recent prospective studies indicate that obesity is an independent risk factor for CVD in women (Manson et al., 1990) and in men (Hubert et al., 1983). Manson et al. (1990) identified obesity as an independent determinant of coronary heart disease, even among middle-aged women who were only mildly to moderately overweight. The authors concluded that as much as 70% of the coronary disease observed among obese women, and 40% of that among women overall, is attributable to overweight.

Other studies have reported that obesity is not an independent risk factor for coronary heart disease. Manson and colleagues attribute this discrepancy to three factors: (1) failure to control for cigarette smokers, who have both higher mortality and lower body weight; (2) failure to take into account the impact of early mortality on longer-range morality trends; and (3) failure to control appropriately for the comorbid risk factors of obesity such as diabetes, hypertension, and hyperglycemia, which are intermediate steps in the etiology (Manson, Stampfer, Hennekens, & Willett, 1987). For example, data from the Framingham Study indicate that for every 10% rise in relative weight, systolic blood pressure rises 6.5 mm Hg, plasma cholesterol 12 mg/dl, and fasting blood glucose 2 mg/dl (Kannel & Gordon, 1979). The *Surgeon General's Report on Nutrition and Health* (U.S. DHHS, 1988) and the National Research Council's *Diet and Health* (Committee on Diet and Health, 1989) provide comprehensive reviews of clinical and epidemiological studies on CVD and obesity that reach similar findings.

To date, no clinical studies have specifically examined the effects of weight loss on morbidity and mortality from CVD. As discussed above, however, obesity is known to affect associated risk factors for CVD, and reduction in body weight is known to improve these health parameters. The positive effects of weight loss on glucose intolerance, insulin resistance, hyperinsulinemia, and hypertension have been discussed previously in this chapter; the remaining sections will address the relationships among obesity, changes in body weight, and other CVD risk factors, including hyperlipidemia, hypertriglyceridemia, and hyperestrogenemia.

Hyperlipidemia

Obesity is associated with an overproduction of cholesterol (Miettinen, 1973). For every excess kilogram of body weight, the rate of cholesterol synthesis increases by 22 mg/day (Schreibman & Deli, 1975). This abnormal production may not be reflected in plasma lipid and lipoprotein levels, and does not necessarily coexist with hyperlipidemia (McNamara, 1987). Indeed, only a marginal relationship has been shown to exist between cholesterol elevation and obesity (Montoye, Epstein, & Kjelsberg, 1966); total cholesterol levels may be elevated or normal. However, the ratio of LDL cholesterol to HDL cholesterol is typically elevated, thus increasing the risk of coronary heart disease. By decreasing total fat and calories, weight loss can have favorable effects on serum lipoprotein levels (Grundy, Mok, Zech, Steinberg, & Berman, 1979; Kesaniemi & Grundy, 1983). Weight gain is associated with a decrease in HDL cholesterol levels (Garrison et al., 1980), whereas weight loss is associated with an increase (Brownell, Bachorik, & Ayerlye, 1982; Sorbris, Petersson, & Nilsson-Ehlle, 1981; Wood et al., 1988). Wood et al. (1988) found that a loss of approximately 5 kg of body fat (equivalent to a 5-8% reduction in initial body weight) over 1 year, whether induced by dieting without exercising or by exercising without dieting, resulted in significant increases in plasma concentrations of HDL cholesterol, HDL_2 cholesterol (which has been associated with a decreased risk of coronary heart disease), and HDL_3 cholesterol. The ratio of total cholesterol to HDL cholesterol also improved with weight loss. Even modest weight loss (5-10%) has been shown to improve both total cholesterol and the more important LDL-HDL ratio (Wood et al., 1988; Sopko et al., 1985; Schwartz, 1987).

Hypertriglyceridemia

Hypertriglyceridemia also ranks as an important risk factor for CVD. Obesity may increase triglyceride levels, partly as a result of associated hyperinsulinemia. Evidence suggests that triglyceride levels are positively related both to weight gain (Albrink, Meigs, & Granoff, 1962) and to circulating insulin levels (Olefsky, Reaven, & Farquhar, 1974). In general, hyperinsulinemia and hypertriglyceridemia are both reversible with weight loss (Olefsky et al., 1974).

Hyperestrogenemia

Obese patients typically have increased estrogen levels, decreased serum testosterone, and an increase in the estrogen-to-testosterone ratio (Kley, Edelmann, & Kruskemper, 1980). Recent evidence supports the theory that hyperestrogenemia is a risk factor for CVD, though the exact mechanism remains unknown (Phillips, 1978). High estrogen levels and an increased estradiol-to-testosterone ratio are associated with hypercholesterolemia, hypertension, and diabetes, all of which are associated with CVD (Amodeo & Messerli, 1986). As with other risk factors for CVD, weight loss is known to reduce plasma estrogen levels (Stanik, Dornfeld, & Maxwell, 1981).

In summary, obesity has been shown by some to be an independent risk factor for CVD, although this is still a matter of debate. Numerous studies have demonstrated that obesity affects many of the other risk factors for CVD, including glucose tolerance, hypertension, and hyperlipidemia. In a review of nutrition and CVD, McNamara (1987) concluded that caloric intake and body weight have the largest single effect on cholesterol synthesis and on the incidence of hyperlipidemia, and that weight reduction is the most effective intervention for reducing hyperlipidemia. Weight reduction is also known to ameliorate other risk factors for CVD—namely, glucose intolerance, insulin resistance, hyperinsulinemia, hypertension, and hyperestrogenemia. Even modest weight losses of 10-20% will improve these risk factors (Blackburn & Kanders, 1987).

Obesity, Weight Loss, and Gallstone Formation

The increased media attention to dieting and symptomatic gallstones has provoked a widespread belief that weight loss causes gallbladder disease. We wish to clarify the relationship between weight loss and gallbladder disease in the obese patient by providing a brief review of the literature. As discussed, obesity is associated with an overproduction of cholesterol (Miettinen, 1973). This increased secretion of cholesterol in the bile leads to supersaturation of bile, and hence to greater risk of gallstone formation (Bennion & Grundy, 1975). Obese individuals develop more symptomatic and asymptomatic gallstones than do normal-weight adults, a trend that rises linearly with body mass index (Maclure et al., 1989). Other risk factors, including age, sex, triglyceride and HDL cholesterol levels, as well as duration of existing silent gallstones, can increase the risk for gallstone formation (Honig & Blackburn, 1991). Dieting—in particular, rapid weight loss—has been reported to increase the risk of gallstones in obese individuals (Broomfield et al., 1988). The mechanisms believed to be responsible for this increased risk include supersaturation of biliary cholesterol and gallbladder stasis, both of which can occur during severe caloric restriction (Liddle, Goldstein, & Saxton, 1989; Bennion & Grundy, 1975). However, weight loss need not lead to gallstone formation in the obese. Diets that (1) provide adequate amounts of protein and fat (i.e., 14 g of protein and 10 g of fat at one meal at least once daily, to ensure adequate gallbladder contraction; Gebhard, Ansel, Peterson, & Stone, 1990); (2) limit weight loss to 2% or less per week; and (3) are 12 weeks or less in duration reduce or eliminate the risk of gallstone formation (Honig & Blackburn, 1991). Reduced-obese patients have, at the cessation of weight loss, a risk of gallstone formation that is comparable to that in the nonobese population (Honig & Blackburn, 1991). Thus, with careful monitoring and appropriate treatment, weight loss can indeed reduce the risk of gallstone formation.

Summary

Obesity is associated with increased risk of several disorders, including hypertension, diabetes, and CVD. Weight loss is known to reduce these risks. Successful treatment of obesity should not be defined as "reduction to desired weight and maintenance of that weight for five years," as has been suggested (Council on Scientific Affairs, 1988, p. 2547). Instead, a 10-20% reduction in initial body weight, with maintenance of at least half of this weight loss over 2-5 years, has been shown to be sufficient to maintain health benefits. This degree of weight loss can ameliorate hypertension, diabetes, and CVD, and can also reduce other risk factors in the obese patient.

State-of-the-art treatment of obesity is comprehensive and includes dietary change, increased physical activity, and other lifestyle modifications (Kanders, Forse, & Blackburn, 1991). Because weight regain represents the major barrier to the management of medically significant obesity, and because weight cycling has been shown to be detrimental to health (Lissner et al., 1991), it is imperative that patients remain in treatment for 1-2 years beyond the period of initial weight loss. After this maintenance phase, an intensive weight loss program may be repeated to reduce body weight further or to minimize recidivism. Future research is needed to isolate factors that promote the long-term control of body weight in the postobese patient. In the meantime, a new criterion of a 10-20% reduction in initial weight in patients with medically significant obesity represents a realistic treatment goal for the majority of patients, and one that will reduce the risk of disease and improve overall health.

References

Albrink, M. J., Meigs, J. W., & Granoff, M. A. (1962). Weight gain and serum triglycerides in normal men. *New England Journal of Medicine, 266*, 484-489.
Amodeo, C., & Messerli, F. H. (1986). Risk for obesity. *Cardiology Clinics, 4*(1), 75-80.
Bennion, L. J., & Grundy, S. (1975). Effects of obesity and caloric intake on biliary lipid metabolism in man. *Journal of Clinical Investigation, 56*, 996-1011.
Blackburn, G. L., Kanders, B. S., Lavin, P., Pontes, M., & Greenberg, I. (1989). Dietary intervention therapy for obese hypertensives. *Circulation, 80*, 284. (Abstract No. 1134)
Blackburn, G. L., & Kanders, B. S. (1987). Medical evaluation of the obese patient with cardiovascular disease. *American Journal of Cardiology, 60*, 556-586.
Broomfield, P. H., Chopra, R., Scheinbaus, R. C., Bonorris, G. G., Silverman, A., Schoenfield, L. J., & Marks, J. W. (1988). Effects of ursodeoxycholic acid and aspirin on the formation of lithogenic bile and gallstones during loss of weight. *New England Journal of Medicine, 319*, 1567-1572.
Brownell, K. D., Bachorik, P. S., & Ayerlye, R. S. (1982). Changes in plasma lipid and lipoprotein levels in men and women after a program of moderate exercise. *Circulation, 65*, 477-484.
Committee on Diet and Health, Food and Nutrition Board, Commission of Life Sciences, National Research Council. (1989). *Diet and health: Implications for reducing chronic disease risk.* Washington, DC: National Academy Press.
Council on Scientific Affairs, American Medical Association. (1988). Treatment of obesity in adults. *Journal of the American Medical Association, 260*, 2547-2551.
Dahl, L. K., Silver, L., & Christie, R. (1958). Role of salt in the fall of blood pressure accompanying reduction of obesity. *New England Journal of Medicine, 258*, 1186-1192.
Defronzo, R. A., Ferrannini, E., & Koivisto, V. (1983). New concepts in the pathogenesis and treatment of noninsulin-dependent diabetes mellitus. *American Journal of Medicine, 74*, 52-81.
D'Eramo, G., Wylie-Rosett, J., & Hagan, J. (1986). Intensity of education in Type II NIDDM: Effect on weight, glycosylated hemoglobin, and knowledge. *Diabetes, 5*, 49A.
Doar, J. W., Wilde, C. E., Thompson, M. E., & Sewell, P. F. (1975). Influence of treatment with diet alone on oral glucose-tolerance test and plasma sugar and insulin levels in patients with maturity onset diabetes mellitus. *Lancet, i*, 1263-1266.
Dustan, H. P. (1983). Mechanisms of hypertension associated with obesity. *Annals of Internal Medicine, 98*(Suppl.), 860-863.
Elihou, H. E., Iaina, A., Gaon, T., Schochat, J., & Modan, M. (1981). Body weight reduction necessary to attain normotension in the overweight hypertensive patient. *International Journal of Obesity, 5*(Suppl. 1), 157-163.
Fagerberg, B., Anderson, O. K., Isaksson, B., & Björntorp, P. (1984). Blood pressure control during weight reduction in obese hypertensive men: Separate effects of sodium and energy restriction. *British Medical Journal, 228*, 11-14.
Farnett, L., Mulrow, C. D., Linn, W. D., Lucey, C. R., & Tuley, M. R. (1991). The J-curve phenomenon and the treatment of hypertension: Is there a point beyond which pressure reduction is dangerous? *Journal of the American Medical Association, 265*, 489-495.

Fitz, J. D., Sperling, E. M., & Fein, H. G. (1983). A hypocaloric high-protein diet as primary therapy for adults with obesity-related diabetes: Effective long-term use in community hospital. *Diabetes Care, 6,* 328-332.

Flood, T. M., Halford, B. N., Coopan, R., & Marble, A. (1985). Dietary management in diabetes. In A. Marble, L. P. Krall, R. G. Bradley, A. R. Christlieb, & J. S. Soeldner (Eds.), *Joslin's diabetes mellitus* (pp. 357-373). Philadelphia: Lea & Febiger.

Garrison, R. J., Kannel, W. B., & Stokes, J. (1985). *CVD Lipid Newsletter, 37,* 7-9. (Abstract No. 50)

Garrison, R. J., Wilson, P. W., Castelli, W. P., Feinleib, M., Kannel, W. B., & McNamara, P. M. (1980). Obesity and lipoprotein cholesterol in the Framingham Offspring Study. *Metabolism, 29,* 1053-1060.

Gebhard, R. L., Ansel, H. J., Peterson, F. J., & Stone, B. G. (1990). Gallbladder emptying stimuli in obese and normal weight subjects. *Hepatology, 12,* 898. (Abstract)

Gordon, T., Castelli, W. P., Hjortland, C., Kannel, L. W., & Dawber, T. R. (1977). Diabetes, blood lipids and the role of obesity in coronary heart disease risk for women: The Framingham Study. *Annals of Internal Medicine, 87,* 393-397.

Greenfield, M., Kolterman, O., Olefsky, J. M., & Reaven, G. M. (1978). The effect of ten days of fasting on various aspects of carbohydrate metabolism in obese diabetic subjects with significant fasting hyperglycemia. *Metabolism, 27,* 1839-1852.

Grundy, S. M., Mok, H. Y., Zech, L., Steinberg, D., & Berman, M. (1979). Transport of very low density lipoprotein triglycerides in varying degrees of obesity and hypertriglyceridemia. *Journal of Clinical Investigation, 63,* 1274-1283.

Hadden, D. R., Montgomery, D. A., Skelly, R. J., Trimble, E. R., Weaver, J. A., Wilson, E. A., & Buchanan, K. D. (1975). Maturity onset diabetes mellitus: Response to intensive dietary management. *British Medical Journal, iii,* 276-278.

Havlik, R. J., Hubert, H. B., Fabsitz, R., & Feinleib, M. (1983). Weight and hypertension. *Annals of Internal Medicine, 98*(Pt. 2), 855-859.

Haynes, A. B., Harper, A. C., & Costley, S. R. (1984). Failure of weight reduction to reduce mildly elevated blood pressure: A randomized trial. *Journal of Hypertension, 2,* 535-539.

Henry, R. R., Wallace, P., & Olefsky, J. M. (1986). Effects of weight loss on mechanisms of hyperglycemia in obese non-insulin-dependent diabetes mellitus. *Diabetes, 35,* 990-998.

Henry, R. R., Wiest-Kent, T. A., & Schaeffer, L. (1986). Very low calorie diet therapy in obese non insulin dependent diabetic and non-diabetic subjects. *Diabetes, 35,* 155-164.

Heyden, S. (1978). The working man's diet. II. Effect of weight reduction in obese patients with hypertension, diabetes, hyperuricemia and hyperlipidemia. *Nutrition and Metabolism, 22,* 141-159.

Honig, J. F., & Blackburn, G. L. (1991). *Practice guidelines for preventing symptomatic gallstones during obesity treatment.* Manuscript submitted for publication.

Hubert, H. B., Feinleib, M., McNamara, P., & Castelli, W. P. (1983). Obesity as an independent risk factor for cardiovascular disease: A 26 year follow-up of participants in the Framingham Study. *Circulation, 67,* 968-977.

Hughes, T. A., Gwynne, J. T., Switzer, B. R., Herbet, C., & White, G. (1984). Effects of caloric restriction and weight loss on glycemic control, insulin release and resistance, and atherosclerotic risk in obese patients with Type II diabetes mellitus. *American Journal of Medicine, 77,* 7-17.

Hypertension Prevention Trial Research Group. (1990). The Hypertension Prevention Trial: Three-year effects of dietary change on blood pressure. *Archives of Internal Medicine, 150,* 153-162.

Istfan, N. W., Plaisted, C. S., Bistrian, B. R., & Blackburn, G. L. (1992). Insulin resistance versus insulin secretion in the hypertension of obesity. *Hypertension, 19*(4).

Joint National Committee (JNC) on Detection, Evaluation, and Treatment of High Blood Pressure. (1988). The 1988 report of the Joint National Committee on Detection, Evaluation, and Treatment of High Blood Pressure. *Archives of Internal Medicine, 148,* 1023-1038.

Kanders, B. S., Blackburn, G. L., Lavin, P. T., & Norton, D. (1989). Weight-loss outcome and health benefits associated with the Optifast Program in the treatment of obesity. *International Journal of Obesity, 13*(Suppl. 2), 131-134.

Kanders, B. S., Blackburn, G. L., Lavin, P. T., Norton, D., Peterson, F. J., & Istfan, N. (1991). *Long-term health effects of obesity treatment with a multidisciplinary very-low-calorie diet program: Change in diabetes and hypertension.* Manuscript submitted for publication.

Kanders, B. S., Forse, A., & Blackburn, G. L. (1991). Method of obesity. In R. E. Rakel (Ed.), *Conn's current therapy 1991* (pp. 524-531). Philadelphia: W. B. Saunders.

Kannel, W. B., Brand, N., Skinner, J. J., Jr., Dawber, T. R., & McNamara, P. (1967). The relation of adiposity to blood pressure and the development of hypertension: The Framingham Study. *Annals of Internal Medicine, 67*, 48-59.

Kannel, W. B., & Gordon, T. (1979). Physiological and medical concomitants of obesity: The Framingham Study. In G. Bray (Ed.), *Obesity in America* (DHEW Publication No. NIH 79-359, pp. 125-163). Washington, DC: U.S. Government Printing Office.

Kaplan, N. M. (1985). Non-drug treatment of hypertension. *Annals of Internal Medicine, 1102*, 359-373.

Kesaniemi, Y. A., & Grundy, S. M. (1983). Increased low density lipoprotein production associated with obesity. *Arteriosclerosis, 3*, 170-177.

Kirschner, M. A., Schneider, G., Ertel, N. H., & Gorman, J. (1988). An eight-year experience with a very-low-calorie formula diet for control of major obesity. *International Journal of Obesity, 12*, 69-80.

Kley, H. K., Edelmann, P., & Kruskemper, H. L. (1980). Relationship of plasma sex hormones to different parameters of obesity in male subjects. *Metabolism, 29*, 1041-1045.

Koch, H., & Knapp, D. A. (1987). *Advance data from vital and health statistics* (DHHS Publication No. PHS 87-1250). Washington, DC: U.S. Government Printing Office.

Langford, H. G., Blaufox, M. D., Oberman, A., Hawkins, C. M., Curb, J. D., Cutter, G. R., Wassertheil-Smoller, S., Pressel, S., Babcock, C., Abernethy, J. D., Hotchkiss, J., & Tyler, M. (1985). Dietary therapy slows the return of hypertension after stopping prolonged medication. *Journal of the American Medical Association, 253*, 657-664.

Leibel, R. L., & Hirsch, J. (1984). Diminished energy requirements in reduced-obese patients. *Metabolism, 33*, 164-170.

Lenfant, C., & Roccella, E. J. (1984). Trends in hypertension control in the United States. *Chest, 86*, 459-462.

Lew, E. A., & Garfinkel, L. (1979). Variations in mortality by weight among 750,000 men and women. *Journal of Chronic Disease, 32*, 563-576.

Liddle, R. A., Goldstein, R. B., & Saxton, J. (1989). Gallstone formation during weight-reduction dieting. *Archives of Internal Medicine, 149*, 1750-1753.

Lissner, L., Odell, P. M., D'Agostino, R. B., Stokes, J., Kreger, B. E., Belanger, A. J., & Brownell, K. D. (1991). Variability of body weight and health outcomes in the Framingham population. *New England Journal of Medicine, 324*, 1839-1844.

Maclure, M. K., Hayes, K. C., Colditz, G. A., Stampfer, M. J., Speizer, F. E., & Willett, W. (1989). Weight, diet, and the risk of symptomatic gallstones in middle-aged women. *New England Journal of Medicine, 321*, 563-569.

MacMahon, S. W., Blacket, R. B., MacDonald, G. J., & Hall, W. (1984). Obesity, alcohol consumption and blood pressure in Australian men and women: The National Heart Foundation of Australia Risk Factor Prevalence Study. *Journal of Hypertension, 2*, 85-91.

MacMahon, S. W., Cutler, J., Brittain, E., & Higgins, M. (1987). Obesity and hypertension: Epidemiological and clinical issues. *European Heart Journal, 8*(Suppl. B), 57-70.

MacMahon, S. W., MacDonald, G. J., Bernstein, L., Andrews, G., & Blacket, R. B. (1985a). A randomized controlled trial of weight reduction and metoprolol in the treatment of hypertension in young overweight patients. *Clinical and Experimental Pharmacology and Physiology, 12*, 267-271.

MacMahon, S. W., MacDonald, G. J., Bernstein, L., Andrews, G., & Blacket, R. B. (1985b). Comparison of weight reduction with metoprolol in treatment of hypertension in young overweight patients. *Lancet, i,* 1233-1236.

MacMahon, S. W., Wilkens, D. E., & MacDonald, G. J. (1986). The effect of weight reduction on left ventricular mass: A randomized controlled trial in young overweight hypertensives. *New England Journal of Medicine, 314,* 334-339.

Mancini, M., Di Biase, G., Contaldo, F., Fischetti, A., Grasso, L., & Mattiolli, P. (1981). Medical complications of severe obesity: Importance of treatment by very-low-calorie diets: Intermediate and long-term effects. *International Journal of Obesity, 5,* 341-352.

Manson, J. E., Colditz, G. A., Stampfer, M. J., Willett, W., Rosner, B., Monson, R. R., Speizer, F. E., & Hennekens, C. H. (1990). A prospective study of obesity and risk of coronary heart disease in women. *New England Journal of Medicine, 322,* 882-889.

Manson, J. E., Stampfer, M. J., Hennekens, C. H., & Willett, W. C. (1987). Body weight and longevity: Reassessment. *Journal of the American Medical Association, 257,* 353-358.

Marks, H. K. (1960). Influence of obesity on morbidity and mortality. *Bulletin of the New York Academy of Medicine, 36,* 296-312.

Maxwell, M. H., Kushiro, T., Dornfeld, L. P., Tuck, M. L., & Waks, A. U. (1984). Blood pressure changes in obese hypertensive subjects during rapid weight loss: Comparison of restricted versus unchanged salt intake. *Archives of Internal Medicine, 144,* 1581-1584.

McLemore, T., & DeLozier, J. (1987). *Advance data from vital and health statistics* (DHHS Publication No. PHS 87-1250). Washington, DC: U.S. Government Printing Office.

McNamara, D. J. (1987). Nutrition and cholesterol metabolism. In R. R. Watson (Ed.), *Nutrition and heart disease* (Vol. 1, pp. 29-44). Boca Raton, FL: CRC Press.

Miettinen, T. A. (1973). Cholesterol production in obesity. *Circulation, 44,* 842-848.

Montoye, J. J., Epstein, F. H., & Kjelsberg, M. O. (1966). Relationship between serum cholesterol and body fatness: An epidemiologic study. *American Journal of Clinical Nutrition, 18,* 397-406.

National Institutes of Health (NIH). (1987). Consensus development conference on diet and exercise in non-insulin-dependent diabetes mellitus. *Diabetes Care, 10,* 639-644.

Oberman, A., Wassertheil-Smoller, S., Langford, H. G., Blaufox, M. D., Davis, B. R., Blaszkowski, T., Zimbaldi, N., & Hawkins, C. M. (1990). Pharmacologic and nutritional treatment of mild hypertension: Changes in cardiovascular risk status. *Annals of Internal Medicine, 112,* 89-94.

Olefsky, J. M., Kolterman, O. G., & Scarlett, J. A. (1982). Insulin action and resistance in obesity and non-insulin dependent Type II diabetes mellitus. *American Journal of Physiology, 243,* E15-E30.

Olefsky, J. M., Reaven, G. M., & Farquhar, J. W. (1974). Effects of weight reduction on obesity: Studies of lipid and carbohydrate metabolism in normal and hyperlipoproteinemic subjects. *Journal of Clinical Investigation, 53,* 64-76.

Phillips, G. B. (1978). Sex hormones, risk factors and cardiovascular disease. *American Journal of Medicine, 65,* 7-11.

Ramsay, L. E., Ramsay, M. H., Hettiarachchi, J., Davies, D. L., & Wichester, J. (1978). Weight reduction in a blood pressure clinic. *British Medical Journal, ii,* 244-245.

Reckless, J. P., Betleridge, D. J., Wu, P., Payne, B., & Galton, D. J. (1978). High density and low density lipoproteins and prevalence of vascular disease in diabetes mellitus. *British Medical Journal, i,* 883-886.

Reaven, G. M. (1988). Role of insulin resistance in human disease. *Diabetes, 37,* 1595-1607.

Reisin, E., Skel, R., Modan, M., Silverberg, D. S., Eliahou, H. E., & Modan, B. (1978). Effect of weight loss without salt restriction on the reduction of blood pressure in overweight hypertensive patients. *New England Journal of Medicine, 298,* 1-6.

Schreibman, P. H., & Deli, R. B. (1975). Human adipocyte cholesterol: Concentration, localization, synthesis and turnover. *Journal of Clinical Investigation, 55,* 986-993.

Schwartz, R. S. (1987). The independent effects of dietary weight loss and aerobic training on high density lipoproteins and apolipoprotein A-I concentrations in obese men. *Metabolism, 36*, 165–171.

Sopko, G., Leon, A. S., Jacobs, D., Foster, N., Moy, J., Kuba, K., Anderson, J. T., Casal, D., McNally, C., & Frantz, T. (1985). The effects of exercise and weight loss on plasma lipids in young obese men. *Metabolism, 24*, 227–236.

Sorbris, R., Petersson, B. G., & Nilsson-Ehlle, P. (1981). Effect of weight reduction on plasma lipoproteins and adipose tissue metabolism in obese subjects. *European Journal of Clinical Investigation, 11*, 491–498.

Stamler, R., Stamler, J., Gosch, F. C., Civinelli, J., Fishman, J., McKeever, P., McDonald, A., & Dyer, A. R. (1989). Primary prevention of hypertension by nutritional-hygienic means: Final report of a randomized, controlled trial. *Journal of the American Medical Association, 262*, 1801–1807.

Stamler, R., Stamler, J., Grimm, R., Gosch, F. C., Elmer, P., Dyer, A., Berman, R., Fishman, J., Van Heel, N., Civinelli, J., & McDonald, A. (1987). Nutritional therapy for high blood pressure: Final report of four year randomized controlled trial—the Hypertension Control Program. *Journal of the American Medical Association, 257*, 1484–1491.

Stanik, S., Dornfeld, L. P., & Maxwell, M. H. (1981). The effect of weight loss on reproductive hormones in obese men. *Journal of Clinical Endocrinology and Metabolism, 53*, 828–832.

Tuck, M. L., Sowers, L., Dornfeld, G., Kledzik, G., & Maxwell, M. (1981). The effect of weight reduction on blood pressure, plasma renin activity, and plasma aldosterone levels in obese patients. *New England Journal of Medicine, 304*, 930–933.

Tyroler, H. A., Heyden, S., & Hames, C. G. (1975). Weight and hypertension: Evans County studies of blacks and whites. In O. Paul (Ed.), *Epidemiology and control of hypertension* (pp. 177–205). New York: Grune & Stratton.

U.S. Department of Health and Human Services (DHHS). (1988). *Surgeon General's report on nutrition and health* (DHHS Publication No. PHS 88-50210). Washington, DC: U.S. Government Printing Office.

VanItallie, T. B. (1979). Obesity: Adverse effects on health and longevity. *American Journal of Clinical Nutrition, 32*(Suppl.), 2723–2733.

Watts, N. B., Spanheimer, R. G., DiGirolamo, M., Gebhart, S. S., Musey, V. C., Siddiq, K, & Phillips, L. S. (1990). Prediction of glucose response to weight loss in patients with non-insulin-dependent diabetes mellitus. *Archives of Internal Medicine, 150*, 803–806.

Wing, R. R., Epstein, L. H., Norwalk, M. P., Koeske, R., & Haag, S. (1985). Behavioral change, weight loss, and physiological improvement in Type II diabetic patients. *Journal of Consulting and Clinical Psychology, 53*, 111–122.

Wing, R. R., Koeske, R., Epstein, L. H., Norwalk, M. P., Booding, W., & Becker, D. (1987). Long-term effects of modest weight loss of Type II diabetic patients. *Archives of Internal Medicine, 147*, 1749–1753.

Wood, P. D., Stefanick, M. L., Dreon, D. M., Frey-Hewitt, B., Garay, S. C., Williams, P. T., Superko, H. R., Fortmann, S. P., Albers, J. J., Vranizan, K. M., Ellsworth, N. M., Terry, R. B., & Haskell, W. L. (1988). Changes in plasma lipids and lipoproteins in overweight men during weight loss through dieting as compared with exercise. *New England Journal of Medicine, 319*, 1173–1179.

10

Very Low Calorie Diets in the Treatment of Type II Diabetes: Psychological and Physiological Effects

RENA R. WING

Diabetes is a major health problem in the United States; it is estimated to affect 12 million individuals and costs $20 billion per year. The major form of diabetes is Type II, or non-insulin-dependent diabetes mellitus (NIDDM), which affects approximately 90% of the diabetic population. This form of diabetes usually occurs in midlife and is strongly associated with obesity.

The treatment of choice for obese Type II diabetic patients is weight loss. However, producing long-term weight loss among diabetic patients, as among nondiabetics, has proven to be very difficult. Very low calorie diets (VLCDs) show promise in the treatment of obese Type II diabetic subjects. These diets appear to be well tolerated by diabetic patients and can produce dramatic improvements in glycemic control. The goal of this chapter is to review the literature on the use of VLCDs in the treatment of Type II diabetes and to highlight directions for future research.

The Link between Obesity and Diabetes

Evidence of the effect of obesity on diabetes comes from various types of research, including the cross-cultural comparisons of West (1978), which show that populations with the greatest prevalence of obesity have the highest prevalence of diabetes. In data from the second National Health and Nutrition Examination Survey (NHANES II), the relative risk of diabetes among overweight individuals aged 20–79 was 2.9 times that of nonoverweight individuals of comparable age (VanItallie, 1985). The effect of obesity was particularly striking among younger individuals. In those aged 20–45, the relative risk of diabetes among the overweight was 3.8 times that of nonoverweight individuals. Among those aged 45–75, the relative risk was 2.1 times that of nonoverweight individuals.

Several prospective studies also have demonstrated a relationship between obesity and the subsequent incidence of diabetes (Knowler, Pettitt, Savage, & Bennett, 1981; Westlund & Nicolaysen, 1972). These studies show a nonlinear relationship between obesity and diabetes. Thus, there is only a modest relationship between weight and diabetes over the majority of the weight distribution, but a substantial increase in diabetes in the most obese individuals (Jarret, 1989).

Body fat distribution, independent of obesity, is also related to Type II diabetes. Vague (1956) reported that upper body obesity (i.e., android obesity) was more prevalent than lower body obesity (i.e., gynoid obesity) in diabetic patients. This finding has been confirmed by others; moreover, upper body obesity has been related prospectively to the incidence of Type II diabetes. In a study of 792 males aged 54 years, who were followed for 13½ years, Ohlson et al. (1985) found that upper body fat distribution and body mass index (BMI) both contributed independently to the probability of developing diabetes. The highest risk of developing diabetes occurred in those men who were in the highest tertile of obesity and the highest tertile of upper body obesity, as measured by the waist-to-hip ratio (Figure 10.1).

Despite the strong relationship between diabetes and obesity, it is clear that not all obese individuals become diabetic and not all diabetic patients are obese. Type II diabetes has a strong genetic component, predisposing individuals to the development of the disease. Recent evidence suggests that obesity and genetic predisposition may interact in determining the risk of diabetes. Data from the Pima Indians (Figure 10.2) show that the incidence of Type II diabetes is greatest in those who are obese and have one or two parents with diabetes (Knowler et al., 1981). Thus, obesity, body fat distribution, and family history of diabetes may all contribute to increasing the risk of Type II diabetes.

Obesity and Complications among Diabetic Patients

Diabetes is a major cause of blindness, kidney disease, and amputations; it is also the seventh leading cause of death in the United States, mainly through its association with coronary heart disease (CHD). However, there has been only limited research on the relationship between obesity and the development of complications among diabetic subjects. Reviewing this literature, Barrett-Connor (1989) concluded that the evidence did not clearly indicate that obesity increased the risk of complications or mortality among diabetic subjects. Pirart (1979) found that obese diabetic subjects had increased retinopathy and nephropathy, compared to leaner diabetics. Although Ballard et al. (1986) replicated this finding for retinopathy, others have failed to find any relationship between obesity and retinopathy or have found a negative relationship (Knowler, Bennett, & Ballintine, 1980; Klein, Klein, Moss, Davis, & DeMets, 1984). In the Framingham Study, obesity combined with diabetes increased

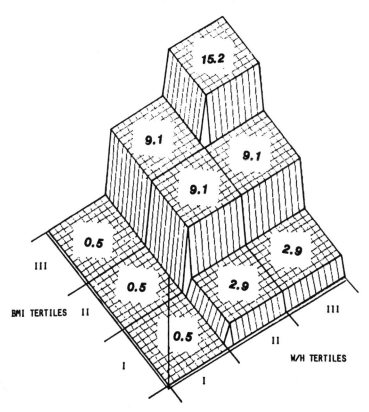

FIGURE 10.1. Percentage probability (isotonized figures) of developing diabetes mellitus during 13.5 years in relation to tertiles of initial body mass index (BMI) and waist-to-hip circumference ratio (W/H). From "The Influence of Body Fat Distribution on the Incidence of Diabetes Mellitus" (p. 1057) by L. O. Ohlson, B. Larsson, K. Svardsudd, L. Welin, J. Eriksson, L. Wilhelmsen, P. Björntorp, & G. Tibblin, 1985, *Diabetes, 34*, 1055-1058. Copyright 1985 by American Diabetes Association. Reprinted by permission.

mortality risk. The mortality ratio for those individuals who were 20-30% above ideal body weight was 2.5 to 3.3 times that of diabetic patients of normal weight. For patients whose weight was ≥40% of ideal body weight, the mortality ratio was 5.2-7.9 times that of normal-weight diabetics. More recently, Manson et al. (1990) reported prospective data on the risk of CHD in 115,886 women aged 30-55, who were followed for 8.5 years. Their results, reprinted in Figure 10.3, showed that the combination of obesity and diabetes markedly increased the risk of fatal and nonfatal CHD combined. Whereas nonobese diabetic subjects had only a twofold risk of CHD compared to nonobese nondiabetics, diabetic women who had a BMI of ≥29 had a 12-fold increase in risk.

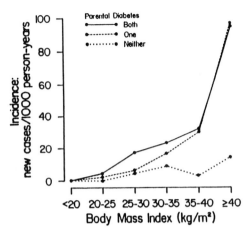

FIGURE 10.2. Age-adjusted incidence of diabetes in Pima Indians according to body mass index. Rates are shown for subjects aged 5 through 44 years with two nondiabetic parents, parents discordant for diabetes, and two diabetic parents. Parents' diabetic status was determined by glucose tolerance testing. From "Diabetes Incidence in Pima Indians: Contributions of Obesity and Parental Diabetes" (p. 152) by W. C. Knowler, D. J. Pettitt, P. J. Savage, & P. H. Bennett, 1981, *American Journal of Epidemiology, 113*, 144–156. Copyright 1981 by *American Journal of Epidemiology*. Reprinted by permission.

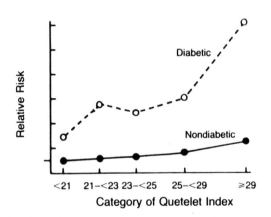

FIGURE 10.3. Relative risks of nonfatal myocardial infarction and fatal coronary heart disease (combined), according to Quetelet index and coronary risk factor status, after adjustment for age and smoking. The reference group comprised the women in the leanest Quetelet index category who did not have the specified coronary risk factor. The diabetic group included women who received their diagnosis at ≥30 years of age. From "A Prospective Study of Obesity and Risk of Coronary Heart Disease in Women" (p. 886) by J. E. Manson, G. A. Colditz, M. J. Stampfer, W. C. Willett, B. Rosner, R. R. Monson, F. E. Speizer, and C. H. Hennekens, 1990, *New England Journal of Medicine, 322*, 882–889. Copyright 1990 by *New England Journal of Medicine*. Reprinted by permission.

The Acute Effect of Weight Loss on Glycemic Control in Type II Diabetes

The majority of studies investigating the effect of weight loss on glycemic control and on the mechanisms of hyperglycemia have utilized VLCDs. Most of these studies have been conducted on metabolic wards, with liquid diets of 300–500 kilocalories (kcal) per day, and have lasted 2–5 weeks. These studies show rapid improvements in glycemic control with VLCDs. For example, Henry and colleagues treated 10 obese Type II diabetic subjects with a 300-kcal/day diet for a period of 36 days (Henry, Wiest-Kent, Scheaffer, Kolterman, & Olefsky, 1986). Weight loss averaged 11.1 kg during this time (loss of 0.28–0.34 kg/day), and fasting glucose decreased from 291 mg/dl to 95 mg/dl. However, the majority of the improvement in fasting blood sugar occurred by day 10, when it had declined to 120 mg/dl. Lipid levels normalized within the 36 days, with triglycerides reduced from 153 to 95 mg/dl and cholesterol from 174 to 129 mg/dl. Insulin levels decreased from 34 to 16 μU/ml, indicating an increase in insulin sensitivity.

The hyperglycemia seen in obese Type II diabetics is due to a combination of decreased insulin secretion, elevated rates of hepatic glucose output (HGO), and peripheral insulin resistance (Kahn & Porte, 1990). Recent studies suggest that each of these mechanisms can be improved with weight loss. Henry, Wallace, and Olefsky (1986) reported that obese subjects with diabetes had elevated levels of HGO, and noted a correlation of .91 between fasting glucose and HGO. When these subjects were placed on a VLCD and restudied after a weight loss of 16.8 kg, they had marked reductions in fasting blood sugar (277 to 123 mg/dl) and marked reductions in HGO (138 to 87 mg $\cdot$ m^{-2} $\cdot$ min^{-1}). Moreover, there was a correlation of .74 between improvements in fasting glucose and decreases in HGO, suggesting that the majority of the change in fasting levels was due to decreased HGO.

The improvement in postprandial hyperglycemia appears to result from decreased peripheral insulin resistance, which in turn is due to improved postreceptor insulin action (Henry, Wallace, & Olefsky, 1986). Although weight loss does not appear to normalize insulin sensitivity (Greenfield, Kolterman, Olefsky, & Reaven, 1978), it does improve sensitivity by 25–70% (Greenfield et al., 1978; Laasko et al., 1988; Hughes, Gwynne, Switzer, Herbst, & White, 1984).

Changes in insulin secretion have also been observed with weight loss. A recent study by Gumbiner et al. (1990) found that weight loss improved the impaired beta cell responsivity to both absolute and incremental changes in blood sugar. Increases in insulin secretion may occur mainly in those with severe hyperglycemia at pretreatment (Stanik & Marcus, 1980).

Although VLCDs produce dramatic improvements in glycemic control, similar effects can be achieved with more modest restriction. Bauman, Schwartz, Rose, Eisenstein, and Johnson (1988) retrospectively evaluated 64 subjects with Type II diabetes who were hospitalized for an average of 23 days and treated with a 909-kcal/day diet. Patients entered treatment weighing 105.9 kg and lost an average of 5.9 kg ($M = 0.27$ kg/day). Weight loss per day was thus not markedly different from that achieved by Henry, Wiest-Kent, et al. (1986) using a 300-kcal/day regimen. Moreover, fasting glucose levels were dramatically improved even with this more moderate diet; fasting levels of plasma glucose decreased from 221 mg/dl at baseline to 122 mg/dl, and 70% of patients achieved fasting levels of <125 mg/dl. At entry, 1 subject was treated with diet only, 21 with drugs, and 42 with insulin; of the 42 subjects on insulin, 40 could be discharged off insulin. Thus, these authors feel that severe caloric restriction is unnecessary to achieve an acute therapeutic response.

Weight Loss versus Calorie Restriction

One of the interesting questions in this area of research is whether calorie restriction or weight loss is responsible for the improvement in glycemic control. As noted above, marked improvements in blood sugar occur within 10 days, before any substantial weight loss has occurred, raising the possibility that it is calorie restriction that is fundamentally important. A study by Henry, Scheaffer, and Olefsky (1985) suggests that calorie restriction and weight loss may both contribute to the improvement in control. Thirty obese subjects with NIDDM were studied over 40 days while consuming a diet of 330 kcal/day. Weight losses averaged 4.6 kg after 10 days, 7.1 kg at 20 days, and 10.5 kg at 40 days. Despite this steady pattern of weight loss, the majority (89%) of the improvement in fasting glucose occurred after 10 days (297 to 158 mg/dl), with a further reduction to 138 mg/dl on day 40. Twelve of the subjects were treated with longer periods of VLCD (40–180 days) and then refed with a weight maintenance diet (25–30 kcal/kg) for 40 days. These subjects lost an average of 17.8 kg during the initial fast and regained 1.5 kg over the 40 days of refeeding. Although they maintained the majority of their weight loss, they experienced worsening of their glycemic control (Figure 10.4). Fasting glucose decreased from 254 mg/dl at baseline to 93 mg/dl after the fast, and then rose to 167 mg/dl by day 40 of refeeding. The level achieved after the refeeding period was thus midway between the other two values, and differed significantly from both, suggesting that both weight loss and calorie restriction may affect glycemic control. The increase in glucose observed during the refeeding period varied markedly among subjects, but was unrelated to the duration of the fast, calories consumed during refeeding, or the magnitude of weight regained. The increase in fasting glucose was, however, significantly related to the increase in HGO.

Further evidence of an effect of calorie restriction, independent of weight loss comes from a recent study (Wing, Marcus, & Bononi, 1990) comparing subjects who consumed 400 kcal/day of high quality protein ($n = 33$) with subjects who were consuming a 1000-kcal/day balanced diet ($n = 17$). Both groups were studied before and after losing 12% of initial body weight (M loss = 12 kg). Thus, subjects were matched for weight loss, but differed in the degree of caloric restriction. Subjects in the two groups had comparable fasting blood sugar at baseline, but those subjects who were treated with the VLCD

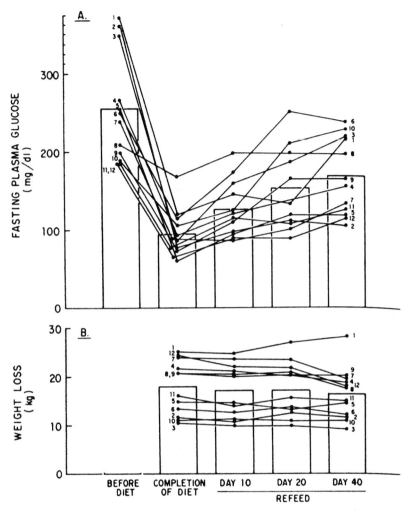

FIGURE 10.4. Individual and mean levels of fasting plasma glucose (A) and corresponding individual and mean alterations in weight loss (B) before and at completion of VLCD and during various intervals of refeeding. From "Glycemic Effects of Intensive Caloric Restriction and Isocaloric Refeeding in Noninsulin-Dependent Diabetes Mellitus" (p. 920) by R. R. Henry, L. Scheaffer, and J. M. Olefsky, 1985, *Journal of Clinical Endocrinology and Metabolism, 61*, 917–925. Copyright 1985 by Endocrine Society. Reprinted by permission.

had significantly ($p < .01$) greater improvements in glycemic control after losing 12 kg (245 to 138 mg/dl) than did subjects on the 1000-kcal/day regimen (240 to 182 mg/dl).

After consuming the VLCD regimen for 12 weeks, subjects in the 400-kcal/day group were gradually returned to a 1000-kcal balanced diet. These subjects continued to lose weight during refeeding and attained an overall weight loss averaging 19.2 kg. However, despite the continued weight loss, their blood sugar levels increased during refeeding (138 to 154 mg/dl). In contrast, in those fed 1000 kcal/day throughout, blood sugars continued to decrease (174 to 153 mg/dl). Thus, the calorie level, independent of weight loss, appears to affect the acute changes in blood sugar.

Further research is needed to define the effects of weight loss versus calorie restriction on glycemic control, and the mechanisms responsible for these effects. It is possible that acute caloric restriction affects glycemic control mainly by ameliorating hepatic insulin resistance. Weight loss, in contrast, may affect glycemic control by increasing insulin secretion and improving skeletal muscle insulin sensitivity.

Short- versus Long-Term Effects of Weight Loss on Glycemic Control

In contrast to the above described studies, which show dramatic improvements in glycemic control, the long-term studies show far more modest effects. This is due in large part to the problem of maintaining weight losses over the long term.

In an earlier publication (Wing, 1985), I reviewed the long-term studies (follow-up $>$ 1 year) that had been done with Type II diabetics. Many of these were uncontrolled clinical studies, and the number of subjects who entered treatment was often not given, making it difficult to evaluate the results. A few of the results are described briefly here. Streja, Boyko, and Rabkin (1981) restudied 66 subjects from an original cohort of 82 subjects. Weight loss averaged 4.1 kg at 2 months and 2.4 kg at 32 months. Subjects experienced significant long-term changes in glycemic control, but the changes were not related to weight loss. In the University Group Diabetes Program (1971) study, subjects randomized to diet plus placebo maintained a 1.6% reduction in body weight over 4¾ years of study, but there was a gradual worsening in glycemic control. Stanik and Marcus (1980) used a 600-kcal/day diet with seven obese hospitalized diabetics. Weight loss averaged 11 kg after 1-3 months on the diet; when followed up a year later, four of the seven had regained their weight. The two subjects who maintained their weight loss had long-term improvements in glycemic control. Thus, a major problem in evaluating the long-term impact of weight loss on glycemic control is the difficulty of producing long-term weight loss.

Behavioral Treatment of Obesity in Type II Diabetes

My associates at the University of Pittsburgh and I have been working to develop an effective treatment program for obese patients with Type II diabetes, and have focused on the use of behavior modification strategies. Behavioral techniques have been shown to improve long-term weight loss in nondiabetic populations (Wing & Jeffery, 1979), and hence might also improve weight loss in Type II diabetic subjects. To examine this, we randomly assigned 53 obese subjects with Type II diabetes to one of three groups (Wing, Epstein, Nowalk, Koeske, & Hagg, 1985). Group 1 was given a behavioral weight control program with 16 weekly sessions, and was provided with a calorie-counting, individualized diet and training in behavior modification techniques. Group 2 was given a nutrition education program. Subjects in this condition also attended 16 weekly meetings and were given comparable, individualized calorie goals. However, their program focused on general nutrition and exercise information, and none of the behavior change strategies (e.g., self-monitoring or problem solving) were taught. The third group was also given nutrition education, but was seen only monthly to more closely approximate usual care.

The major findings of this study were that the behavioral weight control program led to significantly greater weight losses at the end of the 16 weeks (6.3, 3.9, and 2.9 kg for groups 1-3, respectively), but did not affect weight losses at 1-year follow-up (1.8, 3.0, and 3.4 kg, respectively). Fasting glucose and glycosylated hemoglobin (HbA_1), a measure of long-term glycemic control, improved in all three groups from baseline to the end of the 16-week program, but there were no significant differences among groups. Moreover, these improvements were not maintained at the 1-year follow-up. Finally, weight loss was significantly correlated with improvements in glycemic control, with correlation coefficients of .40-.50 at posttreatment and 1 year.

Subsequent studies by our group and others have sought to examine specific components of the behavioral regimen and to improve long-term outcome. Research related to the use of structured exercise, VLCDs and self-monitoring of blood glucose as added components in a behavioral weight loss program will be reviewed below.

Diet and Exercise in the Treatment of Type II Diabetes

Although there have been several studies in nondiabetic subjects suggesting that diet plus exercise improves weight loss compared to diet alone, there have been few studies on this topic with diabetic subjects, and the results have been conflicting. Bogardus et al. (1984) randomly assigned 18 diabetic subjects to either a VLCD alone or a VLCD plus exercise. Weight losses at the end of the 12 weeks were comparable in the two groups (9.9 kg for diet only vs. 11.1 kg for diet plus exercise). Improvements in blood sugar were also comparable. The failure to find an effect of exercise in this study may have been due to the fact that maximum results were achieved with diet only.

In contrast, we found that adding structured exercise to a behavioral weight control program improved both short- and long-term weight losses, compared to a program that focused on diet only (Wing, Epstein, Paternostro-

Bayles, et al., 1988). Thirty subjects were randomly assigned to behavioral treatment programs that focused on either diet only or diet plus exercise. Both conditions attended meetings three times per week for 10 weeks and once per week for the next 10 weeks, and both were given training in behavior modification. All subjects were given an individualized calorie goal, designed to produce a weight loss of 1 kg per week, and were instructed to self-monitor their intake. Subjects in the diet-only group were asked not to change their exercise, whereas subjects in the diet-plus-exercise group were given gradually increasing exercise goals, until they achieved a goal of walking a 3-mile route four times a week. In order to reach this goal, subjects in the diet-plus-exercise group exercised with the group at each of their treatment meetings. The combination of diet plus exercise produced significantly greater weight losses than diet only at each time point studied (Figure 10.5). Improvements in glycemic control, assessed by FBS and HbA_1, were significant at both the 10-week point and a 1-year follow-up, but did not differ between conditions. However, the diet-plus-exercise group was able to achieve these comparable improvements in glycemic control despite greater reductions in oral hypoglycemic medication and insulin. Thirty-eight percent of the patients in the diet only group who started the study on medication had reductions in their medication at 1 year, compared to 83% of the diet-plus-exercise group ($p < .05$).

The only other study to evaluate the long-term effects of diet versus diet plus exercise in the treatment of obese diabetic subjects was conducted by

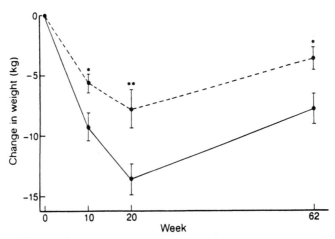

FIGURE 10.5. Changes in weight at weeks 10, 20, and 62 for patients in diet-only (dashed line with dots) and diet-plus-exercise (solid line with dots) groups. *$p < .01$; **$p < .001$. From "Exercise in a Behavioural Weight Control Programme for Obese Patients with Type 2 (Non-Insulin-Dependent) Diabetes" (p. 905) by R. R. Wing, L. H. Epstein, M. Paternostro-Bayles, A. Kriska, M. P. Nowalk, and W. Gooding, 1988, *Diabetologia, 31*, 902–909. Copyright 1988 by Springer-Verlag. Reprinted by permission.

Hartwell, Kaplan, and Wallace (1986). In this study, 66 obese diabetic subjects were randomly assigned to an education control group or to behavior modification programs focusing on either diet, exercise, or diet plus exercise. Subjects in the treatment groups attended 10 consecutive weekly meetings. Weight losses were best in the diet-only group (2.5 kg at the end of 3 months and 1.7 kg at 18 months), but were nevertheless quite modest. In contrast, long-term improvements in glycemic control were best in the diet-plus-exercise condition. Thus, both the Hartwell et al. (1986) and the Wing, Epstein, Paternostro-Bayles, et al. (1988) studies suggest that the combination of diet plus exercise may be helpful in producing long-term improvements in glycemic control in obese diabetic subjects.

Very Low Calorie Diets plus Behavior Modification

Recently, we have been investigating the combination of VLCDs plus behavior modification in the treatment of obese Type II diabetic subjects (Wing, Marcus, Salata, et al.,1991). Thirty-six obese Type II diabetic subjects were randomly assigned to behavior therapy (BT; $n = 19$) or to the combination of BT with a VLCD ($n = 17$). All subjects attended a 20-week behavioral weight control program. Subjects in the BT group consumed a balanced diet of 1000–1500 kcal throughout the 20 weeks. Subjects in the VLCD group consumed a balanced diet of 1000–1500 kcal for weeks 1–4, followed by a VLCD (400 kcal/day of lean meat, fish, or fowl) for weeks 5–12. These subjects gradually increased their consumption of conventional foods during weeks 13–16 and consumed a balanced diet of 1000–1500 kcal/day for weeks 17–20. Both groups consumed a balanced 1000–1500 kcal/day throughout maintenance or until ideal body weight was achieved.

Subjects in the VLCD group had greater improvements in glycemic control than those in BT, both at the end of the 20-week intervention and at a 1-year follow-up. The fasting blood sugar level in the VLCD condition decreased from 254 mg/dl at baseline to 138 mg/dl at week 20 and remained significantly improved at 1 year (186 mg/dl) ($p < .003$) The BT group, on the other hand, had positive initial changes (228 mg/dl at baseline and 167 mg/dl at week 20) but had nonsignificant increases (241 mg/dl) at 1 year. Similar results were obtained with HbA_1.

Interestingly, the superior long-term improvements in glycemic control of VLCD subjects were not due to significant differences in weight loss. Subjects in the VLCD condition lost significantly more weight from pretreatment to week 20 (18.6 kg vs. 10.1 kg, $p < .003$); however, as Wadden and Stunkard (1986) also found, weight losses of the two groups did not differ significantly at 1 year (8.6 kg for VLCD vs. 6.8 kg for BT). The greater improvement in glycemic control in the VLCD group may have derived from increases in insulin secretion produced by the 8-week 400-kcal/day diet. The VLCD subjects had greater decreases in fasting insulin from pretreatment to week 20 than did the BT subjects, as would be appropriate for their lower glucose level. However, the VLCD subjects had higher insulin levels during an oral glucose tolerance test at week 20 and greater area under the insulin curve than the BT subjects, despite lower glucoses, suggesting an increase in beta cell function. Moreover, the VLCD group had greater increases in fasting insulin from posttreatment to 1 year and higher fasting insulin–glucose ratios at 1 year, suggesting that the VLCD produced significant restoration in beta cell capacity, so that subsequent increases in calorie intake and body weight could be effectively dealt with by enhanced insulin output. This is an important finding, deserving further research with more detailed measures of insulin secretion, because it suggests that VLCDs may be of long-term benefit to Type II diabetic subjects.

We also examined the question of the psychological impact of VLCDs in subjects with Type II diabetes (Wing, Marcus, Blair, & Burton, 1991). Subjects were asked to complete the Beck Depression Inventory (BDI) and the State Anxiety subscale of the State–Trait Anxiety Inventory periodically throughout the initial 20 weeks of the program. Scores on both measures were highest at baseline (i.e., before entry into the program) and showed significant decreases from baseline to the refeeding period. There were no differences between the VLCD and BT conditions. Thus, treatment with either diet improved mood state.

Hunger was examined by placing questionnaires in the self-monitoring records and asking subjects to indicate their hunger, preoccupation with thoughts about food, and desire to eat more food than allowed on the diet or to eat different types of food from those allowed on the diet. On each of these measures, scores were highest during the initial month of the program (when all subjects were consuming a balanced diet of 1000–1500 kcal/day) and decreased significantly over the subsequent months on the VLCD and the refeeding interval. Again, the responses of subjects on the VLCD did not differ from those of subjects consuming 1000–1500 kcal/day. This finding is similar to Wadden and colleagues' findings with nondiabetics; the nondiabetic subjects reported less hunger while on a VLCD than while on a 1200-kcal/day diet (Wadden, Stunkard, Day, Gould, & Rubin, 1987). These data suggest that the actual number of calories consumed may not determine subjective feelings of hunger.

A concern that has been raised about strict diets, such as the VLCD, is that these rigid rules will invariably lead to "slips" or lapses, following which patients may experience feelings of guilt and failure, which in turn may lead to relapse. To test this hypothesis, we examined the frequency of "objective" and "subjective" lapses that subjects experienced while on the two different types of diets. Objective lapses were defined as days on which patients' intake was more than 20% above their daily calorie goal. These were tallied from patients' daily self-monitoring records for the first 5 months of treatment. Subjective lapses were defined as a patient's perception that he or she had slipped, lapsed, or gone off the program, independent of the patient's actual calorie intake. These were reported to an independent interviewer who called each patient randomly once a month. The interviewer inquired about lapses in the week prior to the call. These calls were made during months 3–8 of treatment.

There were no significant differences in the frequency of objective or subjective lapses between patients on the two dietary regimens. Patients in the VLCD group exceeded their calorie goals on an average of 2.3% of the days that they monitored during the first 5 months of the program, whereas patients in the BT group exceeded their calorie goals on an average of 1.1% of the days that they monitored during the same period. Similarly, there were no significant differences in the number of months for which patients reported at least one subjective lapse during the previous week (VLCD = 2.4 months vs. BT = 2.0 months). These data suggest that lapses occur with equal frequency in subjects consuming either VLCDs or higher calorie reducing diets.

Self-Monitoring of Blood Sugar and Self-Regulation

Patients with diabetes are now able to monitor their blood sugar with a great deal of accuracy, and could possibly use this information to adjust their subsequent caloric intake and exercise (Wing, Epstein, Nowalk, & Lamparski, 1986). My colleagues and I have tried to teach patients to utilize information about their blood sugar as part of a behavioral weight control program. In our first study on this topic, subjects were randomly assigned to a standard behavioral weight control program or to a behavioral program that included self-monitoring of blood sugar (Wing, Epstein, Nowalk, Scott, Koeske, & Hagg, 1986). In the latter condition, subjects were given visual strips for home glucose monitoring and were asked to measure their glucose nine times per week. Goals for blood sugar were specified, and subjects were instructed to modify their intake and exercise to achieve these goals. Both groups lost weight and had significant improvements in glycemic control. However, no benefits of adding self-monitoring of glucose procedures were observed.

To determine whether the failure to find an effect of self-monitoring was due to insufficient training, we conducted a second study in which subjects were given meters to ensure accurate determination of blood sugar; homework assignments to teach them the effects on blood sugar of specific changes in eating and exercise behaviors; and a point system to indicate the number and types of behavior changes that were required for various levels of hyperglycemia (Wing, Epstein, Nowalk, & Scott, 1988). On average, subjects lost 6 kg during the initial 16-week program and reduced their HbA_1 from 10.5% to 8.65%; however once again, there was no evidence that this training in self-regulation improved treatment outcome compared to the control condition that did not receive training in self-regulation. Detailed analysis revealed that subjects made the specified behavior changes (e.g., walked 1 extra mile or ate 200 kcal less), but these changes did not result in demonstrable changes in glycemic control.

Perhaps a more effective approach would be to use VLCDs in the self-regulation model, as suggested by Atkinson. Atkinson, Berke, Kaiser, and Pohl (1985) studied 15 obese diabetic subjects who had been treated with 1–4 weeks of VLCD. After the VLCD, these subjects were randomized to an experimental group ($n = 6$) or to a control group ($n = 9$). The experimental subjects were told to consume only liquid formula for three meals whenever a premeal blood sugar was greater than 150 mg/dl. This procedure resulted in significant improvements in the maintenance of weight loss and glycemic control. The initial weight losses of the control and experimental groups were comparable (7.3 vs. 6.4 kg, respectively), but at the 6-month follow-up evaluation, the control group maintained a loss of only 1.4 kg as compared to a 4.6-kg loss in the experimental group. Improvements in glycemic control were also better maintained in the experimental group. This interesting use of the VLCD as a maintenance strategy for obese diabetic subjects deserves further investigation.

Thus, it appears from our research that the use of structured exercise and a structured VLCD may both be helpful in the treatment of Type II diabetic subjects. Whether adding self-monitoring of blood glucose to the program improves effectiveness is still unclear. Further studies combining a VLCD with a structured exercise program are needed to determine whether these two approaches used in combination might have additive or synergistic effects on weight loss and/or glycemic control.

Predictors of Weight Loss and Glycemic Control

Because of the difficulty in producing long-term weight loss, it would be helpful to be able to identify at the outset those subjects who will lose the most weight and/or have the greatest improvements in glycemic control. Previous studies with nondiabetics have been unsuccessful in identifying predictors of weight loss, with the exception of gender; men tend to lose more weight than women. In our own research with diabetic subjects, we also found that men lost more weight than women at the end of the initial treatment intervention ($M = 9.5$ kg for men vs. 6.3 kg for women, $p < .0001$) and at a 1-year follow-up ($M = 6.9$ kg for men vs. 3.8 kg for women, $p < .008$) (Wing, Shoemaker, Marcus, McDermott, & Gooding, 1990). These differences remained significant whether BMI or percentage overweight was used. Harris, Davidson, and Bush (1988) suggested that insulin treated patients had poorer weight losses during a 6-week VLCD program than did patients on oral medication or nondiabetic controls. However, the short duration of the study (6 weeks), the small sample size ($n = 7$–12 per group), and the uneven sex ratio make it difficult to interpret these results. We compared weight losses of diabetic subjects treated with diet only ($n = 35$), oral medication ($n = 100$), or insulin ($n = 43$). As seen in Figure 10.6, there were no differences in weight loss at posttreatment (−8.7, −6.7, and −7.4 kg, respectively) or at 1 year (−5.5, −4.1, and −5.5 kg, respectively) (Wing, Shoemaker, et al., 1990). These results

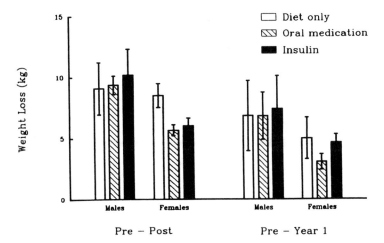

FIGURE 10.6. Effect of gender and diabetes medication on weight loss from pretreatment to posttreatment and pretreatment to a 1-year follow-up. Bars show *SEM*s. From "Variables Associated with Weight Loss and Improvements in Glycemic Control in Type II Diabetic Patients in Behavioral Weight Control Programs" (p. 499) by R. R. Wing, M. Shoemaker, M. D. Marcus, M. McDermott, and W. Gooding, 1990, *International Journal of Obesity*, *14*, 495–503. Copyright 1990 by Macmillan Press Ltd. Reprinted by permission.

should be encouraging to physicians and patients alike, since they suggest that pharmacological treatments for diabetes do not lessen the effectiveness of concomitant behavioral approaches.

We also looked at baseline variables that might predict subsequent improvements in glycemic control (Wing, Shoemaker, et al., 1990). The variable that had the greatest influence on improvements in control was initial blood sugar: Subjects who began the study with fasting blood sugar levels of >200 mg/dl had far greater reductions in blood sugar than subjects with levels of <200 mg/dl, despite equal weight losses. These results contrast with those of Henry et al. (1985), who defined the response to weight loss by the final fasting glucose level rather than by reduction in glucose. With this definition, opposite results were obtained: Those subjects who began the study with the highest initial blood glucose levels continued to have the highest levels after weight loss. Watts et al. (1990) examined the predictors of the glucose response to weight loss in a sample of 135 Type II diabetic subjects, all of whom lost at least 9.1 kg. These authors defined responders as those who achieved a fasting glucose level of <180 mg/dl. With this definition of response, the authors found no effect of initial fasting glucose. Responders and nonresponders were also comparable in age, gender, and initial weight, but responders were closer to their ideal weight at the start of the diet.

Finally, a fourth paper on this topic found that the glycemic response to weight loss (both amount of change and final level) was dependent on the duration of diabetes. Subjects ($n = 8$) who had had diabetes for more than

5 years had less improvement in blood sugar than subjects ($n = 10$) who had had diabetes for less than 2 years, despite comparable weight loss (Nagulesparan, Savage, Bennion, Unger, & Bennett, 1981). The recent-onset and long-duration diabetic subjects began treatment with comparable fasting glucose levels (259 vs. 267 mg/dl, respectively); however, the recent-onset subjects achieved a final fasting glucose level of 119 mg/dl, compared to 175 mg/dl in the long-duration diabetic subjects ($p < .01$), after weight losses of 7.2 kg and 9.8 kg, respectively. In the Wing, Shoemaker, et al. (1990) paper described above, subjects with long-duration diabetes had higher initial glucose levels than recent-onset patients and consequently experienced greater reductions in glucose. Thus, the findings of Nagulesparen et al. (1981) may be due to the selection of subjects with comparable glycemic control at entry and may not be applicable to patients typically seen in clinical settings.

Taken together, these data suggest that the only baseline predictor of weight loss is gender, and that initial blood sugar, duration of diabetes, and distance from ideal body weight may be related to the improvements in glycemic control seen with weight loss. A more successful approach to predicting the glycemic response to weight loss may be to use the initial response to predict the long-term outcome. Watts et al. (1990) noted that responders to weight loss (i.e., those who would achieve a fasting glucose level of <180 mg/dl after a 9.1-kg weight loss) could be predicted from their initial responses to weight reduction. The response after a 2.3-kg weight loss had a 62% positive predictive value of their response to larger weight loss (9.1 kg), and their response after a 4.5-kg weight loss had a 79% predictive value. This is very interesting, because it suggests that individuals who do not show an initial response to weight loss (and hence are probably not responding to calorie restriction) will probably not show a response to subsequent weight loss. These subjects may then be candidates for pharmacological treatment. It will be important in subsequent studies to determine whether the results are similar if larger weight losses are obtained.

Benefits of Modest Weight Loss in Type II Diabetic Patients

In concluding this chapter, it is important to address the issue of whether we should continue to emphasize weight loss as a primary treatment for obese Type II diabetic subjects, given that the initial glycemic responses may be due to calorie restriction rather than weight loss, and that the long-term weight losses in most programs remain modest. The negative side of this argument might best be supported by reference to the study by Watts et al. (1990), described above. These investigators studied 135 patients with Type II diabetes, all of whom had lost 9.1 kg or more within 4 years of their first visit to the diabetes unit. Only 55 of these 135 subjects (41%) achieved fasting glucose levels of <180 mg/dl after weight loss. Thus, weight loss failed to "normalize" glucose levels in the majority of patients. Moreover, information is not presented on the number of patients who failed to achieve a loss of 9.1 kg, but if these patients are also considered, then the value of weight loss for glycemic control becomes very questionable.

Several issues should be raised about this study before it is agreed that weight loss has limited value. First, subjects entered the study with an average fasting glucose of 280 mg/dl; this is a very elevated glucose level and, as noted above, would predict greater change in glucose but higher final levels (i.e., higher than the goal of 180 mg/dl). Second, weight losses were modest (9.1 kg in patients whose initial weight was 94 kg). Finally, this modest weight loss produced significant ($p < .05$) improvements in glucose for the sample as a whole. Blood glucose decreased from 280 mg/dl to 247 mg/dl. Whether such changes would have positive effects on the development of complications is not known, nor is it clear how much the blood glucose would have increased if these subjects had not lost weight.

More positive findings showing a long-term benefit from modest weight loss come from the study by Bauman et al. (1988), also described above. Fifty of the 64 patients in this study were followed up after an average of 19 months (range = 3–40 months). The mean fasting glucose had increased from 122 mg/dl at discharge to 199 mg/dl. Insulin therapy was eventually needed in 13 of the 50 patients, and 26 required oral medication. However, 11 of the subjects could still be maintained on diet only (vs. 1 at baseline), and the fasting glucose level was still below the baseline value of 221 mg/dl. Thus, there was clearly a long-term benefit to the weight loss regimen, but obviously "normalization" of glycemia did not occur. Moreover, neither the magnitude of weight loss nor the amount regained predicted the blood glucose response.

Our own long-term outcome data also suggest positive conclusions about the benefits of modest weight loss. We followed our first 114 diabetic patients for 1 year after treatment (Wing et al., 1987). Table 10.1 shows the weight loss of the subjects and the effects of weight loss on changes in glycemic control, insulin, triglycerides, and high density lipoprotein (HDL) cholesterol. As seen, weight losses were modest, with only 21 subjects losing 6.9 kg or more and 6 subjects losing 13.6 kg or more. However, even these modest weight losses produced significant long-term improvements in glycemic control. Weight losses of 6.9–13.6 kg produced significant decreases in fasting glucose, HbA_1, and insulin levels, suggesting improvements in insulin sensitivity. It also reduced triglycerides and increased HDL cholesterol, thus hopefully reducing the risk of CHD. Moreover, weight losses of 13.6 kg or more produced normalization of these variables, despite the fact that subjects remained 20% above ideal body weight.

We also examined the effect of weight loss on changes in depressive symptomatology in these patients. At pretreatment, scores on the BDI averaged 11.3, and 25% of subjects reported clinically significant dysphoria (BDI scores of ≥ 16). At the end of the treatment, the average BDI score had dropped to 6.5, and only 10% of subjects reported clinically significant depression. BDI

TABLE 10.1. Weight Loss and Improvements in Glycemic Control: CHD Factors

	Weight category (kg)				
	Lost				
	>13.6	6.9–13.6	2.4–6.8	0–2.3	Gained
n	6	21	42	22	23
M/F	3/3	6/15	12/30	7/15	5/18
% of ideal body weight					
Before	159.0	159.0	158.9	158.9	159.2
1 year	120.6	142.7	151.8	156.9	163.7
HbA_1 (%)					
Before	0.097 (9.7)	0.098 (9.8)	0.098 (9.8)	0.098 (9.8)	0.098 (9.8)
1 year	0.071 (7.1)	0.087 (8.7)	0.98 (9.8)	0.104 (10.4)	0.106 (10.6)
Fasting glucose, mmol/L (mg/dl)					
Before	10.3 (186)	10.6 (191)	10.6 (191)	10.6 (191)	10.4 (187)
1 year	6.1 (109)	9.0 (162)	10.3 (185)	10.9 (197)	12.0 (217)
Insulin, pmol/L (μU/ml)					
Before	151 (21.1)	131 (18.2)	131 (18.3)	131 (18.2)	136 (18.9)
1 year	21 (2.9)	75 (10.5)	85 (11.8)	105 (14.6)	107 (14.9)
Triglycerides, mmol/L (mg/dl)					
Before	2.19 (194.4)	2.19 (194.4)	2.15 (190.6)	2.28 (202.3)	2.17 (192.5)
1 year	0.99 (87.3)	1.74 (154.5)	1.87 (165.7)	1.00 (175.9)	2.31 (204.3)
HDL cholesterol, mmol/L (mg/dl)					
Before	0.99 (38.2)	1.00 (38.8)	1.00 (38.8)	0.99 (38.4)	1.00 (38.6)
1 year	1.26 (48.8)	1.07 (41.3)	1.04 (40.3)	0.99 (38.4)	1.03 (39.7)

Note. Adapted from "Long-Term Effects of Modest Weight Loss in Type II Diabetic Patients" by R. R. Wing, R. Koeske, L. H. Epstein, M. P. Nowalk, W. Gooding, and D. Becker, 1987, *Archives of Internal Medicine, 147*, 1749-1753. Copyright 1987 by American Medical Association. Adapted by permission.

scores at 1-year follow-up averaged 8.8, still significantly ($p < .001$) below pretreatment levels, and only 17% reported significant depression.

When we looked at these findings in relationship to magnitude of weight loss, we found that subjects who lost 13.6 kg had significant reductions in depressive symptomatology, as did subjects who lost 6.9–13.6 kg ($p < .01$). Patients who lost less weight and even those who gained weight still reported slight improvements in mood, but these changes were not significant. Thus, participation in the behavioral weight control program appeared to be of benefit to these patients, even if weight losses were limited.

Thus, there appear to be both physical and psychological benefits to weight loss, even if weight losses are modest. Larger weight losses may be needed to "normalize" these variables, as is suggested by our data and by a recent study by Gleysteen, Barboriak, and Sasse (1990). These investigators followed subjects for 5–7 years after gastric bypass surgery. Prior to surgery, six of the patients had diabetes, and three of these required insulin. One year after bypass surgery, blood sugars were normal in all patients, and hypoglycemic medication was not needed by any. At 5-7 years, two of the six patients required oral hypoglycemic medication, but still none of the patients had been returned to insulin.

Finally, a recent study examined the effect of weight loss on mortality in Type II diabetics (Lean, Powrie, Anderson, & Garthwaite, 1990). These authors reviewed the medical records of 233 Type II diabetics (189 of whom were overweight), who had survived at least 1 year from the time of diagnosis. Weight loss in the first year after diagnosis was associated with longer survival time. For the average patient, each kilogram of weight loss was associated with 3-4 months longer survival.

Thus, it appears that weight loss is an important therapeutic approach for obese Type II diabetic patients. The major obstacle in using weight loss as a therapeutic modality is not the fact that weight loss has limited effects on blood sugar, but rather that it is necessary to produce larger weight losses in a broader segment of the diabetic populations in order to see positive long-term effects on blood sugar. VLCDs used in combination with behavior modification and structured exercise, may be helpful in producing these larger weight losses and affecting long-term glycemic control.

Acknowledgment

Preparation of this chapter was supported in part by NIH Grant 29757 awarded from NIDDK to Dr. Rena R. Wing.

References

Atkinson, R. L., Berke, L. K., Kaiser, D. L., & Pohl, S. L. (1985). Effects of very low calorie diets on glucose tolerance and diabetes mellitus in obese humans. In G. L. Blackburn & G. A. Bray (Eds.), *Management of obesity by severe caloric restriction* (pp. 279-299). Littleton, MA: PSG.

Ballard, D. J., Melton, L. J., Dwyer, M. S., Trautmann, J. C., Chu, C. P., O'Fallon, W. M., & Palumbo, P. J. (1986). Risk factors for diabetic retinopathy: A population-based study in Rochester, Minnesota. *Diabetes Care, 9,* 334-342.

Barrett-Connor, E. (1989). Epidemiology, obesity, and non-insulin-dependent diabetes mellitus. *Epidemiological Reviews, 11,* 172-181.

Bauman, W. A., Schwartz, E., Rose, H. G., Eisenstein, H. N., & Johnson, D. W. (1988). Early and long-term effects of acute caloric deprivation in obese diabetic patients. *American Journal of Medicine, 85,* 38-46.

Bogardus, C., Ravussin, E., Robbins, D. C., Wolfe, R. R., Horton, E. S., & Sims, E. A. H. (1984). Effects of physical training and diet therapy on carbohydrate metabolism in patients with glucose intolerance and non-insulin-dependent diabetes mellitus. *Diabetes, 33,* 311-318.

Gleysteen, J. J., Barboriak, J. J., & Sasse, E. A. (1990). Sustained coronary-risk-factor reduction after gastric bypass for morbid obesity. *American Journal of Clinical Nutrition, 51,* 774-778.

Greenfield, M., Kolterman, O., Olefsky, J. M., & Reaven, G. M.(1978). The effect of ten days of fasting on various aspects of carbohydrate metabolism in obese diabetic subjects with significant fasting hyperglycemia. *Metabolism, 27,* 1839-1852.

Gumbiner, B., Polonsky, K. S., Beltz, W. F., Griver, K., Wallace, P., Brechtel, G., & Henry, R. R. (1990). Effects of weight loss and reduced hyperglycemia on the kinetics of insulin secretion in obese non-insulin dependent diabetes mellitus. *Journal of Clinical Endocrinology and Metabolism, 70*, 1594–1602.

Harris, M. D., Davidson, M. B., & Bush, M. A. (1988). Exogenous insulin therapy slows weight loss in type 2 diabetic patients. *International Journal of Obesity, 12*, 149–155.

Hartwell, S. L., Kaplan, R. M., & Wallace, J. P. (1986). Comparison of behavioral interventions for control of type II diabetes mellitus. *Behavior Therapy, 17*, 447–461.

Henry, R. R., Scheaffer, L., & Olefsky, J. M. (1985). Glycemic effects of intensive caloric restriction and isocaloric refeeding in noninsulin-dependent diabetes mellitus. *Journal of Clinical Endocrinology and Metabolism, 61*, 917–925.

Henry, R. R., Wallace, P., & Olefsky, J. M. (1986). Effects of weight loss on mechanisms of hyperglycemia in obese non-insulin-dependent diabetes mellitus. *Diabetes, 35*, 990–997.

Henry, R. R., Wiest-Kent, T. A., Scheaffer, L., Kolterman, O. G., & Olefsky, J. M. (1986). Metabolic consequences of very low calorie diet therapy in obese non-insulin-dependent diabetic and nondiabetic subjects. *Diabetes, 35*, 155–164.

Hughes, T. A., Gwynne, J. T., Switzer, B. R., Herbst, C., & White, G. (1984). Effects of caloric restriction and weight loss on glycemic control, insulin release and resistance, and atherosclerotic risk in obese patients with type II diabetes mellitus. *American Journal of Medicine, 77*, 7–17.

Jarret, R. J. (1989). Epidemiology and public health aspects of non-insulin dependent diabetes mellitus. *Epidemiological Reviews, 11*, 151–171.

Kahn, S. E., & Porte, D. (1990). The pathophysiology of type II (non-insulin-dependent) diabetes mellitus: Implications for treatment. In H. Rifkin & D. Porte (Eds.), *Diabetes mellitus: Theory and practice* (pp. 436–456). New York: Elsevier.

Klein, R., Klein, B. E. K., Moss, S. E., Davis, M. D., & DeMets, D. L. (1984). The Wisconsin Epidemiologic Study of Diabetic Retinopathy: II. Prevalence and risk of diabetic retinopathy when age at diagnosis is less than 30 years. *Archives of Ophthalmology, 102*, 520–526.

Knowler, W. C., Bennett, P. H., & Ballintine, E. J. (1980). Increased incidence of retinopathy in diabetics with elevated blood pressure: A six-year follow-up study in Pima Indians. *New England Journal of Medicine, 302*, 645–650.

Knowler, W. C., Pettitt, D. J., Savage, P. J., & Bennett, P. H. (1981). Diabetes incidence in Pima Indians: Contributions of obesity and parental diabetes. *American Journal of Epidemiology, 113*, 144–156.

Laasko, M., Uusitupa, M., Takala, J., Majander, H., Reijonen, T., & Penttila, I. (1988). Effects of hypocaloric diet and insulin therapy on metabolic control and mechanisms of hyperglycemia in obese non-insulin-dependent diabetic subjects. *Metabolism, 37*, 1092–1100.

Lean, M. E. J., Powrie, J. K., Anderson, A. S., & Garthwaite, P. H. (1990). Obesity, weight loss and prognosis in type 2 diabetes. *Diabetic Medicine, 7*, 228–233.

Manson, J. E., Colditz, G. A., Stampfer, M. J., Willett, W. C., Rosner, B., Monson, R. R., Speizer, F. E., & Hennekens, C. H. (1990). A prospective study of obesity and risk of coronary heart disease in women. *New England Journal of Medicine, 322*, 882–889.

Nagulesparan, M., Savage, P. J., Bennion, L. J., Unger, R. H., & Bennett, P. H. (1981). Diminished effect of caloric restriction on control of hyperglycemia with increasing known duration of type II diabetes mellitus. *Journal of Clinical Endocrinology and Metabolism, 53*, 560–568.

Ohlson, L. O., Larsson, B., Svardsudd, K., Welin, L., Eriksson, H., Wilhelmsen, L., Björntorp, P., & Tibblin, G. (1985). The influence of body fat distribution on the incidence of diabetes mellitus. *Diabetes, 34*, 1055–1058.

Pirart, J. (1979). Do degenerative complications differ between normal-weight and obese diabetics. In J. Vague & P. H. Vague (Eds.), *Diabetes and obesity: Proceedings of the Fifth International Meeting of Endocrinology, Marseilles, June 18–21, 1978* (pp. 270–276). New York: Elsevier.

Stanik, S., & Marcus, R. (1980). Insulin secretion improves following dietary control of plasma glucose in severely hyperglycemic obese patients. *Metabolism, 29*, 346–350.

Streja, D., Boyko, E., & Rabkin, S. W. (1981). Nutrition therapy in non-insulin-dependent diabetes mellitus. *Diabetes Care, 4*, 81–84.
University Group Diabetes Program. (1971). Effects of hypoglycemic agents on vascular complications in patients with adult-onset diabetes. *Journal of the American Medical Association, 218*, 1400–1409.
Vague, J. (1956). The degree of masculine differentiation of obesities: A factor determining predisposition to diabetes, atherosclerosis, gout and uric calculus disease. *American Journal of Clinical Nutrition, 4*, 20–34.
VanItallie, T. B. (1985). Health implications of overweight and obesity in the United States. *Annals of Internal Medicine, 103*, 983–988.
Wadden, T. A., & Stunkard, A. J. (1986). Controlled trial of very low calorie diet, behavior therapy, and their combination in the treatment of obesity. *Journal of Consulting and Clinical Psychology, 54*, 482–488.
Wadden, T. A., Stunkard, A. J., Day, S. C., Gould, R. A., & Rubin, C. J. (1987). Less food, less hunger: Reports of appetite and symptoms in a controlled study of a protein-sparing modified fast. *International Journal of Obesity, 11*, 239–249.
Watts, N. B., Spanheimer, R. G., DiGirolamo, M., Gebhart, S. S.P., Musey, V. C., Siddiq, Y. K., & Phillips, L. S. (1990). Prediction of glucose response to weight loss in patients with non-insulin-dependent diabetes mellitus. *Archives of Internal Medicine, 150*, 803–806.
West, K. M. (1978). *Epidemiology of diabetes and its vascular lesions*. New York: Elsevier.
Westlund, K., & Nicolaysen, R. (1972). Ten-year mortality and morbidity related to serum cholesterol. *Scandinavian Journal of Clinical and Laboratory Investigation, 30*, 1–24.
Wing, R. R. (1985). Improving dietary adherence in patients with diabetes. In L. Jovanovic & C. M. Peterson (Eds.), *Nutrition and diabetes* (pp. 161–186). New York: Alan R. Liss.
Wing, R. R., Epstein, L. H., Paternostro-Bayles, M., Kriska, A., Nowalk, M. P., & Gooding, W. (1988). Exercise in a behavioural weight control programme for obese patients with type 2 (non-insulin-dependent) diabetes. *Diabetologia, 31*, 902–909.
Wing, R. R., Epstein, L. H., Nowalk, M. P., Koeske, R., & Hagg, S. (1985). Behavior change, weight loss and physiological improvements in Type II diabetic patients. *Journal of Consulting and Clinical Psychology, 53*, 111–122.
Wing, R. R., Epstein, L. H., Nowalk, M. P., & Lamparski, D. M. (1986). Behavioral self-regulation in the treatment of patients with diabetes mellitus. *Psychological Bulletin, 99*, 78–89.
Wing, R. R., Epstein, L. H., Nowalk, M. P., & Scott, N. (1988). Self-regulation in the treatment of type II diabetes. *Behavior Therapy, 19*, 11–23.
Wing, R. R., Epstein, L. H., Nowalk, M. P., Scott, N., Koeske, R., & Hagg, S. (1986). Does self-monitoring of blood glucose levels improve dietary compliance for obese patients with type II diabetes? *American Journal of Medicine, 81*, 830–836.
Wing, R. R., & Jeffery, R. W. (1979). Outpatient treatments of obesity: A comparison of methodology and clinical results. *International Journal of Obesity, 3*, 261–279.
Wing, R. R., Koeske, R., Epstein, L. H., Nowalk, M. P., Gooding, W., & Becker, D. (1987). Long-term effects of modest weight loss in type II diabetic patients. *Archives of Internal Medicine, 147*, 1749–1753.
Wing, R. R., Marcus, M. D., Blair, E. H., & Burton, L. R. (1991). Psychological responses of obese type II diabetic subjects to very-low-calorie diet. *Diabetes Care, 14*, 596–599.
Wing, R. R., Marcus, M., & Bononi, P. (1990). Glycemic control after weight loss is affected by how weight loss is achieved. *Diabetes, 39*(Suppl. 1), 50A.
Wing, R. R., Marcus, M. D., Salata, R., Epstein, L. H., Miaskiewicz, S., & Blair, E. H. (1991). Effects of a very low-calorie diet on long-term glycemic control in obese type 2 diabetic subjects. *Archives of Internal Medicine, 151*, 1334–1340.
Wing, R. R., Shoemaker, M., Marcus, M. D., McDermott, M., & Gooding, W. (1990). Variables associated with weight loss and improvements in glycemic control in type II diabetic patients in behavioral weight control programs. *International Journal of Obesity, 14*, 495–503.

11

Psychological Aspects of Obesity and Dieting

PATRICK MAHLEN O'NEIL
MARK P. JARRELL

Obese individuals suffer from a chronic disorder that is at once personally undeniable, publicly visible, and socially scorned. Regardless of the physiological, genetic, and environmental forces that cause obesity, the potential psychological significance of this plight is noteworthy. Further, obese patients in comprehensive weight loss programs must undergo physiological readjustments, major lifestyle changes, and curtailment of an appetitive behavior. Thus, the psychological consequences of dieting and weight loss also deserve examination.

In this chapter, we will discuss the psychological aspects of obesity and its treatment by diet and lifestyle change. Our review of the psychological aspects of obesity will include general psychopathology, personality factors, psychological and behavioral characteristics specific to weight and eating patterns, and body image. The discussion of psychological concomitants of dieting will include mood changes, hunger, and body image; we will also provide a brief discussion of clinical impressions concerning other factors.

Psychological Characteristics of Obese Persons

General Psychopathology and Obesity

The belief that obesity is the result of psychological dysfunction has been widespread, even among health professionals (Maiman, Wang, Becker, Finlay, & Simonson, 1979). Early conceptualizations of obesity focused on aberrant psychological development, an underlying depression or anxiety condition, or inadequate adjustment to life stress (Leon & Roth, 1977). These etiological models do not lend themselves to direct empirical investigation. If, however, obesity is caused by psychological dysfunction, one might expect to find a higher incidence of psychopathology among obese persons than among normal-weight individuals.

Studies conducted on samples drawn from the general population have not found this to be the case (Silverstone, 1968). In fact, two large studies found less anxiety and depression among obese individuals than among normal-weight individuals (Crisp & McGuiness, 1976; Stewart & Brook, 1983). In a review of more than 10 relevant studies, Wadden and Stunkard (1985) concluded that "there is little evidence of increased psychopathology in the obese population as a whole" (p. 1063).

Compared to nonclinical samples, higher levels of psychological distress have been noted among obese individuals seeking treatment for their obesity. Halmi, Long, Stunkard, and Mason (1980) found a lifetime prevalence of 47.5% for any Axis I (noncharacterological) psychiatric diagnosis among morbidly obese patients seeking gastric bypass. This is somewhat higher than comparable prevalence estimates (26–35%) for the general population (Robins et al., 1984).

Leon and Roth (1977) reviewed several studies that used the Minnesota Multiphasic Personality Inventory (MMPI; Hathaway & McKinley, 1951) to assess obese individuals seeking treatment and found elevated scores on the Psychasthenia scale (thought to measure neurotic tendencies), and the Depression scale. Similarly, Wadden and Stunkard (1985) reported that an additional 10 MMPI studies of obese individuals seeking treatment found at least mild elevations on the Depression scale, and less frequently on other clinical scales. As indicated in this latter review, however, it is important to note that these elevations were no greater than those seen among other patients seeking medical or surgical care.

Taken together, the evidence suggests that the obese population as a whole exhibits mental health functioning comparable to that of the general population. Obese persons seeking treatment may show higher levels of general psychopathology than those of community samples, but no higher than those of other medical and surgical patients. Because the prevalence of psychiatric problems is relatively high among patients seeking medical services, it should be expected that any group of patients seeking treatment for their obesity will contain a significant number of persons with past or present psychiatric disorders.

Obesity and Personality Characteristics

Persons of average weight show tremendous interindividual variation on numerous dispositional traits. In general, obese persons have not been found to differ consistently from normal-weight persons on general (i.e., non-weight-related) traits such as masculinity–femininity, locus of control, assertiveness, and self-consciousness (Klesges, 1984; Leon & Roth, 1977). A few studies have found differences on other personality factors, but replication has been scant to nonexistent. As Leon and Roth (1977) concluded, "There appear to be very few personality characteristics unique to obese persons" (p. 134).

Personality type may be viewed as the relative configuration of several individual traits. Comparisons of group MMPI profiles of obese persons have found large within-group variation (Blankmeyer et al., 1990). Numerous profiles are represented within the obese population, even within subgroups of the obese. In a recent study, cluster analysis was used to analyze the MMPIs of 170 obese women applying for gastric bypass surgery (Blankmeyer et al., 1990). Only 55% of this sample had individual profiles that fit any of the five derived prototypical profiles. Further, all of the five derived clusters have emerged in similar MMPI cluster analysis research on other populations, and thus are not unique to the obese.

The obese, therefore, represent a very heterogeneous population with respect to personality types and traits. It appears that the obese differ from each other as much as they differ from normal-weight persons on psychological characteristics not explicitly concerned with weight and eating.

Psychological and Behavioral Characteristics Related to Weight and Eating

Psychological Characteristics

In contrast to the above-described findings with personality variables, differences have been found consistently between obese and nonobese persons on a number of psychological factors and behavioral patterns that relate specifically to weight and eating. For example, Klesges (1984) compared normal-weight and overweight (but not in treatment) college students on general measures of depression, assertiveness, and self-consciousness, and also on measures of these characteristics as they applied specifically to weight and eating. The groups did not differ on any of the global measures. On measures applied to weight and eating, however, overweight subjects were more depressed and self-conscious and less assertive than normal-weight subjects.

O'Connor and Dowrick (1987) presented subjects with a list of self-defeating and/or pessimistic self-statements concerning weight and eating. Compared to normal-weight subjects, overweight subjects engaged in these negative cognitions more frequently and professed a stronger belief in them.

Paine (1982) compared clinically obese, nonclinically obese, and nonobese groups on a measure of characteristic cognitive reactions to dietary transgressions. Obese subjects, especially the clinically obese, were more prone to absolutistic, perfectionistic self-statements than were the nonobese.

Another relevant characteristic is that of restrained eating. The concept had its roots in the work of Nisbett (1972), who suggested that obese people are in a chronic state of energy deficit and are physiologically hungry because they attempt to hold their weight below its biological "set point." Herman and his colleagues (Herman & Mack, 1975; Herman & Polivy, 1980) extended this idea and proposed that the hypothesized distinctive eating behavior of the obese reflected not so much their obesity as their chronic dieting. This chronic restriction of food to control body weight, whether by obese or by average-weight people, has been labeled "restrained eating."

One aspect of restrained eating is "disinhibition" or "counterregulation," which refers to overeating when control is threatened or disrupted or when self-imposed limits on intake are exceeded. Björvell, Rössner, and Stunkard (1986) compared obese groups in treatment, an obese group waiting for treatment, and average-weight women on the Eating Inventory (Stunkard & Messick, 1985). The obese groups scored higher than the average-weight subjects on scales measuring disinhibition and perceived hunger (awareness of and susceptibility to hunger). Citing this and other studies, Stunkard and Wadden (1990) suggest that elevations on these scales are also found among obese persons not seeking treatment.

Eating Behavior

Early behavioral models of obesity and behavioral treatment strategies were based on the premises that obese and average-weight persons differ in their eating styles and that the obese consume more calories than do the normal-weight. The presumed "obese eating style" was distinguished by a faster eating rate, achieved by taking larger and more frequent bites and by chewing food less thoroughly. Direct investigations of these behaviors have not supported such a distinctive eating style (Adams, Ferguson, Stunkard, & Agras, 1978; Kisseleff, Jordan, & Levitz, 1978; Mahoney, 1975; Rosenthal & Marx, 1978; Stunkard & Kaplan, 1977). The only evidence of a characteristic eating style is that obese persons may chew their food less thoroughly and may take larger but not necessarily more frequent bites (Adams et al., 1978; Dodd, Birky, & Stalling, 1976; Drabman, Hammer, & Jarvis, 1977; Gaul, Craighead, & Mahoney, 1975).

Scores of studies have sought to determine the average daily calorie intake of obese and average-weight groups. Reviews of these studies have concluded that despite popular beliefs, there is no convincing evidence that obese persons consume more daily calories than do average-weight persons (Garrow, 1974, 1978a; Wooley, Wooley, & Dyrenforth, 1979). Several studies have suggested that the obese may even consume fewer daily calories (Beaudoin & Mayer, 1953; Johnson, Burke, & Mayer, 1956) and require fewer calories to maintain a given weight (Leibel & Hirsch, 1984).

Despite these studies, it is premature to rule out larger caloric intakes by the obese, for several reasons. For example, most studies have failed to ensure that subjects were in a state of energy balance and were neither gaining nor losing weight. Dieting is more prevalent among the obese than among the nonobese, so obese subjects are more likely to be in a dieting phase when assessed. Also, caloric intake has been found to vary greatly across assessment settings (Coll, Meyer, & Stunkard, 1979; Dodd et al., 1976; Wooley et al., 1979). Finally, the available assessment methods do not appear sufficiently precise to detect small differences in intake that could result in significant long-term weight gain. A daily intake of only 100 kilocalories (kcal) above energy needs will lead, on average, to a 10-pound weight gain over a year. Garrow (1974, 1978b) has concluded that the error of estimate in nearly all studies of daily intake is large enough to allow a difference of this magnitude to escape detection.

Further, obese persons have higher resting metabolic rates (RMRs) than do average-weight persons (James, Bailes, Davies, & Dauncey, 1978; Jéquier & Schutz, 1985; Sjöström, 1985). Because RMR accounts for the majority of total energy expenditure, it is likely that the total daily caloric requirements for weight maintenance are higher for obese persons than for normal-weight persons. Therefore, a failure to find differences in daily caloric intake may reflect problems with assessment methodology and subject reporting. Recent studies using the technique of doubly labeled water to measure 24-hour energy expenditure have suggested that both obese and average-weight persons significantly underestimate their caloric intake, the obese by as much as 40% (Bandini, Schoeller, Cyr, & Dietz, 1990; Schoeller, 1988).

Recently, more attention has been focused on the type of foods eaten by the obese and nonobese to determine whether macronutrient selection affects body composition. Some evidence suggests that the diets of obese persons are higher in fats and lower in carbohydrates (Lindemann, Miller, Wallace, & Niederpruem, 1989). Dietary fat intake is significantly correlated with body fat percentage (Dreon et al., 1988; Lindemann et al., 1989).

Binge Eating

Regardless of whether the obese as a group display any distinctive eating behaviors or eat more calories than average-weight individuals, a subgroup of the obese exhibit a characteristic eating style—binge eating.

Binge eating was first identified by Stunkard (1959) as a distinct eating pattern of potential significance in the obese, characterized by the intake of a large amount of food in a short period of time, followed by severe discomfort and self-condemnation. In 1980, the third edition of the *Diagnostic and Statistical Manual of Mental Disorders* (DSM-III) of the American Psychiatric Association (1980) first acknowledged binge eating as a defining component of a psychiatric disorder—bulimia. Although none of the current DSM-III-R (American Psychiatric Association, 1987) criteria for bulimia nervosa address weight per se, researchers have focused primarily on average-weight or anorectic individuals who binge-eat and purge. Binge eating, however, appears to be very common among the obese. Estimates of the prevalence of "moderate" binge eating among obese individuals seeking treatment range from 23% to 82% (Gormally, Black, Daston, & Rardin, 1982; Keefe, Wyshogrod, Weinberger, & Agras, 1984; Loro & Orleans, 1981; Marcus, Wing, & Lamparski, 1985).

Although no comprehensive studies of the psychological differences of obese binge eaters and their non-binge-eating counterparts have appeared, information from various studies suggests that obese binge eaters (1) report more restrictive dieting standards and feel less capable of maintaining their diets (Marcus, Wing, & Hopkins, 1988); (2) experience more hunger and a higher tendency toward disinhibition of eating (Marcus et al., 1985, 1988); (3) show more emotional disturbances on the MMPI, especially obsessive–compulsive thinking, anxiety, self-doubt, and guilt (Kolotkin, Revis, Kirkley, & Janick, 1987); (4) report more depression (Marcus et al., 1988); and (5) have an increased prevalence of psychiatric disorders, especially affective disorders (Hudson et al., 1988; Marcus, Wing, Ewing, Kern, Gooding, & McDermott, 1990). One study found that clinical samples of bingeing and nonbingeing obese females did not differ on measures of psychopathology; however, both groups were more depressed and histrionic than a group of obese individuals from a nonclinical sample (Prather & Williamson, 1988).

The eating topography of obese binge eaters has received less attention than the binge eating of average-weight bulimics. Although most of the relevant data are anecdotal, the available evidence suggests that the binge-eating behaviors of obese and average-weight individuals are similar (Marcus & Wing, 1987). Caloric estimates based on self-reported intake during binges by the obese range from 1000 to 20,000 kcal (Loro & Orleans, 1981; Stunkard, 1959); typically, calorie-dense or "forbidden" foods are consumed during binges (Marcus & Wing, 1987). The most significant difference in the binges of obese and average-weight people is the usual absence of purging behaviors (i.e., self-induced vomiting, laxative abuse, diuretic abuse) among obese bingers.

Given the apparent prevalence of binge eating among the obese and the detrimental effects binge eating may have on weight loss and weight loss maintenance, it is surprising how little is known about the impact of binge eating on the outcome of obesity treatment. With respect to behavioral programs, the effects of binge status on weight loss have been inconsistent (Marcus & Wing, 1987). Bingers and nonbingers did not differ in their responses to a program combining fluoxetine and behavior modification (Marcus, Wing, Ewing, Kern, McDermott, & Gooding, 1990). Within a very low calorie diet (VLCD) and behavior modification program, one of us found that severe bingers, moderate bingers, and nonbingers did not differ on attrition, weight loss during the VLCD phase, or total weight loss (Jarrell, 1990). There is evidence that bingers show poorer maintenance of behaviorally induced weight loss than do nonbingers (Keefe et al., 1984; Marcus et al., 1988). No data have appeared concerning binge status and maintenance of weight loss following VLCD or pharmacological treatment.

Binge eating in the obese certainly merits more attention from clinicians and researchers. A useful first step would be the development of an operational definition of a "binge" that allows for reliable identification of people whose episodes of overeating have significant effects on psychological functioning and weight. The targeted level of severity should avoid diagnostic thresholds that are either so high as to exclude clinically significant cases or so low as to render the diagnosis meaningless.

In addition to caloric intake, other parameters defining a binge episode may include mood, duration of the episode and reasons for its termination, and experienced degree of control while eating. Further, the diagnosis of binge eating should stipulate the frequency with which bingeing must occur. Currently, the DSM-III-R criteria for bulimia nervosa require a minimum average of two binge episodes per week for at least 3 months (American Psychiatric Association, 1987). Whether this would be an appropriate frequency criterion for defining binge eating in the obese awaits empirical determination.

Body Image

Body image represents the cognitive perception of one's body size and appearance, and the emotional response to these perceptions. Accuracy of perceived body size can be measured by varying the apparent proportions of a visual representation of the subject's body (or of a prototypical body) and having the subject select the variation believed to represent his or her actual proportions. Obese adults have been found to be less accurate than average weight adults in these procedures. Average estimates by obese subjects are 6–12% greater than actual size, whereas estimates of average-weight subjects are within 1–2% of actual size (Collins, 1987; Collins et al., 1987). Indeed, obese subjects are three times as likely to overestimate their body size as are average-weight subjects (Collins et al., 1987).

Obesity during childhood may affect body size estimates in adulthood, even when the person is no longer obese. Counts and Adams (1985) found that among currently average-weight (but weight-conscious) adults, 9 of 17 (53%) of those with a history of childhood obesity overestimated their body size, compared to only 1 of 7 (14%) who had not been obese in childhood.

Some obese persons suffer pronounced negative feelings toward their bodies. Stunkard and Mendelson (1961) described a pattern of body image disparagement that includes "overwhelming preoccupation with one's obesity, often to the exclusion of any other personal characteristics" and "appraisal of one's own body as grotesque and even loathsome, and the consequent feeling that others can look on him only with horror and contempt" (p. 328). It is thought that this extreme derogation of body image is seen almost exclusively in persons with childhood- or adolescent-onset obesity, especially when the clinical picture includes a disturbed family environment, parental criticism of the child's weight, and other neurotic symptoms (Stunkard & Burt, 1967; Stunkard & Mendelson, 1961).

Psychological Changes during Dieting

This section will review findings concerning psychological changes during weight reduction. We will not address the issues of longer-term psychological consequences of substantially reduced body weight, nor the effects of weight regain on psychological functioning.

Mood

Mood changes may be expected concomitants and/or consequences of dieting, reflecting both caloric restriction and weight loss. A review of early studies examining mood changes during weight reduction noted a high incidence of untoward emotional responses (Stunkard & Rush, 1974). However, these studies involved differing weight reduction regimens conducted on an individual basis, prior to the development of behavioral weight control methods. Many studies included selected obese patients who were seen by psychiatrists and/or who had pre-existing psychopathology (Wing, Epstein, Marcus, & Kupfer, 1984).

In stark contrast, mood changes during group behavioral treatment appear consistently more salubrious. Wing et al. (1984) reviewed 10 studies that used objective measures of depression and/or anxiety to assess mood changes during behavioral treatment. None reported increases in depression or anxiety from pretreatment to posttreatment. Six of the 10 studies showed significant reductions in depression or, less frequently, anxiety. Interestingly, these salutary changes were not limited to groups receiving behavioral treatment; positive changes were also noted in response to pharmacotherapy and social pressure. Untreated control subjects did not show positive mood changes, however, suggesting that the improvement shown by other groups was not an artifact and that some degree of active participation in treatment was necessary for improvement in mood to occur.

Mood and Very Low Calorie Diets

VLCDs (providing 800 or fewer kcal/day) have within the past decade become widely used for obese patients who are overweight by about 30% or 20 kg. Table 11.1 summarizes findings from studies that systematically measured changes in levels of depression and/or anxiety during treatment with VLCD.

As can be seen, all but one of these studies reported either no change or an improvement in depression. The studies that reported benign effects all used the Beck Depression Inventory (BDI; Beck, Ward, Mendelson, Mock, & Erbaugh, 1961); pretreatment mean scores were generally in the nondepressed range. The earliest study (Glucksman, Hirsch, McCully, Barron, & Knittle, 1968), which was the only one to report increases in depression, differed from the other studies in that the subjects were described as having pre-existing personality disorders; also, the measures used included staff ratings and the Rorschach test, a global projective measure of psychological functioning.

Table 11.1 also shows the results of VLCD studies that systematically measured changes in anxiety from pre- to posttreatment. Findings are divided

TABLE 11.1. Pre- to Posttreatment Changes in Depression and Anxiety during Treatment with VLCD

Study	n	Treatment	Depression		State anxiety		Trait anxiety	
			Effect	Measure	Effect	Measure	Effect	Measure
Glucksman et al. (1968)	6	VLCD, inpatient	↑	Staff ratings/ Rorschach	↑	Semiweekly staff ratings	↑	Rorschach
Rosen et al. (1982)	8	VLCD (827 kcal), inpatient[a]	No change	BDI	No change	Daily staff ratings	↓	STAI
Wadden et al. (1984)	17	VLCD + behavior therapy	↓	BDI	↓	STAI	↓	STAI
Wadden et al. (1987)	19	VLCD + behavior therapy	↓	BDI	No change	STAI	↓	STAI
Wadden & Stunkard (1986)	15	VLCD alone	No change	BDI	—	—	—	—

Note. BDI, Beck Depression Inventory (Beck et al., 1961); STAI, State–Trait Anxiety Inventory (Spielberger, 1983).
[a]No difference between isocaloric diets with and without carbohydrate.

into those concerned with state anxiety (anxiety at the time of assessment) and those concerned with trait anxiety (a more enduring predisposition to respond with anxiety) (Spielberger, 1983). As can be seen, all but one of the studies found either no change or a reduction in levels of state anxiety and reductions in trait anxiety. Only the aforementioned study by Glucksman et al. (1968) reported an increase in anxiety.

Anxiety and depression during VLCDs do not appear to be influenced by degree of ketogenesis (Rosen, Hunt, Sims, & Bogardus, 1982) or by whether the diet is food-based or formula-based (Wadden, Stunkard, Brownell, & Day, 1985). Despite substantial reduction in serum triiodothyronine (T_3) during VLCD, these changes have not been found to be related to changes in depression (Wadden, Mason, Foster, Stunkard, & Prange, 1990).

As Table 11.1 indicates, the addition of behavior modification to a VLCD program seems to be associated with reductions in depression, whereas levels of depression remain unchanged when VLCDs are used alone. (As noted above, behavioral treatment of obesity without VLCD has often been associated with reduction of depression.) There seems to be no such consistent effect of behavioral treatment on anxiety during consumption of a VLCD.

The method of assessment may influence findings concerning mood changes during weight loss. Smoller, Wadden, and Stunkard (1987) reviewed 35 studies of mood and dieting that had been published over a 35-year period. They categorized the assessment methods as either nomothetic (standardized, objective tests) or idiographic (open-ended, unstructured approaches requiring clinical judgment). All of the studies that used nomothetic methods reported benign changes in mood, whereas all of the idiographic studies reported adverse changes. However, methods of assessment and treatment approach were confounded. All of the studies that reported positive changes included behavioral or medical treatment as well as nomothetic assessment; all studies reporting negative changes included psychiatrically oriented treatments.

Wadden, Stunkard, and Smoller (1986) administered different assessment methods to subjects undergoing VLCD with behavioral modification. More symptoms of dysphoria were reported retrospectively and in open-ended interviews than were reported during concurrent assessment using standardized, objective tests. More frequent assessment also detected more instances of depression; although the group showed significant pre- to posttreatment improvement in mood, weekly assessments indicated that 35% of subjects had a clinically significant increase in depression during at least 1 week of treatment. Further, more frequent assessments may detect transient group-wide increases (Rosen et al., 1982).

Hunger and Related Responses

The extent to which dieters experience hunger and similar responses may be expected to influence adherence and treatment completion (LaPorte & Stunkard,

1990). VLCDs and moderately restrictive diets seem to have different effects on hunger, preoccupation with eating, and responsiveness to food stimuli.

Studies systematically tracking patient self-reports of hunger indicate that over the course of a VLCD, hunger either decreases (Lappalainen, Sjoden, Hursti, & Vesa, 1990; Wadden et al., 1985; Wadden, Stunkard, Day, Gould, & Rubin, 1987) or remains at pretreatment levels (Rosen et al., 1982; Wadden et al., 1985). Transient increases, however, have been observed during the first 1 or 2 weeks of treatment (Rosen et al., 1982). Hunger on a VLCD is lower than that reported on diets of 1200–1600 kcal/day (Lappalainen et al., 1990; Wadden et al., 1987).

Similarly, preoccupation with eating either decreases or remains unchanged during a VLCD and tends to be less than that on a 1200-kcal/day diet (Wadden et al., 1985, 1987). When presented with visual food stimuli, subjects on a VLCD show a diminished self-reported hunger response, whereas subjects on diets of 1200–1600 kcal/day show no change from pretreatment (Lappalainen et al., 1990).

Factors accounting for the generally lower degree of reported hunger on VLCDs remain to be identified. Reductions in hunger have been reported with both high and low ketogenic diets (Rosen et al., 1982), as well as with diets extremely low in caloric and protein content (Lappalainen et al., 1990). It has been suggested that the stimulus-narrowing aspects of VLCDs (fewer food cues and tastes) may limit the perceived desire for food. However, one study found a trend over 4 weeks for subjects on a food-based VLCD to report somewhat less hunger than subjects on a (presumably more monotonous) formula VLCD (Wadden et al., 1985).

Body Image

Little is known about the effects of weight reduction on the components of body image. Glucksman and Hirsch (1961) reported overestimates of body size by six hospitalized patients during and following an inpatient nonbehavioral VLCD program. Notably, these obese patients all had childhood-onset obesity, and all had personality disorders. However, two adult-onset subjects undergoing the same protocol tended to underestimate their body size after weight loss (Grinker, 1973).

Speaker, Schultz, Grinker, and Stern (1983) found that 18 obese adolescent boys, after a weight loss camp, underestimated their body size by 9–14%. Although they were on a 1200-kcal/day diet, the rate of weight loss ($M = 13.3$ kg in 7 weeks) was comparable to that observed on a VLCD.

Recently, we measured body size estimates among patients in a 30-week VLCD and behavior modification program with a 12-week VLCD component. A live video distortion procedure was used, in which each patient viewed himself or herself in a television monitor while the relative width of the patient's image was systematically varied from -52% to $+58\%$ of actual size (Freeman, Thomas, Solyom, & Miles, 1983). The patient noted the point at

Psychological Aspects of Obesity and Dieting

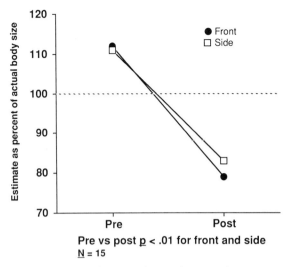

FIGURE 11.1. Body size estimates by female patients before and after treatment with VLCD.

which the image on the monitor corresponded to his or her perceived image; at that time the experimenter recorded the degree and direction of deviation.

Preliminary pre- and posttreatment results for 15 females are shown in Figure 11.1 (O'Neil & Jarrell, 1991). As can be seen, subjects initially overestimated their body size by 12.1% (front view) and 10.6% (side view), consistent with other findings (Collins, 1987; Collins et al., 1987). After treatment, however, and a mean weight loss of 27.0 kg ($SD = 8.0$), patients underestimated their actual size by -21.4% (front view; $t - 6.45, p < .01$) and -17.2% (side view; $t = 4.07, p < .01$). Thus, patients' perceptions of their new body size exaggerated the degree of weight loss. It is interesting to note that 11 of these 15 patients reported onset of obesity before 18 years of age.

Frequently, it has been asserted that patients with childhood-onset versus adult-onset of their obesity display different changes in their body size estimates following weight loss. As can be seen above, the commonly held belief that childhood-onset subjects retain an overly large body image after weight loss is contradicted by our recent data. More research is needed to clarify this issue, as well as the impact of perceptual and affective body image aberrations on weight loss maintenance. Regrettably, the existing literature on these issues has more reference citations than experimental subjects.

Other Effects of Dieting and Weight Loss: Some Clinical Impressions

The preceding section has reviewed changes in psychological factors that have been systematically assessed by empirical studies. However, these are not the only changes to occur among obese persons undergoing weight reduction. We would like to close with a selective survey of benefits and problems that have been observed to accompany weight loss in some of our patients.

Benefits of Weight Loss

Improved physical health is the *raison d'être* of weight loss. The well-known physical benefits such as decreased blood pressure, decreased low density lipoprotein cholesterol, and improved blood glucose control are generally not experienced directly by the patient, but instead are determined by clinical tests. Improvements, however, in other medical conditions have much greater impact on the patient's daily life, and therefore on his or her behavioral and psychological functioning.

A dramatic example of such physically mediated psychological improvement is that of patients with sleep apnea (Jamison, 1988). With weight loss, quality of sleep and oxygenation improve markedly, reducing daytime sleepiness and increasing mental alertness. Patients who previously may have been unable to drive, study, or attend class because of excessive daytime sleepiness and general cognitive sluggishness are able to resume these vital activities. Frequently, the interpersonal behavior of such patients is also greatly enhanced as they become more alert in both appearance and performance.

Likewise, mobility increases as problems with weight-bearing joints abate. Physical stamina and endurance at everyday activities are also improved by increased aerobic capacity and the reduced physical cost of activity. Patients who have been limited in these respects find that their personal world expands as the work and recreational options available to them multiply. Further, they may no longer be physically excluded from certain social activities.

Patients losing significant weight often display increased self-confidence and self-esteem. The affective component of body image may improve, as evidenced when patients begin to dress more stylishly and to invest more time and resources in their appearance with hair styling, manicures, makeup, and the like. Patients also find that opportunities for dating increase as they lose the social handicap of excess weight. With increased self-esteem and reduced social discrimination may come increased assertiveness and optimism and a willingness to take on changes in other life areas, even at some personal risk. More than one patient has expressed the thought that "Once I conquered my weight problem, I felt like I could handle everything else in my life."

Problems with Weight Loss

The thought quoted above is closely akin to a frequently observed problem—the patient's belief that most troubling things in his or her life are attributable to obesity, and the expectation that once the excess weight is lost, all other problems will disappear. Such patients scapegoat their obesity, and when their weight is lost they are disappointed to find, for example, that job and relationship problems remain. This realization may lead to self-examination and requests for professional help, but more often it seems to trigger relapse and weight regain. The patient's expectations concerning the effects of weight loss should be assessed prior to treatment; any unrealistic hopes should be challenged. Excessively unrealistic expectations may argue against admission to treatment.

The equilibria in patients' social relationships may be perturbed both by dieting (with its restriction on eating as a social activity and its demands for different meal choices at home) and by weight loss (which may remove the patient from a socially undesirable category, enhance assertiveness and self-esteem, and increase attention from the opposite sex). These changes can affect friendships as well as romantic relationships, but perhaps none is affected more than marriage. Excess eating may no longer be an available response to marital strife or despair. The spouse of the formerly obese patient may become exceedingly jealous and suspicious, and the patient may no longer be willing to assume a passive, subservient role. If not dealt with, any of these disruptions can bring about a weight regain, often encouraged by the spouse. Verbal abuse or physical abuse (or both) of a now thinner spouse by a jealous partner are not unknown. The complicated marital issues surrounding weight and weight loss are discussed effectively in the tellingly titled *Weight, Sex, and Marriage: A Delicate Balance* (Stuart & Jacobson, 1987).

In a related area, the weight-reduced single patient who finds (usually) herself with greatly improved dating prospects may be forced to face interpersonal problems that were formerly less apparent. One rather simple but personally important issue is that of dating skills deficits; the person whose obesity was a social obstacle to dating has not had the opportunities to learn how to develop and maintain relationships and how to decipher the often confusing interpersonal signals in such dyads. Fears of intimacy may be exposed as opportunities for intimacy increase; the patient who has no means of working through such fears may flee to overeating and return to the safe isolation of obesity. Patients with histories of sexual abuse who have been sexually inactive may experience particularly acute anxiety as they find themselves in sexually charged relationships.

Although group data show generally benign psychological consequences of weight loss, such averages do not capture adequately the experience of the individual patient for whom weight reduction unmasks other psychological problems. The person's obesity may have been a defense that "keeps the world away"; this is seen, for example, in patients who feel that they have not been accountable or responsible in certain areas because of their obesity. As noted earlier, the weight-reduced patient can no longer blame personal discontent or interpersonal difficulties on the world's reaction to obese people. Concomitant psychological problems, such as depression or anxiety disorders, may become more obvious and more severe as the patient rules out eating as a coping strategy and faces a world with more opportunities, and therefore more risks and responsibilities.

The problems described above are not inclusive, nor do they occur in the majority of cases. They are, however, sufficiently prevalent that the clinician should be vigilant. It should be remembered that while they are not unique in this respect, the population of obese individuals seeking treatment contains substantial numbers of persons who are psychologically vulnerable. Members of this group should be identified and should be allowed to undertake a rigorous weight loss regimen only if psychological assessment suggests a favorable risk-benefit ratio. Further, continued contact with the patient after active weight loss is especially important, as many problems do not appear until the patient has been at a reduced weight for several months; by this time, unfortunately, most patients are no longer in contact with their treatment providers.

Acknowledgments

We wish to thank Lynn Byrd, Vicki Brumbelow, and Chris Hobby for assistance with manuscript preparation.

References

Adams, N., Ferguson, J., Stunkard, A. J., & Agras, S. (1978). The eating behaviour of obese and nonobese women. *Behaviour Research and Therapy, 16*, 225-232.

American Psychiatric Association. (1980). *Diagnostic and statistical manual of mental disorders* (3rd ed.) Washington, DC: Author.

American Psychiatric Association. (1987). *Diagnostic and statistical manual of mental disorders* (3rd ed., rev.). Washington, DC: Author.

Bandini, L. G., Schoeller, D. A., Cyr, H. N., & Dietz, W. H. (1990). Validity of reported energy intake in obese and non-obese adolescents. *American Journal of Clinical Nutrition, 52*, 421-425.

Beaudoin, R., & Mayer, J. (1953). Food intakes of obese and nonobese women. *Journal of the American Dietetic Association, 29*, 29-33.

Beck, A. T., Ward, C., Mendelson, M., Mock, J., & Erbaugh, J. (1961). An inventory for measuring depression. *Archives of General Psychiatry, 4*, 561-571.

Björvell, H., Rössner, S., & Stunkard, A. J. (1986). Obesity, weight loss, and dietary restraint. *International Journal of Eating Disorders, 5*, 727-734.

Blankmeyer, B. L., Smylie, K. D., Price, D. C., Costello, R. M., McFee, A. S., & Fuller, D. S. (1990). A replicated five cluster MMPI typology of morbidly obese female candidates for gastric bypass. *International Journal of Obesity, 14*, 235-247.

Coll, M., Meyer, A., & Stunkard, A. J. (1979). Obesity and food choices in public places. *Archives of General Psychiatry, 36*, 795-797.

Collins, J. K. (1987). Methodology for the objective measurement of body image. *International Journal of Eating Disorders, 6*, 393-399.

Collins, J. K., Beumont, P. J. V., Touyz, S. W., Krass, J., Thompson, P., & Philips, T. (1987). Variability in body shape perception in anorexic, bulimic, obese, and control subjects. *International Journal of Eating Disorders, 6*, 633-638.

Counts, C. R., & Adams, H. E. (1985). Body image in bulimic, dieting, and normal females. *Journal of Psychopathology and Behavioral Assessment, 7*, 289-300.

Crisp, A. H., & McGuiness, B. (1976). Jolly fat: Relation between obesity and psychoneurosis in the general population. *British Medical Journal, iii*, 7–9.

Dodd, D. K., Birky, H. J., & Stalling, R. B. (1976). Eating behaviour of obese and normal-weight females in a natural setting. *Addictive Behaviors, 1*, 321–325.

Drabman, R. S., Hammer, D., & Jarvis, G. J. (1977). Eating styles of obese and nonobese black and white children in a naturalistic setting. *Addictive Behaviors, 2*, 83–86.

Dreon, D., Frey-Hewitt, B., Ellsworth, N., Williams, P., Terry, R., & Wood, P. (1988). Dietary fat: Carbohydrate ratio and obesity in middle-aged men. *American Journal of Clinical Nutrition, 47*, 995–1000.

Freeman, R. J., Thomas, C. D., Solyom, L., & Miles, J. E. (1983). Body image disturbances in anorexia nervosa: A reexamination and a new technique. In P. L. Darby, P. E. Garfinkel, D. M. Garner, & D. V. Coscina (Eds.), *Anorexia nervosa: Recent developments in research* (pp. 117–127). New York: Alan R. Liss.

Garrow, J. (1974). *Energy balance and obesity in man*. New York: Elsevier.

Garrow, J. (1978a). *Energy balance and obesity in man* (2nd ed.). New York: American Elsevier.

Garrow, J. (1978b). The regulation of energy expenditure in man. In G. A. Bray (Ed.), *Recent advances in obesity research: II. Proceedings of the Second International Congress on Obesity* (pp. 200–210). London: Newman.

Gaul, D. J., Craighead, W. E., & Mahoney, M. J. (1975). Relationship between eating rates and obesity. *Journal of Consulting and Clinical Psychology, 43*, 123–125.

Glucksman, M. L., & Hirsch, J. (1961). The response of obese patients to weight reduction. *Psychosomatic Medicine, 31*, 1–7.

Glucksman, M. L., Hirsch, J., McCully, R. S., Barron, B. A., & Knittle, J. L. (1968). The response of obese patients to weight reduction. *Psychosomatic Medicine, 30*, 359–373.

Gormally, J., Black, S., Daston, S., & Rardin, D. (1982). The assessment of binge eating severity among obese persons. *Addictive Behaviors, 7*, 47–55.

Grinker, J. (1973). Behavioral and metabolic consequences of weight reduction. *Journal of the American Dietetic Association, 62*, 30–34.

Halmi, K. A., Long, M., Stunkard, A. J., & Mason, E. (1980). Psychiatric diagnosis of morbidly obese gastric bypass patients. *American Journal of Psychiatry, 137*, 470–472.

Hathaway, S., & McKinley, J. (1951). *The Minnesota Multiphasic Personality Inventory manual*. Minneapolis: University of Minnesota Press.

Herman, C. P., & Mack, D. (1975). Restrained and unrestrained eating. *Journal of Personality, 43*, 647–660.

Herman, C. P., & Polivy, J. (1980). Restrained eating. In A. J. Stunkard (Ed.), *Obesity* (pp. 208–225). Philadelphia: W. B. Saunders.

Hudson, J. I., Pope, H. G., Wurtman, J., Yurgelun-Todd, D., Mark, S., & Rosenthal, N. E. (1988). Bulimia in obese individuals. *Journal of Nervous and Mental Disease, 176*, 144–152.

James, W. P. T., Bailes, J., Davies, H. L., & Dauncey, M. J. (1978). Elevated metabolic rates in obesity. *Lancet, i*, 1122–1125.

Jamison, A. O. (1988). Obesity and sleep-disorder breathing. *Annals of Behavioral Medicine, 10*, 107–112.

Jarrell, M. P. (1990). *Obese binge eaters: Toward a more comprehensive understanding*. Unpublished doctoral dissertation, University of Mississippi.

Jéquier, E., & Schutz, Y. (1985). Does a defect in energy metabolism contribute to human obesity? In J. Hirsch & T. B. VanItallie (Eds.), *Recent advances in obesity research: IV. Proceedings of the Fourth International Congress on Obesity* (pp. 76–81). London: John Libbey.

Johnson, M. L., Burke, B. S., & Mayer, J. (1956). Relative importance of inactivity and overeating in the energy balance of obese high school girls. *American Journal of Clinical Nutrition, 4*, 37–44.

Keefe, P. H., Wyshogrod, D., Weinberger, E., & Agras, W. S. (1984). Binge eating and outcome of behavioural treatment of obesity: A preliminary report. *Behaviour Research and Therapy, 22*, 319–321.

Kissileff, H. S., Jordan, H. H., & Levitz, L. S. (1978). Eating habits of obese and normal weight humans. *International Journal of Obesity, 2*, 379.

Klesges, R. C. (1984). Personality and obesity: Global versus specific measures. *Behavior Therapy, 6*, 347–356.

Kolotkin, R. L., Revis, E. S., Kirkley, B., & Janick, L. (1987). Binge eating in obesity: Associated MMPI characteristics. *Journal of Consulting and Clinical Psychology, 55*, 872–876.

Lappalainen, R., Sjoden, P. O., Hursti, T., & Vesa, V. (1990). Hunger/craving responses and reactivity to food stimuli during fasting and dieting. *International Journal of Obesity, 14*, 679–688.

LaPorte, D. J. & Stunkard, A. J. (1990). Predicting attrition and adherence to a very low calorie diet: A prospective investigation of the Eating Inventory. *International Journal of Obesity, 14*, 197–206.

Leibel, R. C., & Hirsch, J. (1984). Diminished energy requirements in reduced-obese patients. *Metabolism, 33*, 164–170.

Leon, G. R., & Roth, L. (1977). Obesity: Psychological causes, correlations, and speculations. *Psychological Bulletin, 84*, 117–139.

Lindemann, A. K., Miller, W. C., Wallace, J., & Niederpruem, M. (1989). Diet composition, caloric intake, and exercise in relation to body fat. *Medicine and Science in Sports and Exercise, 21*(Suppl.), 599. (Abstract No. 591)

Loro, A. D., & Orleans, C. S. (1981). Binge eating in obesity: Preliminary findings and guidelines for behavioral analysis and treatment. *Addictive Behaviors, 6*, 155–166.

Mahoney, M.J. (1975). The obese eating style: Bites, beliefs, and behavior modification. *Addictive Behaviors, 1*, 47–53.

Maiman, L. A., Wang, V. L., Becker, M. H., Finlay, J., & Simonson, M. (1979). Attitudes toward obesity and the obese among professionals. *Journal of the American Dietetic Association, 74*, 331–336.

Marcus, M. D., & Wing, R. R. (1987). Binge eating among the obese. *Annals of Behavioral Medicine, 9*, 23–27.

Marcus, M. D., Wing, R. R., Ewing, L., Kern, E., Gooding, W., & McDermott, M. (1990). Psychiatric disorders among obese binge eaters. *International Journal of Eating Disorders, 9*, 69–77.

Marcus, M. D., Wing, R. R., Ewing, L., Kern, E., McDermott, M., & Gooding, W. (1990). A double-blind, placebo-controlled trial of fluoxetine plus behavior modification in the treatment of obese binge-eaters and non-binge-eaters. *American Journal of Psychiatry, 147*, 876–881.

Marcus, M. D., Wing, R. R., & Hopkins, J. (1988). Obese binge eaters: Affect, cognitions, and response to behavioral weight control. *Journal of Consulting and Clinical Psychology, 55*, 433–439.

Marcus, M. D., Wing, R. R., & Lamparski, D. M. (1985). Binge eating and dietary restraint in obese patients. *Addictive Behaviors, 10*, 163–168.

Nisbett, R. E. (1972). Hunger, obesity, and the ventromedial hypothalamus. *Psychological Review, 79*, 433–453.

O'Connor, J., & Dowrick, P. W. (1987). Cognitions in normal weight, overweight, and previously overweight adults. *Cognitive Therapy and Research, 11*, 315–326.

O'Neil, P. M., & Jarrell, M. P. (1991, August). *Body image changes during a very low calorie diet.* Paper presented at the meeting of the American Psychological Association, San Francisco.

Paine, P. M. (1982). Investigation of the abstinence violation effect in an obese population. *Dissertation Abstracts International, 42*, 3434B–3435B. (Abstract)

Prather, R. C., & Williamson, D. A. (1988). Psychopathology associated with bulimia, binge eating, and obesity. *International Journal of Eating Disorders, 31*, 429–440.

Robins, L. N., Helzer, J. E., Weissman, M. M., Orvaschel, H., Gruenberg, E., Burke, J. D., & Regier, D. A. (1984). Lifetime prevalence of specific psychiatric disorders in three sites. *Archives of General Psychiatry, 41*, 949–958.

Rosen, J. C., Hunt, D. A., Sims, E. A. H., & Bogardus, C. (1982). Comparison of carbohydrate-containing and carbohydrate-restricted hypocaloric diets in the treatment of obesity: Effects on appetite and mood. *American Journal of Clinical Medicine, 36,* 463-469.

Rosenthal, B. S., & Marx, R. D. (1978). Differences in eating patterns of successful and unsuccessful dieters, untreated overweight and normal weight individuals. *Addictive Behaviors, 3,* 129-134.

Schoeller, D. A. (1988). Measurement of energy expenditure in free-living humans by using doubly labeled water. *Journal of Nutrition, 118,* 1278-1289.

Silverstone, J. T. (1968). Psychological aspects of obesity. *Proceedings of the Royal Society of Medicine, 61,* 371-375.

Sjöström, L. (1985). A review of weight maintenance and weight changes in relation to energy metabolism and body composition. In J. Hirsch & T. B. VanItallie (Eds.), *Recent advances in obesity research: IV. Proceedings of the Fourth International Congress on Obesity.* London: John Libbey.

Smoller, J., Wadden, T., & Stunkard, A. J. (1987). Dieting and depression: A critical review. *Journal of Psychosomatic Research, 31,* 429-440.

Speaker, J. G., Schultz, C., Grinker, J. A., & Stern, J. S. (1983). Body size estimation and locus of control in obese adolescent boys undergoing weight reduction. *International Journal of Obesity, 7,* 73-83.

Spielberger, C. D. (1983). *Manual for the State-Trait Anxiety Inventory.* Palo Alto, CA: Consulting Psychologists Press.

Stewart, A. L., & Brook, R. H. (1983). Effects of being overweight. *American Journal of Public Health, 73,* 171-178.

Stuart, R. B., & Jacobson, B. (1987). *Weight, sex, and marriage: A delicate balance.* New York: Norton.

Stunkard, A. J. (1959). Eating patterns and obesity. *Psychiatry Quarterly, 33,* 284-292.

Stunkard, A. J., & Burt, V. (1967). Obesity and the body image: II. Age at onset of disturbances in the body image. *American Journal of Psychiatry, 123,* 1443-1447.

Stunkard, A. J., & Kaplan, D. (1977). Eating in public places: A review of reports of the direct observation of eating behavior. *International Journal of Obesity, 1,* 89-101.

Stunkard, A. J., & Mendelson, M. (1961). Disturbances in body image of some obese persons. *Journal of the American Dietetic Association, 38,* 328-331.

Stunkard, A. J., & Messick, S. (1985). The three-factor eating questionnaire to measure dietary restraint, disinhibition, and hunger. *Journal of Psychosomatic Research, 29,* 71-83.

Stunkard, A. J., & Rush, J. (1974). Dieting and depression reexamined: A critical review of reports of untoward responses during weight reduction for obesity. *Annals of Internal Medicine, 81,* 526-533.

Stunkard, A. J., & Wadden, T. A. (1990). Restrained eating and human obesity. *Nutrition Review, 48*(2), 78-86.

Wadden, T. A., Mason, G., Foster, G. D., Stunkard, A. J., & Prange, A. J. (1990). Effects of a very low calorie diet on weight, thyroid hormones and mood. *International Journal of Obesity, 14,* 249-258.

Wadden, T. A., & Stunkard, A. J. (1985). Social and psychological consequences of obesity. *Annals of Internal Medicine, 103,* 1062-1067.

Wadden, T. A., & Stunkard, A. J. (1986). Controlled trial of very low calorie diet, behavior therapy, and their combination in the treatment of obesity. *Journal of Consulting and Clinical Psychology, 54,* 482-488.

Wadden, T. A., Stunkard, A. J., Brownell, K. D., & Day, S. C. (1984). Treatment of obesity by behavior therapy and very low calorie diet: A pilot investigation. *Journal of Consulting and Clinical Psychology, 52,* 692-694.

Wadden, T. A., Stunkard, A. J., Brownell, K. D., & Day, S. C. (1985). A comparison of two very-low-calorie diets: Protein-sparing-modified fast versus protein-formula-liquid diet. *American Journal of Clinical Nutrition, 41,* 533-539.

Wadden, T. A., Stunkard, A. J., Day, S. C., Gould, R. A., & Rubin, C. J. (1987). Less food, less hunger: Reports of appetite and symptoms in a controlled study of a protein-sparing modified fast. *International Journal of Obesity, 11,* 239-249.

Wadden, T. A., Stunkard, A. J., & Smoller, J. W. (1986). Dieting and depression: A methodological study. *Journal of Consulting and Clinical Psychology, 54,* 869-871.

Wing, R. R., Epstein, L. H., Marcus, M. D., & Kupfer, D. J. (1984). Mood changes in behavioral weight loss programs. *Journal of Psychosomatic Research, 28,* 189-196.

Wooley, S. C., Wooley, O. W., & Dyrenforth, S. R. (1979). Theoretical, practical, and social issues in behavioral treatment of obesity. *Journal of Applied Behavior Analysis, 12,* 3-25.

PART FOUR

CLINICAL USE OF VERY LOW CALORIE DIETS

12

Medical Evaluation and Monitoring of Patients Treated by Severe Caloric Restriction

RICHARD L. ATKINSON

Severe caloric restriction as a strategy for weight reduction is very attractive to obese patients because it induces rapid weight loss. However, the physiological and pathophysiological consequences of severe caloric restriction mandate a greater degree of medical concern and monitoring than do other types of weight reduction programs. Since starvation is no longer viewed as a therapeutic option for obesity, this chapter will focus on very low calorie diets (VLCDs). The discussion will include a definition and the criteria for use of a VLCD; the initial evaluation; components of a comprehensive weight reduction program; monitoring during a VLCD; transition from a VLCD to a maintenance diet; and the role of a VLCD in long-term weight maintenance. I attempt to present opposing viewpoints, in addition to my own recommendations for use of a VLCD.

Definition of Very Low Calorie Diets

The term "very low calorie diet" has been used to define a variety of different diets with calorie levels between 0 and 800 kilocalories (kcal)/day. An "official" definition was devised in 1979 by an expert panel under the auspices of the Life Sciences Research Office of the Federation of American Societies for Experimental Biology, which was convened following the report of 60 fatalities in persons who consumed collagen-based "liquid protein" diets (Life Sciences Research Office [LSRO], 1979). This panel declared that diets containing less than 800 kcal/day are VLCDs. The use of fixed calorie levels, however, to define low calorie diets or VLCDs ignores the differences among individuals and cannot be defended on a physiological basis. A more rationale definition would be based on the number of calories required per kilogram of lean body mass, since lean body mass correlates best with daily energy expenditure. It is not practical, however, to measure lean body mass in individual patients; hence, I base calorie prescriptions on the medium frame "desirable" weight as defined by the Metropolitan Life Insurance Company (1959). In an arbitrary fashion, I define a VLCD as one that provides up to 10 kcal/kg of "desirable" body weight. Thus, for an "average" female 64 inches tall, with a "desirable" weight of about 55 kg, a VLCD would provide 550 kcal/day or fewer. It should be noted that these definitions deal only with calorie levels. As will be discussed below, essential nutrients must be carefully considered to ensure adequate intake.

Criteria for Use of Very Low Calorie Diets

Because VLCDs cause significant physiological changes and untoward side effects, many practitioners believe that they should be used with caution and according to strict criteria (Atkinson, 1989; Blackburn & Bray, 1985; Fisler & Drenick, 1987; Palgi et al., 1985; Wadden, Stunkard, & Brownell, 1983). Efforts to establish criteria for use of VLCDs evoke intense debate, and conservative medical opinion holds that the diets should be used only under a physician's supervision. The adverse health consequences of VLCDs are discussed elsewhere in this volume; in brief summary, however, VLCDs cause initial negative nitrogen balance, electrolyte changes, and profound changes in glucose metabolism and insulin levels (Atkinson, 1989; Wadden et al., 1983). Patients on a VLCD are prone to attacks of gout, gallbladder disease, and perhaps cardiac arrhythmias, leading some physicians to set very strict criteria for the use of these diets (Atkinson, 1989; Blackburn & Bray, 1985; Broomfield et al., 1988; U.S. Department of Health, Education and Welfare [DHEW], 1978; Fisler & Drenick, 1987; Lantigua, Amatruda, Biddle, Forbes, & Lockwood, 1980; Liddle, Goldstein, & Saxton, 1989; Palgi et al., 1985; Sours et al., 1981; Wadden et al., 1983). Such criteria limit VLCDs to patients who are at least 50% over "ideal" body weight and who have no cardiac, renal, hepatic, or other systemic disease (LSRO, 1979; Wadden et al., 1983; Wadden, VanItallie, & Blackburn, 1990). According to conservative criteria, angina is also a contraindication, although some physicians believe that angina may be an indication for VLCDs, since symptoms may improve rapidly upon initiation (Vertes, 1985). Clearly, malignant arrhythmias and unstable angina are absolute contraindications to VLCDs (de Silva, 1985).

Advanced renal disease is a contraindication because VLCDs cause negative nitrogen balance and require a high nitrogen intake to limit protein loss, both of which may further compromise renal function. Adequate documentation of the effects of VLCDs on short- and long-term renal function is lacking, but many investigators believe that a creatinine level over 2 mg/dl is a contraindication for VLCDs. Some believe that any elevation of creatinine precludes the use of these diets. Documentation of permanent adverse effects of VLCDs on hepatic function is also lacking, but abnormalities in liver function tests during consumption of VLCDs are well known (Andersen, in press). These abnormalities return to baseline when the diet is terminated.

Major systemic diseases, particularly those causing protein wasting, are absolute contraindications to VLCDs, as are drugs that cause protein wasting. A history of gout is also an absolute contraindication unless the patient is willing to take medication to lower uric acid. Uric acid rises dramatically during consumption of VLCDs, but I have never seen an attack of gout in a patient who did not have a previous history of gouty attacks (Atkinson, Russ, Ciavarella, Owsley, & Bibbs, 1984).

Patients on drugs must be carefully evaluated, especially drugs that cause electrolyte abnormalities. Insulin or oral hypoglycemic agents, antihypertensive agents, and psychotropic drugs may have adverse effects or exacerbate side effects of patients on a VLCD. Patients with a history of noncompliance to medical regimens or with emotional disorders that might affect compliance should be carefully evaluated before a VLCD is started.

A summary of contraindications for use of VLCDs is presented in Table 12.1. Of note is the criterion of body weight. I believe that VLCDs should not be used in patients less than 20% over "ideal" body weight. This figure is lower than the figure of 30–50% overweight used by many investigators, who argue that the 20% criterion is too low and is not safe (Wadden et al., 1990). One rationale for this position is that there is evidence that leaner individuals lose more protein than do the more obese (Forbes & Drenick, 1979). However, protein losses may be estimated incorrectly, depending on the method used

TABLE 12.1. Contraindications for Use of Very Low Calorie Diets

1. Absolute contraindications
   a. Malignant arrhythmias
   b. Unstable angina
   c. Pregnancy or lactation
   d. Protein-wasting diseases (e.g., lupus, Cushing's syndrome)
   e. Major system failure (e.g., liver failure, renal failure)
   f. Drug therapy causing protein wasting (e.g., steroids, antineoplastic agents)
   g. Body weight less than 20% over "desirable" (body mass index < 25)
   h. Gout or history of gout, not on medication
2. Relative contraindications
   a. Congestive heart failure
   b. Drug therapy with potassium-wasting diuretics, adrenergic-stimulating agents
   c. Young age (prepuberty)
   d. Electrolyte abnormalities
   e. History of eating disorder
   f. Body weight less than 50% over "desirable" (body mass index < 30)
   g. History of failure of compliance with medical regimen
3. Cautions
   a. Angina or history of heart disease
   b. Presence of systemic disease
   c. History of psychiatric or emotional disorder
   d. Chronic drug therapy (insulin, oral hypoglycemics, anti-inflammatory agents, psychotropic agents, etc.)

(Coxon et al., in press; Hegsted, 1978). In addition, the degree of nitrogen loss depends on total calorie intake, as well as the total quantity and quality of protein intake (Fisler & Drenick, 1987). Thus, a definitive number cannot be recommended for either calorie or protein intake, since these must be individualized according to the patient and the source of the nutrients. Fisler and Drenick (1987) reported that intakes of 66 g/day of good quality protein gave a less negative nitrogen balance than the lower levels of intake that were tested. Thus, very low calorie levels (10 kcal/kg of "desirable" weight or less) should be used with caution if daily intake of protein is less than 66 g.

Modern commercial VLCD formulations with adequate protein, vitamins, and minerals have been used by millions of people, with and without physician supervision or approval. The lack of reports to the Food and Drug Administration of deaths or serious side effects suggests that these diets may be safer than previously believed. The etiology of the deaths and arrhythmias reported with the use of "liquid protein" diets in the late 1970s is unclear and may have been due to a peculiarity of those formations. In addition, deaths in obese patients on "liquid protein" were compared to the expected death rate for the normal population (U.S. DHEW, 1978; Sours et al., 1981). Since obesity itself is associated with an increased risk of death, the death rate reported for obese patients on "liquid protein" diets was almost certainly overestimated. Thus, I am willing to allow patients with only modest obesity to consume a VLCD, as long as the diet is part of a long-term program for weight maintenance and patients are adequately supervised. It should be reiterated that this is not the opinion of all experts in the field.[1]

Initial Evaluation of Patients

History

A thorough history is the most important part of this evaluation. In addition to a medical history, information about obesity, body weight changes, and food intake patterns is critical. The examiner should ask when obesity or overweight first appeared, as well as inquire about changes in body weight over the years, lifetime maximum weight, events associated with rapid weight gain or loss, and (for females) effects of pregnancy on weight. A history of known complications of obesity should be obtained, and questions should be asked to identify any unrecognized complications. Complications that frequently have not been

---

[1]*Editors' note*: We believe that it is absolutely essential that patients receive an extensive medical evaluation to determine their appropriateness for treatment by a VLCD, and that they be monitored by a physician while consuming the diet. Moreover, we believe that VLCDs should be limited to persons who are a minimum of 30% overweight. Mildly obese persons spare fat-free mass less satisfactorily during severe caloric restriction than do the markedly obese. In addition, the mildly obese can be successfully treated by the safer and less expensive approach of a 1200-kcal/day diet combined with lifestyle modification.

recognized by the patient are sleep apnea, diabetes mellitus, hypertension, gallbladder disease, gout, and hyperlipidemia. Sleep apnea deserves special mention, since it is common among the obese and frequently is not recognized. The major symptoms include morning headache, daytime hypersomnolence, restless sleep, nightmares, nocturnal awakening with dyspnea, and dramatically loud snoring. Family members may give a history of apneic episodes if asked. A suspicious history for sleep apnea mandates referral to a sleep laboratory for evaluation.

Other items of importance in the history include documentation of prior attempts to lose weight and their success. The examiner should ask about the use of drugs for weight loss and prior attempts to lose weight using a VLCD. Total weight lost with each attempt and time to regain weight should be noted.

The family history is important, including heights and weights of immediate family members and presence of any complications of obesity. Patients should be asked to try to identify any special problems or risk factors that perpetuate obesity or cause weight regain. Patients may be reluctant to talk about emotional or social factors, so special attention should be paid to these issues. Specific questions should be asked about use and abuse of alcohol or any unusual eating habits or patterns, since VLCDs should be used with extreme caution in patients with a history of alcoholism or eating disorder. Finally, a thorough review of systems must be taken to identify any evidence of endocrine or metabolic disease as an occult etiology of obesity, and to identify any systemic disease that might affect the treatment program (e.g., cardiac disease, arthritis, etc.).

Physical Examination

A complete physical examination is necessary, with attention to details specific to obesity, complications of obesity, or factors that might affect the treatment program. Evidence of hypertension or diabetes should be sought. The upper airway (tonsils, adenoids, uvula) should be checked for evidence of airway narrowing, particularly if symptoms of sleep apnea are present. Evidence of dental problems, skin breakdown in intertriginous areas, varicose veins or calf tenderness (for thrombophlebitis), peripheral edema, and venous stasis changes may be more common in obese patients. Conditions that might affect the treatment or exercise program, such as flat feet, arthritis, and varus or valgus deformities of the feet or legs, should be determined.

Laboratory Tests

Laboratory tests I recommend include (1) a complete blood count and differential; (2) a chemistry panel including electrolytes, glucose, renal and liver function tests, uric acid, cholesterol, and triglycerides; (3) thyroid function tests; (4) urinalysis; and (5) an electrocardiogram (EKG). Because cardiac arrhythmias are a potential danger of VLCDs, a serum magnesium level is also useful. Heavy alcohol intake may cause magnesium loss in the urine, predisposing the patient to arrhythmias. Further evaluation is indicated for anemia, abnormal white blood cell count, and elevated hepatic or renal function tests.

Careful consideration must be given before starting a VLCD with a patient with abnormalities of any of these tests. An elevated uric acid level should alert the physician to evaluate the patient for a history of gout and to follow the individual more closely on the VLCD for any evidence of an acute attack of gout. If there is any evidence from the history or physical exam of cardiac arrhythmias or angina, a cardiac stress test may be useful before starting an exercise program. Since any exercise program must be started very slowly anyway, the cost-benefit ratio of stress testing must be evaluated. I should note that some investigators do not believe that all of these laboratory tests are indicated, but it is prudent to obtain them in the presence of massive obesity or any evidence of a complication of obesity.

Components of a Comprehensive Weight Program Using a Very Low Calorie Diet: An Overview

The elements of a comprehensive weight reduction program are discussed elsewhere in this volume, but a brief summary is provided here for reference to medical evaluation and monitoring. Nutrition education is critical when a VLCD is used, especially if a commercial formula diet is not employed. Patients must understand the importance of ingesting adequate quantities of essential vitamins and minerals, and obtaining these from food is difficult on a VLCD. Since long-term use of a VLCD is not possible, patients should be given dietary education about the transition period from VLCD to regular food, and the necessity for lifelong modification of eating habits.

Behavioral techniques must be taught for short-term adaptation to the VLCD and for long-term weight maintenance. Many programs that employ a VLCD teach behavioral techniques for long-term weight maintenance while patients are on the VLCD. I believe that this is a mistake and that such training should be withheld until patients resume consumption of a maintenance diet. Alternatively, it should be provided before patients start the VLCD.

Exercise is a critical component of a long-term weight reduction program. Investigators disagree, however, concerning whether exercise provides additional benefit during consumption of the VLCD. Phinney and colleagues showed that peak aerobic power and submaximal endurance were not affected on a high protein VLCD after the initial period of adaptation to ketone utilization (Phinney et al., 1980; Phinney, LaGrange, O'Connell, & Danforth, 1988). In reviewing a number of studies, however, Phinney (in press) noted that VLCDs providing low protein intakes may be associated with decreased exercise performance and that exercise probably does not increase nitrogen retention unless protein intake is low.

The final component of a comprehensive weight reduction program is the psychological support and encouragement provided by the multidisciplinary team of professionals. The initial weight reduction caused by the natriuresis and diuresis on a VLCD is exciting for patients. Education and support are required, however, when the rate of loss slows or when patients reach a plateau on the VLCD or gain a small amount of weight. The possibility of fluid retention and "stairstep" weight loss (periods of rapid loss followed by periods of no loss) must be explained to patients. Since marked food restriction may increase the tendency to binge-eat (Keys, Brozek, Henschel, Mickelsen, & Taylor, 1950), patients must be warned of this and preventive strategies formulated. Finally, extensive psychological support and encouragement are needed when patients terminate the VLCD. Patients must be warned in advance of the possibility of rapid weight gain, due to refilling of the gut with food and to the sodium and water retention occurring with carbohydrate ingestion. Binge eating during this time is common, so patients need closer attention.

Initiation of the Diet

The first 2 weeks of a VLCD are a time of great physiological change and stress, so following patients closely during this time is desirable. Hunger is the first symptom noted by most patients, and is greatest during the first week. The reason why hunger tends to diminish after the first week is unclear, although some investigators attribute the decline to the rise in serum ketones. Other studies suggest that hunger diminishes even in the absence of ketosis (Rosen, Hunt, Sims, & Bogardus, 1982).

Most VLCDs are low to very low in carbohydrate (CHO) and fat, while relatively high in protein. Since CHO is the preferred substrate for the brain, red blood cells, and renal medulla, the body defends the level of blood glucose vigorously. Thus, during the first 24–48 hours in which a VLCD is consumed, glycogen stores in the liver are mobilized to support the blood sugar. Glucose cannot be made from endogenous or exogenous fat, and liver glycogen supplies are limited to about 1 day's energy needs. Once liver glycogen is depleted, blood sugar would fall without an alternate source of glucose production. Gluconeogenesis from protein is the only alternative, and protein catabolism accelerates as liver glycogen is depleted. Muscle is the main source of protein for gluconeogenesis, but other organs, such as the lungs and heart, also have negative protein balance during the first 1–2 weeks of consumption of the VLCD. All VLCDs, whatever their total daily intake of protein, cause negative nitrogen balance during this time (Fisler & Drenick, 1987). Since protein is critical, however, for structure and function in the body, there is gradual adaptation to utilizing ketones and fatty acids from fat as the major fuel source for most of the body, including the brain. Patients need to be educated about these changes and followed carefully during this period to encourage them not to "cheat" on their diet by eating additional CHO, since this seems to enhance hunger and may lead to additional cheating.

Patients with Medical Complications

Patients who enter a VLCD with complications of obesity or other health problems may require special care, particularly if they are on medication. Potassium-losing diuretics are contraindicated on a VLCD. Hypertensive patients should be taken off such drugs and followed carefully. Several visits per week may be required initially to check blood pressure. Since weight loss alone reduces blood pressure (Reisin et al., 1978), such drugs are rarely needed while the patient remains on the VLCD. When the patient discontinues the VLCD, however, drug therapy may need to be restarted. Diabetics receiving treatment must also be followed closely. Since elevated blood glucose levels fall rapidly on a VLCD (Atkinson & Kaiser, 1985; Genuth, Castro, & Vertes, 1974), insulin or oral hypoglycemics should be cut in half or discontinued. Even high doses of insulin may be discontinued without problems in the vast majority of obese patients who consume a VLCD. Patients *must* check their blood sugars at home with glucose-testing strips or meters. It is wise to measure ketone levels as well, since rare cases of diabetic ketoacidosis have been reported. Patients may call in to report daily blood sugar and ketone levels rather than visiting the office or clinic.

Patients on drug treatment for both diabetes and hypertension must be followed extremely carefully, especially if they are on beta-blocking agents. These drugs may mask symptoms of hypoglycemia. Such patients should have hypoglycemic agents stopped, and they should check blood sugars several times daily. Alternately, the beta blocker may be stopped and blood pressure monitored or another agent started. There is no substitute for adequate patient education about the complications of obesity and the problems that may be encountered on a VLCD.

Rapid Weight Loss

Patients also need to be educated about the rapid weight loss that occurs with VLCDs. Weight losses of 2–7 kg during the first week on a VLCD are common, and I once observed a massively obese patient with edema who lost 24.5 kg during this time. This rapid weight loss raises false expectations about longer-term weight loss and the time that will be needed to lose all excess weight. Patients should be told that several factors cause an accelerated weight loss during their initial consumption of the VLCD, and that this rate of loss will slow to about 1–2 kg per week. Gut fill of food and feces accounts for about 0.5 to 2 kg of weight, and when intake decreases to very small amounts of low fiber food, gut fill decreases correspondingly. Of more importance are the diuresis and natriuresis of fasting (Boulter, Hoffman, & Arky, 1973; DeHaven, Sherwin, Hendler, & Felig, 1982; Saudek, Boulter, & Arky, 1973; Scheen, Luyckx, Fossion, & Lefebvre, 1983). The low CHO intake results in a tendency for lowered blood glucose, and thus insulin levels decrease (Atkinson & Kaiser, 1985). Insulin is a sodium-retaining hormone, and lower levels promote a natriuresis (Boulter et al., 1973; DeHaven et al., 1982). Furthermore, glucagon levels rise with the low CHO intake and the necessity to defend the blood sugar. Glucagon is a natriuretic hormone, and thus accelerates sodium loss (Saudek et al., 1973). Glucagon also increases fatty acid metabolism and ketone formation in the liver. Some of the ketones are excreted in the urine, and since they are negatively charged anions, they require positively charged cations to be excreted to maintain neutrality (Scheen et al., 1983). Sodium and potassium are the major cations excreted initially with the ketones. As sodium levels fall, mineralocorticoid secretion increases to preserve sodium stores, and this accelerates potassium excretion. Potassium also is lost when glycogen is mobilized, since 0.45 mmol of potassium are bound per gram of glycogen (Coxon et al., in press). Within a few days, ammonium ions become the major cation excreted to preserve acid–base balance, but patients remain prone to sodium and particularly potassium loss throughout the VLCD.

Schedule of Monitoring

The numerous changes, both physiological and psychological, that occur early in a VLCD make this one of the most critical periods for medical observation and psychological support. Some programs see patients briefly each day during the VLCD, whereas others have weekly visits. I recommend weekly visits for the first 2 weeks, then visits every other week during the VLCD.

Duration of Dieting

The number of weeks that patients should be allowed to stay on a VLCD is also controversial. Many programs allow massively obese patients to remain on VLCD for extended periods of 6 months or longer. In the past, I have limited time on a VLCD to 12 weeks, but this is a conservative position. Moyer and colleagues performed Holter monitoring and repeated stress tests on 24 patients on VLCDs for a period of 6 weeks and found no evidence of arrhythmias (Moyer, Holly, Amsterdam, & Atkinson, 1989). Neither Weigle, Callahan, Fellows, and Greene (1989) nor Doherty et al. (1991) observed a significant increase in arrhythmias in patients who dieted for 95 and 112 days, respectively. These data, along with those from other studies that have shown no cardiac problems, suggest that VLCDs can be used safely for at least 16 weeks (Amatruda, Biddle, Patton, & Lockwood, 1983; McLean Baird, 1985; Phinney et al., 1983; Ramhamadany et al., 1989). The average length of time before death for the people who died on the "liquid protein" diets of the 1970s was about 5 months, with a range of 2–8 months (U.S. DHEW, 1978; Sours et al., 1981). However, there has not been an excess of deaths reported with modern formulas, which provide protein of high biological value; this finding supports the use of VLCD for periods longer than 12 weeks.

Another rationale for allowing patients to remain on a VLCD for more extended periods is that they may not lose as much weight during a second period of VLCD (Smith & Wing, 1991). This may be due to a metabolic adaptation or to difficulty in adhering to the VLCD during a second diet. On the other hand, patients should not be allowed to reduce below their "desirable" weight. Patients who continue to lose after achieving "desirable" weight should be carefully evaluated for any signs of an eating disorder.

Treatment Personnel

There is diversity of opinion as to the makeup of the health care team for patients who consume a VLCD. At one extreme are programs that insist that a physician assess the patient at each visit. At the other extreme are commercial diet plans sold over the counter or by lay salespersons; some of these require no physician involvement.

I strongly believe that all persons considering the use of a VLCD should receive a thorough medical examination to determine their appropriateness for such treatment. With patients who pass this initial examination, I take the somewhat controversial position that trained nonphysician health professionals, working under supervision, can provide adequate care at a lower cost. The problems that arise in obese patients who consume a VLCD are routine and generally not life-threatening. Nurses, nurse practitioners, and dietitians can be trained to recognize unusual physical and emotional problems that require referral to a physician or mental health professional (Atkinson & Kaiser, 1981; Atkinson et al., 1977, 1984). Patients may be discussed with the physician at periodic chart review sessions or more frequently, as needed. Over 1000 patients were treated without significant problems by nurses and dietitians under my supervision (Atkinson & Kaiser, 1981). These therapists spend about 1 hour per visit with each patient, treating them individually and in small groups at a cost far lower than would be possible with physician visits.

This concern for cost containment extends also to the issue of providing multidisciplinary care by a team which includes not only a physician or nurse, but a behavioral psychologist, dietitian, and exercise physiologist. Logically, programs that include a variety of trained health professionals should produce better short- and long-term results than those programs that do not include multidisciplinary care, but this has not been shown conclusively. There is some evidence that a comprehensive behavioral program improves the maintenance of weight loss 1-2 years after treatment (Pavlou, Krey, & Steffee, 1989; Sikand, Kondo, Foreyt, Jones, & Gotto, 1988; Wadden & Stunkard, 1986). Few commercial studies, however, have published data on their results, and the intensive programs at academic centers may have little relationship to nonacademic programs. Weight losses 3-5 years after treatment by VLCD are generally small or not significantly different from baseline for the vast majority of people, regardless of the depth of the health care team (Wadden, Sternberg, Letizia, Stunkard, & Foster, 1989; Wadden, Stunkard, & Liebschutz, 1988). Further research is clearly needed to determine the most cost-effective approach to treatment.

Medical Monitoring during the Diet

Review of Information with the Patient

At each visit during patients' consumption of a VLCD, certain information must be obtained. Measurements of weight, blood pressure, and pulse should be recorded; patients should also be questioned specifically about symptoms of known major complications of VLCDs, such as cardiac dysfunction, gallbladder disease, gout, syncopal episodes, and electrolyte deficiencies (e.g., arrhythmias, angina, dyspnea, abdominal pain, joint pain, syncope or faintness, muscle cramps or weakness, etc.). Therapists should ask about compliance with the diet, presence of any physical symptoms in addition to those listed above, and any emotional problems or new life stressors since the last visit. Any new drug use (including over-the-counter drugs) and any visits to physicians or other health care professionals should be elicited. The rate of weight loss should be followed carefully. After the initial period of diuresis, weight loss greater than 2 kg per week may signal that the patient is not eating the prescribed amount of VLCD, may be starving to achieve more rapid loss, or may be developing anorectic behavior. All diabetic patients should be on home glucose monitoring (at least once daily), and these records must be reviewed.

Laboratory Tests

There is no agreement on the appropriate laboratory tests that should be ordered at each visit. I am conservative and obtain a complete blood count, chemistry panel (e.g., SMA-20), serum magnesium, and an EKG rhythm strip at each weekly or biweekly visit. Many physicians feel that obtaining these tests once monthly is adequate. In my experience, the need to alter care on the basis of these tests is infrequent. An elevated uric acid level in the absence of symptoms is not an indication for initiation of medication. High uric acid levels usually drop to or toward normal after 3–4 weeks on a VLCD. Obviously, if symptoms of gout appear, the patient must be treated, and consideration should be given to stopping the VLCD if symptoms are not quickly controlled. Low potassium levels are occasionally seen and should prompt the therapist to inquire about the use of diuretics. Many patients have access to diuretics from previous treatment for hypertension or from relatives, and they may self-medicate when they reach a plateau period during the VLCD. Others may forget or neglect to tell the physician at the time of the initial physical exam that they are on a diuretic. Some patients who have been on diuretics and discontinue them upon initiation of the VLCD may have low total body potassium reserves and may require supplementation. Finally, as noted above, potassium is lost as a consequence of alterations of mineralocorticoid secretion, glycogen breakdown, and preservation of acid–base balance.

An occasional patient with a borderline hematocrit (usually a female) will have a slow drop in hematocrit on a VLCD and fall into the anemic range. Such patients should be checked for any evidence of gastrointestinal blood loss, and an iron supplement may be started. Since iron preparations may be irritating to the gastric or intestinal mucosa, they should be taken with a meal or serving of formula diet.

Since EKG rhythm strips may miss arrhythmias present on Holter monitoring (Lantigua et al., 1980), the physician should not become falsely complacent if the patient has cardiac symptoms and a normal rhythm strip. A 24-hour Holter monitor test is indicated if cardiac arrhythmia symptoms (e.g., tachycardia, palpitations, etc.) appear or become more frequent, and the physician should consider stopping the VLCD. The presence of a prolonged QTc interval has been thought to predispose individuals to cardiac arrhythmias (Blackburn & Bray, 1985; U.S. DHEW, 1978; Fisler & Drenick, 1987; Lantigua et al., 1980; Sours et al., 1981); therefore, appearance of this finding on the EKG rhythm strip mandates careful evaluation and may be an indication for stopping the VLCD.

Terminating the Diet

The transition period to a regular diet is perhaps the most dangerous time during a VLCD. The mineral and electrolyte changes that occur at initiation of a VLCD are reversed at termination. With increased CHO intake, insulin levels rise, resulting in sodium retention and concomitant water retention. The combination of increased CHO and insulin drives potassium and phosphorus into the cells, and there is danger of low blood levels of these substances. The "refeeding syndrome" is well known (Keys et al., 1950), and about 40% of the deaths that occurred with the "liquid protein" diets came during the early part of the refeeding period (U.S. DHEW, 1978; Sours et al., 1981). The transition to a more normal diet should be carried out gradually. I use a powdered formula diet mixed with water for the VLCD. During the transition period, the formula diet is mixed with milk, increasing the calories from about 450 to 800 kcal/day for about 1 week. At week two, regular food (about 500 kcal) is added for one meal per day, then two meals per day, and finally back to three meals per day over about 7–10 days. Lactose-intolerant patients cannot use this regimen and must go through the transition with regular food. Other programs initiate refeeding over variable periods as long as 12 weeks (Genuth et al., 1974; Kirschner, Schneider, Ertel, & Gorman, 1988; Palgi et al., 1985).

Psychological problems also occur with termination of the VLCD. Patients may develop a false sense of accomplishment and believe that their problem with obesity is solved. They may drop out of the treatment program and resume previous eating habits. The cessation of weight loss and occasional rapid weight gain that occurs even in compliant patients (due to gut fill and water retention) can be very discouraging. Binge eating may appear, perhaps because of the loss of rigid discipline of the VLCD, but also because of physiological forces. Keys et al. (1950) reported that bingeing lasted up to 2 years in their normal volunteers who consumed a 1500-kcal diet for 6 months. This excessive feeding behavior can be seen in animals who have been starved, and probably represents a form of defense of body weight. Patients need to be informed of what to expect and given added support with frequent visits during this time. These problems are minimized by a gradual increase in calorie intake as described above.

Because of the physiological and psychological problems that appear, patients should be seen weekly for the first 2–4 weeks or longer upon termination of the VLCD. This should be a time of intensified education, encouragement, and psychological support. The potential for mineral and electrolyte abnormalities mandates that laboratory tests be performed at each visit. Appearance of an arrhythmia or congestive heart failure should be treated as a medical emergency. At a minimum, if arrhythmias occur, a 24-hour Holter monitor test should be performed and the diet strictly monitored. It may be wise to decrease the consumption of CHO if symptoms occur. Careful evaluation and replacement of potassium, magnesium, and phosphorus is mandatory if symptoms occur. Binge eating should be diagnosed and treated aggressively.

Long-Term Care and Weight Cycling

A comprehensive program of diet, exercise, and lifestyle modification is necessary for long-term weight maintenance, as described elsewhere in this volume. If this strategy fails and the patient regains weight, pressure inevitably is brought upon the health care team to allow the patient to go back on a VLCD. Some investigators and commercial programs suggest that repeated cycles of VLCD are a reasonable strategy for long-term weight maintenance. In recent years, there has been concern that weight cycling may be detrimental to long-term health (Brownell, 1989). The data supporting this hypothesis are skimpy and contradictory (Blackburn et al., 1989; Brownell, 1989; Brownell, Steen, &

Wilmore, 1987; Lissner, Andres, Muller, & Shimokata, 1990; Prentice et al., in press; Prentice, Whitehead, Roberts, & Paul, 1981; Steen, Oppliger, & Brownell, 1988; van Dale & Saris, 1989). Many investigators speculate that weight cycling will increase body fatness. Few human studies have been done, but animal studies do not support this hypothesis (Prentice et al., in press). Prentice et al. (in press) have shown that Gambian natives who go through periods of limited food supplies each year during the agricultural cycle do not have evidence of increased weight gain or adiposity. There may well be a more rapid weight gain of lost weight with repeated cycles and a slower weight loss with dieting, but these appear to be acute, not long-term, changes. Recent studies suggest that weight change is associated with an increased incidence of coronary artery disease and mortality (Lissner et al., 1991). Further studies are necessary to determine whether the potential adverse effects of cycles of weight loss and regain outweigh the acute favorable improvements in health bestowed by weight loss.

References

Amatruda, J. M., Biddle, T. L., Patton, M. L., & Lockwood, D. H. (1983). Vigorous supplementation of a hypocaloric diet prevents cardiac arrhythmias and mineral depletion. *American Journal of Medicine, 74*, 1016-1022.

Andersen, T. (in press). Liver and gallbladder disease before and after very low calorie diet. *American Journal of Clinical Nutrition*.

Atkinson, R. L. (1989). Low and very low calorie diets. *Medical Clinics of North America, 73*, 203-215.

Atkinson, R. L., Greenway, F. L., Bray, G. A., Dahms, W. T., Molitch, M. E., Hamilton, K., & Rodin, J. (1977). Treatment of obesity: Comparison of physician and nonphysician therapists using placebo and anorectic drugs in a double-blind trial. *International Journal of Obesity, 1*, 113-120.

Atkinson, R. L., & Kaiser, D. L. (1981). Nonphysician supervision of a very-low-calorie diet: Results in over 200 cases. *International Journal of Obesity, 5*, 237-241.

Atkinson R. L., & Kaiser, D. L. (1985). Effects of calorie restriction and weight loss on glucose and insulin levels in obese humans. *Journal of the American College of Nutrition, 4*, 411-419.

Atkinson, R. L., Russ, C. S., Ciavarella, P. A., Owsley, E. S., & Bibbs, M. L. (1984). A comprehensive approach to outpatient obesity management. *Journal of the American Dietetic Association, 84*, 439-444.

Blackburn, G. L., & Bray, G. A. (Eds.). (1985). *Management of obesity by severe caloric restriction*. Littleton, MA: PSG.

Blackburn, G. L., Wilson, G. T., Kanders, B. S., Stein, L. J., Lavin, P. T., Adler, J., & Brownell, K. D. (1989). Weight cycling: The experience of human dieters. *American Journal of Clinical Nutrition, 49*(Suppl. 5), 1105-1109.

Boulter, P. R., Hoffman, R. S., & Arky, R. A. (1973). Pattern of sodium excretion accompanying starvation. *Metabolism, 22*, 675-683.

Broomfield, P. H., Chopra, R., Sheinbaum, R. C., Bonorris, G. G., Silverman, A., Schoenfield, L. J., & Marks, J. W. (1988). Effects of ursodeoxycholic acid and aspirin on the formation of lithogenic bile and gallstones during loss of weight. *New England Journal of Medicine, 319*, 1567-1572.

Brownell, K. D. (1989). Weight cycling. *American Journal of Clinical Nutrition, 49*(Suppl. 5), 937.

Brownell, K. D., Steen, S. N., & Wilmore, J. H. (1987). Weight regulation practices in athletes:

Analysis of metabolic and health effects. *Medicine and Science in Sports and Exercise, 19*, 546-556.

Coxon, A. Y., Kreitzman, S. N., Morgan, W. D., Johnson, P. G., Compston, J. E., Eston, R., & Howard, A. N. (in press). Change in body composition and energy balance on VLCD: A multicenter study. *American Journal of Clinical Nutrition.*

DeHaven, I., Sherwin, R., Hendler, R., & Felig, P. (1982). Nitrogen and sodium balance and sympathetic-nervous-system activity in obese subjects treated with a low-calorie protein or mixed diet. *New England Journal of Medicine, 302*, 477-482.

de Silva, R. A. (1985). Ionic, catecholamine and dietary effects on cardiac rhythm. In G. L. Blackburn & G. A. Bray (Eds.), *Management of obesity by severe caloric restriction* (pp. 183-204). Littleton, MA: PSG.

Doherty, J. U., Wadden, T. A., Zuk, L., Letizia, K. A., Foster, G. D., & Day, S. C. (1991). Long-term evaluation of cardiac function in obese patients treated by very-low-calorie diet: A controlled clinical study of patients without underlying cardiac disease. *American Journal of Clinical Nutrition, 53*, 854-858.

Fisler, J. S., & Drenick, E. J. (1987). Starvation and semistarvation diets in the management of obesity. *Annual Review of Nutrition, 7*, 465-484.

Forbes, G. B., & Drenick, E. J. (1979). Loss of body nitrogen on fasting. *American Journal of Clinical Nutrition, 32*, 1570-1574.

Genuth, S. M., Castro, J. H., & Vertes, V. (1974). Weight reduction in obesity by outpatient semistarvation. *Journal of the American Medical Association, 230*, 987-991.

Hegsted, D. M. (1978). Assessment of nitrogen requirements. *American Journal of Clinical Nutrition, 31*, 1669-1677.

Keys, A., Brozek, J., Henschel, A., Mickelsen, O., & Taylor, H. L. (1950). *The biology of human starvation* (2 vols.). Minneapolis: University of Minnesota Press.

Kirschner, M. A., Schneider, G., Ertel, N. H., & Gorman, J. (1988). An eight-year experience with a very-low-calorie formula diet for control of major obesity. *International Journal of Obesity, 12*, 69-80.

Lantigua, R. A., Amatruda, J. M., Biddle, T. L., Forbes, G. B., & Lockwood, D. H. (1980). Cardiac arrhythmias associated with a liquid protein diet for the treatment of obesity. *New England Journal of Medicine, 303*, 735-738.

Liddle, R. A., Goldstein, R. B., & Saxton, J. (1989). Gallstone formation during weight-reduction dieting. *Archives of Internal Medicine, 149*, 1750-1753.

Life Sciences Research Office (LSRO). (1979). *Research needs in management of obesity by severe caloric restriction* (Contract No. FDA 223-75-2090). Washington, DC: Federation of American Societies for Experimental Biology.

Lissner, L., Andres, R., Muller, D. C., & Shimokata, H. (1990). Body weight variability in men: Metabolic rate, health and longevity. *International Journal of Obesity, 14*, 373-383.

Lissner, L., Odell, P. M., D'Agostino, R. B., Stokes, J., Kreger, B. E., Belanger, A. J., & Brownell, K. D. (1991). Variability of body weight and health outcomes in the Framingham population. *New England Journal of Medicine, 324*, 1839-1844.

McLean Baird, I. (1985). Ambulatory monitoring of obese subjects on normal and very low calorie diets. In G. L. Blackburn & G. A. Bray (Eds.), *Management of obesity by severe caloric restriction* (pp. 215-222). Littleton, MA: PSG.

Metropolitan Life Insurance Company. (1959). Metropolitan height and weight tables. *Statistical Bulletin of the Metropolitan Life Insurance Company, 40*, 1-4.

Moyer, C. L., Holly, R. G., Amsterdam, E. A., & Atkinson, R. L. (1989). The effects of cardiac stress during a very low calorie diet and exercise program in obese women. *American Journal of Clinical Nutrition, 50*, 1324-1327.

Palgi, A., Read, J. L., Greenberg, I., Hoefer, M. A., Bistrian, B. R., & Blackburn, G. L. (1985). Multidisciplinary treatment of obesity with a protein-sparing modified fast: Results in 668 outpatients. *American Journal of Public Health, 75*, 1190-1194.

Pavlou, K. N., Krey, S., & Steffee, W. P. (1989). Exercise as an adjunct to weight loss and maintenance in moderately obese subjects. *American Journal of Clinical Nutrition, 49,* 1115-1123.

Phinney, S. D. (in press). Exercise during and after very low calorie dieting. *American Journal of Clinical Nutrition.*

Phinney, S. D., Bistrian, B. R., Kosinski, E., Chan, D. P., Hoffer, L. J., Rolla, A., Schachtel, B., & Blackburn, G. L. (1983). Normal cardiac rhythm observed during hypocaloric diets of varying carbohydrate content. *Archives of Internal Medicine, 143,* 2258-2261.

Phinney, S. D., Horton, E. S., Sims, E. A. H., Hanson, J. S., Danforth, E., Jr., & LaGrange, B. L. (1980). Capacity for moderate exercise in obese subjects after adaptation to a hypocaloric ketogenic diet. *Journal of Clinical Investigation, 66,* 1152-1161.

Phinney, S. D., LaGrange, B. M., O'Connell, M., & Danforth, E., Jr. (1988). Effects of aerobic exercise on energy expenditure and nitrogen balance during very low calorie dieting. *Metabolism, 37,* 758-765.

Prentice, A. M., Jebb, S. A., Goldberg, G. R., Coward, W. A., Murgatroyd, P. R., Poppitt, S. D., & Cole, T. J. (in press). Effects of weight cycling on body composition. *American Journal of Clinical Nutrition.*

Prentice, A. M., Whitehead, R. G., Roberts, S. B., & Paul, A. A. (1981). Long-term energy balance in child-bearing Gambian women. *American Journal of Clinical Nutrition, 34,* 2790-2799.

Ramhamadany, E., Dasgupta, P., Brigden, G., Lahiri, A., Raftery, E. B., & McLean Baird, I. (1989). Cardiovascular changes in obese subjects on very low calorie diet. *International Journal of Obesity, 13*(Suppl. 2), 95-99.

Reisin, E., Abel, R., Modan, M., Silverberg, D. S., Eliahou, H. E., & Modan, B. (1978). Effect of weight loss without salt restriction on the reduction of blood pressure in overweight hypertensive patients. *New England Journal of Medicine, 298,* 1-6.

Rosen, J. C., Hunt, D. A., Sims, E. A. H., & Bogardus, C. (1982). Comparison of carbohydrate-containing and carbohydrate-restricted hypocaloric diets in the treatment of obesity: Effects on appetite and mood. *American Journal of Clinical Nutrition, 36,* 463-469.

Saudek, C. D., Boulter, P. R., & Arky, A. R. (1973). The natriuretic effect of glucagon and its role in starvation. *Journal of Clinical Endocrinology and Metabolism, 36,* 761-765.

Scheen, A. J., Luyckx, A. S., Fossion, A., & Lefebvre, P. J. (1983). Effect of protein-supplemented fasting on the fuel-hormone response to prolonged exercise in obese subjects. *International Journal of Obesity, 7,* 327-337.

Sikand, G., Kondo, A., Foreyt, J. P., Jones, P. H., & Gotto, A. M. (1988). Two-year follow-up of patients treated with a very low calorie diet and exercise training. *Journal of the American Dietetic Association, 88,* 487-488.

Smith, D. E., & Wing, R. R. (1991). Diminished weight loss and behavioral compliance during repeated diets in obese patients with type II diabetes. *Health Psychology, 10,* 373-383.

Sours, H. E., Frattali, V. P., Brand, C. D., Feldman, R. A., Forbes, A. L., Swanson, R. C., & Paris, A. L. (1981). Sudden death associated with very low calorie weight reduction regimens. *American Journal of Clinical Nutrition, 34,* 453-461.

Steen, S. N., Oppliger, R. A., & Brownell, K. D. (1988). Metabolic effects of repeated weight loss and regain in adolescent wrestlers. *Journal of the American Medical Association, 260,* 47-50.

U.S. Department of Health, Education and Welfare (DHEW). (1978, May-July). *Liquid protein and sudden cardiac death—an update* (FDA Drug Bulletin, Vol. 8, No. 3). Washington, DC: U.S. Government Printing Office.

van Dale, D., & Saris, W. H. M. (1989). Repetitive weight loss and weight regain: Effects on weight reduction, resting metabolic rate, and lipolytic activity before and after exercise and/or diet treatment. *American Journal of Clinical Nutrition, 49,* 409-416.

Vertes, V. (1985). Clinical experience with a very low calorie diet. In G. L. Blackburn & G. A. Bray (Eds.), *Management of obesity by severe caloric restriction* (pp. 349-358). Littleton, MA: PSG.

Wadden, T. A., Sternberg, J. A., Letizia, K. A., Stunkard, A. J., & Foster, G. D. (1989). Treatment of obesity by very low calorie diet, behavior therapy, and their combination: A five year perspective. *International Journal of Obesity, 13*(Suppl. 2), 39–46.

Wadden, T. A., & Stunkard, A. J. (1986). A controlled trial of very low calorie diet, behavior therapy, and their combination in the treatment of obesity. *Journal of Consulting and Clinical Psychology, 4*, 482–488.

Wadden, T. A., Stunkard, A. J., & Brownell, K. D. (1983). Very low calorie diets: Their efficacy, safety, and future. *Annals of Internal Medicine, 99*, 675–684.

Wadden, T. A., Stunkard, A. J., & Liebschutz, J. (1988). Three- year follow-up of the treatment of obesity by very low calorie diet, behavior therapy, and their combination. *Journal of Consulting and Clinical Psychology, 6*, 925–928.

Wadden, T. A., VanItallie, T. B., & Blackburn, G. L. (1990). Responsible and irresponsible use of very-low-calorie diets in the treatment of obesity. *Journal of the American Medical Association, 263*, 83–85.

Weigle, D. S., Callahan, D. B., Fellows, C. L., & Greene, H. L. (1989). Preliminary assessment of very low calorie diets by conventional and signal-averaged electrocardiography. *International Journal of Obesity, 13*, 691–697.

13

Behavioral Assessment and Treatment of Markedly Obese Patients

THOMAS A. WADDEN
GARY D. FOSTER

This chapter describes the behavioral assessment and treatment of markedly obese individuals seeking weight loss by very low calorie diet (VLCD). The chapter is divided into two sections, the first of which describes the initial evaluation of patients. The second section discusses the principles of behavioral treatment and outlines a typical course of therapy.

Section One: Initial Evaluation

Patients seeking treatment by VLCD must undergo an extensive medical evaluation, as described by Atkinson in Chapter 12 of this volume, to ensure that they are free of contraindications to such therapy. They should receive an additional evaluation to determine whether they have any behavioral (i.e., psychological/psychiatric) complications that would contraindicate treatment by this method. Little has been written about this latter evaluation (Agras et al., 1976; Brownell, 1981; Wadden, 1985). In the absence of research findings, we will describe the goals and methods of a clinical interview developed over the past decade at the University of Pennsylvania. This assessment has five principal goals:

1. Obtaining a psychosocial history.
2. Assessing the etiology of the patient's obesity.
3. Identifying behavioral contraindications to treatment.
4. Determining goals of therapy.
5. Preparing patients for treatment.

These goals and the accompanying methods of assessment are highly interrelated in many cases, as will be seen.

Psychosocial Evaluation

Too frequently, practitioners initiate weight reduction therapy without knowing the persons whom they plan to treat. Obesity may well be some patients' most salient attribute, but all persons have other, more important characteristics, which should be explored in an initial interview. Thus, the first 15 to 20 minutes of the assessment should be devoted to getting to know the patient. The interview should provide the practitioner with an understanding of the patient's (1) intimate relationships (i.e., with parents, partner, children, and friends) and social functioning; (2) satisfaction with work; (3) general strengths and weaknesses; (4) methods of coping; and (5) current life goals. From the beginning, the practitioner should attempt to understand how weight affects and is affected by these factors, and what life changes the patient anticipates with weight loss.

Psychological inventories generally do not predict weight loss or attrition from therapy (Wilson, 1985). We, however, routinely administer the Beck Depression Inventory (BDI; Beck, Ward, Mendelson, Mock, & Erbaugh, 1961), the Minnesota Multiphasic Personality Inventory (MMPI; Hathaway & McKinley, 1951), and other instruments before treatment, having found that they alert us to personality and/or emotional factors that may emerge during weight reduction. Moreover, these tests may be useful in identifying contraindications to treatment, as discussed in a later section.

In addition to assessing the patient's current psychosocial functioning, the practitioner must address several questions related specifically to weight loss. The goal of this assessment is to determine whether the patient is motivated to lose weight, has realistic expectations of treatment, and is free of major life stressors that would disrupt weight control efforts.

1. *Why has the patient decided to lose weight now?* Although this question may be answered rather perfunctorily (e.g., "Because I am overweight and want to look better"), the practitioner should remember that the patient probably has been obese for many months, if not years, and something has recently happened to motivate the patient to enter treatment. Overweight persons frequently seek therapy because of poor physical health, prodding by a spouse or employer, or hopes that their social life and job opportunities will improve. In many cases, patients have experienced disappointment, sadness, anger, or other feelings, which should be examined before weight loss is initiated.

It is particularly important that the patient be relatively free of major life stressors when undertaking weight loss. We have found that protracted stress in intimate or professional relationships, as well as life crises (i.e., death of parent, financial problems, etc.), disrupt an individual's ability to diet (Wadden & Letizia, Chapter 16, this volume). In such cases, patient and practitioner should discuss the desirability of delaying therapy until the patient's stress has been resolved.

2. *For whom is the patient losing weight?* In most cases, patients appropriately indicate that they wish to lose weight for themselves, to feel better

physically and psychologically. The prognosis for treatment is poor, however, in cases in which a patient appears for treatment solely because of "doctor's orders" or a partner's insistence. In the former case, it is important to determine whether the patient has a realistic understanding of the weight problem, its health implications, and the role that he or she must play in weight control. Therapy will only be successful if patients take "ownership" of their treatment. In the second case, the practitioner should meet with the patient and partner to determine what issues are being played out in the weight arena. These may include avoidance of intimacy, testing of love, or attempts to separate from a domineering partner.

3. *What is the social context in which the patient will diet?* Weight loss does not occur in a vacuum. The weights, eating habits, and attitudes of a patient's family members and friends are likely to affect the patient's weight control efforts. These factors should be reviewed in the interview. We frequently ask, "What did your partner (or friends) do that helped you lose weight the last time you dieted? What did your partner (or friends) do that hindered your weight loss efforts?" Family meetings may be appropriate in cases in which family members appear to thwart the patient's weight control efforts.

4. *What are the patient's specific goals of treatment, and are they realistic?* Many persons wish to lose weight as a means to another goal. If these goals, such as finding a new relationship or job, can be articulated at the outset of treatment, patient and practitioner can evaluate whether they are realistic and, if necessary, plan additional steps to achieve them. Some overweight persons, for example, are shy and unassertive, as are many persons of average weight. Thus, no matter how well they look after losing weight, their social lives are unlikely to improve, particularly if they are hoping for someone "to just notice me." Social skills training, psychotherapy, and other interventions may be appropriate here.

In summary, the psychosocial assessment should provide a brief sketch of who the person is, identify why she or he has decided to lose weight at this time, and search for personal and social factors that may facilitate or hinder weight control.

Type and Etiology of Obesity

The practitioner also must use the interview to determine the type and etiology of the patient's obesity. This determination is important for establishing realistic treatment goals and for selecting appropriate interventions. Laboratory tests, such as described by Atkinson in Chapter 12, may provide definitive findings concerning etiology in some cases. At present, however, the most useful information is frequently obtained from a careful weight and dieting history and from an assessment of the patient's eating and exercise habits. This information can be helpful in determining the extent to which the patient's obesity is attributable primarily to biological as opposed to behavioral factors.

Biological Factors

Stunkard's (1984) classification (Table 13.1; see also Chapter 2, this volume) is a simple threefold one of mild, moderate, and severe obesity, characterized by body weights that are 20–40%, 41–100%, and more than 100% overweight, respectively. As shown in Table 13.1, persons 20–40% overweight usually have hypertrophic obesity (i.e., increase in fat cell size) with approximately normal fat cell number (Leibel, Berry, & Hirsch, 1983; Sjöström, 1980). These persons generally have a good prognosis for reaching "ideal" weight, because cell hypertrophy is reversible (Sjöström, 1980).

As body fat increases to two or more times the normal amount (which usually occurs by 40% or more overweight), the probability increases that the patient's adipose tissue is characterized not only by increased fat cell size but also by increased cell number (i.e., hyperplasia) (see Figure 13.1). Markedly obese persons may have as many as 50 to 150 billion fat cells, as compared with 25 to 35 billion in persons of average weight (Leibel et al., 1983). Most reports indicate that fat cell number is irreversible, although there are exceptions (Naslun, Hallgren, & Sjöström, 1988). Thus, even with weight reduction, patients with severe, hyperplastic obesity may still have two to three times the normal fat cell number and a fat mass increased by the same proportion. Successfully treated patients may thus remain 50% or more overweight (Mason, 1987; Sjöström, 1980).

Determination of fat cell size and number is inaccessible to most practitioners. These values, however, can be estimated, as can the contribution of biological factors (i.e., genetics) to the weight problem by obtaining a careful history in which patients describe their weights at 5-year intervals from infancy to the present. We have patients complete a weight and dieting history, such as that developed by Agras et al. (1976), prior to the interview so that this

TABLE 13.1. Classification of Obesity

Type	Classification of obesity		
	Mild	Moderate	Severe
Percentage overweight	20–40%	41–100%	>100%
Prevalence (among obese women)	90.5%	9.0%	0.5%
Pathology	Hypertrophic	Hypertrophic, hyperplastic	Hypertrophic, hyperplastic
Complications	Uncertain	Conditional	Severe
Treatment	Behavior therapy	Low calorie diet and behavior therapy	Surgery

Note. From "The Current Status of Treatment for Obesity in Adults" (p. 158) by A. J. Stunkard, 1984, in A. J. Stunkard and E. Stellar (Eds.), *Eating and Its Disorders* (pp. 157–183). New York: Raven Press. Copyright 1984 by Raven Press. Reprinted by permission.

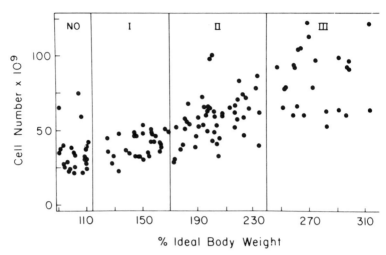

FIGURE 13.1. The relationship between fat cell number (in billions) and percent of ideal body weight (as determined by the 1959 Metropolitan Life Insurance Co. height and weight tables). I, II, and III refer to three groups of subjects with increasing severity of obesity. NO refers to nonobese subjects. From "Biochemistry and Development of Adipose Tissue in Man" (p. 27) by R. L. Leibel, E. M. Berry, and J. Hirsch, 1983, in H. L. Conn, E. A. DeFelice, and P. Kuo (Eds.), *Health and Obesity* (pp. 21-48). New York: Raven Press. Copyright 1983 by Raven Press. Reprinted by permission.

information can be obtained with maximal efficiency. The history should provide answers to the following questions:

1. *When did the patient first become significantly overweight?* Childhood onset and adolescent onset of obesity are generally associated with greater body weight as an adult and with increased fat cell number (Sjöström, 1980; Wadden, 1987). Conversely, weight gain in adulthood in previously average-weight persons may not be associated with marked increases in fat cell number, particularly if the gain is limited to approximately 30% of ideal weight. Persons with childhood onset of their obesity can lose significant amounts of weight but frequently fall short of reaching ideal weight, as noted previously.

2. *Does the patient have a family history of obesity?* Obesity is under substantial genetic control, with studies of identical twins reared apart yielding heritability estimates as great as 0.66 to 0.70 (Stunkard, Harris, Pedersen, & McClearn, 1990). The family history should provide clues to the possible influence of genetic factors. If neither parent is obese, the likelihood of the child's becoming obese is only 8%. If one parent is obese, the likelihood jumps to 40%, and if both parents are overweight, the probability of the child's becoming obese is an astonishing 70% (Gurney, 1936). We have found that the markedly overweight patient with a positive family history of obesity, as well as

childhood onset, almost invariably has hyperplastic obesity (Wadden, 1987). The independent contributions here of weight, age of onset, and genetics are not known.

3. *What is the patient's dieting history?* Persons who are moderately or severely overweight and regain weight rapidly following treatment are likely to have excess fat cell number (Krotkiewski, Sjöström, Björntorp, Carlgren, & Smith, 1977; Sjöström, 1980). Thus, a history of weight loss and regain may be a marker for hyperplastic obesity, independent of any possible contribution of weight cycling to increased adiposity.

In summary, the practitioner can expect to find normal fat cell number in mildly overweight persons who have become obese in adulthood. Persons previously of normal weight who have become moderately or severely obese as adults may display increased fat cell number, but probably not to the same degree as persons of similar weight with childhood onset and a family history of obesity. As described later, information from this history is useful for selecting an appropriate goal weight.

Behavioral Factors

Assessment of the patient's current dietary and caloric intake, as well as eating and exercise habits, is critical to determining appropriate areas for intervention. If the practitioner works as part of a multidisciplinary team, much of this assessment may be conducted by a dietitian (McNulty, Chapter 14, this volume) and an exercise physiologist (Fox, Chapter 15, this volume). Assessment of these behaviors can be facilitated by the use of a structured recall, prospective diaries, and other methods. In addition, these behaviors are assessed continuously throughout treatment by having patients keep food and exercise diaries.

This component of the initial assessment should answer the following questions (Brownell & Wadden, 1991):

1. Does the patient report overeating?
2. What is the patient's pattern of food intake (i.e., number of meals a day, times and places of eating, degree of snacking, etc.)?
3. What is the composition of the diet (i.e., approximate percentage of calories from carbohydrate, protein, and fat)?
4. Does the patient report difficulty in handling particular foods or eating-related situations?
5. Is binge eating a problem? How is it defined, and what thoughts, emotions, and other events are associated with it? Does the patient compensate for binges by vomiting or using laxatives?
6. What is the patient's general level of physical activity, and what attitudes are held toward activity?
7. What physical activities does the patient engage in on a regular basis and with what frequency, duration, and intensity?

Answers to these questions should begin to provide greater understanding of whether the patient's obesity is attributable primarily to increased energy intake, decreased energy output, or both. The practitioner may wish to request an assessment of resting metabolic rate (RMR) (Feurer & Mullen, 1986) in those cases in which patients report gaining weight on low caloric intakes (Tremblay, Seale, Almeras, Conway, & Moè, 1991). Although some patients do have low energy requirements (Foster et al., 1988; Geissler, Miller, & Shah, 1987), recent research using the technique of doubly labeled water suggests that both obese and nonobese individuals significantly underestimate their daily caloric intake, the obese by as much as 40% (Bandini, Schoeller, Cyr, & Dietz, 1990; Prentice et al., 1986; Schoeller, 1988). Measurement of RMR can thus confirm the presence of a low caloric intake, or, alternatively, can alert patient and practitioner to the need for more careful assessment of food intake.

Psychological and Behavioral Contraindications to Treatment

In the process of assessing psychosocial function and the etiology of the patient's obesity, the practitioner must continually search for conditions that might contraindicate weight reduction, and specifically the use of a VLCD. Moreover, contraindications to the patient's participation in group therapy, if it is being considered, must also be ruled out.

There is little research on behavioral and psychosocial contraindications to weight reduction, either by a VLCD or by a more conventional diet of 1200 kilocalories (kcal)/day. As such, the recommendations that follow represent our best clinical judgment but are not supported by research findings, which simply are lacking at present.

Behavioral Contraindications to Very Low Calorie Diet

Behavioral and psychiatric contraindications to treatment by VLCD include the following:

1. *Bulimia nervosa.* Patients with bulimia nervosa—binge eating associated with loss of control and subsequent compensation (i.e., vomiting, laxative abuse, etc.)—should not be treated by a VLCD. (For criteria for bulimia nervosa, see the American Psychiatric Association's [1987] *Diagnostic and Statistical Manual of Mental Disorders*, 3rd edition, revised [DSM-III-R].) Binge eating is likely to disrupt the patient's adherence to the diet, and could be associated during the refeeding period with serious consequences, including death (VanItallie & Abraham, 1985). Purging will alter electrolyte balance. The severe caloric restriction imposed by VLCDs is likely to exacerbate bulimia nervosa (Polivy & Herman, 1985). Persons who have recovered from this disorder should probably avoid VLCDs in favor of treatment by a conventional diet of 1200-1500 kcal/day, composed of conventional foods.

Patients who engage in binge eating without purging may be appropriate for treatment, provided that their history suggests that they can adhere to the diet (Wadden, Foster, & Letizia, in press). Such persons, however, are more likely than obese nonbingers to be depressed (Marcus, Wing, & Hopkins, 1988; Marcus, Wing, & Lamparski, 1985). They also may be more likely to drop out of treatment once the VLCD is terminated (Wadden, Foster, & Letizia, in press). Thus, they should be monitored carefully throughout treatment.

Research is needed to determine the best method of treating binge eaters who wish to lose weight. The most favorable course may be to address the binge eating first, using cognitive–behavioral techniques, and then to tackle the weight problem (Telch, Agras, Rossiter, Wilfley, & Kenardy, 1990). Adjunct pharmacotherapy, particularly with one of the serotonin reuptake inhibitors, may also prove beneficial with some patients (Marcus et al., 1990).

Patients can be screened for binge eating with the Binge Eating Scale (Gormally, Black, Daston, & Rardin, 1982). The interview should be used to clarify the extent to which patients suffer from this condition or the more serious problem of bulimia nervosa.

2. *Major depressive episode.* Patients experiencing a major depressive episode (as defined by DSM-III-R criteria) should not be accepted for treatment by VLCD. These diets are associated with alterations in thyroid hormones and metabolism (Wadden, Mason, Foster, Stunkard, & Prange, 1990), which may mimic changes associated with severe depression (Whybrow, Prange, & Treadway, 1969). Thus, dieting could exacerbate depression in some persons (Stunkard & Rush, 1974). Persons taking lithium to control a bipolar disorder (manic–depressive illness) are generally thought to be inappropriate for VLCD because of the difficulty in maintaining an appropriate blood level of the drug (Bistrian, 1978). We are aware of several practitioners, however, who have successfully treated such patients.

We routinely screen patients with the BDI (Beck et al., 1961) and/or the MMPI. Persons who score in the clinically significant range of depression are examined at greater length to determine the factors responsible for their mood disturbance. In most cases, it is appropriate to refer the patient for treatment of the depression first and to address the weight problem subsequently. In some individuals, however, it is clear that their weight problem is the principal cause of their dysphoria. Weight loss in behavioral programs frequently results in rapid improvements in mood in such persons (Smoller, Wadden, & Stunkard, 1987).

3. *Acute psychiatric disorder.* Patients experiencing an acute psychiatric disorder, including anxiety and psychosis, are inappropriate for treatment by VLCD and perhaps by conventional diet therapy. The distress associated with the psychiatric disorder is likely to disrupt adherence to the diet, whereas the deprivation of dieting may exacerbate mental health. The primary psychiatric disorder should be treated before weight reduction is considered.

We encourage practitioners, however, to rely upon their clinical judgment and knowledge of the specific individual in deciding when it is appropriate to initiate weight reduction therapy in a patient with a psychiatric condition. We have successfully treated for their obesity, using diets providing 500-1200 kcal/day, patients who received concomitant treatment for obsessive-compulsive disorder, schizophrenia, bipolar disorder, and dysthymia. In all cases, however, patients had been diagnosed with the psychiatric disorder for several months (or years) and had had sufficient time and treatment to adapt to it. Thus, the decision to provide weight reduction therapy rests in large part upon whether the psychiatric disorder is acute or longstanding.

4. *Substance abuse disorders.* VLCDs also are inappropriate for persons who suffer from substance abuse disorders, including the abuse of alcohol, barbiturates, cocaine, and marijuana. Patients should be encouraged to seek treatment of their substance abuse disorder first, after which they can address their obesity.

Tobacco use is not a contraindication to treatment by VLCD. Patients, however, should not be advised to stop smoking during weight reduction therapy, because the psychological and physiological changes (including weight gain) associated with smoking cessation are likely to disrupt adherence to the program (Williamson et al., 1991). Patients who wish to stop smoking should be advised to do so several months before or after undertaking weight loss. Smoking, in most cases, is a far greater risk to health than is obesity.

Possible Behavioral Contraindications to Very Low Calorie Diet

Possible behavioral contraindications to treatment by VLCD include the following:

1. *History of dieting-induced depression.* Persons who report that they became significantly depressed during a previous diet should be carefully evaluated to determine factors surrounding the untoward episode (Stunkard & Rush, 1974). Since past behavior is frequently the best predictor of future behavior, these persons should be closely monitored if accepted for treatment by either a VLCD or a conventional reducing diet.

2. *Life crisis.* Persons experiencing marked stress resulting from marital or vocational problems, illness or death of loved ones, or other untoward events may not be good candidates for weight reduction. We found in a recent study that the more adverse life events patients experienced at the time of enrolling in treatment, the more likely they were to discontinue therapy prematurely (Wadden & Letizia, Chapter 16, this volume). Patients are more likely to have difficulty meeting the demands of a rigorous weight reduction program if their concentration and emotional energies are taxed by a life crisis. Such persons should consider delaying treatment until they have resolved the untoward life event. If patients insist, however, that they can meet the demands of treatment, they should be allowed to enroll. Some report that weight is the one thing they can control in a life that otherwise feels out of control.

3. *Financial considerations.* The practitioner should determine whether the patient can afford a full course of therapy by VLCD and lifestyle modification. This is an important consideration, given the high cost of such treatment and the poor long-term outcome that patients experience with early discontinuation from treatment (Kaplan & Atkins, 1987). Other treatment options should be explored if patient and practitioner cannot find the means for the patient to receive the full course of therapy.

Contraindications to Group Behavioral Treatment

Much of the weight reduction therapy offered in university and hospital clinics incorporates group treatment, the benefits and deficits of which are discussed in a later section of this chapter. When conducting the initial interview, practitioners must remember that they are selecting patients not only for weight reduction therapy, but also for group treatment. Thus, it is important to consider how each individual will "fit" in the group and to consider possible negative effects that an individual might have upon the group process (Yalom, 1975).

Behavioral contraindications to group treatment include the following:

1. *Antipathy to group care.* A practitioner should take seriously a patient's statement that he or she has a strong aversion to group treatment. The clinician should explore the patient's dislike of such therapy, which may derive from the mistaken belief that participants will be forced to "bare their souls." In such a case, the practitioner should describe the difference between group treatment for obesity and the more traditional group psychotherapy with which the patient has confused it. Patients who continue to have negative feelings after such discussion should not be encouraged to participate in a group program; individual treatment and other options should be explored.

2. *Markedly inappropriate behavior.* Persons who display markedly inappropriate behavior do not make good group members. Thus, individuals who show evidence of a thought disorder, are very hostile in the initial interview, or are extremely withdrawn are likely to have an unfavorable effect upon the group. In some cases, one very negative patient can disrupt an entire group, causing discontent and attrition (Yalom, 1975). Practitioners should trust their instincts. If the clinician finds the patient's behavior troublesome or annoying, in all likelihood the group members also will. In some cases, it may be useful to refer the patient to a colleague for additional evaluation in order to confirm the practitioner's perception of the patient's troublesome behavior.

3. *Episodic attendance.* Persons who indicate that they will miss three or more consecutive treatment sessions or 20% or more of the total visits are not good candidates. Their poor attendance prevents adequate medical monitoring during consumption of the VLCD, disrupts their learning, and demoralizes other group members. Persons who cannot attend group sessions regularly should be considered for individual treatment. If individual care

cannot be arranged, a patient should be encouraged to alter business or vacation plans to meet the requirements of treatment or to wait until his or her calendar is clear.

Possible Behavioral Contraindications to Group Treatment: Personality Disorders

Patients with significant personality disorders are difficult to treat in individual therapy and even more difficult to manage in a group treatment program. This is particularly true of persons presenting with narcissistic or borderline personality disorders (as defined in the DSM-III-R). Narcissistic persons often display a grandiose sense of self-importance or uniqueness and may demand unlimited attention from friends and health professionals. They frequently dominate group sessions with stories of their problems or accomplishments and dislike sharing the spotlight. They tend to be insensitive toward the needs of other group members. Persons with a borderline personality disorder are very emotionally labile; they frequently show marked changes in mood from minute to minute (despair to euphoria, adulation of staff to denigration). Their behavior may be impulsive, unpredictable, and occasionally self-destructive (i.e., suicidal gestures, self-mutilations, etc). Such patients frequently complain that they do not "know" who they are.

Individuals with personality disorders may be difficult to identify in an initial 60- to 90-minute interview; such persons are likely to be socially appropriate, if not charming, in order to gain acceptance in treatment. In cases in which a prospective patient is currently receiving or has recently completed psychotherapy, it is both useful and professionally appropriate to contact the patient's treatment provider, who can provide information concerning the patient's difficulties and prognosis. This individual also should be consulted concerning whether weight reduction therapy is appropriate for the patient at present, as well as concerning the patient's likelihood of successful weight loss. The practitioner should obtain written consent to contact the patient's psychotherapist after having discussed the desirability of doing so.

The practitioner, either intentionally or by oversight, is likely to accept for group treatment a number of individuals with personality disorders. Our experience indicates that these persons will lose weight as successfully as other group members. If, however, these persons disrupt treatment sessions, the practitioner must act quickly to manage the patient's behavior and arrange for individual therapy, as needed. We have found that individual therapy is best provided by a practitioner other than the group leader.

Summarizing Findings and Identifying Goals of Treatment

Once the practitioner has a preliminary understanding of the patient's weight problem and prognosis for treatment, he or she should briefly summarize the relevant findings. The patient, in turn, should be given ample opportunity to comment and ask questions.

Summary of Findings

Highlights from the interview can be summarized using the acronym "BEST Treatment," in which

    B = biological predisposition
    E = environmental factors (i.e., eating and exercise habits)
    S = social support and psychological status
    T = timing (i.e., propitious time to diet, motivation, etc.)

Thus, the practitioner might begin the summary by stating: "I've enjoyed speaking with you, Mrs. Smith, about your weight history, eating, and exercise habits, and the other topics that we discussed. Now I would like to share some of my impressions with you, which are based upon what you have told me."

Biological Predisposition. "You have been overweight since you were in elementary school, and you noted that your mother had a serious weight problem all of her life, as did her mother. Thus, it is possible that you inherited a tendency toward obesity—a tendency that probably makes weight control more difficult for you than the next person. It's important that you understand, however, that a genetic tendency toward obesity does not mean that you are destined to be overweight. You still can control your weight by diet and exercise, although it will probably be harder for you than other people" (as discussed by Price & Stunkard, 1989).

Environmental Factors. "You indicated that you are very sedentary; you drive to work, sit at a desk most of the day, and rarely engage in purposeful exercise. In some ways, I'm glad to hear that, because it means that you should be able to help control your weight by increasing your physical activity—both your lifestyle activity at the office and around the house, as well as your planned activity such as walking or swimming. Increased physical activity plays an important role in any weight control program.

"In terms of your eating habits, you reported that you do not overeat at meal time but have trouble snacking after dinner, into the late evening. You indicated that you don't feel that you lose control while snacking, but find yourself repeatedly returning to the kitchen while watching television. It will be important to determine how many calories you consume in this fashion during the evening and for us to find ways to limit your snacking."

The practitioner would continue by summarizing findings from other areas, such as the patient's psychosocial functioning, anticipation of help or hindrance from significant others in losing weight, and the desirability of undertaking weight control at present. Throughout the summary, and particularly at its conclusion, the practitioner should give the patient plenty of opportunity to respond and ask questions. Thus, the summary should reveal that the practitioner has listened carefully to the patient and welcomes the patient's response to the findings presented.

Further Evaluation. If weight reduction is indicated, the practitioner should initiate a discussion of this topic and the patient's goals of treatment. In the case, however, of a patient who requires further evaluation because of possible contraindications, the practitioner should provide a summary of findings and then identify the issue requiring further assessment. The clinician should avoid the use of alarmist language and indicate that further consultation is desired to ensure that the patient receives the most appropriate treatment possible. The practitioner should expect some patients to be upset about the need for further evaluation and should invite them to discuss their feelings.

Contraindications. In the case of a patient with clear contraindications to treatment by VLCD, the practitioner should explain why weight reduction (or a VLCD, in particular) is not appropriate for the patient. The emphasis should be placed on how the treatment program is not appropriate for the patient, rather than vice versa. In all cases, the patient should be provided a referral to obtain the care that is required. When appropriate, the patient should be invited to contact the practitioner when the primary disorder has been resolved.

Identifying Goals of Treatment

The practitioner and patient are likely to have discussed, at the outset of the interview, the patient's goals in seeking treatment. Patients frequently report very similar goals: "I want to lose weight and feel better about myself." Thus, the anticipated benefits of therapy should be clarified, once it is clear that the patient is appropriate for weight reduction therapy.

Weight Loss Goals. Selection of a weight loss goal and/or goal weight is an issue that must be addressed. Patients frequently enter treatment desiring to obtain a specific weight. It is very important to determine how this "goal weight" was selected and whether it is realistic. Careful review of the weight history should help in identifying a reasonable goal weight. As a general rule, the goal weight should be no lower than the patient's lowest weight since age 21 that was maintained for at least 1 year. Thus, a woman who is currently 40 years old and 110 kg should set a goal weight of no less than 75 kg, if that is her lowest weight since age 21 (Brownell & Wadden, 1991). Moreover, the practitioner might suggest that the patient initially select as a target reducing her initial weight by 10–20%. A weight loss of this magnitude is frequently sufficient to control medical complications associated with obesity, such as hypertension and diabetes (Kanders & Blackburn, Chapter 9, this volume).

Patients may be discouraged by the practitioner's suggestion of a relatively high goal weight or modest weight loss. It is important, however, that the clinician shape realistic expectations for treatment from the outset. Avoiding discussion of weight loss goals is not helpful. In the absence of explicit goals, patients adhere to their implicit and often unrealistic goals and become very demoralized when they fail to reach them.

Psychosocial Benefits. Anticipated psychosocial benefits of treatment should be discussed in the same detail as weight loss. As noted earlier, many patients seek weight loss as means to other goals, such as securing an intimate relationship or a promotion at work, in addition to wanting to look better and being able to purchase from a wider selection of more attractive clothing. The likelihood should be assessed that, with successful weight loss, the patient will obtain each of the desired benefits; these should be recorded on a sheet of paper. Were such benefits obtained with prior weight loss? The practitioner also should discuss the additional steps that the patient can take to increase the likelihood of obtaining the desired goals.

Preparing Patients for Treatment

Following discussion of the goals of weight reduction, patients should be given a brief overview of their treatment options, with an assessment of the strengths and weaknesses of each approach. (This is "Treatment" in the acronym "BEST Treatment.") Discussion of relevant options can be guided by the conceptual scheme provided by Brownell and Wadden (1991), shown in Figure 13.2. This scheme suggests classes of treatment that are likely to be appropriate, as well as matching factors, which are used to select the best treatment fit for each patient.

The use of the most conservative approach—a conventional reducing diet of 1000–1200 kcal/day, combined with a comprehensive program of lifestyle modification—should be considered with all markedly obese individuals. Patients should have tried this approach at least twice before being considered for a VLCD. Similarly, patients 100% or more above ideal body weight who have been treated by VLCD two or more times may wish to consider surgical intervention, as described by Kral (Chapter 21, this volume).

In the course of selecting the most appropriate care, it is important to review patients' previous weight loss experiences to determine what worked, what went wrong, and what can be done to improve the chances of long-term success. Many individuals bring negative expectancies to therapy, based upon their previous encounters. It is critical that patients believe that the proposed therapy offers new hope, as well as instruction and skills that will facilitate weight loss. Alternatively, patients must believe that they can now apply themselves to the proposed therapy in a manner that they previously could not.

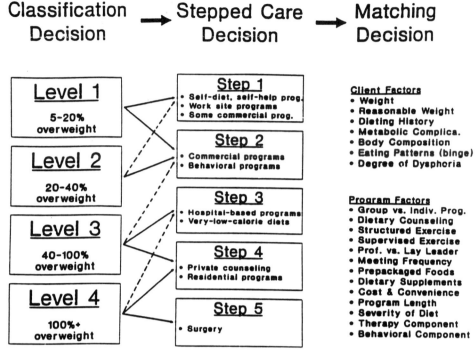

FIGURE 13.2. A conceptual scheme showing the three-stage process in selecting a treatment for an individual. The first step, the "classification decision," divides individuals according to percentage overweight into four levels. This level dictates which of the five steps would be reasonable in the second stage, the "stepped care decision." This indicates that the least intensive, costly, and risky approach will be used from among alternative treatments. The third stage, the "matching decision," is used to make the final selection of a program, and is based on a combination of client and program variables. The dashed lines with arrows between the classification and stepped care stages show the lowest level of treatment that may be beneficial, but more intensive treatment is usually necessary for people at the specified weight level. From "The Heterogeneity of Obesity: Fitting Treatments to Individuals" (p. 162) by K. D. Brownell and T. A. Wadden, 1991, *Behavior Therapy*, 22, 153–177. Copyright 1991 by Association for Advancement of Behavior Therapy. Reprinted by permission.

Overview of Treatment

Having selected the most appropriate treatment, the practitioner should briefly describe the typical course of such therapy. We provide patients with a written description of treatment in the context of obtaining their informed consent to participate in our clinical trials. Many indicate that written material is very useful, because it can be shared with family and friends.

This is an appropriate time to describe the requirements of treatment. Thus, patients should understand that they will be asked to complete weekly homework assignments, which include keeping a diet diary, participating in an exercise program, and recording thoughts and emotions that facilitate or hinder weight control efforts. The frequency and length of treatment visits should be specified, and the schedule of medical monitoring should be reiterated. If group treatment is being considered, the requirements of this therapy should be reviewed, so that the patient will be prepared to be an active and productive group member.

This is also the time to inform patients that treatment will address primarily weight control behaviors, with only limited attention to more personal issues such as low self-esteem or troubled relationships with intimate others. The practitioner should discuss the possible benefits of adjunctive psychotherapy or other therapy with patients who report that they will need more help, as appropriate (Brownell & Wadden, 1991).

Patients should be invited to share their thoughts and concerns about the treatment program outlined and to rate the degree to which they think that they will be successful. The practitioner should respond to a patient's concerns or misunderstandings about treatment and note any assistance available to the patient to cope with an anticipated problem.

Long-Term Care

Regardless of the length of the initial treatment prescribed, the practitioner should emphasize throughout the interview that marked obesity is a chronic disorder requiring long-term care. Patients should leave the initial interview with the understanding that after they have lost weight they will need to participate in a formal program of weight maintenance, as described by Perri (Chapter 19, this volume). As one of our patients remarked, "People need to realize that it's not over when the thin lady sings." Thus, beginning with the initial interview, the practitioner should emphasize the need for long-term care.

Conducting the Interview

A practitioner must obtain a formidable amount of information in the initial interview in a brief period. In addition, he or she must convey interest in the patient by giving the individual ample opportunity to raise questions and concerns. We have found that the following steps help to ensure that the interview is conducted with maximal efficiency and benefit. We usually allow 60 to 90 minutes for this assessment.

1. Following the patient's contacting our clinic and a brief telephone interview, we mail patients test materials (i.e., BDI, Binge Eating Scale, weight and dieting history, eating and exercise habits questionnaire) to complete before their clinic interview. Patients are asked to return the materials by mail or to bring them to the interview. Thus, before meeting a patient, a practitioner can briefly review the materials to identify clinical issues requiring further examination.

We have observed informally that patient completion of these questionnaires and punctual attendance at the initial interview are markers for adherence and attendance during treatment. Persons who fail to complete the questionnaires satisfactorily often dislike and fail to complete diet diaries and other homework assignments. This issue should be addressed with patients in the initial interview.

2. Many persons come to the initial interview feeling ashamed and anxious. They feel ashamed of their inability to control their weight and worry that they will fail in treatment again. They also frequently wonder whether the practitioner will be sensitive to their problems and treat them respectfully, or instead will make disparaging comments about their appearance and character. Thus, patients use the initial interview to conduct their own assessment of the practitioner.

3. In response to the patient's probable anxiety described above, we find it useful to structure the interview in the following manner. We begin by welcoming the patient and asking whether he or she had any difficulty finding our clinic. We next explain the purpose of the visit in terms such as these: "Mrs. Smith, during our meeting today, I want to get to know you better and learn about the causes of your weight problem and what we can do to help you with it. We will learn more about your weight history and your eating and exercise habits by reviewing the results of the questionnaires that you completed. Thanks very much for completing them. You did a very thorough job. Do you have any questions about any of the tests that you completed?"

We respond to any questions that the patient may have, and then talk briefly about either the patient's work, family, or social activities. We try to select what appears to be a conflict-free topic that the patient can discuss without significant difficulty (i.e., we avoid sensitive issues until greater rapport has been established). For example, "I read in one of your questionnaires that you are an accountant. Tell me about your work." Although such discussion may resemble social chit-chat, it nevertheless provides an opportunity to learn about the patient's satisfaction with work and the degree of stress associated with it. Moreover, it provides the practitioner an opportunity to observe the patient's mood and language, as well as comfort level in describing aspects of daily life (as is required in group treatment).

Following the discussion of this and related topics, we turn our attention to the patient's weight and dieting histories, followed by an examination of eating and exercise habits. This information can be reviewed selectively, as can that concerning level of depression and psychosocial functioning, depending upon responses to the questionnaires.

4. We attend at all times throughout the interview to possible contraindications to treatment by VLCD or group therapy (if the latter approach is to be used). We frequently use a checklist to ensure that all contraindications are ruled out, and try to make this determination relatively early in the interview. If contraindications are discovered, the remaining time can be used to identify

appropriate care for the patient. If the patient is free of contraindications, the practitioner can use the remaining time to explore the issues that appear to be most salient to the patient's weight problem.

5. Patients should leave the interview feeling that they have learned something about their weight problem and its causes. They also should leave with a clear understanding of the course of the proposed therapy, if weight reduction is to be undertaken.

6. We believe that the initial interview is best conducted by a mental health professional (i.e., psychologist, psychiatrist, social worker, or mental health counselor) who is also knowledgeable of the causes and treatment of obesity. Mental health practitioners are better able to judge than are other health professionals (e.g., dietitian, exercise specialist, physician) whether patients have significant behavioral or psychiatric complications that require treatment or that might be affected by weight reduction therapy. Mental health practitioners, however, should be aware that the initial behavioral interview described here differs markedly from the psychosocial interview conducted with persons typically seeking psychiatric care. The interview must address the weight-specific issues enumerated above.

In cases in which persons without training in mental health choose to conduct the initial behavioral interview, they should have a working relationship with a psychologist or psychiatrist with whom they can consult concerning behavioral issues. On occasion, they will need to refer patients to a mental health professional for further evaluation.

Section Two: Principles of Behavioral Treatment

This section will review the principles of the behavioral treatment of obesity. Our goal is not to provide a list of all the techniques used in treatment, but rather to review the assumptions of behavioral treatment and some of its distinguishing characteristics. Several other sources provide a detailed description of behavioral techniques (Stunkard & Berthold, 1985; Wadden & Bell, 1990).

The goal of behavioral treatment is to help obese individuals identify and modify inappropriate eating, exercise, and thinking habits that contribute to their weight problem. We should note at the outset that not all obese people have inappropriate eating and exercise habits (Wadden & Bell, 1990). Nevertheless, behavioral treatment may provide patients a set of skills with which to control their obesity, regardless of its etiology.

Behavioral treatment makes extensive use of the functional analysis of behavior (Brownell & Wadden, 1986). Eating and exercise habits are analyzed to determine their covariation with a variety of stimuli, such as times, places, activities, thoughts, emotions, and other people. For example, after a period of self-monitoring, a patient identified that her eating was often triggered by or associated with feelings of frustration at work. This frustration led to unwanted snacking at the work station, subsequent distress about eating out of control, and eventually more eating. Once the patient had identified the events that led to inappropriate eating, she used problem-solving skills to develop alternative methods of coping with the difficulty (Black, 1987; Black & Scherba, 1983). In this case, she discussed her frustration with a supportive colleague and eventually confronted the individual who she believed was contributing to her difficulties.

Hallmarks

Behavioral treatment has several distinguishing hallmarks. First, it is goal-directed. It specifies very clear goals for therapy in terms that can be easily measured. This is true whether the goal is walking three times per week, lengthening meal time by 5 minutes, or decreasing the number of self-critical comments. Specification of goals facilitates problem solving and the assessment of treatment outcome.

Second, treatment focuses on changing behaviors per se. Thus, it differs from a psychoanalytic approach, which focuses on the dynamics underlying behavior. For example, behavioral treatment emphasizes recording food intake rather than exploring past causes of "orality." Such a behaviorally oriented approach enables treatment to remain on task and concentrate on the *behaviors* most directly related to weight control.

Third, treatment is process-oriented. It is more than helping people to decide what they want to accomplish; it is helping them find ways to change. In cases in which behavior is not implemented, attention is devoted to finding new strategies or to removing roadblocks. After prolonged or significant difficulty in changing a behavior, treatment may examine issues similar to those discussed in more dynamically oriented therapy. This step, however, is only taken when more direct methods to change behavior are not successful. Behavioral treatment is the most useful approach, in our opinion, because in addition to providing a compendium of weight control skills, its efficacy has been documented in numerous controlled research studies (Brownell & Wadden, 1986).

Mechanics of Treatment

Behavioral treatment has evolved into a set of fixed interventions, which are described in detail elsewhere (Stunkard & Berthold, 1985; Wadden & Bell, 1990). This "package," which includes extensive instruction in nutrition and exercise, has been developed for convenience on the basis of standardized research protocols. Such a standard package, however, cannot take the place of the individual analysis of behavior.

Group versus Individual Care

Behavioral treatment can be delivered in the context of either individual or group therapy. Individual therapy provides greater opportunity to tailor treatment to patients' specific needs. We believe, however, that there are several advantages to group treatment. First, it is a great source of support, creating an atmosphere of camaraderie as patients share a common experience (such as a VLCD) together. Second, groups help patients to see that they are not alone with their difficulties; this can be a very healing experience (Yalom, 1975). Third, group treatment produces larger weight losses than individual treatment, even among patients who express a preference for individual treatment (Renjilian, Perri, Nezu, McKelvey, & Schein, 1990). Fourth, group treatment requires less practitioner time per patient, making it cost-effective. The optimum group size is 6 to 10, and we believe that no group should exceed 12 members. Larger groups prevent patients from receiving the individual attention they need.

Individual treatment is probably best used as an adjunct to group therapy. Individual sessions enable the patient and practitioner to focus on issues that cannot be adequately addressed in the group, such as prolonged difficulty in changing behavior or stressful life events. Individual treatment is not equivalent to psychotherapy; it remains goal-directed and behaviorally oriented, focusing on weight control issues. The length of the sessions is usually 30 to 60 minutes.

Length and Structure of Treatment

Most behavioral treatment programs that incorporate a VLCD last 4 to 6 months and meet weekly. The length of the various phases of treatment is reviewed later in this chapter. Treatment is often delivered in a time-limited fashion. Having a clear end to therapy helps patients pace themselves and allocate resources (Wadden, Foster, Letizia, & Stunkard, in press). The length of each session is 75 to 90 minutes. Groups of shorter duration will prevent the group from accomplishing its didactic, interactional, and problem-solving functions.

Groups function most productively when they are closed. This means that all patients begin treatment together and that no new members are admitted after the first few weeks. Adding new members throughout treatment disrupts group cohesion. In addition, a curriculum of behavior change that builds on the previous session's material is difficult to administer when patients are at different stages of treatment. It is difficult, for example, to address the concerns of patients entering the first week of refeeding when others are still consuming a VLCD as their sole source of nutrition. Although no controlled comparisons exist, studies that have employed a time-limited, closed-group approach (Wadden, Foster, Letizia, & Stunkard, in presss) have reported significantly less attrition than those that have employed open groups and allowed patients to continue treatment indefinitely (Kirschner, Schneider, Ertel, & Gorman, 1988; Hovell et al., 1988).

Treatment Providers

Group treatment is usually provided by a behavioral psychologist or other mental health professional. As a general rule, practitioners should have at least master's-level training in psychology (or a related discipline) and experience in behavior therapy, group therapy, and weight control. The group leader often works with patients as part of a multidisciplinary team that includes a dietitian, exercise physiologist, and physician.

Ultimately, behavioral treatment is provided by the patient. Patients become students of their own behavior, identify problems, and implement strategies to change them. Effective treatment results in patients' becoming experts on their own eating, exercise, and thinking habits.

Appropriate Patients

Behavioral treatment is best suited for patients with inappropriate eating and exercise habits, in whom cognitive and emotional factors exacerbate weight control efforts. As noted previously, however, research shows that not all overweight patients have inappropriate eating and exercise habits (Wadden & Bell, 1990). These latter patients may still benefit from behavioral treatment as a result of acquiring a set of weight control skills. Whatever the cause of their obesity, patients must still employ skills to control their food intake and increase their energy expenditure.

For some, these skills may not be enough. This is especially true for patients who have become overweight as the result of psychological trauma, including rape or physical abuse (Felitti, 1991). As noted in the assessment section, these patients may benefit from psychotherapy, either before or as an adjunct to weight control treatment. In short, we believe that the skills taught in behavioral programs are necessary but not always sufficient to assure a favorable outcome. Treatment is more successful with some individuals than with others, but, despite great effort, researchers have been only modestly successful in identifying the patients who will benefit the most. Predictors of weight loss and attrition from therapy are discussed by Wadden and Letizia in Chapter 16 of this volume.

Treatment by Very Low Calorie Diet and Lifestyle Modification: A Clinical Approach

This section describes the use of behavioral techniques combined with a VLCD. The behavioral methods are very similar to those used with a 1200-

kcal/day diet (Brownell & Wadden, 1986; Stunkard & Berthold, 1985; Wadden & Bell, 1990); the major difference is that the stages of treatment are more clearly delineated as patients progress through various phases of caloric restriction. A typical program of VLCD and lifestyle modification lasts 4 to 6 months, although the length of treatment will vary, depending on the duration for which the VLCD is consumed. Most programs can be characterized by four distinct phases: (1) introduction; (2) VLCD; (3) refeeding period; and (4) stabilization. Each stage has its own behavioral challenges and goals. The primary behavioral techniques and common clinical issues of each phase are described below.

Introductory Phase

Many programs employ an initial 1- to 4-week period during which patients are instructed to reduce their caloric intake to 1200–1500 kcal/day (Palgi et al., 1985; Wadden & Stunkard, 1986; Wing et al., 1991). This time is used to prepare patients behaviorally and emotionally for the VLCD. It is a time of great anticipation and, occasionally, anxiety for patients. The two primary behavioral goals during this period are self-monitoring and preparing for severe caloric restriction.

Self-Monitoring. Patients are instructed to record all foods and beverages that they consume as they attempt to reduce their intake to 1200–1500 kcal/day (Brownell, 1991). Self-monitoring is begun at this time because it reinforces the importance of recording food intake throughout treatment. In addition, this information is useful to the dietitian and patient in making meal plans after the VLCD. Adherence to record keeping during the initial weeks of treatment also predicts weight loss over the next 6 months of treatment (Hartman, Wapner, & Saxton, 1990).

Preparing the Environment. The second and more important goal of this "readiness" period is to prepare patients for the VLCD. Much of this information is didactic and covers medical information, such as expected symptoms and their treatment, fluid intake, and the nature of the diet to be consumed. In addition, patients are asked to "clean house" to make the physical environment (e.g., home and workplace) conducive to adhering to a VLCD. This is accomplished by removing candy dishes from end tables, banishing troublesome foods from the home, purchasing noncaloric beverages, and similar behaviors. For patients who plan to consume a VLCD of conventional foods, this is also a time to prepare portions of lean meat, fish, or fowl, which can be frozen and used at a later date.

Obtaining Support. Patients also are asked at this time to discuss the VLCD with family and friends. Patients are encouraged to have family members review all of the written materials concerning the program. More importantly, patients should identify the specific behaviors that family and friends can perform to assist the patient during the VLCD. Thus, some patients may request that family members not snack around them or may ask spouses to be responsible for all food preparation during the VLCD. Whatever the request, it should be specific, so that both the family members and the patients are clear about the expectations for support. Some programs invite family members to a group session during the initial weeks of treatment to assist partners and patients in developing supportive strategies.

Normalizing Eating Habits. Some patients respond to the anticipation of the VLCD by engaging in a series of "last suppers." These typically consist of overeating "bad" foods that patients will not be able to consume during the VLCD. Although it is appropriate to consume some special foods before the VLCD, patients should be discouraged from having extravagant meals. This can be accomplished by acknowledging the impulse to go on an eating binge, but discussing its likely psychological and physical consequences. Thus, any special meals should be carefully planned with the staff's assistance.

Group Sessions and Clinical Issues. Many tasks must be accomplished during the initial group meetings, including introducing patients, establishing norms for appropriate behavior, and discussing the important issue of confidentiality. These initial group sessions are much more didactic than later sessions, because of the large amount of information that has to be conveyed about consuming the VLCD safely. Group interaction should be encouraged wherever possible, but it will take time to develop.

These initial weeks of treatment are, in some ways, the most difficult for patients, who are eager to start the VLCD and may resist what they perceive as a "waiting" period. A major appeal of a VLCD is its quick weight loss, so it is not surprising that any delay is met with disappointment. This is particularly true of patients who have not been adequately prepared for this introductory period. Imagine the frustration of a patient who expects to begin a VLCD tomorrow, but is told that he or she is about to start a 4-week introductory period. Alerting patients at an orientation meeting to the rationale for and nature of the introductory period minimizes frustration and enables patients to pace themselves for the beginning of the VLCD.

Patients' eagerness to "get started" is mixed with anxiety about their ability to adhere to the VLCD. It is common to hear questions such as "Will I be able to survive on only 500 calories a day?" and "Will I be restricted to a liquid diet for 12 weeks?" Patients should be encouraged to voice their concerns in the group sessions so that they can be addressed directly, rather than being left to the "expertise" of the waiting room group or the patients' imaginations. This is also an appropriate time to underscore the patients' role in ensuring safe and successful weight loss by their consuming adequate calories and fluid, participating in medical monitoring, and initiating behavior change. Giving patients realistic expectations about symptoms and weight loss will also minimize their anxiety. Some programs invite former patients to talk to the group about their initial VLCD experience to allay these pre-VLCD "jitters."

Confidentiality is an issue that is often overlooked in obesity treatment. As already indicated, weight control treatment is not psychotherapy, but it does involve a therapeutic relationship in which sensitive issues are discussed. We believe that it is important to explicitly discuss at the first treatment session the nature and limits of confidentiality. Practitioners should assure patients that everything said in the group sessions will be held strictly confidential among the professional staff. No information about patients will be communicated to persons outside of the weight control program (including health care professionals) without the patients' written consent.

Patients should be informed that practitioners on the patients' treatment team will share information with each other in providing comprehensive care. This prevents patients from "splitting" staff members by asking practitioners not to share certain information with each other and thus potentially pitting one practitioner against another. We believe that all information that directly concerns a patient's adherence, progress, and health in the program should be shared among practitioners. There are times, however, when a patient may request strict confidentiality, and it should be considered. For example, a patient is entitled, in our opinion, to limit the number of staff members who are told about a history of sexual abuse or other historical information. Conversely, all staff members should be informed about a patient's consuming less than the prescribed amount of the VLCD.

Practitioners should ask patients to respect each other's confidentiality as well, and illustrate why it is important. Confidentiality should extend, at a minimum, to not disclosing participants' last names and not discussing issues of a sensitive nature. Patients should be encouraged to discuss their feelings about the need for confidentiality. The practitioner's task is to help the group achieve a working consensus on this issue.

Another task of the first session is to decide upon the parameters for discussing weekly weight changes. Patients frequently differ in their desire to discuss this issue. There are several options. One is to have patients report their weight losses (or gains) at the beginning of each session as they "check in" for the week. Another is not to discuss weight during the group session. A third is to permit the discussion of weight change but not to make it mandatory. We find the last option the most satisfactory; it allows patients who want to discuss their weight losses to do so without forcing those who would rather not. We do, however, require all participants to discuss their eating and exercise habits and other issues addressed in the weekly homework assignments.

Very Low Calorie Diet

The introductory phase described above is typically followed by a fixed period of VLCD ranging from 8 to 16 weeks (Wadden & Stunkard, 1986; Wing et al., 1991), although some programs encourage patients to continue the VLCD until a prescribed goal weight is achieved (Kirschner et al., 1988). The excitement and gratification that patients and practitioners experience during the VLCD can mask the significant behavioral tasks during this period.

Continued Self-Monitoring. Patients are encouraged to continue their self-monitoring while consuming the VLCD. Frequently, they are not inclined to do so because their diet varies so little, especially if they are consuming a liquid VLCD. The rationale for recording food intake during the VLCD is threefold. First, it assists patients in developing self-monitoring as a habit. It is critical that patients monitor their food intake when the VLCD is terminated and they increase the variety and palatability of their diet. Second, even when consuming the VLCD, patients can still learn much about their eating by recording the times, places, activities, and emotions that are associated with the desire to eat. Conditioned eating habits, such as having a snack before bed each night, become very apparent during the VLCD. Third, recording food intake during the VLCD helps ensure that patients consume adequate calories and fluids. In particular, patients cannot afford to miss a serving of protein, given the importance of protein in preserving lean tissue (Yang & VanItallie, Chapter 4, this volume). Similarly, adequate fluid must be consumed to prevent dehydration.

Stimulus Control. Self-monitoring can assist patients in learning the techniques of stimulus control, which consist of limiting exposure to cues that prompt eating (such as the sight of food or watching TV). Patients should be encouraged to regard their VLCD as food (which it is) and practice stimulus control behaviors, such as limiting the times and places associated with eating, storing food out of sight, eating in a designated place, and limiting the activities associated with eating. Practicing appropriate eating behaviors three to five times a day during the consumption of the VLCD will facilitate patients' performance of these behaviors when they resume consumption of a conventional diet. One patient's story illustrates how eating behavior during the VLCD can generalize to more conventional eating. One week during refeeding, Susan reported that she was consuming several of her meals standing up in the kitchen. It turned out that this was the exact spot (next to the blender) where she had prepared and consumed her liquid VLCD for the previous 12 weeks.

Identification of Hunger. Another task during the VLCD is the identification of different types of hunger. Since VLCDs are typically associated with feelings of satiety and mild anorexia (Rosen, Gross, Loew, & Sims, 1985; Wadden, Stunkard, Day, Gould, & Rubin, 1987), this period provides an excellent opportunity for patients to distinguish between physical and psychological hunger. Patients will experience physical hunger when they delay a scheduled meal, but most often they will experience psychological hunger prompted by some external stimulus. Identifying the difference between the two types of hunger and the conditions that are associated with each should help extinguish psychological hunger.

Increasing Physical Activity. Patients are encouraged to increase their physical activity as soon they adapt to the VLCD, which usually occurs in 2 to 3 weeks. This activity consists, for most patients, of a program of moderate walking, since more intense exercise during a VLCD is associated with further reductions in RMR (Phinney, LaGrange, O'Connell, & Danforth, 1988). Patients are also encouraged to increase lifestyle activity, such as parking further from store entrances and using steps instead of escalators. It is important to make physical activity a habit as soon as possible, given the strong association between regular exercise and long-term weight control (Kayman, Bruvold, & Stern, 1990; Pavlou, Krey, & Steffee, 1989). Helping patients select reasonable goals and enjoyable activities will increase long-term adherence, as discussed by Fox (Chapter 15, this volume).

Group Sessions and Clinical Issues. Group meetings during the VLCD are used to discuss patients' adherence to the diet and to identify any difficulties they may have. Each session, two or three patients are asked to review in detail with the group their food intake and physical activity. This practice is continued throughout treatment. It provides both individual feedback for the selected patients and practice for other group members in analyzing and solving eating- and exercise-related difficulties.

Patients who have trouble adhering to the diet during the first 2 weeks are asked to see the practitioner before or after group for a brief (i.e., up to 15-minute) individual session. We find that excluding from the group session detailed discussions of nonadherence helps set a strong norm for adherence and keeps morale high. After this 2-week period, patients can discuss their difficulties in adhering, provided that they do not elaborate upon the foods consumed. Detailed descriptions of such "forbidden" foods often stimulate other group members' appetites. It is important to create an atmosphere in which adherence problems can be addressed without glorifying them.

The most frequent clinical issue that arises during the VLCD, in addition to adherence to the diet, is disappointment with weight loss. Despite consuming 800 kcal/day or fewer, many patients (usually women) will eventually have a week in which they lose little if any weight. Some patients will exhibit a very idiosyncratic pattern of weight loss (e.g., every other week). In patients who are adhering to the diet, this irregularity is typically due to shifts in water balance, especially near the time of menstruation.

It is critical to acknowledge the frustration that patients experience when they do not lose weight. Such frustration increases the risk of nonadherence, as patients are likely to feel that "all of the work isn't worth it." Thus, staff members should be sensitive to patients' frustration at the weekly weigh-in. Nonjudgmental statements such as "That must be really frustrating," or "You must be disappointed," are much more helpful than accusations such as "Did you stick to the diet this week?" or "Try harder next week." Examining the weight losses of all patients before the group may help the practitioner detect those patients who are distressed about their weight or who are having adherence difficulties.

Even if practitioners suspect nonadherence, but patients do not report it, it is best first to acknowledge the disappointment of dieting all week and losing less weight than expected. Practitioners can then underscore the weak relation that exists between weight loss and behavior change in the short term (Brownell & Stunkard, 1978); review the factors that temporarily affect body weight (e.g., humidity, time of day, fluid intake, salt intake); and remind patients of the large weight losses that they achieved the first few weeks because of water loss. All of the factors that influence body weight should be reviewed before the initiation of the VLCD to provide realistic weight loss expectations. Patients who fail to lose weight for 2 or more consecutive weeks require further support. In addition, the practitioner should review patients' diet and exercise records with them to determine whether their adherence is satisfactory.

Patients often experience feelings of euphoria and omnipotence while consuming the VLCD, as a result of losing weight quickly and receiving positive feedback on their success (e.g., compliments, smaller clothing sizes, changes on the scale). It can be difficult, under these circumstances, to convince patients that they need to work on fundamental lifestyle changes. It is important to acknowledge patients' significant success, while still emphasizing that lifestyle change requires more than a change in menu.

Patients also may display some "magical thinking" regarding their practitioners, the treatment program, or the diet. They frequently say things such as "This is the best program in the world," or "I couldn't stick to any other diet before this." While it is nice to hear praise, this also is a time to underscore the patients' role in changing behavior. The diet, program, or practitioner did not adhere to an eating plan and lose weight; the patients did. Having patients acknowledge their active role in treatment helps increase their self-efficacy and minimizes the perception of treatment providers as rescuers.

Practitioners also experience a variety of emotions while patients are consuming the VLCD. They, like patients, are excited about the significant weight losses and the ease with which they are achieved. Practitioners are likely to hear plenty of praise about their clinical skills and how much they have helped patients. This praise and success can lead practitioners to experience the same euphoria and omnipotence as patients. It is not uncommon to think, "This is it; maybe I really have cured this patient's obesity." These feelings are soon tempered by seeing the difficulties that patients have in changing their lifestyle behaviors (i.e., being assertive, self-monitoring, asking for support). The challenge for the practitioner is to balance enthusiastic support with realistic expectations.

The Refeeding Period: A Time of Transition

Following the VLCD, patients increase their caloric intake over 2 to 6 weeks until it reaches approximately 1200–1500 kcal/day. Patients begin to increase both the level and variety of their caloric intake during the "refeeding" (i.e., transition) period, as described by McNulty (Chapter 14, this volume). It is a period marked by increased anxiety and numerous behavioral challenges.

Nutrition Education. During refeeding, patients begin an intensive period of nutrition education. This includes information about caloric and nutrient density, identification of types of fat, meal planning, and low fat cooking. This information is best presented by a dietitian experienced in working with overweight patients. Even for patients who already have a high degree of nutritional sophistication, the challenge of how to translate this knowledge into practice remains. In general, the more practical the instruction (e.g., cooking demonstrations, supermarket tours), the better.

Stimulus Narrowing. Another behavioral challenge for patients during transition is portion control. The transition from a very fixed, bland diet to one that includes a variety of foods is difficult for most patients and may be most challenging for those who have consumed a liquid VLCD, as compared with a diet of lean meat, fish, and fowl.

Some clinicians (Berkowitz, 1990) advocate the use of a stimulus-narrowing approach which limits patients' food choices, particularly in the initial weeks of refeeding. A limited menu is thought to minimize sensory stimulation and make adherence easier. Although the concept of stimulus narrowing was derived, in part, from Rolls's (1979) studies on sensory-specific satiety, no controlled research has been performed to test this approach following a VLCD. It is generally accepted, however, that adherence is improved and anxiety is lessened by gradually introducing foods into the diet over a 4- to 6-week period. It is our experience that patients have difficulty adhering to a rigid menu beyond this period.

More Stimulus Control. The transition to a greater variety of foods provides the opportunity to focus on behaviors associated with food selection, preparation, and consumption. A principal task during this time is to increase the patients' ability to prepare a variety of foods in a healthy manner, as discussed by McNulty in Chapter 14. One such skill is shopping for food. Patients require information on supermarket layouts, reading labels, making grocery lists, and storing foods in the home (Brownell, 1991; Stunkard & Berthold, 1985; Wadden & Bell, 1990). Once the food is purchased, they require instruction in preparing meals using minimal amounts of fat. Although some of this instruction (e.g., steaming vegetables, making recipe substitutions for fat/sugar, stir-frying) may seem mundane, it will help patients make permanent changes in their eating habits.

An additional set of skills involves the distribution and consumption of foods. Thus, patients are instructed in eating slowly, leaving some food on the plate, pausing before selecting additional portions, eating in a designated place, and removing serving dishes from the table (Brownell, 1991; Stunkard &

Berthold, 1985; Wadden & Bell, 1990). Those patients who have consumed a food-based VLCD will already have had an opportunity to practice some of these skills, such as eating slowly and serving foods appropriately.

Group Sessions and Clinical Issues. Group sessions during the refeeding period are used to review patients' eating and exercise behavior. By this time, patients should be able to provide constructive feedback to fellow group members. The practitioner should encourage direct communication among members, rather than having all communication proceed through the practitioner.

At least half of each session during this period is devoted to nutrition education topics, typically presented by a dietitian. Since the dietitian may be new to the group, the practitioner should inform the dietitian about group members and any relevant clinical issues. Whenever two practitioners lead a group together, they should meet briefly before the session to review the critical points to be covered and the person to address them.

Patients are likely to feel anxious and, in some cases, even angry during the refeeding period. The anxiety is prompted, in part, simply by the change in the dietary regimen. Patients frequently begin to wonder whether they will be as successful during this transition as they were during the VLCD. They fear that even a slight increase in caloric intake will diminish weight loss significantly. They also question their ability to handle their former nemesis, food. They attribute some of their success during the VLCD to the fact that they did not have to make food choices. This questioning of competence stems from a history of other weight control efforts that failed once "the diet" was over. (Patients in our clinic have attempted an average of five diets, which resulted in a total weight loss [and regain] of 55 kg, before beginning our treatment program; Wadden, Bartlett, et al., in press.) It also stems from the common belief that the VLCD, not the patients, was responsible for the successful weight loss. Some patients also may be angry because they have been asked to stop using a method of dieting (i.e., VLCD) that has worked so well. It is common to hear statements such as "I finally found something that works and now you want to take it away from me." Finally, patients may be angry because they feel they have not reached their goal weight.

There are several ways to respond to the marked anxiety and anger that patients may experience. The first is to acknowledge that their feelings are understandable. Patients should be given plenty of opportunity to discuss their reactions to discontinuing the VLCD and resuming consumption of conventional foods—a discussion that should "decharge" these emotions somewhat and give the practitioner a chance to address the underlying issues. We suggest that this discussion be initiated during the last month of the VLCD. We caution, however, that in preparing patients for the transition period, the practitioner should avoid reviewing the refeeding protocol in detail. Such a review may prompt some patients to begin refeeding early, since it's only "a few weeks away."

Once their fears and worries have been aired, patients' concerns can be addressed in a more rational manner. For example, the practitioner should underscore that the patients, not the VLCD, have been responsible for the excellent weight loss. The same behaviors that were successful during the VLCD (i.e., self-monitoring, planning, stimulus control) will serve patients well during the refeeding period. The practitioner should indicate that the transition is gradual (4 to 6 weeks) and involves very few choices.

Patients may fail to lose weight the first week or two of refeeding, but this is primarily because of the increased consumption of carbohydrate with its attendant fluid retention. Patients should be apprised of this fact in order to alleviate their fears that they will not be able to lose weight without a VLCD. We find that mathematically illustrating the expected difference in weight loss between the VLCD and the refeeding diet helps minimize anxiety. For example, doubling caloric intake from 400 to 800 kcal/day slows weight loss by only 0.3 kg/week. Patients also frequently find it reassuring for a former patient who has made a successful transition from the VLCD to address the group.

The time immediately following the VLCD is one at which patients are at high risk for attrition from treatment (Wadden, Foster, Letizia, & Stunkard, in press). Attending to patients' psychological needs and normalizing their concerns helps to limit dropouts. If patients do not stay in treatment through transition and stabilization, they are more likely to regain weight than are those who complete the full course of therapy (Wadden & Stunkard, 1986). For these reasons, we suggest that at least one-quarter of the group time during the last two sessions of the VLCD and the first two sessions of the refeeding period be allotted to discussion of patients' emotional reactions to this transition.

Binge eating is a clinical problem that deserves special attention. Depending on the criteria used, between 23% and 70% of patients who seek treatment of their obesity engage in binge eating, consuming large quantities of food in a short period of time (Loro & Orleans, 1981; Marcus et al., 1985, 1988; Telch et al., 1990; Wadden, Foster, & Letizia, in press). Some investigators believe that binge eating is precipitated by episodes of severe dietary deprivation (Polivy & Herman, 1985), as simulated by the consumption of a VLCD. Thus, VLCDs may present a risk for exacerbating binge eating in patients who already display it, as well as inducing the disorder in persons who were free of it prior to the VLCD. The refeeding period is thought to be the period of greatest risk for binge eating as patients resume consumption of conventional foods, which may include heretofore avoided impulse items such as cookies, cakes, salty foods, and ice cream.

There has been little research on the occurrence of binge eating during treatment by a VLCD. What evidence is available suggests that binge eaters will lose as much weight as nonbingers, but may be at increased risk of discontinuing treatment following termination of the VLCD (Wadden, Foster, & Letizia, in press). More research is needed on the topic. In the meantime, practitioners should try to minimize the occurrence of binge eating during the refeeding period by inviting patients to talk about their food-related fantasies, so that they do not feel compelled to act them out. Patients should be assured that they will have an opportunity to consume their favorite foods again, but that consumption of these foods will be planned carefully with the group leader and dietitian.

Consuming a large amount of food after a period of VLCD is likely to be associated with significant stomach discomfort. Consequently, some patients may decide to compensate by purging or by using laxatives or diuretics. The electrolyte imbalance caused by these behaviors is especially serious in the time following the VLCD (VanItallie & Abraham, 1985). It is important, therefore, to work with these patients intensively to control the bingeing, and to monitor carefully whether any purging is occurring. A first step with these patients is to increase the caloric intake to 1200–1500 kcal/day rather than attempting to maintain a restricted intake (Telch et al., 1990). Such cases of binge eating with purging are rare in our experience, but they require prompt attention.

Stabilization

Stabilization is the period in which patients attempt to stabilize their caloric intake and weight. This period usually lasts 6 to 10 weeks, focuses on the behaviors and cognitions necessary for long-term weight control, and, regrettably, is the only instruction in weight maintenance that most patients will receive.

Cognitive Restructuring. There are several therapeutic challenges during this time. Among the most difficult are identifying and modifying inappropriate thoughts related to eating. The most prevalent cognitive style following a period of VLCD is "all-or-none thinking." In some ways, consumption of a VLCD promotes all-or-none thinking as a model of success. Patients who consume only the foods prescribed are the most successful. During the stabilization period, however, the key to success is being able to see shades of gray along a continuum of success. An example of this ability is in the categorization of foods. An all-or-none thinker categorizes foods as "good" or "bad" on the basis of their caloric content, fat and sugar content, or some other factor. A more appropriate categorization of foods recognizes that none are inherently "good" or "bad." It is possible to eat and enjoy virtually any food, provided that it is consumed in appropriate quantities within the context of a balanced diet.

Lapse versus Relapse. Sooner or later, all patients will overeat or consume foods that they had not intended to. For many patients, the first dietary indiscretion brings with it a host of negative self-statements such as "Here I go again, I haven't changed at all," or " I've blown it; I have absolutely no willpower." Patients should be told to expect such dietary slips and to examine their thoughts and emotions in response to them. One useful distinction is the difference between a lapse and a relapse. It is important for patients to realize that lapses—dietary slips—are an expected and natural part of reasonable eating. Everyone has lapses; nobody is perfect. Although most patients can accept this lack of perfection in other aspects of their lives (such as work performance, relationships, or driving skills), they can be the harshest of self-critics concerning their eating. Lapses need to be viewed for what they are—temporary slips from which recovery is possible. Rather than passing final judgment on their eating behavior in such terms as "I'm a total failure," patients should be encouraged to examine what contributed to their lapses and find ways to prevent future such episodes.

By contrast, relapse is a return to a previous state or condition from which recovery is difficult and/or unlikely. It is characterized by a lack of hope. It is important to note that the difference between a lapse and relapse is not a quantitative one; the distinction is based more on attribution than on behavior. Some patients may experience "relapse" cognitions after only one lapse; others may have several lapses in a week, yet continue to record their food intake, to exercise, and to practice other weight control behaviors. The interested reader should consult Marlatt and Gordon (1985) for a more detailed discussion of this distinction.

Recovering from Overeating. Since may patients have formerly responded to overeating episodes with the relapse cognitions described above, they have been diverted from learning the behaviors required to recover from these episodes. The most useful techniques include removing themselves from the risky situation and setting short-term goals to avoid eating. Worksheets that guide patients through the recovery in a step-by-step fashion (see Figure 13.3) provide structure at a critical time when patients typically feel out of control and despondent.

Future Plans. A final task of the stabilization period is making plans for future weight control. It is important that patients develop a program of weight loss maintenance, because weight regain is highly likely in the absence of such a program (Perri, Chapter 19, this volume). For some, maintenance may involve a weekly weigh-in and review of dieting and exercise records at home, while others may enroll in a formal, structured program. Patients should commit their program to writing approximately 3 weeks before the end of treatment and should review it with the practitioner in a brief, individual meeting. The tone of this meeting should be supportive, not threatening. It is *not* helpful to coerce patients into formal weight maintenance programs with threats of "You're likely to regain your weight if you do not join a program." Some patients may be drained emotionally or financially after 6 months of intensive weight reduction and require a break. Thus, the practitioner must help patients develop a maintenance program that meets their particular needs and resources. This is an appropriate time to review previous weight maintenance efforts and to identify the skills that will be required for long-term success.

RECOVERING FROM AN OVEREATING EPISODE

Well, it's happened. You've overeaten. You feel lousy about it. You're probably angry with yourself. You may be scared. All of these feelings are understandable.

Remember, it's what you do after overeating that's important, not the fact that you've overeaten. Everyone overeats from time to time. So, what are you going to do now that you've overeaten?

1. Remove yourself immediately from the situation in which you have overeaten. In what room will you feel safe? Where do you want to go?

   Describe where you will go: _____

2. Stay cool by talking to yourself appropriately. Watch out for negative, automatic thoughts. Describe what you'll say to yourself to stay cool and rational:

   _____
   _____

3. Set an initial goal of not eating for 15 minutes. Determine an activity you can engage in during this time. When the first 15 minutes have passed, check the box indicating that you have accomplished your goal of not eating. Set another goal of not eating for 15 minutes and describe the activity you'll engage in during this time. Check the box after this period has passed. Continue this practice until it is time for your next meal.

GETTING PAST THE BAD MOMENTS AFTER OVEREATING

Time (min)	Activity you engaged in	Check here that you didn't eat
0–15		
16–30		
31–45		
46–60		
61–75		
76–90		

Congratulations. You made it!

4. Are you feeling calmer now about your eating? Are you feeling more in control of your eating? You probably are. If you are, there are a couple of things that you should do now.

   First, dispose of the foods on which you overate. Flush them down the toilet, put them down the garbage disposal, or run water over them and throw them in the trash.

   Describe how you will dispose of the troublesome food:

   _____

   Second, you should determine how many calories you consumed during your overeating episode. You probably won't want to do this, but more than likely, your fantasies about the number of calories you consumed are far worse than the realities of your overeating.

   Even if you have not kept your diet diary for several days, calculate the number of calories that you just ate. Then, determine how much weight you will gain from this overeating episode.

   If you ate _____ excess calories, you will gain _____ lb. of fat.

200	1/17
500	1/7
700	1/5
1200	1/3
1750	1/2
2000	4/7
2500	5/7

   It's unlikely that you will ever eat more than 2500 calories in a single overeating episode. Even if you did eat this much, you can see that you would gain only slightly more than ½ pound of fat. You can certainly live with this small amount.

Don't weigh yourself immediately after eating. Your weight will be up by several pounds as a result of the physical weight of the foods you have eaten. Wait at least 24 hours after overeating to weigh yourself. If you can, wait 48 hours.

5. You may not want to eat your next meal after having overeaten. You may feel that you need to starve yourself in order to make up for your binge. You may feel that you don't deserve to eat. Resist these impulses to starve or condemn yourself. Starving yourself after a binge only sets you up to binge again.

    It's important that you eat your next scheduled meal. It doesn't have to be a big meal, but do eat something. You should eat a minimum of 250 calories.

    Indicate what you will eat for your next meal.

FOOD	CALORIES

6. After you have finished eating for the day, total the number of calories that you have consumed. Expect the calories to be higher than normal. That's OK. Remember, it's what you do after overeating that's important.

    How many calories did you eat today? _____

    By how many calories did you overeat? _____

    Now, it's time to find a few ways to make up for your overeating episode. You'll need to eat a few less calories for the next few days and moderately increase your physical activity during this time. Be careful not to overexert yourself. Describe your plan for doing so.

Day	Number of calories I'll cut out of my diet	Meals when I'll do this	Number of extra calories I'll burn in exercise

7. You've done a good job of recovering from your overeating episode. Congratulations!

    The final step is to prevent such episodes from occurring again. When you are fully relaxed, try to determine the factors that contributed to your overeating episode. Concentrate on how, when, and where instead of on why. Try to answer these questions.

    Where did I overeat? _____
    What time of day was it? _____
    What foods did I eat? _____
    Where did I get the food? _____
    What were the serving sizes? _____
    What people were present? _____
    How did I feel before overeating? _____

    What prevented me from stopping my eating sooner? _____

    How did I finally stop myself? _____

8. Use this space to describe how you will handle this situation if it occurs again. Be specific.

    _____
    _____
    _____
    _____
    _____
    _____

FIGURE 13.3. Worksheet for recovering from overeating episode. From *The OPTIFAST Core Program Patient Manual* (pp. 205–207) by Sandoz Nutrition Corporation, 1987, Minneapolis: Author. Copyright 1987 by Sandoz Nutrition Corporation. Reprinted by permission.

An important part of any plan for future weight control is setting "caution" markers that, when reached, call for a prompt, corrective response. For example, patients may identify a maximum acceptable weight (Bandura & Simon, 1977) that is 1-3 kg above their current weight. If this weight is reached, the patient should immediately engage in a set of predetermined behaviors, which might include consuming a 1200-kcal/day diet, increasing exercise by 30 minutes per week, or contacting the clinic. These caution markers and accompanying interventions can be used to correct eating and exercise behaviors. Finally, "clinic" markers should be established that, when reached, call for outside help. For example, if patients regain 5 kg or more, they should contact the clinic or another formal program to get the help they need in reversing the weight gain. These primary and secondary interventions should be outlined in writing during the last month of treatment.

Group Sessions and Clinical Issues. The group sessions continue to focus on eating and exercise habits, but include an increased emphasis on modifying maladaptive thinking habits. This is accomplished by spending less time reviewing food records and more time analyzing records of thoughts. Homework sheets should be designed to identify the precipitating events (such as overeating by 500 kcal) associated with automatic irrational thoughts (such as "I've blown it"), which need to be reformulated into a rational thought (such as "I can recover from this if I start now"). Identifying automatic cognitions is difficult for some patients, who simply report that they do not have any thoughts. The practitioner should encourage these patients to work backwards from the feeling they experience (which most can easily identify) to the thoughts that underlie them. Readers interested in cognitive therapy should consult Beck's writing on this topic (Beck, 1976; Beck, Rush, Shaw, & Emery, 1979).

Perhaps the practitioner's most critical task during the last weeks of treatment is to convince patients to seek professional help if they regain a significant amount of weight. Patients are frequently hesitant to seek such help because they feel ashamed and embarrassed about their weight regain. They need to understand that it is preferable to seek help after a 5-kg weight gain than to wait until they have gained 25 kg. Practitioners should indicate that they will admire patients for seeking help, given the shame, guilt, and other obstacles they have to overcome to do so. Follow-up treatment is not a sign of failure; on the contrary, it is a sign of courage and good sense.

Some patients are likely to feel sad or anxious about ending treatment. They have become very attached to their treatment providers, their fellow group members, and the structure that the weekly meeting provides. The practitioner should encourage patients to express these feelings and acknowledge that they are understandable. Some participants will cope with these emotions by exchanging phone numbers to keep in contact with each other or by continuing to hold group sessions outside of the clinic—practices that we do not discourage.

Maintenance

Weight Loss versus Weight Maintenance

The length of maintenance programs following a VLCD varies. Some are open-ended and offered on a "for life" basis. Others are time-limited with options for renewal. Most maintenance programs meet every other week or monthly, as a means to encourage patients to become less dependent on the treatment providers and to assume more of the monitoring functions usually provided by clinic visits (i.e., weigh-ins and review of diet and exercise records).

It is important to note that the behavioral challenges of weight maintenance are quite different from the skills required to lose weight. Table 13.2 outlines some of the principal differences. Perhaps the most critical difference concerns the foods consumed. As mentioned previously, success during the VLCD and transition periods is related to the ability to avoid conventional foods, whereas long-term success is dependent upon the ability to consume conventional foods in a controlled manner, to decrease the consumption of foods high in fat and sugar, and to master troublesome foods (on which the individual may have previously binged).

Most of the strategies used in a formal maintenance program are an amplification of the cognitive and behavioral work begun in the stabilization

TABLE 13.2. Comparison of Behaviors and Reinforcement Associated with Losing Weight versus Maintaining a Weight Loss

Weight loss	Maintenance of weight loss
The goal of treatment is to lose a large amount of weight, after a prolonged period of weight gain.	The goal of treatment is to lose small amounts of weight, as small increases in weight occur.
The dieter's principal strategy is to *avoid* eating all of the foods that have caused the weight problem.	The dieter's principal task is to learn to eat troublesome foods in a controlled fashion (mastery) and to eat new foods, low in fat and calories.
Treatment is time-limited, usually 15 to 25 weeks.	Treatment is ongoing and lifelong.
The dieter receives support from the diet program and from family and friends.	The dieter receives little or no support from professionals or family members.
Weight loss is highly reinforcing; it is very noticeable and pleasing to dieters and their families.	Maintenance of weight loss is not reinforcing; dieters forget about their accomplishments, as do their family members.
Dieters do not have to exercise to lose weight.	Exercise appears to be critical to maintenance of weight loss.

Note. From "Obesity" (p. 465) by T. A. Wadden and S. T. Bell, 1990, in A. S. Bellack, M. Hersen, and A. E. Kazdin (Eds.), *International Handbook of Behavior Modification and Therapy* (2nd ed., pp. 449–473). New York: Plenum. Copyright 1990 by Plenum Publishing Corporation. Reprinted by permission.

period. The advantage of the maintenance period is that practitioners are able to help patients cope with difficulties as they occur. For example, it is likely during a 6-month maintenance program that patients will gain weight or have significant overeating episodes. Working with patients' behaviors and cognitions while they experience these difficulties is more helpful than addressing hypothetical scenarios.

Reversing Small Weight Gains

Perri (Chapter 19, this volume) has provided a detailed review of weight maintenance strategies. We, however, will briefly review one skill that is critical to long-term weight control—reversing small weight gains. Teaching patients the skills required to reverse small weight gains is difficult for several reasons. First, patients do not initially believe that they will regain weight. Second, even when they do gain weight, they stop weighing themselves, which prompts further gain. Third, they rationalize that "I'll lose the weight when I get around to it. I can lose 5 pounds with no trouble. I've just lost 50." Alternatively, they may feel that all is lost and fall into a precipitous relapse. Helping patients to identify small weight gains and to reverse them quickly through behavioral, nutritional, and exercise interventions will increase patients' confidence in managing their weight. It provides a set of skills—responding to weight gain—that no other program has provided them. That is because after successful weight loss, treatment typically ends when, instead, it should just be beginning.

Primary and Secondary Prevention of Relapse

We find that teaching patients a two-step approach to maintenance is helpful. The first step—primary prevention—involves upkeep skills that they need to perform on a weekly or monthly basis (i.e., monitoring of weight, exercise, and food intake) to prevent weight regain. These upkeep skills are similar to those of changing the oil and obtaining state inspections to ensure the long-term maintenance of a car. Crisis skills (i.e., secondary prevention) call for immediate intervention and are used to prevent a problem from worsening. Examples include taking steps to recover from an overeating episode or seeking additional treatment after a 5-kg weight gain. These efforts are similar to fixing a flat tire before the axle is damaged, or attending to an overheated engine before the engine block cracks. Having this two-step gives patients a framework for monitoring their weight, eating, and exercise, and for responding to overeating episodes and other difficulties.

A Final Recommendation

Regardless of the patient's degree of obesity or the course of treatment selected, there is an important fact that should not be overlooked: Overweight persons should be treated with respect and compassion (Wadden, 1985). In so many cases, they have been ridiculed, scorned, and rejected—not only by passing strangers, but by family and friends. Each time that they have lost weight and regained it, they have lost a little more self-respect and gained greater feelings of shame and inadequacy. Thus, the very prospect of undertaking another weight reduction program is frightening to many patients, for it may be just another encounter with failure.

Heath care providers, like the public at large, harbor a host of negative stereotypes toward the obese, which are likely to be aroused when patients fail to lose weight. In some cases, patients will have followed treatment recommendations to the letter but will have failed to reduce. In other cases, they will have had difficulty adhering to recommendations and will have gained weight during treatment. In neither case, however, can the practitioner afford to blame the patient for the lack of progress. It is unfair to blame patients for the fact that we do not fully understand the nature and causes of obesity, or for the fact that we have failed to develop treatments that are universally effective.

Instead, practitioners should examine the feelings that they experience in working with unsuccessful patients, for they are often the same ones experienced by the patients: frustration, anger, and sadness. In many cases, the greatest service that the practitioner can perform is to allow patients to verbalize their feelings and to respond empathically to them. Particularly with those persons who cannot lose weight, the goal of treatment is to help them recover their lost self-esteem and to realize that they can live rich and fulfilling lives, regardless of their weight.

References

Agras, W. S., Ferguson, J. M., Greaves, C., Qualls, B., Rand, S. C., Ruby, J., Stunkard, A.J., Taylor, C. B., Werne, J., & Wright, C. (1976). A clinical research questionnaire for obese patients. In B. J. Williams, S. Martin, & J. P. Foreyt (Eds.), *Obesity: Behavioral approaches to dietary management* (pp 168–176). New York: Brunner/Mazel.

American Psychiatric Association. (1987). *Diagnostic and statistical manual of mental disorders* (3rd ed., rev.). Washington, DC: Author.

Bandini, L. G., Schoeller, D. A., Cyr, H. N., & Dietz, W. H. (1990). Validity of reported energy intake in obese and nonobese adolescents. *American Journal of Clinical Nutrition, 52*, 421–425.

Bandura, A., & Simon, K. M. (1977). The role of proximal intentions in self-regulation of refractory behavior. *Cognitive Therapy and Research, 1*, 177–193.

Beck, A. T. (1976). *Cognitive therapy and the emotional disorders*. New York: International Universities Press.

Beck, A. T., Rush, A. J., Shaw, B. F., & Emery, G. (1979). *Cognitive therapy of depression*. New York: Guilford Press.

Beck, A. T., Ward, C., Mendelson, M., Mock, J., & Erbaugh, J. (1961). An inventory for measuring depression. *Archives of General Psychiatry, 4*, 561–571.

Berkowitz, R. (1990, November). *Stimuli-narrowing: A behavioral strategy for controlled eating*. Paper presented at the Sandoz Nutrition Postgraduate Seminar, Atlanta.

Bistrian, B. R. (1978). Clinical use of a protein sparing modified fast. *Journal of the American Medical Association, 240*, 2299–2302.

Black, D. R. (1987). A minimal intervention program and problem-solving for weight control. *Cognitive Therapy and Research, 11*, 107–120.

Black, D. R., & Scherba, D. S. (1983). Contracting to problem-solve versus contracting to practice behavioral weight loss skills. *Behavior Therapy, 14*, 100–109.

Brownell, K. D. (1981). Assessment of eating disorders. In D. H. Barlow (Ed.), *Behavioral assessment of adult disorders* (pp. 329–404). New York: Guilford Press.

Brownell, K. D. (1991). *The LEARN program for weight control*. Dallas: American Health.

Brownell, K. D., & Stunkard, A. J. (1978). Behaviour therapy and behaviour change: Uncertainties in programs for weight control. *Behaviour Research and Therapy, 16*, 301.

Brownell, K. D., & Wadden, T. A. (1986). Behavior therapy for obesity: Modern approaches and better results. In K. D. Brownell & J. P. Foreyt (Eds.), *Handbook of eating disorders: Physiology, psychology, and treatment of obesity, anorexia, and bulimia* (pp. 180–197). New York: Basic Books.

Brownell, K. D., & Wadden, T. A. (1991). The heterogeneity of obesity: Fitting treatments to individuals. *Behavior Therapy, 22*, 153–177.

Felitti, V. J. (1991). Long-term medical consequences of incest, rape, and molestation. *Southern Medical Journal, 84*, 328–331.

Feurer, D., & Mullen, J. L. (1986). Measurement of energy expenditure. In J. Rombeau & J. Caldwell (Eds.), *Parenteral nutrition* (pp. 224–236). Philadelphia: W. B. Saunders.

Foster, G. D., Wadden, T. A., Mullen, J. L., Stunkard, A. J., Wang, J., Feurer, I. D., Pierson, R. N., Yang, M.-U., Presta, E., VanItallie, T. B., Lemberg, P. S., & Gold, J. (1988). Resting energy expenditure, body composition, and excess weight in the obese. *Metabolism, 37*, 467–472.

Geissler, C. A., Miller, D. S., & Shah, M. (1987). The daily metabolic rate of the post-obese and the lean. *American Journal of Clinical Nutrition, 45*, 914–920.

Gormally, J., Black, S., Daston, S., & Rardin, D. (1982). The assessment of binge eating severity among obese person. *Addictive Behaviors, 7*, 47–55.

Gurney, R. (1936). Hereditary factor in obesity. *Archives of Internal Medicine, 57*, 557–562.

Hartman, W., Wapner, D., & Saxton, J. (1990, November). *A simple procedure to identify persons at risk for dieting failure*. Paper presented at the 24th Annual Conference of the Association for Advancement of Behavior Therapy, San Francisco.

Hathaway, S., & McKinley, J. (1951). *The Minnesota Multiphasic Personality Inventory manual*. Minneapolis: University of Minnesota Press.

Hovell, M. F., Koch, A., Hofstetter, C. R., Cipan, C., Faucher, P., Dellinger, A., Borok, G. Forsythe, A., & Felitti, V. J. (1988). Long-term weight loss maintenance: Assessment of a behavioral and supplemented fasting regimen. *American Journal of Public Health, 78*, 663–666.

Kaplan, R. M., & Atkins, C. J. (1987). Selective attrition causes overestimation of treatment effects in studies of weight loss. *Addictive Behaviors, 12*, 297–303.

Kayman, S., Bruvold, W., & Stern, J. S. (1990). Maintenance and relapse after weight loss in women: Behavioral aspects. *American Journal of Clinical Nutrition, 52*, 800–807.

Kirschner, M. A., Schneider, G., Ertel, N. H., & Gorman, J. (1988). An eight-year experience with a very-low-calorie formula diet for control of major obesity. *International Journal of Obesity, 12*, 69–80.

Krotkiewski, M., Sjöström, L., Björntorp, P., Carlgren, G., & Smith, U. (1977). Adipose tissue cellularity in relation to prognosis for weight reduction. *International Journal of Obesity, 1*, 395–416.

Leibel, R. L., Berry, E. M., & Hirsch, J. (1983). Biochemistry and development of adipose tissue in man. In H. L. Conn, E. A. De Felice, & P. Kuo (Eds.), *Health and obesity* (pp. 21–48). New York: Raven Press.

Loro, A. D., Jr., & Orleans, C. S. (1981). Binge eating in obesity: Preliminary findings and guidelines for behavioral analysis and treatment. *Addictive Behaviors, 6*, 155–166.

Marcus, M. D., Wing, R. R., Ewing, L., Kern, E., Gooding, W., & McDermott, M. (1990).

Psychiatric disorders among obese binge eaters. *International Journal of Eating Disorders, 9*, 69-77.

Marcus, M. D., Wing, R. R., & Hopkins, J. (1988). Obese binge eaters: Affect, cognitions, and response to behavioral weight control. *Journal of Consulting and Clinical Psychology, 56*, 433-439.

Marcus, M. D., Wing, R. R., & Lamparski, D. M. (1985). Binge eating and dietary restraint in obese patients. *Addictive Behaviors, 10*, 163-168.

Marlatt, G. A., & Gordon, J. R. (Eds.). (1985). *Relapse prevention: Maintenance strategies in the treatment of addictive behaviors.* New York: Guilford Press.

Mason, E. E. (1987). Morbid obesity: Use of vertical banded gastroplasty. *Surgical Clinics of North America, 67*, 521-537.

Naslun, I., Hallgren, P., & Sjöström, L. (1988). Fat-cell weight and number before and after gastric surgery for morbid obesity in women. *International Journal of Obesity, 12*, 191-197.

Palgi, A., Read, J. L., Greenberg, I., Hoffer, M. A., Bistrian, B. R., & Blackburn, G. L. (1985). Multidisciplinary treatment of obesity of protein-sparing modified fast: Results in 688 outpatients. *American Journal Public Health, 75*, 1190-1194.

Pavlou, K. N., Krey, S., & Steffee, W. P. (1989). Exercise as an adjunct to weight loss and maintenance in moderately obese subjects. *American Journal of Clinical Nutrition, 49*, 1115-1123.

Phinney, S. D., LaGrange, B. M., O'Connell, M., & Danforth, E., Jr. (1988). Effects of aerobic exercise on energy expenditure and nitrogen balance during very low calorie dieting. *Metabolism, 37*, 758-765.

Polivy, J., & Herman C. P. (1985). Dieting and bingeing: A causal analysis. *American Psychologist, 40*, 193-201.

Prentice, A. M., Black, A. E., Coward, W. A., Davies, H. L., Goldberg, G. R., Murgatroyd, P. R., Ashford, J., Sawyer, M., & Whitehead, R. G. (1986). High levels of energy expenditure in obese women. *British Medical Journal, 292*, 983-987.

Price, R. A., & Stunkard, A. J. (1989). Commingling analysis of obesity in twins. *Human Heredity, 39*, 121-135.

Renjilian, D. A., Perri, M. G., Nezu, A. M., McKelvey, W. F., & Schein, R. L. (1990, August). *Individual versus group therapy for obesity: Matching clients with treatments.* Paper presented at the annual convention of the American Psychological Association, New Orleans.

Rolls, B. J. (1979). How variety and palatability can stimulate appetite. *Nutrition Bulletin, 5*, 78-86.

Rosen, J. C., Gross, J., Loew, D., & Sims, E. A. H. (1985). Mood and appetite during minimal-carbohydrate and carbohydrate-supplemented hypocaloric diet. *American Journal of Clinical Nutrition, 42*, 371-379.

Sandoz Nutrition Corporation. (1987). *The OPTIFAST Core Program patient manual.* Minneapolis: Author.

Schoeller, D. A. (1988). Measurement of energy expenditure in free-living humans by using doubly labeled water. *Journal of Nutrition, 118*, 1278-1289.

Smoller, J. W., Wadden, T. A., & Stunkard, A. J. (1987). Dieting and depression: A critical review. *Journal of Psychosomatic Research, 31*, 429-440.

Sjöström, L. (1980). Fat cells and body weight. In A. J. Stunkard (Ed.), *Obesity* (pp. 72-100). Philadelphia: W. B. Saunders.

Stunkard, A. J. (1984). The current status of treatment for obesity in adults. In A. J. Stunkard & E. Stellar (Eds.), *Eating and its disorders* (pp. 157-183). New York: Raven Press.

Stunkard, A. J., & Berthold, H. C. (1985). What is behavior therapy? A very short description of behavioral weight control. *American Journal of Clinical Nutrition, 41*, 821-823.

Stunkard, A. J., Harris, J. R., Pedersen, N. L., & McClearn, G. E. (1990). The body mass index of twins who have been reared apart. *New England Journal of Medicine, 322*, 1483-1487.

Stunkard, A. J., & Rush, J. (1974). Dieting and depression reexamined: A critical review of reports of untoward responses during weight reduction for obesity. *Annals of Internal Medicine, 81*, 526–533.

Telch, C. F., Agras, W. S., Rossiter, E., Wilfley, D., & Kenardy, J. (1990). Group cognitive-behavioral treatment for the non-purging bulimic: An initial evaluation. *Journal of Consulting and Clinical Psychology, 58*, 629–635.

Tremblay, A., Seale, J., Almeras, N., Conway, J., & Moe, P. (1991). Energy requirements of a postobese man reporting a low energy intake at weight maintenance. *American Journal of Clinical Nutrition, 54*, 506–508.

VanItallie, T. B., & Abraham, S. (1985). Some hazards of obesity and its treatment. In J. Hirsch & T. B. VanItallie (Eds.), *Recent advances in obesity research: IV* (pp. 1–19). London: John Libbey.

Wadden, T. A. (1985). Treatment of obesity in adults: A clinical perspective. In P. A. Keller & L. G. Ritt (Eds.), *Innovations in clinical practice: A sourcebook* (Vol. 4, pp. 127–152). Sarasota, FL: Professional Resource Exchange.

Wadden, T. A. (1987, April). *Factors affecting the treatment of obesity*. Paper presented at the Sandoz Nutrition Postgraduate Seminar, Scottsdale, AZ.

Wadden, T. A., Bartlett, S. J., Letizia, K. A., Foster, G. D., Stunkard, A. J., & Conill, A. (in press). Relationship of dieting history to resting metabolic rate, body composition, eating behavior, and subsequent weight loss. *American Journal of Clinical Nutrition*.

Wadden, T. A., & Bell, S. T. (1990). Obesity. In A. S. Bellack, M. Hersen, & A. E. Kazdin (Eds.), *International handbook of behavior modification and therapy* (2nd ed., pp. 449–473). New York: Plenum.

Wadden, T. A., Foster, G. D., & Letizia, K. A. (in press). Response of obese binge eaters to treatment by behavior therapy and very-low-calorie diet. *Journal of Consulting and Clinical Psychology*.

Wadden, T. A., Foster, G. D., Letizia, K. A., & Stunkard, A. J. (in press). A multi-center evaluation of a proprietary weight reduction program for the treatment of marked obesity. *Archives of Internal Medicine*.

Wadden, T. A., Mason, G., Foster, G. D., Stunkard, A. J., & Prange, A. J. (1990). Effects of a very low calorie diet on weight, thyroid hormones, and mood. *International Journal of Obesity, 14*, 249–258.

Wadden, T. A., & Stunkard, A. J. (1986). A controlled trial of very-low-calorie diet, behavior therapy and their combination in the treatment of obesity. *Journal of Consulting and Clinical Psychology, 54*, 482–486.

Wadden, T. A., Stunkard, A. J., Day, S. C., Gould, R. A., & Rubin, C. J. (1987). Less food, less hunger: Reports of appetite and symptoms in a controlled study of a protein sparing modified fast. *International Journal of Obesity, 11*, 239–249.

Whybrow, P. C., Prange, A. J., & Treadway, C. R. (1969). Mental changes accompanying thyroid gland dysfunction. *Archives of General Psychiatry, 20*, 48–63.

Williamson, D. F., Madans, J., Anda, R. F., Kleinman J. C., Giovino, G. A., & Byers, T. (1991). Smoking cessation and severity of weight gain in a national cohort. *New England Journal of Medicine, 324*, 739–745.

Wilson, G. T. (1985). Psychological prognostic factors in the treatment of obesity. In J. Hirsch & T. B. VanItallie (Eds.), *Recent advances in obesity research: IV* (pp. 301–311). London: John Libbey.

Wing, R. R., Marcus, M. D., Salata, R., Epstein, L. H., Miaskiewicz, S., & Blair, E. H. (1991). Effects of a very-low-calorie diet on long-term glycemic control in obese Type II diabetics. *Archives of Internal Medicine, 151*, 1334–1340.

Yalom, I. (1975). *The theory and practice of group psychotherapy* (2nd ed.). NewYork: Basic Books.

14

Nutritional Counseling during Severe Caloric Restriction and Weight Maintenance

SUZANNE McNULTY

Nutrition is the cornerstone of the treatment of obesity. Dietitians and nutritionists have traditionally used a balanced diet of 1000–1500 kilocalories (kcal)/day to treat overweight individuals, with a resulting weight loss of about 0.5 kg per week (Brownell, 1982; Brownell & Jeffery, 1987; Foreyt et al., 1982). This approach is the treatment of choice for mildly obese individuals, but may not produce adequate weight losses in persons 30% or more overweight (Stunkard, 1984). Thus, during the past decade, dietitians have increasingly found themselves working as members of multidisciplinary teams to provide treatment of marked obesity by very low calorie diet (VLCD) and lifestyle modification (Wadden, VanItallie, & Blackburn, 1990).

VLCDs are not well received by some dietitians because of the perception that the diets violate the principles of sound nutrition and may be associated with serious health complications (Rock & Coulston, 1988). Such misgivings are understandable, but generally are not supported by a thorough review of the research literature (Kanders, Plaisted, Greenberg, & Blackburn, 1988). Thus, a diet of 1000–1500 kcal/day should be used as the first step of treatment with all obese individuals. A VLCD, however, should be considered with those persons who have repeatedly failed to lose weight on conventional diets and must reduce their weight to control health complications.

This chapter reviews the nutritional assessment and treatment of persons participating in a program of VLCD and lifestyle modification. The goal is to provide an overview of the dietitian's responsibilities in working as a member of a multidisciplinary team. These responsibilities overlap, in many cases, with those of the behavioral psychologist as described by Wadden and Foster (Chapter 13, this volume).

Initial Evaluation

Prior to treatment, the dietitian should evaluate the patient's dietary habits, using assessment tools that may include (1) a 24-hour recall; (2) a dietary history; and (3) a 3-day prospective record of food intake. These tools provide information concerning the patient's appropriateness for treatment by VLCD, as well as guidance in modifying the patient's dietary intake over the course of therapy.

Twenty-Four-Hour Recall

A 24-hour dietary recall provides a retrospective account of the types and amounts of food eaten and their times of consumption. This method has high reliability, due to the short period of time covered, although it does not account for variations in diet related to work schedules, holidays, seasonality, and days of the week (Bray, Zachary, Brahms, Atkinson, & Oddie, 1978; Gersovitz, Madden, & Smiciklas-Wright, 1978). Thus, the practitioner should always inquire whether the day selected is representative of the patient's usual dietary intake.

Dietary History

A dietary history, such as that developed by Willett and colleagues, evaluates longstanding food preferences and consumption habits covering periods of a year or longer (Willett, Reynolds, Cottrell-Hoehner, Sampson, & Browne, 1987; Willett et al., 1988). Information obtained by these self-report questionnaires provides reliable estimates of the patient's daily consumption of calories, protein, carbohydrate, fat, and several micronutrients.

Taken together, the 24-hour recall and the dietary history can help to determine the degree to which the patient's obesity is attributable to the excess consumption of calories and/or fat. Thus, it is not uncommon for some obese women to report a caloric intake of only 1200 kcal/day, while others of the same weight report intakes of 3000 kcal/day or more. Measurement of resting metabolic rate is frequently useful in the former group of patients to confirm their low energy requirements (Feurer & Mullen, 1986). Increased physical activity, rather than dietary modification, is critical for persons with low caloric requirements.

The dietary history may also serve to alert the dietitian to nutritional deficiencies, such as low iron or calcium, which can be further assessed by biochemical assays. Attention to such issues is necessary not only before but also during treatment, since VLCDs and weight loss may be associated with changes in minerals and electrolytes. Evaluation of nutritional status is one of several cases in which it is important that the dietitian have a close working relationship with the physician monitoring the patient's physical health.

Three-Day Food Record

The dietitian may also wish to obtain a prospective, 3-day food record from patients prior to their beginning treatment. This method, which is particularly useful with persons who provide an incomplete dietary history, captures the times and places of eating, in addition to the quality and quantity of foods consumed. It should provide a more representative assessment of normal dietary intake than does the 24-hour recall method, provided that a patient is instructed to "follow your normal eating habits."

Use of the food record also helps to assess the patient's ability to comply with the self-monitoring of dietary intake that is required throughout treatment. Persons who are unable to complete a 3-day food record prior to treatment, when motivation is usually high, are unlikely to keep adequate records during the 20 or more weeks of therapy. The dietitian should discuss in detail the difficulties encountered by persons who report that they "hate" to keep diet diaries. Record keeping is critical to a patient's safe completion of the VLCD, and informal observation suggests that it is also a predictor of weight maintenance.

Summary of Evaluation

Information from all three sources should be used to derive an estimate of the patient's daily caloric intake, the composition and nutritional adequacy of the diet, the patient's nutrition awareness, and the appropriateness of the baseline diet for long-term weight control. This information will be used to help individualize the patient's meal plan following consumption of the VLCD. The dietitian can also use the initial evaluation to explore the patient's readiness to try new foods that are low in fat and calories, such as poultry and fish.

The dietitian and psychologist should consult in cases in which either professional suspects that the patient has an eating disorder, whether it is the night eating syndrome, bulimia nervosa, binge eating without compensation, or another abnormal pattern of food intake (Wadden & Foster, Chapter 13, this volume). Patients should be asked whether they experience difficulty with binge eating and related problems, with the expectation that a significant percentage will answer affirmatively. Marcus, Wing, and Lamparski (1985) found that 46% of patients in a behavioral weight loss program reported problems with binge eating, although they did not meet the criteria for bulimia nervosa (i.e., binge eating followed by compensation in the form of vomiting, excessive exercising, or laxative abuse).

Bulimia nervosa is a clear contraindication to treatment by VLCD, as discussed by Wadden and Foster (Chapter 13, this volume). Binge eating per se does not appear to be a contraindication, although bingers may experience increased anxiety and troubled eating during the refeeding period after the VLCD. These problems can be minimized by providing patients with additional support and guidance during the transition from the VLCD to consumption of conventional foods.

The Orientation Period

In most programs, patients consume a diet of 1000–1500 kcal/day for 1 to 4 weeks before beginning the VLCD (Palgi et al., 1985). This introductory period provides an opportunity for patients to lower their calorie intake gradually, which in turn promotes a slow diuresis. The immediate introduction of a VLCD may be associated with rapid losses of water, with attendant complications.

This orientation period also provides patients ample time to prepare for the VLCD, and thus maximize their success. Preparation includes (1) discussing the VLCD and its requirements with family and friends; (2) removing problem foods from the home; (3) purchasing noncaloric fluids and a blender in which to mix the liquid diet (if one is used); and (4) developing a daily meal plan that identifies when and where the VLCD will be consumed. Nutrition education during this phase is usually very brief and is limited to suggestions on how to decrease the portion size of foods and to limit the daily intake of fat to 30% of calories.

The orientation period is also an excellent time to introduce the use of food records (i.e., diet diaries). Clinical observations suggest that the earlier patients start to develop this skill, the more likely they are to retain it during the VLCD and during the more difficult refeeding period. It is not necessary at this early stage for patients to worry about the precise portion size or caloric content of the foods that they consume. These skills can be sharpened later in treatment.

The Very Low Calorie Diet

It is difficult and perhaps inadvisable for the dietitian to provide traditional instruction in nutrition education while patients consume the VLCD. Discussion of macronutrient selection, meal planning, and other topics is likely to fall on deaf ears, because patients are preoccupied at this time in trying to avoid the consumption of conventional foods. Moreover, discussion of conventional foods could increase patients' difficulty in adhering to the VLCD. Nevertheless, the dietitian has several important responsibilities during this phase of treatment; these include (1) selecting an appropriate diet for patients, and (2) counseling them on their fluid intake and consumption of the diet.

Selecting a Diet

Most VLCDs currently provide 400–800 kcal daily and at least 40 g of protein (Wadden, Stunkard, & Brownell, 1983). The quality and quantity of protein provided is the most important nutritional component that the dietitian should evaluate. There is universal agreement that the protein should be of high biological value, as provided by lean meat, fish, and fowl or by calcium caseinate and pasteurized egg whites, as found in powdered-protein liquid diets (Bistrian, 1978; Blackburn, Bistrian, & Flatt, 1975; Genuth, 1979; Wadden et al., 1983).

Investigators do not agree, however, concerning the amount of protein that should be provided; thus, recommendations vary widely from clinic to clinic and country to country. Table 14.1 shows that the amounts recommended by advisory committees of several European countries vary by as much as 30 g daily. A British task force recommended in 1987 that women receive no fewer than 400 kcal and 40 g of protein daily, and men no fewer than 500 kcal and 50 g of protein daily (Committee on Medical Aspects of Food Policy, 1987).

Though it is not conclusive, the bulk of the evidence indicates that the greater the protein intake, the better the preservation of lean body mass (Blackburn et al., 1975; Hoffer, Bistrian, Young, Blackburn, & Matthews, 1984; Scalfi et al., 1987). Thus, caution suggests that patients should be prescribed a minimum 1.2 g of protein daily per kilogram of ideal body weight (Bistrian, 1978). This is equivalent, for persons of average height, to approximately 70 g daily for women and 90 g daily for men. Tall and/or very active individuals are likely to require larger amounts (Apfelbaum, Fricker, & Igoin-Apfelbaum, 1987).

TABLE 14.1. VLCD Status in European Countries

Country	kcal	Protein (g)	Fat (g)	EFA (g)	Carbohydrates (g)
Denmark	330	34	3	—	44
Spain	330	34	3	—	44
France	390	30.6	4	2.3	57
Federal Republic of Germany	717	51	—	7	99
Switzerland	900	60	—	—	100

Note. EFA, essential fatty acids. From "Very-Low-Calorie Diets: Future Perspectives" (p. 13) by J. R. Munro and I. Stolarek, 1989, *International Journal of Obesity*, *13*, 11–15. Copyright 1989 by Macmillan Press Ltd.. Reprinted by permission.

Type of Diet

Powdered-Protein, Formula Diets

The vast majority of persons in the United States treated by a VLCD consume one of the powdered-protein, formula diets that are commercially produced. These diets are mixed with water and consumed three to five times daily in liquid form. The three most popular diets in this country provide approximately 30–50 g of carbohydrate daily, small amounts of fat, and 100% of the recommended dietary allowances (RDAs) for vitamins, minerals, and trace elements (where established) (see Table 14.2). The diets vary in taste and palatability, but all can be improved by mixing them with extracts, spices, and noncaloric fluids such as diet colas. The diets usually also have a thicker texture and better taste when mixed with ice in an electric blender. The dietitian should demonstrate how the diets can be prepared in either a shaker or blender.

Protein-Sparing Modified Fast

Patients can obtain equivalent amounts of dietary protein by consuming a diet of lean meat, fish, and fowl, which is often referred to as a "protein-sparing modified fast" (PSMF) (Blackburn et al., 1975). Thus, the patient might select three servings daily from the protein sources shown in Table 14.3. As with the liquid diet, consumption of all other foods is prohibited. The PSMF must,

TABLE 14.2. Some Diet Formulas

Product	kcal/day	Protein (g)	Carbohydrates (g)	Fat (g)	Cost ($)[a]
HMR 500[b]	520	50	79	1	25.20
70+[b]	520	70	63	1	25.20
800[b]	800	80	97	10	28.70
Medifast 55	435	55	45	4	20.00
70	462	70	37	3	25.00
Plus	848[c]	98	60	24	16.00
OPTIFAST 70	420	70	30	2	[d]
800	800	70	100	13	[d]

Note. From The Medical Letter 1989, 31 (787), 22–23. Copyright 1989 by Medical Letter, Inc. Reprinted by permission.

[a]Cost to the doctor for a week's supply of packets containing powdered supplement. Complete programs involve additional costs.

[b]HMR products are also called Complement 100, 70+, and 800.

[c]Formula provides 374 kcal; the rest come from a single meal of 8 ounces of meat, fish, or fowl, plus 2 cups of salad.

[d]Packets of OPTIFAST are only available as part of a core 26-week program including a patient manual, weekly classes, physician visits, and lab tests. Total cost to the patient averages $2000–$2500.

Nutritional Counseling

TABLE 14.3. Examples of Foods Provided by a Protein-Sparing Modified Fast (PSMF)

Food	Protein (oz)	Calories (kcal)	Protein (g)
White-meat turkey, roasted without skin	3	135	25.0
White-meat chicken, roasted without skin	3	142	26.7
Tuna, drained, packed in water	3	135	30.0
Lean ground beef, broiled	3	230	21.0
Cod, broiled, no fat added	4	117	25.3
Shrimp, boiled, no fat added	4	132	27.4

however, be supplemented with approximately 2–3 g daily of potassium and a multivitamin. Calcium supplementation may also be required (Bistrian, 1978).

These two approaches produce comparable weight losses (Wadden, Stunkard, Brownell, & Day, 1985). Proponents of the liquid diets contend that this approach fosters better dietary adherence, because conventional foods can be avoided altogether. Moreover, the inclusion of vitamins and minerals ensures that patients receive adequate potassium, and the inclusion of small amounts of carbohydrate reduces the large diuresis (and electrolyte loss) that accompanies consumption of VLCDs (DeHaven, Sherwin, Herdler, & Felig, 1980; Wadden et al., 1983).

Proponents of PSMF argue that this approach fosters better long-term behavior change, because patients continue to consume conventional foods throughout treatment (Wadden et al., 1983). Thus, the patient can continue to purchase and prepare foods during the period of supplemented fasting, which should facilitate a smooth transition during the refeeding period. There is also evidence that the PSMF is associated with greater reductions in hunger and cravings than are the liquid diets (Wadden et al., 1985). In addition, the PSMF may be less disruptive of social interactions involving food.

Food and Fluid Intake

The dietitian should carefully review with patients the appropriate methods for preparing the diet selected. Liquid diets require minimal effort, as noted above. Persons, however, who choose a PSMF will need instruction in low fat cooking in order to minimize the number of calories introduced in preparing their protein servings. Thus, these foods generally should be baked, boiled, or broiled. Lemon juice, soy sauce, and other low fat condiments can be used to enhance flavor.

Adherence to the VLCD will be facilitated by helping patients develop a schedule for consuming their meals. The PSMF is usually consumed in three daily servings, and thus can be eaten in lieu of the customary breakfast, lunch, and dinner meals. Liquid diets are usually consumed five times daily. A total of three servings can be consumed at breakfast, lunch, and dinner, with the addition of a serving in the late afternoon and another in the late evening. This schedule should be adjusted to accommodate persons who do not customarily eat breakfast, as well as those who report increased hunger or tiredness at particular times of the day. For each daily meal, patients should indicate when and where they will consume it and how the meal will be prepared. Persons who work outside of the home may have to make special arrangements for consuming their lunch and late afternoon meals.

Full Protein Intake

It is imperative that patients consume the prescribed amount of protein each day, to ensure that they achieve and maintain positive nitrogen balance (VanItallie, 1978). The dietitian should explain the critical role of protein in the diet and discourage patients from skipping meals in order to increase their weight loss. Such practice only increases the likelihood that fat-free mass, rather than fat, will be lost. Deaths related to the consumption of the liquid protein diets of 1976–1977 may have been partially attributable to patients' sparing use of the diets in order to increase the velocity of their weight loss (VanItallie, 1978).

Fluid Intake

Patients must drink a minimum of 2 L daily of noncaloric fluid during consumption of the VLCD, in order to prevent dehydration, electrolyte imbalance, and other complications (Bistrian, 1978; Fisler & Drenick, 1987; Genuth, 1979; Maagøe, 1967; Wadden et al., 1983). Water is the preferred fluid, but the daily intake may include diet soda, coffee, tea, and other noncaloric beverages. Patients should be instructed in reading labels to ensure that the fluid is calorie-free (i.e., less than 1 kcal/6 ounces) and relatively low in sodium (in the case of persons with hypertension). The dietitian may wish to demonstrate the volumes of a variety of glasses and other containers during the first few sessions to familiarize patients with measurement. Patients also may find it helpful to put a 2-L pitcher of water in the refrigerator each morning with the goal of emptying it by bedtime.

Ensuring a Safe Diet

The safe administration of the VLCD is dependent upon the provision of rigorous medical supervision, as described by Atkinson (Chapter 12, this volume), and upon the limitation of the diet to 12 to 16 weeks (Wadden et al., 1990). The dietitian and psychologist can contribute to the safe consumption of the diet by reviewing food records with patients to ensure adequate intake of protein and water. Diet diaries should be reviewed with patients during weekly visits to the extent that time allows. The dietitian may also wish to collect diaries at the end of the meeting, review them, provide brief written comments, and return them to patients at the following week's visit. Written feedback underscores that the information that patients record in their diet diaries is important and of interest to staff members. The dietitian and psychologist may also inquire about the patient's health during the previous week and communicate any concerns to the program physician.

The dietitian should also monitor weight losses carefully to determine when patients fall below 20% overweight. This will occur primarily in lighter individuals who begin treatment only 30–50% overweight. Some investigators believe that caloric intake should be increased significantly once patients reduce below 20% overweight (VanItallie, 1988). This recommendation is based upon findings that when subjected to severe caloric restriction, mildly obese individuals (i.e., less than 30% overweight) do not preserve fat-free mass as well as the more overweight (Forbes, 1987; Forbes & Drenick, 1979). This is perhaps the principal reason why VLCDs are limited to persons who are a minimum of 30% overweight. Weight loss may slow somewhat as caloric intake is increased, but the composition of the weight loss should be more favorable than on a more severely restricted diet.

The Refeeding Period

The refeeding period, in which patients gradually resume consumption of a conventional diet, is challenging for patients and dietitians alike. Patients frequently display one of three behaviors at this time. Many leave treatment immediately after the VLCD, believing that they have achieved their weight loss goals and will have few problems with weight maintenance. Others plead with the practitioner to remain on the VLCD for another month or so, because "it is the best thing that has ever happened to me." A third group of individuals, perhaps more honest and realistic than those in the first two groups, verbalize that they are very anxious about ending the VLCD and fear that they will start bingeing and regain their weight. Thus, the dietitian's most important work begins when patients are fleeing treatment, criticizing the program for not extending the VLCD, or feeling too anxious to think rationally. Such situations are clearly not conducive to learning!

For these reasons, the dietitian should begin to discuss the refeeding period—its purpose and patients' reactions to it—at least 3 weeks prior to its scheduled initiation. Patients should be advised that the refeeding period is highly structured, as is the VLCD, and that they should encounter few difficulties if they follow the recommended guidelines. The dietitian, as well as other staff members, should also reiterate that the refeeding diet must be adhered to carefully in order to prevent any complications, such as refeeding edema. Patients should be given ample opportunity to ask questions and voice their concerns.

Overview of Refeeding

The goal of the refeeding period is to return the patient from a VLCD, containing only small amounts of carbohydrate, to a diet of at least 1000–1200 kcal/day, with ample carbohydrate. There is no research to indicate the optimal length of refeeding, but in most programs it is accomplished in 4 to 6 weeks (Bistrian, 1978; Palgi et al., 1985). The refeeding diet differs, depending upon whether a PSMF or a liquid diet has been used. With the PSMF, the patient slowly adds fruits and vegetables, breads and cereals, and a small fat portion—in that order—while continuing to consume lean meat, fish, or fowl as the protein source. With time, skim milk is used to replace one of the protein servings, usually that consumed for breakfast. Refeeding after a liquid diet follows the same principles, but patients must gradually replace servings of the formula diet with lean meat, fish, or fowl, in addition to gradually increasing their consumption of carbohydrates and fats.

Caloric intake is increased each week by 100–150 kcal/day until it reaches approximately 1000–1200 kcal/day. In addition to calories, the dietitian should carefully monitor the intake of carbohydrates. If they are introduced too quickly, patients may experience marked fluid retention, electrolyte imbalance, and abdominal discomfort (Atkinson, 1986; Bistrian, 1978; Genuth, 1979). Some evidence suggests that marked overconsumption of carbohydrates (i.e., binge eating) during refeeding can precipitate cardiac arrhythmias and pancreatitis (VanItallie & Abraham, 1985).

Facilitating Refeeding

The dietitian can take several steps to facilitate adherence during the refeeding period:

1. Providing patients with an overview of the entire refeeding protocol so that they will know what to expect over the several weeks. The dietitian also should determine whether patients understand the rationale for the protocol. It is designed to: (a) ensure their safety; (b) increase feelings of self-control and minimize unwanted binge eating; and (c) prevent undesired weight gain. Patients should be prepared for the possibility that they will not lose weight (or will show a small gain) during the first 2 weeks of refeeding—an occurrence that is attributable to the consumption of large amounts of dietary carbohydrate.

2. Allowing patients to discuss their food-related fantasies prior to beginning refeeding. Patients frequently have a secret plan for how they will terminate the VLCD. Such plans may include a trip to the neighborhood ice cream parlor or bakery, a meal in a fine restaurant, or a reunion with missed cakes and candies. All of these plans are appropriate when undertaken at the end of the refeeding period—not the beginning. Thus, patients should be informed that they will have an opportunity for their special celebration at the end of refeeding and that staff members will be happy to help them plan it.

3. Limiting patients' food choice. Although there is little research on the topic, clinical experience suggests that refeeding is facilitated by limiting patients' food choices during this 4- to 6-week period. This can be accomplished by assigning specific foods for each meal during the first 1 to 2 weeks of refeeding. If instead, a Chinese menu is used, in which patients are allowed to choose vegetable, fruit, bread, and protein servings, the number of selections in each category should be limited to two or three during the first few weeks.

Patients frequently indicate that one of the greatest benefits of a VLCD is the reduction in the number of food choices that they must make. They identify this as a factor allowing them to lose weight on a VLCD when they cannot do so on a traditional 1200-kcal/day diet. They also report that they feel overwhelmed when presented with long lists of foods from which to select their refeeding diet. Thus, the dietitian should slowly introduce new foods (and choices) over the course of refeeding and the subsequent period in which a conventional diet is consumed.

4. Discussing meal selection and preparation. The dietitian should review patients' diet histories, 3-day food records, and other materials before the refeeding period, to determine patients' likes and dislikes and any food allergies. This information can be used to individualize a patient's refeeding diet. To facilitate meal preparation, the dietitian also may wish to instruct patients in the use of scales and measuring cups and spoons, and in methods of preparing foods without fat.

Nutrition Education

The refeeding period is an ideal time in which to instruct patients in the essentials of sound nutrition. This instruction can begin with a discussion of the major macronutrients—protein, carbohydrate, and fat. The dietitian should explain the role played by each macronutrient in ensuring good health and identify common foods that contain it. This task is perhaps best accomplished by discussing each macronutrient as it is introduced into the refeeding diet. Thus, the function as well as the common sources of protein might be discussed first, since this macronutrient has played such a prominent role during the VLCD. The role of carbohydrate can be discussed as breads and cereals are introduced into the refeeding diet, and that of fat as it is introduced in the latter stages.

The information presented should be practical rather than technical. It is not necessary for patients to understand the chemical structure of the various macronutrients. Instead, they should be able to identify the best sources of each macronutrient and the amounts of each that need to be consumed daily. Thus, sources of protein that are low in fat should be identified, as should sources of complex carbohydrates. Patients also should be informed of the different types of dietary fat (i.e., saturated, monounsaturated, and polyunsaturated), their effects on health, and common sources of each. Cholesterol and dietary fiber should be discussed in a similar manner.

Other topics to be covered include the importance of vitamins, minerals, and trace elements, and common sources of these. It is critical that patients be provided with practical rather than technical information about these topics. Practical information is that which patients can use when shopping for groceries and/or preparing meals.

Supermarket Shopping Tactics

Initiation of the refeeding diet may mark a return to grocery shopping for many patients who have avoided it while consuming the VLCD. This shopping can be both intimidating and overwhelming, given that many supermarkets contain over 10,000 foods (Wadden & Brownell, 1984). The dietitian should discuss food shopping with patients to determine their skills and concerns (Brownell, 1991). The following points should be raised in the course of this discussion:

1. Before shopping for groceries, patients should first plan their meals for the week and then make a list of the foods they need to purchase. They should not enter the market without this list.

2. Most supermarkets keep fresh foods (i.e., dairy, meats, fruits, and vegetables) on the outside aisles of the store. The inner aisles are reserved for canned and packaged foods. It may be possible to skip some of the inner aisles (which display cookies, chips, sodas, etc.).

3. Impulse items, including candies, cakes, and other snacks, are usually displayed at the ends of the aisles and at the checkout counter. Thus, patients should beware of making last-minute purchases while the groceries are being bagged. Retailers' profits rely heavily upon the purchase of impulse items. They know very well that shoppers make 50% of their purchases on impulse while roaming the store (Point of Purchase Advertising Institute, 1978).

4. "Convenience" stores should be avoided, since they specialize not in convenience but in impulse and junk foods. Specialty stores (such as farmers' markets or butcher shops) may be less expensive in the long run, since they reduce impulse buying.

5. Patients should always shop on a full stomach. Shopping when hungry is likely to result in the purchase of impulse items.

6. Patients should shop with a friend if this practice facilitates weight control efforts. Children usually undermine such efforts by requesting items that are not on the grocery list.

The dietitian may wish to include a group shopping trip during the refeeding period. Such trips help to illustrate, in concrete terms, the importance of planning meals, making a shopping list, and using caution once inside the supermarket.

Weight Maintenance

Patients decide, after completing the refeeding diet, whether they wish to lose more weight or to concentrate instead on maintaining the loss that they have achieved. Those who have not reached "goal" weight frequently elect to continue dieting. The various options, and the merits of each, should be discussed at length with patients. Patients electing to reduce further should not anticipate a loss of more than 0.5 kg per week, the size of the loss associated with a conventional reducing diet of 1000–1500 kcal/day.

Once patients have identified their goals, the dietitian must help them select an appropriate diet, composed of conventional foods. Daily caloric requirements based on the patient's sex, age, weight, height, and activity level may be determined with the aid of tables or equations (Harris & Benedict, 1919). These tables or equations, however, are not entirely accurate when applied to obese individuals (Foster et al., 1988). Thus, caloric adjustments may be necessary in response to weight gain or loss. When possible, the patient's resting energy expenditure should be measured (Feurer & Mullen, 1986).

Ensuring a Balanced Diet

To ensure a balanced diet, it is necessary to instruct patients in two methods of food selection—an exchange plan and calorie counting.

Exchange Plan

Since dietitians are very familiar with the exchange plan developed jointly by the American Dietetic Association and the American Diabetes Association, it will not be discussed in detail here. The following information should be reviewed with patients:

1. Foods included in each group.
2. Serving size for foods in each group.
3. Nutrients provided by foods in each group.
4. Calories typically contained in foods in each group.
5. Number of servings allowed from each group.

The manner in which the exchange plan is organized can be explained to patients by reference to the refeeding diet, with which they are familiar. Thus, discussion of the meat group would include a review of the refeeding diet's protein foods, the calories and nutrients provided by the foods, and the number of servings allowed. It also is helpful to discuss mixed foods, which contain components from more than one food group; most persons have difficulty categorizing such items, which include pizza, lasagna, and casseroles.

Patients frequently feel overwhelmed by the exchange system in their initial attempts to use it. They should be forewarned of this possibility and encouraged to give themselves a couple of weeks to "get the hang of it."

Calorie Counting

Patients will have counted calories during the VLCD and refeeding diet, and thus should be familiar with this approach. The dietitian should restate the importance of weighing and measuring foods during the first few weeks in order to determine their caloric content. In addition, patients should be instructed not to worry if they cannot determine precisely the calories contained in some foods. They should make their best guess in such cases.

Although patients may be knowledgeable about calorie counting, they may not be aware of the guidelines for selecting a variety of foods to ensure a balanced diet. They should be instructed to make selections so that approximately 50% of their daily caloric intake is derived from carbohydrate, 15-20% from protein, and 30% or less from fat (Select Committee on Nutrition and Human Needs, 1977). Most patients consume adequate amounts of protein and carbohydrate. They need assistance, however, in reducing their consumption of fat, which (they should be reminded) contains approximately two and one-half times as much energy as the two other major macronutrients. This discussion should include an examination of the caloric density of common foods and the desirability of consuming foods that are filling but calorically dilute. The dietitian may wish to use food models to demonstrate the increased quantities of food that patients can consume if they select items which are calorically dilute rather than dense. Alternatives to frequently consumed calorically dense foods should be identified.

Selecting an Approach

The benefits and disadvantages of the exchange plan and of calorie counting should be discussed at length. Some patients may dislike the exchange plan because it appears rigid or requires too much time to master, while others may enjoy working with the food groups. Still others may find the exchange plan quite easy as compared with the sometimes tedious chore of looking up the calories in all foods consumed. A 1-week trial of each method may help undecided patients make a choice.

A few patients, immediately following the refeeding period, may report that they are too anxious to begin a new meal plan. They may ask to continue the refeeding diet. This diet, while balanced, is very restrictive; in many cases, patients who wish to continue it may be trying to avoid making food choices. The dietitian should listen empathically to these patients and work with them to find an agreeable solution. Continued use of the refeeding diet for a brief time is certainly acceptable. Patients, however, should be encouraged to add a few new selections each week, to ensure that the diet includes a variety of foods by the end of the maintenance period. Otherwise, patients will finish treatment ill prepared to consume conventional foods.

Resources Required during Maintenance

A good calorie guide is an essential tool for weight control. Thus, the dietitian should recommend several, which range in price and in the detail provided. Guides that list the macronutrient components of foods are particularly useful. Patients with high cholesterol levels may require more extensive guides, which list the amounts of cholesterol and saturated and unsaturated fat contained in foods. Several guides also provide information concerning fast and frozen foods.

The ability to read food labels is also critical to long-term weight control. Food labels include variable amounts of information, ranging from a list of the principal ingredients to the number of grams of fat derived from saturated, monounsaturated, and polyunsaturated fat. Government efforts are currently underway to require food manufacturers to provide specific information rather than permitting voluntary disclosure, as is the current practice. In cases in which labels describe only the principal ingredients, patients need strategies for determining the approximate caloric value of the food. In addition, patients should be informed of the numerous terms commonly used on labels to describe sugar, fat, and preservatives.

The dietitian should review with patients the labels from several foods, to test their ability to determine the number of calories from fat, protein, and carbohydrate. Moreover, patients should be able to evaluate the degree to which each food contributes to sound nutrition and health. They also should recognize the questionable practices of many food manufacturers who state with pride that their products (such as potato chips) are cholesterol-free, despite containing large amounts of saturated fat (which are likely to increase serum cholesterol levels).

Planning Meals and Serving Food

Meal planning involves determining what to eat, when to eat, and how much time to set aside for preparation. Clearly, patients' schedules impinge upon their ability to plan meals, and therefore these must be considered when structuring the maintenance regimen. Some patients will not have the time to prepare low calorie meals every day and may be tempted at times to eat fast-food items. Suggestions for these patients may include preparing several days' meals at one time and packaging them in single servings. This method requires self-control, and patients who often eat while cooking or are tempted by a stocked refrigerator may find it easier to purchase frozen, low calorie meals.

Weight control efforts are also aided by serving and eating food in an appropriate manner (Brownell, 1991). Serving foods properly provides a pleasant dining experience, increases awareness of the foods consumed, and fosters greater feelings of self-control. Patients should find some of the following suggestions helpful:

1. Eat only while seated. (Despite the perception that foods eaten on the run or while standing in front of the kitchen sink contain fewer calories, they do not!)

2. Consume all foods from a plate or napkin. Do not eat any foods directly from containers (e.g., ice cream) or bags (e.g., cookies or potato chips).

3. Take medium-sized portions. A second portion can be taken after a 15-minute wait if hunger persists.

4. Use smaller plates and glasses. (This practice does create the illusion of having more food to eat.)

5. Leave some food on the plate. This practice helps to break the compulsion reported by some patients to eat whatever is before them.

6. Return serving dishes to the kitchen once everyone has had an initial serving. Those wishing seconds can serve themselves away from the table.

7. Clear the table after eating. Scrape plates directly into the disposal (or garbage pail) and put away leftovers immediately.

8. Try to avoid arguments while eating. Emotional distress prevents people from enjoying their meals and is likely to precipitate unwanted eating in some.

Review of Food Records

The dietitian should periodically review patients' diet diaries to determine whether they are consuming a well-balanced diet and whether they are experiencing any unvoiced problems. The federal government considers nutrient intake adequate if a diet contains at least two-thirds of the RDAs (Allen & Gadson, 1984; National Academy of Sciences, 1989). It is considered difficult to meet 100% of the RDAs in diets containing fewer than 1200 kcal without careful selection or supplementation (Smoller, Wadden, & Brownell, 1988). Two nutrients requiring careful consideration are iron and calcium. Supplementation or additional food sources rich in iron and calcium may be required.

To foster greater self-reliance, patients should be encouraged to review their own diet diaries on a daily basis. The dietitian can help patients to develop this skill by reviewing their records with them and pointing out the areas of concern.

Cooking Demonstrations

Many patients have the misconception that low calorie foods must be bland, boring, and generally unappetizing. This perception increases the belief that weight control must be associated with feelings of deprivation. In-class cooking demonstrations can be used to demonstrate that a low fat, weight maintenance diet can be both satisfying and fun to prepare. Thus, the dietitian should prepare several meals in group sessions to illustrate how to reduce calories in recipes and to add flavor with spices and other seasonings. For instance, a recipe that requires heavy cream can be prepared using evaporated skim milk, whereas sauces that require flour are just as tasty if cornstarch is used.

It is important to encourage patients to experiment with recipes—old and new—in order to prevent monotony and boredom and a possible reversion to former eating habits. Such experimentation can be facilitated by the dietitian's presenting a new recipe each week in the group session and inviting patients to share one of their favorite meals. Information on low calorie cookbooks and cooking classes is also helpful.

Cooking demonstrations also provide an opportunity to practice, *in vivo*, appropriate methods of serving and eating food. Thus, foods prepared during the treatment session may be consumed by group members while they practice behaviors such as eating slowly and leaving food on their plates.

Special Topics

All persons are routinely confronted by a number of eating-related situations that thwart efforts at weight control. This section briefly reviews some of the challenges most frequently encountered.

High Calorie "Problem" Foods

Many patients report that they have several favorite foods on which they frequently overeat. Such "problem" foods may include ice cream, cookies, chocolate, cakes, potato chips, and corn chips. The dieter may try to avoid these foods completely, only to find that such deprivation leads to binge eating (Polivy & Herman, 1985). What is the best strategy for dealing with such foods?

As a general rule, any food—no matter what the calorie or fat content—can be included in the diet at least occasionally. Patients, however, must carefully plan the consumption of such foods; the following guidelines should help:

1. The patient should make sure that the food fits into the day's calorie allotment. Thus, it is permissible to consume 300 kcal of ice cream, provided that the patient has reserved the calories to do so or has made clear plans to exercise and reduce calories the next day.

2. High calorie foods should be purchased in small quantities if they are to be eaten at home. Preferably, they should be consumed outside of the home (e.g., at a restaurant, ice cream parlor, etc.).

3. Foods should be eaten in an appropriate manner. Thus, they should be served on a plate or napkin and eaten slowly (to enhance enjoyment).

4. Patients should anticipate wanting more of the food after eating the prescribed amount. This experience is quite common. They should engage in another activity immediately after eating; the craving for the food usually decreases within a few minutes.

Many persons find that they continue to have trouble with certain foods, even when they follow these steps. Some report that it is easier to avoid problem foods altogether than to try to eat them in a controlled fashion. This strategy may be useful if applied to one or two problem foods. Patients, however, certainly should not be encouraged to avoid all of their favorite foods.

Eating Out

Approximately 57% of women and 69% of men surveyed in a study in 1985 indicated that they ate at least one meal outside of the home the previous day (U.S. Department of Agriculture, 1985a, 1985b). Thus, our nation is increasingly eating out and eating on the run. Eating out may present a special problem for overweight individuals. It is, therefore, critical that the dietitian provide patients with methods to eat appropriately on such occasions.

Planning is the key to eating a healthy meal out. Before heading out the door, patients should consider the restaurant to which they are going and the types of foods that it serves. Restaurants offering a large variety of foods that can be prepared to order facilitate weight control efforts to a far greater degree than do fast-food establishments. Patients also should think about the meal that they wish to consume and calculate its approximate number of calories. Steps should be taken to ensure that the meal fits into the daily caloric allotment. Finally, it is important for patients not to starve themselves before going out. Excessive hunger is likely to lead to excessive eating.

Once at the restaurant, tactics that prove helpful include the following:

1. Asking for a glass of water immediately upon being seated.
2. Ordering first to avoid being influenced by the decisions of others.
3. Forgoing a cocktail in favor of dessert, or vice versa.
4. Refusing bread and butter.
5. Asking for salad dressing on the side.
6. Avoiding items with sauces and gravies.
7. Sharing entrees or desserts.
8. Ordering extra vegetables.

An optimal way to instruct patients in eating out is to plan a group meal at a restaurant, at which all of these skills can be practiced. In addition, the dietitian may wish to share with group members the menus from several local restaurants. Menus can be examined to determine the selections that are most likely to facilitate (or thwart) weight control efforts.

Holidays and Parties

Food is often associated with celebrations. Holiday cookies, Thanksgiving dinners, and wedding and birthday cakes are all examples of foods that are closely associated with special occasions. Even promotions and graduations are celebrated with a special luncheon or dinner. Thus, patients need help in preparing for both expected and unexpected social occasions that involve food.

If the occasion is known in advance, patients may use several techniques to prepare for it. They should allot a given number of calories for the occasion and adjust their eating and exercise accordingly before and after the occasion. They may also bring their own low calorie substitutes to a party or ask the host if such foods will be available.

At both expected and unexpected events, patients should try to occupy themselves with something other than food. Stimulating conversation or vigorous dancing is a good substitute for eating. Drinking low calorie beverages instead of alcohol will help control eating, as will avoiding "party" tables on which foods are displayed. Patients who feel particularly vulnerable to overeating at a party should remember that they have the option of not going! A quick course in assertiveness training may be necessary to help patients deal with demanding hosts or friends.

Alcohol Consumption

Patients who drank alcohol before the VLCD may feel apprehensive about consuming it during the maintenance period. Most know that alcoholic beverages (particularly mixed drinks) are high in calories, and that having one cocktail often leads to several. The dietitian should review the caloric content of popular alcoholic drinks. Alcohol, like calorically dense foods, may be included in a maintenance diet if it is consumed in moderation. Thus, preparation for drinking alcohol involves the same techniques used for eating high calorie "problem" foods, discussed earlier. Patients should be forewarned that alcohol is likely to disinhibit their dietary restraint. Thus, after one or two drinks, they will be more likely to crave and eat any number of high fat foods within their reach (i.e., potato chips, peanuts, etc.). Thus, consumption of alcoholic beverages presents a significant challenge to weight control efforts.

Resource Training

Patients must be prepared to use every available resource in meeting the challenge of long-term weight control. The ability to evaluate nutrition-related information and determine who is qualified to give nutritional advice is a resource that holds unlimited potential. Today's health-conscious consumer will have a difficult time determining who is qualified to give nutritional advice. Never before has so much misinformation been propagated by persons pretending to have training in nutrition. Thus, the dietitian should review the basic guidelines to which all qualified nutritionists adhere:

1. Dietitians and nutritionists should have a strong academic background, as reflected by a degree from a regionally accredited institution of higher learning.
2. Nutrition is a science, not a miracle cure.
3. The nutrients that the body requires are found in the foods that we eat.
4. Consumers should avoid practitioners with something to sell.
5. Sound nutrition is *not* based on testimony.

Patients also must be able to evaluate the nutrition information found in various print and audiovisual materials. The dietitian should invite patients during group sessions to share and discuss materials they may already have accumulated. A variety of sources should be examined, including cookbooks, product pamphlets, and magazine articles.

Patients should be directed to reliable sources of nutrition information, which may include the following:

1. The federal government
   - U.S. Department of Health and Human Services
   - Food and Drug Administration, Office of Consumer Affairs
   - U.S. Department of Agriculture Extension Services
   - Human Nutrition Information Service
2. State health departments
3. County, city, and local health departments
4. Associations
   - American Cancer Society
   - American Dietetic Association
   - American Diabetes Association
   - American Heart Association
   - Society for Nutrition Education

These are just a few of the nutrition resources available. Ideally, the dietitian should provide patients with a list of the resources available in the area, complete with addresses and phone numbers. The steps above will provide patients the skills necessary to assess the soundness of the numerous nutritional claims encountered each day.

Summary

As long as obesity continues to be a major health problem, dietary therapy will play a major role in its treatment. Obese individuals must be carefully screened and guided into programs that meet their nutritional needs and produce sufficient weight loss to maintain motivation. Successful programs must also provide instruction in skills required to maintain weight loss.

Potential candidates for VLCDs must realize that these programs are not for everyone. Guidelines proposed by the American Dietetic Association (1990) require that patients meet the following criteria:

1. At least 30% overweight, with a minimum body mass index of 32.
2. Free from contraindicated medical conditions (pregnancy or lactation; cancer; hepatic disease; renal failure; active cardiac dysfunction; or severe psychological disturbances).
3. Committed to establishing new eating and lifestyle behaviors that will facilitate the maintenance of weight loss.
4. Committed to taking the time to complete both the weight loss and weight maintenance components of a program.

A comprehensive VLCD program can provide safe and effective weight loss. The key to the success of such regimens does not lie in the diet supplement; it resides in the education and support provided by a team of highly trained professionals. The dietitian can help patients to become nutrition experts. The information that patients learn and the skills that they develop can translate into a lifetime of healthy eating and, with continued effort, long-term weight control.

References

Allen, J., & Gadson, K. (1984). Food consumption and nutritional status of low income households. *National Food Review, 26*, 27-29.

American Dietetic Association. (1990). Position of the American Dietetic Association: Very low calorie weight loss diets. *Journal of the American Dietetic Association, 90*, 722-726.

Apfelbaum, F., Fricker, J., & Igoin-Apfelbaum, L. (1987). Low and very low calorie diets. *American Journal of Clinical Nutrition, 45*, 1126-1134.

Atkinson, R. (1986). Very low calorie diets: Getting sick or remaining healthy on a handful of calories. *Journal of Nutrition, 116*, 918-920.

Bistrian, B. R. (1978). Clinical use of a protein sparing modified fast. *Journal of the American Medical Association, 240*, 2299-2302.

Blackburn, G. L., Bistrian, B. R., & Flatt, J. P. (1975). Role of a protein sparing modified fast in a comprehensive weight reduction program. In A. N. Howard (Ed.), *Recent advances in obesity research: Proceedings of the First International Congress on Obesity* (pp. 279-281). London: Newman.

Bray, G. A., Zachary, B., Brahms, A. T., Atkinson, R. L., & Oddie, T. H. (1978). Eating patterns of massively obese individuals. *Journal of the American Dietetic Association, 72*, 24-27.

Brownell, K. D. (1982). Obesity: Understanding and treating a serious prevalent and refractory disorder. *Journal of Consulting and Clinical Psychology, 50*, 821-840.

Brownell, K. D. (1991). *The LEARN program for weight control*. Dallas, TX: American Health.

Brownell, K. D., & Jeffery, R. W. (1987). Improving long-term weight loss: Pushing the limits of treatment. *Behavior Therapy, 18*, 353-374.

Committee on Medical Aspects of Food Policy. (1987). *Report of the working group on very low calorie diets: The use of very low calorie diets in obesity*. London: Her Majesty's Stationery Office.

DeHaven, J., Sherwin, R., Herdler, R., & Felig, P. (1980). Nitrogen and sodium balance and sympathetic nervous system activity in obese subjects treated with a low calorie protein or mixed diet. *New England Journal of Medicine, 302*, 477-482.

Feurer, I. D., & Mullen, J. L. (1986). Measurement of energy expenditure. In J. Rombeau & M. Caldwell (Eds.), *Clinical nutrition* (pp. 224-236). Philadelphia: W. B. Saunders.

Fisler, J. S., & Drenick, E. J. (1987). Starvation and semi-starvation diets in the management of obesity. *Annual Review of Nutrition, 7*, 465-484.

Forbes, G. B. (1987). Lean body mass—body fat interrelationships in humans. *Nutrition Review, 45*, 225-231.

Forbes, G. B., & Drenick, E. J. (1979). Loss of body nitrogen on fasting. *American Journal of Clinical Nutrition, 32*, 1570-1574.

Foreyt, J. P., Mitchell, R. E., Garner, D. T., Gee., M., Scott, L. W., & Gotto, A. M. (1982). Behavioral treatment for obesity: Results and limitations. *Behavior Therapy, 13*, 153-161.

Foster, G. D., Wadden, T. A., Mullen, J. L., Stunkard, A. J., Wang, J., Feurer, I. D., Pierson, R. N., Yang, M.-U., Presta, E., VanItallie, T. B., Lemberg, P. S., & Gold, J. (1988). Resting energy expenditure, body composition and excess weight in the obese. *Metabolism, 37*, 467-472.

Genuth, S. (1979). Supplemented fasting in the treatment of obesity and diabetes. *American Journal of Clinical Nutrition, 32*, 2579-2586.

Gersovitz, M., Madden, J. P., & Smiciklas-Wright, H. (1978). Validity of the 24-hour dietary recall and seven-day record for group comparisons. *Journal of the American Dietetic Association, 73*, 48-55.

Harris, J. A., & Benedict, F. G. (1919). *A biometric study of basal metabolism in man* (Publication No. 279). Washington, DC: Carnegie Institute.

Hoffer, L. J., Bistrian, B. R., Young, V. R., Blackburn, G. L., & Matthews, D. E. (1984). Metabolic effects of very low calorie weight reduction diets. *Journal of Clinical Investigations, 73*, 750-758.

Kanders, B. S., Plaisted, C. S., Greenberg, I., & Blackburn, G. L. (1988). Very low calorie diets [Letter to the editor]. *Journal of the American Dietetic Association, 260*, 905.

Maagøe, H. (1967). Changes in blood volume during absolute fasting with and without sodium chloride administration. *Metabolism, 16*, 133-138.

Marcus, M. D., Wing, R. R., & Lamparski, D. M. (1985). Binge eating and dietary restraint in obese patients. *Addictive Behaviors, 10*, 163-168.

Munro, J. F., & Stolarek, I. (1989). Very-low-calorie diets: Future perspectives. *International Journal of Obesity, 13*, 11-15.

National Academy of Sciences. (1989). *Recommended dietary allowances* (10th ed.). Washington, DC: Author.

Palgi, A., Read, J. L., Greenberg, I., Hoffer, M. A., Bistrian, B. R., & Blackburn, G. L. (1985). Multidisciplinary treatment of obesity with a protein-sparing modified fast: Results in 688 outpatients. *American Journal of Public Health, 75*, 1190-1194.

Point of Purchase Advertising Institute. (1978). *Dupont consumer buying habits study*. New York: Author.

Polivy, J., & Herman, C. P. (1985). Dieting and bingeing: A causal analysis. *American Psychologist, 40*, 193-201.

Rock, C. L., & Coulston, A. M. (1988). Weight control approaches: A review by the California Dietetic Association. *Journal of the American Dietetic Association, 88*, 44-48.

Scalfi, L., Contaldo, F., Borrelli, R., De Caterina, M., Spagnuolo, G., Alfieri, R., & Mariani, M. (1987). Protein balance during very low calorie diets for the treatment of severe obesity. *Annals of Nutrition and Metabolism, 31*, 154-159.

Select Committee on Nutrition and Human Needs, U.S. Senate. (1977). *Dietary goals for the United States* (2nd ed.). Washington, DC: U.S. Government Printing Office.

Smoller, J. W., Wadden, T. A., & Brownell, K. D. (1988). Popular and very low calorie diets in the treatment of obesity. In R. T. Frankle & M.-U. Yang (Eds.), *Obesity and weight control*. Rockville, MD: Aspen.

Stunkard, A. J. (1984). The current status of treatment of obesity in adults. In A. J. Stunkard & E. Steller (Eds.), *Eating and its disorders* (pp. 157-174). New York: Raven Press.

U.S. Department of Agriculture. (1985a). *Nationwide food consumption survey: Continuing survey of food intakes by individuals, women 19-50 years and their children, 1 day* (NFCS CSFII Report No. 85-1). Washington, DC: U.S. Government Printing Office.

U.S. Department of Agriculture. (1985b). *Nationwide food consumption survey: Continuing survey of food intakes by individuals, men 19-50 years, 1 day* (NFCS CSFII Report No. 85-3). Washington, DC: U.S. Government Printing Office.

VanItallie, T. B. (1978). Liquid protein mayhem. *Journal of the American Medical Association, 240*, 140-141.

VanItallie, T. B. (1988). Obesity. In K. M. Jeejeebhoy (Ed.), *Current therapy and nutrition* (pp. 314-324). Toronto: Decker.

VanItallie, T. B., & Abraham, S. (1985). Some hazards of obesity and its treatment. In J. Hirsch & T. B. VanItallie (Eds.), *Recent advances in obesity research: IV. Proceedings of the Fourth International Congress on Obesity* (pp. 1-19). London: John Libbey.

Wadden, T. A., & Brownell, K. D. (1984). The alteration of eating and nutrition habits in healthy population. In J. B. Matarazzo, M. Miller, S. M. Weiss, A. Herd, & S. Weiss (Eds.), *Behavioral health: A handbook of health education and disease prevention* (pp. 608-631). New York: Wiley.

Wadden, T. A., Stunkard, A. J., & Brownell, K. D. (1983). Very low calorie diets: Their efficacy, safety, and future. *Annals of Internal Medicine, 99*, 675-684.

Wadden, T. A., Stunkard, A. J., Brownell, K. D., & Day, S. C. (1985). A comparison of two very-low-calorie diets: Protein-sparing-modified fast versus protein liquid formula diet. *American Journal of Clinical Nutrition, 41*, 533-539.

Wadden, T. A., VanItallie, T. B., & Blackburn, G. L. (1990). Responsible and irresponsible use of very-low-calorie diets in the treatment of obesity. *Journal of the American Medical Association, 263*, 83-85.

Willett, W. C., Reynolds, R. D., Cottrell-Hoehner, S., Sampson, L., & Browne, M. L. (1987). Validation of a semi-quantitative food frequency questionnaire: Comparison with a 1-year diet record. *Journal of the American Dietetic Association, 87*, 43-47.

Willett, W. C., Sampson, L., Browne, M. L., Stampfer, M. J., Rosner, B., Hennekens, C. H., & Speizer, F. E. (1988). The use of a self-administered questionnaire to assess diet four years in the past. *American Journal of Epidemiology, 127*, 188-199.

15

A Clinical Approach to Exercise in the Markedly Obese

KENNETH R. FOX

Exercise is increasingly recognized as a critical component in the treatment of obesity (Bray, 1990; Thompson, Jarvie, Lahey, & Cureton, 1982). Several studies, in fact, suggest that it is the single best determinant of weight loss maintenance (Pavlou, Krey, & Steffee, 1989; van Dale, Saris, & ten Hoor, 1990). Despite these benefits, markedly overweight individuals frequently have difficulty in developing a meaningful program of physical activity. A possible solution to this problem may be found in the design and delivery of exercise strategies that are appropriate to the needs of this particular group.

This chapter is divided into two sections. The first provides an overview of the research on the benefits of exercise for weight control and disease prevention. The second section discusses methods of helping the markedly obese to develop a program of physical activity that will facilitate long-term weight control.

A Rationale for Exercise in Obesity Treatment

It is not possible in this brief chapter to review fully the literature on the benefits of exercise with the markedly obese. At the risk of oversimplifying a complex issue, this review is designed to provide answers to the following three questions:

1. Can exercise promote weight loss and its maintenance?
2. Can exercise reduce the risk and symptoms of disease?
3. Can exercise contribute to well-being?

Exercise, Weight Loss, and Maintenance of Weight Loss

Exercise and Weight Loss

There is ample evidence that increased exercise produces weight loss in the obese (Bray, 1990). Not surprisingly, in comparison with moderate to severe dietary restrictions, weight loss resulting from exercise is slow and rarely exceeds 2 kg/month. However, such amounts are significant over several months and suggest that regular, purposeful exercise can make an important long-term contribution to weight control. The weight loss reported in most studies can be largely accounted for by the total calories expended by the training program. A prolonged increase in thermogenesis following acute bouts of exercise is unlikely to be achieved by the obese, at least in the first 6 months of exercise, because of the intensity and duration of activity required (Brehm, 1988).

When combined with dietary restriction, exercise only marginally increases weight loss, and some studies have shown no effect for exercise. However, there is usually a wide range of responses to diet and exercise training. This variance, accompanied by the small number of subjects in many studies, reduces statistical significance and often masks the underlying trend that exercise becomes more effective with time (van Dale, 1988). The full effects of an exercise program on weight loss may not be apparent until 8 to 12 weeks into the program (Belko, Van Loan, Barbieri, & Mayclin, 1987; Wood et al., 1988). Reasons for this latency are not clear, but a period of adaptation may be required to overcome compensatory lethargy (Weigle, Sande, Iverius, Monsen, & Brunzell, 1988), and glycogen loading may mask early weight loss (Warwick & Garrow, 1981).

It is important to note that weight loss achieved by diet plus exercise results in a greater loss of fat and better preservation of lean body tissue than does weight reduction by diet alone (Pavlou, Steffee, Lerman, & Burrows, 1985; Pavlou, Whatley, et al., 1989; Wood et al., 1988). This may result in a higher posttreatment resting metabolic rate (RMR) in the exercising group than in the diet-alone group (Frey-Hewitt, Vraizan, Dreon, & Wood, 1990), and it may have important implications for weight stabilization. There is also some indication that the process of increased activity itself stimulates metabolic activity above sedentary levels (Molé, 1990). Generally, these exercise effects are stronger when dietary restriction is less severe (Hill et al., 1989; Pavlou, Whatley, et al., 1989). Exercise is not able to prevent the loss of lean body tissue that accompanies the consumption of a very low calorie diet (VLCD) and may exacerbate it if training progresses too rapidly (Phinney, LaGrange, O'Connell, & Danforth, 1988). There are six or more studies in this area with very conflicting results (Donnelly, Jakicic, & Gunderson, 1991).

The impact of exercise seems to be stronger in males than in females (Pavlou, Krey, & Steffee, 1989; van Dale, 1988; van Dale, Saris, Schoffelen, & ten Hoor, 1987). This may be due either to the increased propensity of males to maintain or increase lean body tissue through exercise, or to their characteristic abdominal fat distribution. In addition, there is some indication that hyperplasic obesity is less responsive than hypertrophic obesity to exercise (Krotkiewski & Björntorp, 1986), which may also be linked to differences in fat distribution. On the other hand, some adults with childhood-onset obesity (usually associated with hyperplasia) have demonstrated considerable long-term success with exercise (Gwinup, 1975).

Contradictory evidence can be found for many of these statements, highlighting the need for programs of research that sequentially manipulate variables related to diet, exercise, and subject characteristics. Until that time, the studies reviewed suggest that in the case of markedly obese individuals, who often need to lose weight to control medical complications, restriction of energy intake rather than increased expenditure is required to induce a rapid weight loss. The markedly obese are not capable of expending the amount of energy required to produce significant weight loss. However, it seems appropriate that light to moderate exercise be encouraged at all stages of treatment in order to help patients to adapt physiologically and behaviorally for the longer-term benefits of exercise.

Exercise and Weight Loss Maintenance

Substantial evidence shows that a program of regular physical activity is a key factor to promoting sustained weight loss (Marston & Criss, 1984; Pavlou, Krey, & Steffee, 1989; Stalonas, Johnson, & Christ, 1978; van Dale et al., 1990). In the recent study by van Dale et al. (1990), all subjects who maintained their exercise program or began one during follow-up were moderately successful in sustaining weight loss at 26 months. Over 70% of those who had not exercised during treatment or who had ceased to exercise during follow-up regained at least 75% of their lost weight. Pavlou and colleagues demonstrated that subjects who had received 8 weeks of dietary restriction and supervised exercise, and who had continued to expend the equivalent of 1500 kilocalories (kcal)/week, were successful in sustaining most of their weight loss at 18 months (Pavlou, Krey, & Steffee, 1989). Of those persons originally treated by diet alone, only those who began to exercise during the maintenance period avoided regaining weight. It should be noted, however, that subjects in this study were male police officers who initially averaged only 22% above ideal body weight.

Although the association between exercise and sustained weight loss is strong, identification of the mechanisms by which exercise facilitates maintenance of weight loss is problematic. It is clear that the continuation of regular exercise is the critical factor, because subjects regain weight without it. This would point toward a physiological explanation, with the increased energy expenditure associated with exercise or the effects of exercise on lean body mass and RMR as possible answers. However, studies have not controlled for subjects' performance of other weight-related behaviors (i.e., keeping a diet diary, eating a low fat diet) during maintenance, and it is possible and perhaps likely that subjects who exercise also control their dietary intake more satisfactorily.

Exposure to exercise treatment does not guarantee success, as large percentages of patients stop exercising after treatment. Furthermore, instruction in exercise is not essential for success, given findings that some subjects treated by diet alone have initiated exercise programs on their own and maintained their weight loss (Pavlou, Krey, & Steffee, 1989). However, the vast majority of persons who maintain a program of physical activity receive extensive exercise supervision during treatment (Craighead & Blum, 1989; Pavlou, Krey, & Steffee, 1989; van Dale et al., 1990). Such supervision probably has a combined physiological and psychological impact, with factors such as improved fitness, reduced discomfort, and increased feelings of personal control making long-term adherence more likely.

Exercise and Risk Reduction

The association between sedentary lifestyles and increased risk of morbidity from coronary heart disease is well established (Blackburn & Jacobs, 1988; European Atherosclerosis Society, 1987; Leon, Connett, Jacobs, & Rauramaa, 1987; Paffenbarger, Hyde, Wing, & Hsieh, 1986). Recently, an analysis of 43 studies (Powell, Thompson, Caspersen, & Kendrick, 1987) concluded that physical inactivity is an independent risk factor, almost on a par for relative risk with smoking, hypertension, and hyperlipidemia. In addition, the role of increased physical fitness, which is in large part due to higher activity levels, was recently examined by Blair et al. (1989). Over 10,000 men and 3,000 women were measured for aerobic fitness and followed for an average of 8 years. A strong graded relationship was observed between cardiovascular fitness and reduced mortality, as previously reported (Ekelund et al., 1988; Sobolski et al., 1987); this relationship was independent of age, gender, or other risk factors. The greatest difference in risk was observed between persons in the lowest fitness category (the condition of almost all markedly obese subjects) and those in the middle category.

Harris and colleagues, in a report for the U.S. Preventive Services Task Force, concluded that the negative impact of inactivity on health warranted its being targeted as a primary risk factor, with appropriate public health interventions led by physicians and related health professionals (Harris, Caspersen, DeFriese, & Estes, 1989). This sentiment has been echoed by others (Blackburn & Jacobs, 1988; Koplan, Caspersen, & Powell, 1989). Thus, programs for the obese should target low activity levels as an independent risk factor, comparable to hypertension or high cholesterol, and should seek to promote gradual increases in lifestyle behavior that are associated with modest improvements in aerobic fitness. Increased physical activity may also contribute to the alleviation of other risk factors, most of which are elevated among the obese (Manson et al., 1990).

Lipid Profile

The effect of exercise on blood lipids has recently been summarized by Wood and Stefanick (1990). Cross-sectional comparisons between active and inactive individuals show higher levels in active persons of high density lipoprotein

(HDL) cholesterol, and reduced triglyceride and very low density lipoprotein (VLDL) levels. Controlled trials of exercise in healthy adults have also shown reductions in lipid profiles, which are greater in studies lasting more than 3 months. There are also signs of a dose–response relationship above a threshold level of activity. Similar results have been found with obese men (Pavlou, Krey, & Steffee, 1989; Schwartz, 1987). Studies with obese women have been less successful (Bray, 1990), although Pavlou, Whatley, et al. (1989) found greater reductions in triglycerides and total cholesterol in a diet and exercise condition versus a diet-only condition. Exercise did not increase HDL cholesterol, a result that was attributed to the limitation of the study to only 8 weeks. Improved lipid profiles in the obese appear to be mediated by weight loss, with dietary control and increased aerobic exercise being equally effective (Wood et al., 1988).

Hypertension

Aerobic exercise can produce small reductions in systolic and diastolic blood pressure in some people with essential hypertension (Hagberg, 1990). In addition, the association between increased activity and reduced hypertension appears to be even greater among those at high risk because of their obesity (Paffenbarger, Wing, Hyde, & Jung, 1983). Although it is well established that weight loss in the obese is associated with a proportional decrease in hypertension, the independent role of exercise is not well established. However, Krotkiewski et al. (1979) observed lower blood pressures in obese women who exercised without losing weight, and no studies have reported chronic increases in blood pressure that are a result of exercise.

Insufficient evidence is available to show that the effect of exercise on blood lipids and hypertension in the obese is any stronger than that found in the general population. It appears that during obesity treatment, improvements in health are attributable to weight loss, which is more likely to be achieved by dietary manipulation than by exercise. The effect of exercise on these factors is likely to become more apparent as weight loss slows, as exercise becomes more extensive, and as the emphasis is turned toward weight maintenance.

Glucose Tolerance and Insulin Sensitivity

Insulin sensitivity and glucose uptake are increased with acute bouts of exercise, and are also improved by long-term exercise training in normal and diabetic patients (Vranic & Wasserman, 1990). Improvements appear to be attributable to the acute effects of exercise rather than to improved fitness, since the effects are observed within a few days of initiating activity and disappear when activity is discontinued. This pattern has also been demonstrated in obese subjects, independent of weight loss (Horton, 1988).

To summarize, the recognition of inactivity as a *primary* coronary risk factor among the obese is long overdue. For this reason alone, exercise needs to be considered an integral component of treatment. Exercise is also effective at all points of treatment in the improvement of insulin sensitivity and glucose uptake in the obese. It also holds increasing value for reducing hypertension and improving blood lipid profiles as weight loss slows. Other potential benefits of exercise yet to be fully explored with the obese include protection against osteoporosis, promotion of smoking cessation, reduction in incidence of low back pain, and reduced reactivity to stress.

Exercise and Enhanced Well-Being

One of the major contributions of exercise and improved physical fitness is the potential to improve the quality of life. Epidemiological evidence shows that increased physical activity is associated with psychological well-being, especially in overweight persons (Hayes & Ross, 1986). A growing literature demonstrates that exercise and the resultant changes in fitness can initiate a broad range of mental health benefits (Biddle & Mutrie, 1991; Morgan & Goldston, 1987), and exercise is increasingly used to treat such problems as stress and depression (Brown, 1990).

Acute Benefits Derived from Exercise

Among the strongest effects of exercise consistently reported by subjects is the "feeling good" phenomenon (see Biddle & Fox, 1989, for a summary). This may be experienced as a sense of accomplishment or as a "healthy glow," resulting in a release of muscular tension, reduced anxiety, or enhanced mood. The origins of these effects have been difficult to isolate; thermogenesis, endogenous opiates, changes with brain wave patterns, and mental diversion have been suggested. The issue is complicated further by the possibility of interactions between subjects' current fitness levels and the type and intensity of exercise selected (Steptoe & Cox, 1988). However, there is good evidence to show that some of these acute psychological benefits are available with exercise of low to moderate intensity, which is accessible to the obese (Martinsen, Medhus, & Sandvik, 1985; Steptoe & Bolton, 1988). Our own research (Fox & Dirkin, 1989) with markedly obese patients receiving outpatient treatment revealed that they experienced numerous benefits, such as relaxation and a sense of accomplishment, even in the early stages of exercise adoption.

Chronic Benefits Derived from Exercise

The obese often experience significant improvements in their psychosocial adjustment as they lose weight, and as yet it is impossible to apportion these changes to the weight loss itself, dietary change, increased exercise, or the effects of improved fitness. However, long-term participation in exercise often results in increased self-esteem (Sonstroem & Morgan, 1989), particularly in those who begin with low esteem. The effect may originate from several sources, and it is not known to what extent an improvement in muscular or aerobic fitness is required to obtain improvements. Changes in specific aspects of physical self-perception, such as body image or perceived strength, accompany different types of exercise programs (Fox & Corbin, 1989). These may or may not accurately reflect actual change in physiological parameters. In a previously sedentary population that had completed a 6-month aerobic exercise program, improvements in perceived shape, appearance, and weight were correlated with weight change, but not with improvements in aerobic fitness (King, Taylor, Haskell, & DeBusk, 1989). On the other hand, specific improvements in self-efficacy and body image have been shown to be related to changes in muscular conditioning occurring with weight training programs (Ewart, 1989; Tucker, 1983). It may be possible that muscular improvement provides more direct bodily feedback.

These sources of psychological enhancement probably contribute to an improvement in global self-esteem, but the improvement may result equally from other changes, such as the sense of empowerment experienced with greater command over lifestyle, renewed hope, new coping skills, sense of ability to cope, or factors associated with greater social support and involvement. Furthermore, the increased functional capacity that can result from exercise in the obese (e.g., see Gillett & Eisenmann, 1987; Pavlou, Whatley, et al., 1989) may improve quality of life by providing access to more socially rewarding experiences. Unfortunately, most of these outcomes have not been measured in the obese undergoing exercise treatment.

Clearly, more research is required in this complex yet important area. Given the initially low levels of fitness, lower self-esteem (particularly in the physical domain of body image and perceived fitness), reduced social contact, and the stresses of social discrimination experienced by many obese people (Wadden & Stunkard, 1985), the potential for improving psychological health through exercise has to be given careful consideration. In addition, the strong association between increased physical activity and long-term weight control may be mediated by some of these psychological outcomes.

Summary

The preceding overview illustrates that although exercise can contribute to losses of weight and fat, its impact in comparison to marked dietary restriction is limited. Exercise can be successful in reducing weight in the long run, but clinicians may judge that immediate drastic reduction in weight is desirable. This dictates a reliance on methods such as gastric surgery or VLCD as a means of creating weight loss. However, although the mechanisms are not fully identified, it cannot be denied that patients who do well with exercise greatly improve their chances of long-term weight stabilization.

When viewed from a more holistic perspective (Blundell, 1984), exercise also holds great potential for long-term reductions in the risk of disease and early death. Inactivity should be regarded as a risk factor in itself, and exercise has a favorable effect on other risk factors, including blood lipid profile, glucose tolerance and insulin sensitivity, and (to a lesser extent) hypertension. This becomes increasingly important as weight loss slows down. Finally, regular exercise and improvements in physical fitness have great potential for improving the long-term prognosis for patients' psychological health and quality of life.

Increasing Physical Activity in the Obese

It is now clear that multiple factors contribute to obesity (Wadden & Bell, 1990), and there is general agreement that exercise should play an important role in the multidisciplinary treatment of this disorder (Council on Scientific Affairs, 1988). Unfortunately, clear guidelines are not yet available for clinicians who wish to incorporate an exercise component in obesity treatment. This is a complex matter, because the benefits of exercise are diverse, and different treatment outcomes may require particular formulas in terms of the type, frequency, duration, intensity, and setting of physical activity. Interventions designed to maximize weight loss or increases in fitness, for example, may conflict with the need for strategies to develop long-term exercise adherence. A careful prioritization of desired outcomes is needed in order to select the most effective approach.

The Exercise Adherence Problem

Given the potential of exercise to facilitate sustained weight loss and improved health, efforts to improve patient adherence to exercise regimens must be given top priority at all stages of treatment. Adherence to exercise is a clear public health problem (Dishman, 1988), as less than 50% of the public engages in regular, purposeful physical activity (Canada Fitness Survey, 1983; Stephens, Jacobs, & White, 1985; Sports Council of Great Britain, 1982). Obese people tend to avoid vigorous activity (Blair & Buskirk, 1987; Meyers, Stunkard, Coll, & Cooke, 1980) and are the least likely population to make long-term changes in activity (Bain, 1985). Once exercise is started, the obese are among the first to drop out of formal programs (Bain, 1985; Dishman, 1981), in part because they initially have very low levels of physical conditioning and are susceptible to joint discomfort and problems of exertion.

In addition, many obese persons have negative attitudes toward exercise because of previous unfavorable experiences, and many report low exercise self-efficacy and limited exercise expertise (Fox & Dirkin, 1989; Fox, Mucci, & Dirkin, 1990). Thus, some studies have shown higher attrition rates with obesity treatments that include exercise (van Dale, 1988), and most studies have shown poor long-term maintenance of exercise (Gwinup, 1975; MacKeen, Franklin, Nicholas, & Buskirk, 1983; Perri, McAdoo, McAllister, Lauer, & Yancey, 1986; van Dale et al., 1990). This generally disappointing record suggests that encouraging the obese to adopt and adhere to an exercise program poses serious challenges. On the other hand, many obese people, including those with early-onset obesity (Gwinup, 1975), have demonstrated that they *are* able to maintain exercise as a lifestyle habit (Hill et al., 1989; Pavlou, Krey, & Steffee, 1989).

Traditionally, exercise programs have focused on maximizing weight loss or fitness rather than adherence. Thus, there is a clear need for exercise specialists, psychologists, and other practitioners to identify behavioral, psychosocial, and psychophysiological factors that will promote habitual exercise in the obese (Council on Scientific Affairs, 1988). Besides our own research with obese adults receiving a multidisciplinary treatment (Fox & Dirkin, 1989; Fox et al., 1990), only three other studies have specifically investigated factors affecting attitudes toward and adherence to exercise in overweight women (Bain, Wilson, & Chaikind, 1989; Gillett, 1988; Grimes, 1986). There has been no research on this topic with obese males. Other than the information provided by these studies, practitioners are left to generalize findings from other populations, to make inferences from intervention studies with other health behaviors, and to lean heavily on clinical experience in their attempts to develop exercise protocols that facilitate long-term increases in physical activity.

Commitment to Exercise: A Model to Guide Program Design

Figure 15.1 presents a simplistic, sequential model designed to provide a framework for understanding and increasing patients' commitment to exercise. It illustrates the importance of psychosocial and behavioral factors in designing programs for lifetime maintenance of exercise and fitness. Patients bring to treatment a host of individual characteristics, both psychological and physical, that may influence present and future exercise behaviors. These include their previous exercise experience; their opinions concerning the nature of exercise; their weight and dieting history; and their body type, personality, and family background. These factors produce a complex personal equation, similar to a cost–benefit analysis, that will determine current psychological commitment (Level 1) to the goal of increasing exercise.

A colleague and I found that beliefs regarding the negative and positive aspects of exercise, as well as measures of exercise-related self-efficacy, correlated moderately with the current degree of exercise in overweight patients receiving treatment for their obesity (Fox & Dirkin, 1989). These findings are in line with those from other populations whose physical activity has been studied (Godin & Shephard, 1990; Toshima, Kaplan, & Ries, 1990), and with motivation theory in general (Bandura, 1982; Harter, 1990). These factors may

Exercise in the Markedly Obese

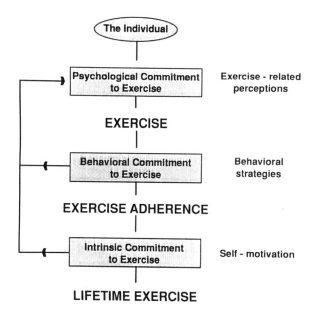

FIGURE 15.1. A model of commitment to exercise.

represent the approach tendency of the obese to exercise. Once prompted, early success should produce positive feedback and strengthen the decision to exercise. Conversely, of course, experiences that are perceived to be embarrassing or physically unpleasant will trigger avoidance behavior. It follows that well-designed programs should utilize strategies to increase patients' exercise expertise and confidence.

Establishing a program of regular physical activity requires more than confidence or a strong belief system. When busy schedules dictate the prioritization of time, exercise adherence may be continually undermined. It is possible to enhance behavioral commitment (Level 2) to exercise through techniques such as goal setting, self-monitoring, time management, stimulus and reinforcement control, preparation for relapse, and provision of social support. Although these strategies have been used extensively with dietary modification, they have not been widely applied to exercise behavior.

The most consistent exercisers appear to be intrinsically committed because of the "feeling good" phenomenon described earlier (Level 3). These acute benefits may eventually be sufficiently rewarding to lead the individual to exercise on a daily basis. It is not known how long it takes to reach this level of commitment, and we might expect several impediments in the obese. However, the limited evidence available indicates that many patients experience some of these benefits (Fox & Dirkin, 1989; Gillett, 1988; Grimes, 1986). The primary objective of an exercise program for the markedly obese is to help them through potential psychosocial and behavioral barriers until the intrinsic benefits of exercise become more apparent.

Exercise Program Design

With direction from this model, it is possible to identify elements of treatment that may (1) enhance the likelihood of increased activity, (2) sustain this activity as a permanent lifestyle change, and (3) maximize the resultant physiological and psychological benefits for obese patients.

The Negotiated Exercise Plan

The evolution of exercise programming has been dominated by the prescriptive biomedical guidelines provided by the American College of Sports Medicine (ACSM), originally proposed in 1978, and recently updated (ACSM, 1990). These guidelines specify the frequency, intensity, and duration of exercise required for the improvement and maintenance of cardiovascular fitness, but the guidelines have also been adopted in exercise settings devoted to disease reduction, rehabilitation, and health promotion.

Fahlberg and Fahlberg (1990) have criticized this prescriptive model, arguing that the paternalistic mode of delivery encourages dependency and actually discourages independent lifestyle change. These authors recommend negotiating an exercise plan with the patient in lieu of the traditional exercise prescription—an approach that appears particularly suited to the needs of the obese. The negotiated exercise plan implies a sharing of information between advisor and patient, and a gradual transfer of program ownership. Passive patients become active participants in designing programs, which are tailored according to past experiences, current fitness and weight status, exercise needs, personal preferences, expectations, and constraints. Exercise leaders exchange the role of the "white-coated" medic for that of an activity counselor. Words such as "compliance" and "reliance" are replaced by "achievement" and "empowerment," and there is a gradual change in emphasis from disease prevention to positive health enhancement. Flexibility and customization are key features and are required to accommodate the range of physiological and psychological differences in an obese population.

Exercise Quantification

Although the negotiated exercise plan takes better account of individual needs, there is still a need to determine guidelines regarding the amount and type of exercise required to achieve treatment objectives. Although the ACSM (1986) guidelines have been almost universally accepted, even for high risk groups, their focus on aerobic fitness as an outcome makes them inappropriate as the foundation of treatment for the markedly obese. Potential problems arise because of the emphasis placed on a threshold level of exercise intensity (usually 60% of maximum heart rate) necessary for improvement in maximum oxygen consumption ($\dot{V}O_2$max). This goal requires heart rate to be monitored during exercise sessions in order to ensure that exercise is achieving threshold intensity. Unfortunately, the concept of an exercise threshold may (1) encourage some obese people to overexercise; (2) create a further perceptual barrier to exercise, since many obese persons tend to avoid even moderately intense exercise (Bain et al., 1989; Blair & Buskirk, 1987; Brownell, Stunkard, & Albaum, 1980); and (3) convey the message that lower intensity exercise has no value. A major objective for the obese is increased energy expenditure, and all movement, regardless of its intensity, makes a valuable contribution. Moreover, large improvements in coronary risk (Powell, 1988) and mental health (Martinsen et al., 1985) can be achieved with exercise of low intensity.

Striving for higher levels of aerobic fitness may be appropriate for those obese individuals who are successful in treatment and wish further challenges during the weight loss maintenance phase. However, it is but one program objective, and improvements in muscular and aerobic function will emerge gradually as patient and practitioner concentrate on the process of increasing physical activity.

The Activity Pathway

The concept of an activity continuum or pathway (see Figure 15.2) is preferable to that of an exercise threshold or target zone. This model emphasizes gradual progression, over a period of months to even years, from a sedentary person toward the more active, fitter, and leaner person that most obese people wish to become. Increased activity provides the basis of success. This emphasis fits well

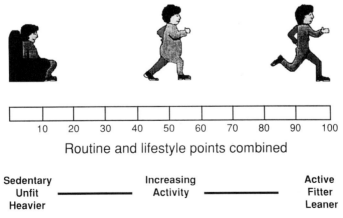

FIGURE 15.2. The activity pathway.

with the evidence that large reductions in coronary risk occur in sedentary individuals who adopt only modestly active lifestyles. This model acknowledges that all movement, including routine daily activity, increases energy expenditure and provides psychosocial benefits. It eliminates perceptual barriers regarding exercise requirements and accommodates all individuals regardless of initial activity levels, and hence is more "exerciser friendly." The model provides the basis for a personal exercise plan that incorporates short- and long-term goals and progress in monitoring activity. Improvements in fitness occur eventually and enhance the patient's desire to exercise. Such improvements, however, are not the primary goal of treatment.

Patterns and Modes of Activity

The exercise program should be designed to maximize the patient's opportunities for movement. However, some patients may wish to include such goals as anxiety reduction, improved abdominal conditioning, increased flexibility, or greater weight loss. The exercise specialist and patient can establish priorities using the negotiated exercise plan, which takes into consideration individual needs and desires. Obese exercisers have reported that finding the right program is a crucial element of success (Grimes, 1986).

For practitioners and patients who may be disconcerted by such a flexible approach, the following three-pronged approach to increasing activity may prove helpful. There is overlap among the three activity categories, but they are conceptualized as separate, as they may have acquired their own motivational and perceptual "set" by patients.

1. *Increase daily lifestyle physical activity.* Although not all obese people are less physically active than their leaner counterparts (Prentice, Black, Murgatroyd, Goldberg, & Coward, 1989), there appears to be considerable opportunity for increase (Blair & Buskirk, 1987; Prentice et al., 1985). Patients should be encouraged to log and analyze their daily and weekly activity patterns and to introduce blocks of movement progressively into their schedules. Examples include climbing stairs, parking the car at the far end of the shopping center, or manually washing the car. The obese have an advantage with weight-bearing activity, as moving their extra weight, regardless of speed, results in greater energy expenditure. When viewed in the long term, small changes can make a big difference. For example, an obese woman weighing 90 kg who walks (2 mph) rather than sits for 30 minutes each day will expend the caloric equivalent of approximately 5–6 kg of fat per year.

2. *Develop a program of exercise.* Ultimately, practitioners would like patients to adopt a regular exercise routine involving large muscle group activity. This will help establish lifetime exercise habits that will eventually improve maintenance of weight loss and aerobic fitness.

In order to establish an exercise habit, the initial part of the program should focus on increasing the frequency of the activity (see Figure 15.3). The exercise should be performed at low intensities (40–50% of maximum heart

	FREQUENCY	DISTANCE	SPEED
1	2 - 3 day	½ - 1 mile	30 mins/mile
2	3 - 4 days	½ - 1 mile	30 mins/mile
3	5 - 6 days	½ - 1 mile	30 mins/mile
4	5 - 6 days	1 - 1½ miles	30 mins/mile
5	5 - 6 days	1½ - 2 miles	30 mins/mile
6	5 - 6 days	2 - 3 miles	30 mins/mile
7	5 - 6 days	2 - 3 miles	Introduce intervals of brisker walking.

FIGURE 15.3. An example of progression in a walking program.

rate) and for relatively short durations (between 10 and 30 minutes), depending on previous experience and perceptions of exertion. Over a period of weeks, frequency should be increased to five or six sessions per week. Injury rate should remain low if progression is gradual. Once this routine is established, the duration of each exercise bout can be increased within the constraints dictated by family and work commitments. When the patient feels ready, usually after several months, and when any severe dietary restriction is completed, intervals of higher intensity exercise (such as brisk striding or even jogging) may be introduced into sessions.

The type of activity is an issue of individual choice, but should involve large muscle groups with rhythmical isotonic contraction. Walking, not surprisingly, appears to be the most popular choice among the obese (Fox et al., 1990). It provides the most natural progression from a sedentary lifestyle, and success can be achieved by a high percentage of severely obese people. In a study by Foss and coworkers, 80% of extremely obese subjects managed to build up to 2 miles of walking per day within 8 weeks (Foss, Lampman, & Schteingart, 1976). Walking is convenient, is inexpensive, and can be done at home—all factors associated with increased adherence. It also has the advantage of spreading the work over large muscle groups (see Round Table Report, 1986). It is weight-bearing, which is advantageous for energy expenditure. Care must be taken to avoid chafing and joint and foot problems, particularly with obese diabetics.

Stationary cycling eliminates some of the problems of weight-bearing activity, especially if a comfortable seat is used. In addition, it can be performed indoors and in private. Drawbacks include complaints of boredom, as well as the requirement of relatively high intensity exertion in specific leg muscles, which may limit output. Rowing machines provide a balanced workout between the upper and lower body; however, the hip flexion involved can be uncomfortable for obese people.

Extra body fat makes the obese buoyant in water, which may make swimming and other water activities attractive. Water exercise also eliminates joint-bearing stress and reduces the chance of injury. Exercise-induced heat stress is reduced because of the cooling effect of the water (Sheldahl, 1986), and venous return is enhanced by the effects of water pressure. A combined program of swimming laps and pool calisthenics provides a well-balanced workout. Unfortunately, swimming appears to be a surprisingly infrequent choice among the obese, perhaps because of embarrassment, inconvenience, or poor swimming skills.

Recently, increased attention has been given to weight training as an alternative mode of exercise. Caution has usually been urged in working with high risk populations because of the high intensities involved with specific muscle groups, resulting in an acute rise in blood pressure. A recent symposium (see Stewart & Keleman, 1989) investigated the use of resistance weight training with coronary-prone populations. A general consensus was reached that low intensity (30-50% repetition maximum) weight training is safe for this group and can have a positive effect on some risk factors and improve muscular and aerobic fitness. Weight training is also associated with psychological benefits in obese males (Short, DiCarlo, Steffee, & Pavlou, 1984). There is no apparent reason why two or three low intensity, circuit-type weight training sessions, as suggested here, should not be included in an exercise routine for the obese. This relatively unexplored mode of exercise may facilitate retention of fat-free mass as patients lose weight (Ballor, Katch, Becque, & Marks, 1988).

Regardless of the activity selected, patients should include time in their programs for adequate warm-up and cool-down. Exercises should also be included that will improve flexibility and conditioning of important postural muscle groups, such as the abdominals.

3. *Increase recreational physical activity.* Patients should analyze how they spend their leisure time. Avenues can be explored that will encourage recreational time to be increasingly activity-based. This may mean introducing new hobbies and pastimes, such as gardening, social dancing, and some of the less vigorous sports (e.g., bowling). Even spending more time with one's children and/or grandchildren will increase activity, as well as strengthen family ties. An individual's use of leisure time is frequently a good indicator of social adjustment and quality of life.

Developing Exercise Confidence and Commitment

These three activity categories represent targets by which obese patients can gauge their progress in becoming leaner, fitter, and healthier individuals. These goals will only be achieved, however, by patients' overcoming psychological and behavioral barriers to physical activity.

Physical Activity and Identity

Campbell (1984) has described human motivation in terms of seeking out opportunities to experience self-esteem. Clearly, the odds are stacked against obese individuals' choosing exercise and physical activity as statements of self-worth. Their weight and its complications are likely to have led them to experience increasing failure and helplessness in this domain. Ironically, the avoidance of exercise and health clubs could be regarded as a reasonable strategy for preserving mental if not physical health. Our own data (Fox et al., 1990) with obese adults entering treatment show that although global self-esteem appears to be normal, perceived aspects of the physical self (such as perceptions of attractiveness, physical conditioning, and sports competence) are very low, even though some of these attributes are highly valued. (Perceived physical strength, not surprisingly, is quite high.) These low perceived competencies may partially explain their reports of low levels of physical activity, with fewer than 25% engaging in purposeful exercise (mainly walking) more than twice per week.

Yet, in order to help patients become intrinsically motivated lifetime exercisers, it is important that they regard activity as a potential means of achievement. Numerous successes may be required in order to initiate an upward spiral. Evidence suggests that once individuals begin to identify themselves as exercisers, they accentuate their positive experiences with activity and eventually seek out opportunities to express their new identity (Kendzierski, 1990; Rosenberg, 1982). This may be reflected by wearing new clothing, reading exercise literature, and mixing with similarly minded groups of people. Clinicians may act as catalysts in this process by helping the obese toward early successful exercise experiences.

Counteracting the Media and Culture

The media's image of exercise has confused what is fundamentally a health-related behavior with athletic performance and sport. Exercise success is defined by categories of physical prowess, measured by running the fastest and farthest or lifting the most weight. The use of exercise in advertising to convey a sleek and slender image has also confounded glamour with exercise, and it is hardly surprising that people fall prey to the circular argument that in order to take part in aerobic dance, they have to look like aerobic dance instructors! These unobtainable false standards serve only to increase the helplessness and futility experienced by many obese people.

In order to raise initial expectations, the clinician must first give patients the opportunity to discuss, analyze, and break down the stereotypes associated with exercise. Appropriate role models are needed (Bandura, 1982). All exercise materials should feature obese subjects, and guest appearances or videos of successful obese exercisers discussing the trials and triumphs of physical activity may be beneficial.

Redefining Exercise Success

One way of making exercise success available to the obese is to redefine it. The "activity pathway" accommodates three important concepts. It establishes a place for all people, regardless of initial fitness/activity level. Bain et al. (1989) report that many overweight people still believe that in exercise there is "no gain without pain." The activity pathway indicates that any and all increases in activity are important. It also defines success in terms of the process of developing an exercise program, measured primarily in terms of the time committed to exercise, rather than as the product of improved physical performance.

There is a great temptation to judge exercise success solely in terms of fitness improvement or weight loss, with the result that testing is scheduled at regular intervals. This practice has significant shortcomings. It may encourage overexertion, because optimal fitness requires higher exercise intensities than are initially appropriate. There is also no guarantee that improvements will be made, since fitness and trainability are partly genetically determined. The results may discourage further exercise. Finally, testing is often laboratory-based and does little to promote exercise independence.

On the other hand, occasional fitness testing, conducted at intervals of at least 6 weeks, can be beneficial. Fitness improvements will indicate that the exercise program is having a positive effect and will increase motivation. An alternative approach is to teach patients simple tests that they can perform at home, and to encourage them to tune in to changes in perceived exertion required to complete such tasks as climbing stairs or walking around the block. The limitations of testing should be clearly acknowledged to patients, and the information should substantiate rather than replace the successes indicated by increased exercise and physical activity.

Increasing Exercise Expertise

The low confidence of the obese in the exercise setting may arise in part from their lack of expertise. Our own research indicates that patients entering treatment lack confidence in their knowledge of exercise, and report that they have received little technical support in the past. Other research (Gillett, 1988; Grimes, 1986) shows that many obese women are concerned about the safety of exercise.

Classes are now available in many schools and universities (some are required for graduation) that aim to promote exercise expertise and health-related attitudes, confidences, and exercise behavior (Corbin, Laurie, Gruger, & Smiley, 1984; Slava, Laurie, & Corbin, 1984), but their recent appearance makes their exposure to the majority of the obese unlikely. The obese are also the least likely to volunteer for such programs when offered in the community.

Effective treatment clearly requires an education component that addresses the specific needs of the obese exerciser. Space does not permit a detailed description, but the package should prepare the patient for safe and effective exercise with the overall aim of promoting "exercise independence." Patients should understand the benefits of exercise for health and weight loss maintenance. They should also learn exercise-related skills, such as the use of heart rate monitoring and ratings of perceived exertion for tuning in to their body's reaction to exercise. They should learn how to exercise correctly, when and when not to exercise, how to increase exercise quantity safely, and how to avoid and recover from injury.

This list is by no means exhaustive, and the logistics of on-site instruction in exercise, whether individual or group, must be addressed. The low levels of confidence and expertise among the obese warrant this approach. The only means of ensuring that early exercise experiences are positive is through instruction by a competent leader who is thoroughly grounded in the physiological and psychological problems of the obese exerciser.

Establishing Exercise Patterns

Patients must be assisted in establishing an exercise routine within the context of a schedule that is constrained by other pressing priorities. The following represents a selection of behavioral strategies applied in a variety of therapeutic settings and designed to establish behavior change. Their effectiveness has received support from research (see Biddle & Mutrie, 1991; Knapp, 1988; Wankel, 1987), but not necessarily from research with an obese population.

Decision Making and Problem Solving

Exercise commitment has been addressed by using a decision balance sheet procedure (Wankel, 1984; Wankel & Thompson, 1977). The potential exerciser is encouraged to list the perceived personal benefits of exercise as well as the costs, with a view toward balancing the equation in favor of exercise. Strategies for increasing the likelihood of experiencing benefits, introducing new incentives, and eliminating some of the negative consequences or barriers to exercise can then be identified and put into operation. In addition to helping patients understand and come to terms with the multitude of variables that contribute to their approach–avoidance tendency, the process encourages self-direction and a problem-solving orientation. Patients and clinicians have also found the tool to be useful for stimulating group discussion.

Goal Setting

The concept of the activity pathway allows obese patients at any level of functional capacity to progress toward increased movement through the planning of short- and long-term goals. The greatest success occurs when patients set goals that are written down and measurable (Dubbert & Wilson, 1984). Some studies have indicated that the dangers of absolutism are overcome if some flexibility is built into the goal system, so that minor lapses can be accommodated without discouragement.

Goals should be designed to meet the specific objectives identified through the negotiated exercise plan. This chapter has suggested three categories of activity, and patients might set short- and long-term goals for each. An example of a short-term exercise goal might be "I will walk for 30 minutes before lunch this week on Monday, Wednesday, and Friday." Similarly, patients might introduce a new activity, such as washing the car manually each Saturday morning. The long-term goal might be eight consecutive Saturdays of car washing, in the hope of encouraging new habits. Note that these goals are behavioral rather than performance-based.

Monitoring Progress

The effectiveness of a well-designed program relies on a good system of recording achievement. Exercise monitoring increases adherence in home-based programs (Juneau et al., 1987; King, Taylor, Haskell, & DeBusk, 1988). Charts can be designed that accommodate patients' weekly plans and achievements. At the start of the week, patients can record on a monitoring card their exercise routine and activity program for the week. On completion, sessions can be signed by the exerciser and a friend or spouse. A points system can be devised that allows the quantification of the week's behavioral achievements, and scores can be recorded on a cumulative activity graph. The record can be kept in a highly visible place to act as a reminder and invite comments by colleagues or family.

Although some patients find record keeping tedious, especially in combination with dietary monitoring, it may enhance motivation in individuals. Technology is also beginning to streamline record keeping, as heart rate monitors, programmable watches, and computer software capable of producing daily and weekly printouts are increasingly widely available (see Rogers et al., 1987).

Promoting Routine Exercise

Quite often, the difference between exercising or not lies at the mercy of changes in daily priorities. For this reason, many successful exercisers eliminate the decision-making process by assigning an exercise hour that they consider untouchable or sacred. From a behavioral perspective, this tends to work best if sessions occur at the same time and in the same place each day. Eventually, environmental cues or reminders develop around the routine and act as a stimulus to exercise (see Knapp, 1988). A lunchtime walking session, for example, may be prompted by a clock on the wall, the first pangs of late morning hunger, or a colleague passing the office window on his or her way to exercise.

In the early stages, exercise reminders such as these can be intentionally built into the schedule. Patients have suggested such strategies as leaving exercise clothes by their bed at night, ready for an early morning walk, or posting reminders on a refrigerator door or in a lunchpack. The ideal situation for many is a daily exercise routine that becomes as automatic as brushing one's teeth or having dinner. However, others may be more successful with a degree of flexibility, in order to accommodate changes in their schedules, their moods, or the weather, and thus avoid feelings of failure and guilt.

Often the most difficult part of an exercise session involves the first step from the comfort of an armchair to the front door. Once this step is taken, sessions are likely to be completed. Patients can be encouraged to recognize and discuss this problem, and to plan "foot-out-of-the-door strategies" that might help overcome their initial inertia. Completion of a decision balance sheet devoted to this specific problem may prove to be an excellent group activity for sharing ideas.

Support Systems

Social support is predictive of better exercise adherence (King & Frederiksen, 1984; Wankel, 1984). Several forms of social support have been identified (Albrecht & Adelman, 1984), each of which can be applied to exercise. These include praise; challenge and motivation; informational and technical support that might be provided by an exercise leader; the camaraderie and informal contracting that occur among exercise partners; or the nonjudgmental ear of a friend willing to listen to exercise problems. Efforts must also be taken to minimize the negative effects of those who undermine the exerciser.

Exercise, therefore, rarely takes place in a social vacuum. It is influenced by and affects the behavior of others. This brings into question the relative merits of a supervised group exercise program versus a home-based, individual program.

Supervised Groups. Group instruction has potential to combine the technical and motivational skills of an exercise specialist with the sharing and friendship that frequently occur among patients (Wankel, Yardley, & Graham, 1985). Programs designed specifically for the obese have produced adherence rates as high as 94% (Gillett, 1988), with social support suggested as a primary reason for program success. Obese women prefer to exercise with women of similar weights (Bain et al., 1989). No data are available to indicate the preferences of obese males.

Supervised exercise groups are less convenient than home-based programs, and their main disadvantage is their tendency to encourage program dependence. Groups often have a limited lifespan, and unless provisions are made for a gradual transition to individually based programs, few individuals continue to exercise when programs terminate (Martin et al., 1984). There is no reason why group exercise sessions should not form *part* of an exercise program. The danger arises when exercise adherence becomes dependent upon the group's continuation.

Individually Directed Exercise. The majority of middle-aged adults prefer to exercise on their own, outside of a formal program (Iverson, Fielding, Crow, & Christenson, 1985; King et al., 1989). The added convenience and control offered by exercising at home or at the worksite may facilitate long-term adherence and achievement of a major objective—that of exercise independence. It is, however, unreasonable to expect obese individuals to develop a home-based program without assistance, since exercise contracts that provide minimal support yield low adherence rates (Craighead & Blum, 1989; Pavlou, Krey, & Steffee, 1989).

Several strategies can be useful to support home-based exercise programs, including the help of spouse and family at home or colleagues at work (Wankel et al., 1985). The exercisers should be encouraged to review weekly records with these persons. The use of a buddy system initiates an informal social contract to exercise. King et al. (1989) have achieved high adherence rates over a 6-month period with home-based exercise, using a phone contact support system. It is possible that weekly group discussions devoted to sharing exercise experiences could achieve similar success.

Preventing Relapse

Brownell, Marlatt, Lichtenstein, and Wilson (1986) have discussed the need for relapse prevention with addictive behaviors. Although there are conceptual differences between relapse to an inactive state (as with exercise relapse) and relapse to an active state (as with drug taking or eating larger quantities), there is sufficient commonality to apply relapse prevention techniques to exercise management (King & Frederiksen, 1984; Knapp, 1988). Situations that disrupt an exercise routine, such as vacations, business trips, or visitors to the home, are sometimes predictable. The practitioner can help patients to prepare contingency plans for these situations.

Often exercise relapse occurs through a gradual decline in activity, represented by fewer sessions per week, rather than through an abrupt halt. The use of cumulative activity records with predetermined "inactivity threshold alarms" may help to cue the patient and prompt a reaction, in much the same way that threshold weights appear to have some impact in weight management (Stuart & Guire, 1978). Patients also can be encouraged to design and adopt appropriate recovery programs following illness or injury, so that temporary lapses do not become permanent exercise relapses.

The preceding discussion has acknowledged that the adoption and maintenance of a physically active lifestyle are by no means easy tasks. Even when they are totally convinced of the benefits and in command of the necessary expertise, confidence, and resources, both obese and lean individuals often find that their daily priorities work against permanent change. Thus, treatment must continually evaluate the priority assigned to exercise and must examine the process by which a program of physical activity is developed.

Administrative Concerns and Strategies

The incorporation of an exercise component into a clinic- or hospital-based program for the severely obese raises a number of administrative issues regarding costs, safety, personnel, resources, and facilities.

Safety Issues

In the case of high risk patients such as the severely obese, particularly those who present with symptoms, a medical evaluation is required to determine each patient's capacity to exercise. Increased obesity may increase the risk of injury, but this is likely only if the exercise program progresses too rapidly and at too high an intensity. Few persons in the general population sustain injury when they adhere to the low to moderate activities suggested here (Koplan, Siskovick, & Goldbaum, 1985), and for a fair assessment, these rates have to be compared with injuries inflicted while not exercising. No data are available for the obese.

The risk of a coronary event is greater during vigorous than during mild activity (Siskovick, 1990), and is substantially greater in the obese than in the nonobese, as well as in persons with pre-existing illness. Thus, special consideration must be taken with obese patients with coronary disease, diabetes, and other illnesses. However, when the potential health benefits are considered, the evidence for exercise even with symptomatic patients is convincing.

Exercise Stress Testing. The decision to recommend exercise for a severely obese patient will depend ultimately on the physician's judgment. There has been considerable debate regarding the general value of exercise stress tests, and in particular their ability to predict future exercise-induced coronary events (Harris et al., 1989; Shephard, 1984; Sox, Littenberg, & Garber, 1989). Present guidelines from the ACSM (1986) would imply that a stress test is required for all obese patients because of their risk of coronary heart disease. Physicians should consider both sides of the issue. Stress testing itself poses a risk, requires more exertion than is advocated in the exercise program itself, is potentially threatening and unpleasant for patients, and increases the cost of treatment. Shephard (1984) comments that even in high risk adults, a stress test will not predict those who will experience a coronary event. Furthermore, in the event of a positive test result, in most cases physicians would still be forced to make decisions regarding the risks versus benefits of a low intensity walking program. However, stress tests may be useful in identifying symptom-free exercise intensity.

Exercise and Very Low Calorie Diets. Currently there is no evidence that a low to moderate intensity (60% ($\dot{V}O_2$ max or less) exercise program cannot be undertaken while patients consume a VLCD (Davis & Phinney, 1990; Phinney et al., 1980; Walberg, Ruiz, Tarlton, Hinkle, & Thye, 1988). Most studies have indicated that aerobic endurance can be retained or improved, even under conditions of low carbohydrate intake. Evidence presented earlier suggests that there are several potential benefits to exercising while dieting. However, large exercise demands that involve high intensity aerobic or anaerobic activity should be avoided, because muscle glycogen may be temporarily depleted. In addition, exercise should be avoided in the first 2 weeks of a VLCD, and progression should be particularly slow in order to accommodate the demands of adaptation. Although exercise is generally advocated, special considerations have also been indicated for obese patients with Type II diabetes (Horton, 1988).

The Design and Delivery of a Quality Exercise Component

A complete exercise program for the obese should incorporate several elements. An initial evaluation that includes an assessment of exercise history, current activity patterns, exercise-related self-perceptions, and knowledge levels will provide valuable information; along with weight-related data, it might be used for grouping similar patients for exercise.

The provision of opportunities for learning and experiencing safe and effective exercise techniques is essential. Small group settings promise to be an effective forum for addressing exercise motivation and adherence problems. One-to-one guidance is required for designing and implementing negotiated exercise plans. The provision of on-site exercise facilities and regular group exercise sessions designed specifically for the obese promises to be of great advantage. Continued contact with patients beyond the first phase of treatment will enhance long-term adherence to exercise.

As with all clinical work, expertise in leadership ultimately determines the quality of the program (Martin et al., 1984; Wankel, 1984). This chapter has deliberately emphasized the need for a psychosocial and behavioral approach to exercise programming. Specialists are required who not only are well grounded in the applied aspects of exercise physiology concerning obesity, but possess educational and counselling skills, as well as a background in motivational psychology.

Finally, progress rests on constant reappraisal and adjustment. Many of the concepts and techniques suggested in this chapter are untried and untested with obese populations. They must be evaluated to determine their success in meeting treatment objectives. Traditional outcomes such as degree of weight loss and/or aerobic fitness should be replaced by the promotion of long-term adherence to a program of modest physical activity that improves health and well-being.

Acknowledgment

Appreciation is extended to Stuart Biddle for his comments on an earlier draft of this chapter.

References

Albrecht, T. L., & Adelman, M. B. (1984). Social support and life stress: New directions for communication research. *Human Communication Research, 11*, 3-22.

American College of Sports Medicine (ACSM). (1986). *Guidelines for graded exercise testing and exercise prescription* (3rd ed.). Philadelphia: Lea & Febiger.

American College of Sports Medicine (ACSM). (1990). The recommended quantity and quality of exercise for developing and maintaining cardiorespiratory and muscular fitness in healthy adults. *Medicine and Science in Sports and Exercise, 22*, 265-274.

Bain, L. L. (1985). A naturalistic study of student's responses to an exercise class. *Journal of Teaching in Physical Education, 5*, 2-12.

Bain, L. L., Wilson, T., & Chaikind, E. (1989). Participant perceptions of exercise programs for overweight women. *Research Quarterly for Exercise and Sport, 60*, 134-143.

Ballor, D. L., Katch, V. L., Becque, M. D., & Marks, C. R. (1988). Resistance weight training during caloric restriction enhances lean body weight maintenance. *American Journal of Clinical Nutrition, 47*, 19-25.

Bandura, A. (1982). Self-efficacy mechanism in human agency. *American Psychologist, 37*, 122-147.

Belko, A. Z., Van Loan, M., Barbieri, T. F., & Mayclin, P. (1987). Diet, exercise, weight loss, and energy expenditure in moderately overweight women. *International Journal of Obesity, 11*, 93-104.

Biddle, S. J. H., & Fox, K. R. (1989). Exercise and health psychology: Emerging relationships. *British Journal of Medical Psychology, 62*, 205-216.

Biddle, S. J. H., & Mutrie, N. (1991). *Psychology of physical activity and exercise: A health-related perspective*. New York: Springer-Verlag.

Blackburn, H., & Jacobs, D. R. (1988). Physical activity and the risk of coronary heart disease. *New England Journal of Medicine, 319*, 1217-1219.

Blair, D., & Buskirk, E. R. (1987). Habitual daily energy expenditure and activity levels of lean and adult-onset and child-onset obese women. *American Journal of Clinical Nutrition, 45*, 540-550.

Blair, S. N., Kohl, H. W., Paffenbarger, R. S., Clark, D. G., Cooper, K. H., & Gibbons, L. W. (1989). Physical fitness and all-cause mortality. *Journal of the American Medical Association, 262*, 2395-2401.

Blundell, J. E. (1984) Behaviour modification and exercise in the treatment of obesity. *Postgraduate Medical Journal, 60*(Suppl. 3), 37-49.

Bray, G. A. (1990). Exercise and obesity. In C. Bouchard, R. J. Shephard, T. Stephens, J. R.

Sutton, & B. D. McPherson (Eds.), *Exercise, fitness, and health* (pp. 497-510). Champaign, IL: Human Kinetics.

Brehm, B. A. (1988). Elevation of metabolic rate following exercise: Implications for weight loss. *Sports Medicine, 6*, 72-78.

Brown, D. R. (1990). Exercise, fitness, and mental health. In C. Bouchard, R. J. Shephard, T. Stephens, J. R. Sutton, & B. D. McPherson (Eds.), *Exercise, fitness, and health* (pp. 607-626). Champaign, IL: Human Kinetics.

Brownell, K. D., Marlatt, G. A., Lichtenstein, E., & Wilson, G. T. (1986). Understanding and preventing relapse. *American Psychologist, 41*, 765-782.

Brownell, K. D., Stunkard, A. J., & Albaum, J. M. (1980). Evaluation and modification of activity patterns in the natural environment. *American Journal of Psychiatry, 137*, 1540-1545.

Campbell, R. N. (1984). *The new science: Self-esteem psychology.* Lanham, MD: University Press of America.

Canada Fitness Survey. (1983). *Fitness and lifestyle in Canada.* Ottawa: Health and Welfare Canada.

Corbin, C. B., Laurie, D. R., Gruger, C., & Smiley, B. (1984). Vicarious success experience as a factor influencing self-confidence, attitudes, and physical activity of adult women. *Journal of Teaching in Physical Education, 4*, 17-23.

Council on Scientific Affairs, American Medical Association. (1988). Treatment of obesity in adults. *Journal of the American Medical Association, 260*, 2547-2551.

Craighead, L. W., & Blum, M. D. (1989). Supervised exercise in behavioral treatment for moderate obesity. *Behavior Therapy, 20*, 49-59.

Davis, P. G., & Phinney, S. D. (1990). Differential effects of two very low calorie diets on aerobic and anaerobic performance. *International Journal of Obesity, 14*, 779-788.

Dishman, R. K. (1981). Biologic influences on exercise adherence. *Research Quarterly for Exercise and Sport, 52*, 143-159.

Dishman, R. K. (Ed.). (1988). *Exercise adherence: Its impact on public health.* Champaign, IL: Human Kinetics.

Donnelly, J. E., Jakicic, J., & Gunderson, S. (1991). Diet and body composition: Effect of very low calorie diets and exercise. *Sports Medicine, 12*(4), 237-249.

Dubbert, P. M., & Wilson, G. T. (1984). Goal setting and spouse involvement in the treatment of obesity. *Behavior Research and Therapy, 22*, 227-242.

Ekelund, L., Haskell, W. L., Johnson, J. L., Whaley, F. S., Criqui, M. H., & Sheps, D. S. (1988). Physical fitness as a predictor of cardiovascular mortality in asymptomatic North American men. *New England Journal of Medicine, 319*, 1379-1384.

European Atherosclerosis Society. (1987). Strategies for the prevention of coronary heart disease: A policy statement of the European Atherosclerosis Society. *European Heart Journal, 8*, 77-88.

Ewart, C. K. (1989). Psychological effects of resistive weight training: Implications for cardiac patients. *Medicine and Science in Sports and Exercise, 21*, 683-688.

Fahlberg, L. L., & Fahlberg, L. A. (1990). From treatment to health enhancement: Psychosocial considerations in the exercise components of health promotion programs. *The Sport Psychologist, 4*, 168-179.

Foss, M. L., Lampman, R. M., & Schteingart, D. (1976). Physical training program for rehabilitating extremely obese patients. *Archives of Physical Medicine and Rehabilitation, 57*, 425-429.

Fox, K. R., & Corbin, C. B. (1989). The Physical Self-Perception Profile: Development and preliminary validation. *Journal of Sport and Exercise Psychology, 11*, 408-430.

Fox, K. R., & Dirkin, G. R. (1989, June). *Psychological orientation to exercise in adults attending extended obesity treatment.* Paper presented at the annual conference of the North American Society for the Psychology of Sport and Physical Activity, Akron, OH.

Fox, K. R., Mucci, G. W., & Dirkin, G. R. (1990). Exercise psychology of obese adults attending clinical treatment: An ongoing longitudinal study. *Journal of Sports Sciences, 8*, 70. (Abstract).

Frey-Hewitt, B., Vraizan, K. M., Dreon, D. M., & Wood, P. D. (1990). The effect of weight loss by dieting and exercise on resting metabolic rate in overweight men. *International Journal of Obesity, 51*, 167-172.

Gillett, P. A. (1988). Self-reported factors influencing exercise adherence in overweight women. *Nursing Research, 37*, 25-29.

Gillett, P. A., & Eisenmann, P. A. (1987). The effect of an intensity aerobic dance program on aerobic capacity of middle-aged overweight women. *Research in Nursing and Health, 10*, 383-390.

Godin, G., & Shephard, R. J. (1990). Use of attitude-behaviour models in exercise promotion. *Sports Medicine, 10*, 103-121.

Grimes, M. J. (1986). The motivations and experiences of obese women who exercise: A phenomenological investigation. *Dissertation Abstracts International, 47*(4), 1723B.

Gwinup, G. (1975). Effect of exercise alone on the weight of obese women. *Archives of Internal Medicine, 135*, 676-680.

Hagberg, J. M. (1990). Exercise, fitness, and hypertension. In C. Bouchard, R. J Shephard, T. Stephens, J. R. Sutton, & B. D. McPherson (Eds.), *Exercise, fitness, and health* (pp. 455-466). Champaign, IL: Human Kinetics.

Harris, S. S., Caspersen, C. J., DeFriese, G. H., & Estes, E. H. (1989). Physical activity counseling for healthy adults as a primary preventive intervention in the clinical setting. *Journal of the American Medical Association, 261*, 3590-3598.

Harter, S. (1990). Causes, correlates, and the functional role of global self-worth: A lifespan perspective. In J. Kolligan & R. Sternberg (Eds.), *Perceptions of competence and incompetence across the lifespan* (pp. 67-98). New Haven, CT: Yale University Press.

Hayes, D., & Ross, C. E. (1986). Body and mind: The effect of exercise, overweight, and physical health on psychological well-being. *Journal of Health and Social Behavior, 27*, 387-400.

Hill, J. O., Schlundt, D. G., Sbrocco, T., Sharp, T., Pope-Cordle, J., Stetson, B., Kaler, M., & Heim, C. (1989). Evaluation of an alternating-calorie diet with and without exercise in the treatment of obesity. *American Journal of Clinical Nutrition, 50*, 248-254.

Horton, E. S. (1988). Exercise and diabetes mellitus. *Medical Clinics of North America, 72*, 1301-1321.

Iverson, D. C., Fielding, J. E., Crow, R. S., & Christenson, G. M. (1985). The promotion of physical activity in the United States population: The status of programs in medical, worksite, community, and school settings. *Public Health Reports, 100*, 212-224.

Juneau, M., Rogers, F., DeSantos, V., Yee, M., Evans, A., Boln, A., Haskell, W. L., Taylor, C. B., & DeBusk, R. F. (1987). Effectiveness of self-monitored, home-based, moderate-intensity exercise training in middle-aged men and women. *American Journal of Cardiology, 60*, 60-70.

Kendzierski, D. (1990). Exercise self-schemata: Cognitive and behavioral correlates. *Health Psychology, 9*, 69-82.

King, A. C., & Frederiksen, L. W. (1984). Low-cost strategies for increasing exercise behavior: Relapse preparation training and social support. *Behavior Modification, 8*, 3-21.

King, A. C., Taylor, C. B., Haskell, W. L., & DeBusk, R. F. (1988). Strategies for increasing early adherence to long-term maintenance of home-based exercise training in healthy middle-aged men and women. *American Journal of Cardiology, 61*, 628-632.

King, A. C., Taylor, C. B, Haskell, W. L., & DeBusk, R. F. (1989). Influence of regular aerobic exercise on psychological health: A randomized controlled trial of healthy middle-aged adults. *Health Psychology, 8*, 305-324.

Knapp, D. N. (1988). Behavioral management techniques and exercise promotion. In R. K. Dishman (Ed.), *Exercise adherence: Its impact on public health* (pp. 203-236). Champaign, IL: Human Kinetics.

Koplan, J. P., Caspersen, C. J., & Powell, K. E. (1989). Physical activity, physical fitness and health: Time to act. *Journal of the American Medical Association, 262*, 2437.

Koplan, J. P., Siskovick, D. S., & Goldbaum, G. M. (1985). The risks of exercise: A public view of injuries and hazards. *Public Health Reports, 100*, 189-194.

Krotkiewski, M., & Björntorp, P. (1986). Muscle tissue in obesity with different distribution of adipose tissue. Effects of physical training. *International Journal of Obesity, 10,* 331-334.

Krotkiewski, M., Mandroukas, K., Sjöström, L., Sullivan, L., Wetterqvist, H., & Björntorp, P. (1979). Effects of long-term physical training on body fat, metabolism, and blood pressure in obesity. *Metabolism, 28,* 650-658.

Leon, A. S., Connett, J., Jacobs, D. R., & Rauramaa, R. (1987). Leisure-time physical activity levels and risk of coronary heart disease and death: The multiple risk factor intervention trial. *Journal of the American Medical Association, 258,* 2388-2395.

MacKeen, P. C., Franklin, B. A., Nicholas, W. C., & Buskirk, E. R. (1983). Body composition, physical work capacity and physical activity habits at 18-month follow-up of middle-aged women participating in an exercise intervention program. *International Journal of Obesity, 7,* 61-71.

Manson, J. E., Colditz, G. A., Stampfer, M. J., Willett, W. C., Rosner, B. R., Monson, R. R., Speizer, F. E., & Hennekens, C. H. (1990). A prospective study of obesity and risk of coronary heart disease in women. *New England Journal of Medicine, 322,* 882-889.

Marston, A. R., & Criss, J. (1984). Maintenance of successful weight loss: Incidence and prediction. *International Journal of Obesity, 8,* 435-439.

Martin, J. E., Dubbert, P. M., Katell, A. D., Thompson, J. K., Raczynski, J. R., Lake, M., Smith, P. O., Webster, J. S., Sikora, T., & Cohen, R. E. (1984). Behavioral control of exercise in sedentary adults: Studies 1 through 6. *Journal of Consulting and Clinical Psychology, 52,* 795-811.

Martinsen, E. W., Medhus, A., & Sandvik, L. (1985). Effects of aerobic exercise on depression: A controlled study. *British Medical Journal, 291,* 109.

Meyers, A. W., Stunkard, A. J., Coll, M., & Cooke, C. J. (1980). Stairs, escalators, and obesity. *Behavior Modification, 4,* 355-359.

Molé, P. A. (1990). Impact of energy intake and exercise on resting metabolic rate. *Sports Medicine, 10,* 72-87.

Morgan, W. P., & Goldston, S. E. (1987). *Exercise and mental health.* Washington, DC: Hemisphere.

Paffenbarger, R. S., Hyde, R. T., Wing, A. L., & Hsieh, C. C. (1986). Physical activity, all-cause mortality, and longevity of college alumni. *New England Journal of Medicine, 314,* 605-613.

Paffenbarger, R. S., Wing, A. L., Hyde, R. T., & Jung, D. L. (1983). Physical activity and incidence of hypertension in college alumni. *American Journal of Epidemiology, 117,* 245-257.

Pavlou, K. N., Krey, S., & Steffee, W. P. (1989). Exercise as an adjunct to weight loss and maintenance in moderately obese subjects. *American Journal of Clinical Nutrition, 49,* 1115-1123.

Pavlou, K. N., Steffee, W. P., Lerman, R. H., & Burrows, B. (1985). Effects of dieting and exercise on lean body mass, oxygen uptake, and strength. *Medicine and Science in Sports and Exercise, 17,* 466-471.

Pavlou, K. N., Whatley, J. E., Jannace, P.W., DiBartolomeo, J. J., Burrows, B. A., Duthie, E. A. M., & Lerman, R. H. (1989). Physical activity as a supplement to a weight-loss dietary regimen. *American Journal of Clinical Nutrition, 49,* 1110-1114.

Perri, M. G., McAdoo, W. G., McAllister, D. A., Lauer, J. B., & Yancey, D. Z. (1986). Enhancing the efficacy of behavior therapy for obesity: Effects of aerobic exercise and a multicomponent treatment maintenance program. *Journal of Consulting and Clinical Psychology, 54,* 670-675.

Phinney, S. D., Horton, E. S., Sims, E. A. H., Hanson, J. S., Danforth, E., & LaGrange, B. M. (1980). Capacity for moderate exercise in obese subjects after adaptation to a hypocaloric ketogenic diet. *Journal of Clinical Investigations, 66,* 1152-1161.

Phinney, S. D., LaGrange, B. M., O'Connell, M., & Danforth, E. (1988). Effects of aerobic exercise on energy expenditure and nitrogen balance during very low calorie dieting. *Metabolism, 37,* 758-765.

Powell, K. E. (1988). Habitual exercise and public health: An epidemiological view. In R. K.

Dishman (Ed.), *Exercise adherence: Its impact on public health* (pp. 15-39). Champaign, IL: Human Kinetics.

Powell, K. E., Thompson, P. D., Caspersen, C. J., & Kendrick, J. S. (1987). Physical activity and the incidence of coronary heart disease. *Annual Review of Public Health, 8*, 253-287.

Prentice, A. M., Black, P. R., Murgatroyd, G. R., Goldberg, G. R., & Coward, W. A. (1989). Metabolism or appetite: Questions of energy balance with particular reference to obesity. *Journal of Human Nutrition and Dietetics, 2*, 95-105.

Prentice, A. M., Coward, W. A., Davies, H. L., Murgatroyd, P. R., Goldberg, G. R., Black, A. E., Sawyer, M., Ashford, J., & Whitehead, R. G. (1985). Unexpectedly low levels of energy expenditure in healthy women. *Lancet, i*, 1419-1422.

Rogers, F., Juneau, M., Taylor, C. B., Haskell, W. L., Kraemer, H. C., Ahn, D. K., & DeBusk, R. F. (1987). Assessment by a microprocessor of adherence to home-based moderate-intensity sedentary middle-aged men and women. *American Journal of Cardiology, 60*, 71-75.

Rosenberg, M. (1982). Psychological selectivity in self-esteem formation. In M. Rosenberg & H. B. Kaplan (Eds.), *Social psychology of the self-concept* (pp. 535-546). Arlington Heights, IL: Harlan Davidson.

Round Table Report. (1986). Walking for fitness. *Physician and Sportsmedicine, 14*, 144-159.

Schwartz, R. S. (1987). The independent effects of dietary weight loss and aerobic training on high density lipoproteins and apolipoprotein A-I concentrations in obese men. *Metabolism, 36*, 165-171.

Sheldahl, L. M. (1986). Special ergometric techniques and weight reduction. *Medicine and Science in Sports and Exercise, 18*, 25-30.

Shephard, R. J. (1984). Can we identify those for whom exercise is hazardous? *Sports Medicine, 1*, 75-86.

Short, M. A., DiCarlo, S., Steffee, W. P., & Pavlou, K. N. (1984). The effects of physical conditioning on self-concept of adult obese males. *Physical Therapy, 64*, 194-198.

Siskovick, D. S. (1990). Risks of exercising: Sudden cardiac death and injuries. In C. Bouchard, R. J. Shephard, T. Stephens, J. R. Sutton, & B. D. McPherson (Eds.), *Exercise, fitness, and health* (pp. 707-713). Champaign, IL: Human Kinetics.

Slava, S., Laurie, D. R., & Corbin, C. B. (1984). Long-term effects of a conceptual physical education program. *Research Quarterly for Exercise and Sport, 55*, 161-168.

Sobolski, J., Kornitzer, M., de Backer, G., Dramaix, M., Abramowicz, M., Degre, S., & Drenolin, H. (1987). Protection against ischemic heart disease in the Belgian Physical Fitness Study: Physical fitness rather than physical activity? *American Journal of Epidemiology, 125*, 601-610.

Sonstroem, R. J., & Morgan, W. P. (1989). Exercise and self-esteem: Rationale and model. *Medicine and Science in Sports and Exercise, 21*, 329-337.

Sox, H. C., Littenberg, B., & Garber, A. M. (1989). The role of exercise testing in screening for coronary heart disease. *Annals of Internal Medicine, 110*, 456-469.

Sports Council of Great Britain. (1982). *Sport in the community: The next ten years.* London: Author.

Stalonas, P. M., Johnson, W. G., & Christ, M. (1978). Behavior modification for obesity: The evaluation of exercise, contingency management and program adherence. *Journal of Consulting and Clinical Psychology, 46*, 463-469.

Stephens, T., Jacobs, D. R., Jr., & White, C. C. (1985). A descriptive epidemiology of leisure-time physical activity. *Public Health Reports, 100*, 147-158.

Steptoe, A., & Bolton, J. (1988). The short-term influence of high and low intensity physical exercise on mood. *Psychology and Health, 2*, 91-106.

Steptoe, A., & Cox, S. (1988). Acute effects of aerobic exercise on mood. *Health Psychology, 7*, 329-340.

Stewart, K. J., & Keleman, M. H. (Chairs). (1989). Symposium: Resistive weight training: A new approach to exercise for cardiac and coronary disease prone populations. *Medicine and Science in Sports and Exercise, 21*, 667-697.

Stuart, R. B., & Guire, K. (1978). Some correlates of the maintenance of weight loss through behavior modification. *International Journal of Obesity, 2*, 225–235.
Thompson, K. J., Jarvie, G. J., Lahey, B. B., & Cureton, K. J. (1982). Exercise and obesity: Etiology, physiology, and intervention. *Psychological Bulletin, 91*, 55–79.
Toshima, M. T., Kaplan, R. J., & Ries, A. L. (1990). Experimental evaluation of rehabilitation in chronic obstructive pulmonary disease: Short-term effects on exercise endurance and health status. *Health Psychology, 9*, 237–252.
Tucker, L. A. (1983). Effect of weight training on self-concept: A profile of those influenced most. *Research Quarterly for Exercise and Sport, 54*, 389–397.
van Dale, D. (1988). *Diet and exercise in the treatment of obesity.* Maastricht, The Netherlands: University of Limburg.
van Dale, D., Saris, W. H. M., Schoffelen, P. F. M., & ten Hoor, F. (1987). Does exercise give an additional effect in weight reduction regimens? *International Journal of Obesity, 14*, 347–360.
van Dale, D., Saris, W. H. M., & ten Hoor, F. (1990). Weight maintenance and resting metabolic rate 18-40 months after a diet/exercise treatment. *International Journal of Obesity, 14*, 347–360.
Vranic, M., & Wasserman, D. (1990). Exercise, fitness, and diabetes. In C. Bouchard, R. J. Shephard, T. Stephens, J. R. Sutton, & B. D. McPherson (Eds.), *Exercise, fitness, and health* (pp. 467–490). Champaign, IL: Human Kinetics.
Wadden, T. A., & Bell, S. T. (1990). Obesity. In A. S. Bellack, M. Hersen, & A. I. Kazdin (Eds.), *International handbook of behavior modification and therapy* (2nd ed., pp. 449–473). New York: Plenum.
Wadden, T. A., & Stunkard, A. J. (1985). Social and psychological consequences of obesity. *Annals of Internal Medicine, 103*, 1062–1067.
Walberg, J. L., Ruiz, V. K., Tarlton, S. L., Hinkle, D. E., & Thye, F. W. (1988). Exercise capacity and nitrogen loss during a high or low carbohydrate diet. *Medicine and Science in Sport and Exercise, 20*, 34–43.
Wankel, L. M. (1984). Decision-making and social support strategies for increasing exercise involvement. *Journal of Cardiac Rehabilitation, 4*, 124–135.
Wankel, L. M. (1987). Enhancing motivation for involvement in voluntary exercise programs. In *Advances in motivation and achievement: Vol. 5. Enhancing motivation* (pp. 239–286). Greenwich, CT: JAI Press.
Wankel, L. M., & Thompson, C. E., (1977). Motivating people to be physically active: Self-persuasion vs. balanced decision-making. *Journal of Applied Social Psychology, 7*, 332–340.
Wankel, L. M., Yardley, J. K., & Graham, J. (1985). The effects of motivational interventions upon the exercise adherence of high and low self-motivated adults. *Canadian Journal of Applied Sports Science, 10*, 147–156.
Warwick, P. M., & Garrow, J. S. (1981). The effect of addition of exercise to a regime of dietary restriction on weight loss, nitrogen balance, resting metabolic rate and spontaneous activity in three obese women in a metabolic ward. *International Journal of Obesity, 5*, 25–32.
Weigle, D. S., Sande, K. J., Iverius, P., Monsen, E. R., & Brunzell, J. D. (1988). Weight loss leads to a marked decrease in non-resting energy expenditure in ambulatory human subjects. *Metabolism, 37*, 930–936.
Wood, P. D., & Stefanick, M. L. (1990). Exercise, fitness and atherosclerosis. In C. Bouchard, R. J. Shephard, T. Stephens, J. R. Sutton, & B. D. McPherson (Eds.), *Exercise, fitness, and health* (pp. 409–423). Champaign, IL: Human Kinetics.
Wood, P. D., Stefanick, M. L., Dreon, D. M., Frey-Hewitt, B., Garay, S., Williams, P. T., Superko, H. R., Fortmann, S. P., Albers, J. J., Vranizan, K. M., Ellsworth, N. M., Terry, R. B., & Haskell, W. L. (1988). Changes in plasma lipids and lipoproteins in overweight men during weight loss through dieting as compared with exercise. *New England Journal of Medicine, 319*, 1173–1179.

16

Predictors of Attrition and Weight Loss in Patients Treated by Moderate and Severe Caloric Restriction

THOMAS A. WADDEN
KATHLEEN A. LETIZIA

Clinicians and researchers have long sought to identify predictors of weight loss. This quest is understandable. The identification of patients at risk of not losing weight would allow practitioners to monitor such persons more carefully during treatment, as well as to consider alternative therapies with them. Patients, in some cases, might be spared the expense of thousands of dollars if their test profiles suggested that they would not benefit from a particular approach.

This chapter reviews predictors of weight loss and attrition from therapy in persons treated by conventional reducing diets and very low calorie diets. Of the two variables, we believe that attrition is the more important. An individual who loses 7.5 kg may not experience as many health benefits as one who loses 15 kg, but both persons will benefit far more than a third individual who discontinues treatment after only 3 weeks. It is extremely unlikely that dropouts will lose weight on their own. Moreover, such persons are likely to be demoralized when leaving therapy, and this could create barriers to their seeking future treatment.

Given the correlation between attrition from therapy and smaller weight losses (Wadden, Foster, & Letizia, 1991), some might argue that it is unnecessary to study these two variables separately. This might be true if it were not for the fact that most investigators do not include data from dropouts in their search for predictors of weight loss. In most cases, predictor variables have been examined only in subjects who completed treatment. Moreover, an individual who discontinues treatment after 1 month and a weight loss of 5 kg is likely to differ in important ways from an individual who loses only 5 kg over 15 weeks but attends treatment regularly.

Senior authorship is shared equally by the authors.

We begin this chapter by reviewing predictors of attrition and methods to improve retention in therapy. This is followed by an examination of predictors of weight reduction and treatment interventions to improve weight loss. We also discuss correlates of weight maintenance, a more thorough discussion of which is provided by Perri (Chapter 19, this volume).

Factors Predicting Attrition

There have been relatively few studies of attrition from weight reduction therapy. Reasons for this include the fact that investigators frequently view attrition as an embarrassment that reflects negatively on the quality of their treatment. Thus, some studies do not report attrition data or mention them only in passing. A second problem is that attrition is usually less than 20% in research trials, which makes it hard to study. Thus, it is difficult to identify correlates of attrition in a study, for example, in which only 7 of 50 subjects discontinued treatment prematurely. Samples of this size are likely to be too small to yield significant findings. Given the importance of attrition to clinical care, we hope that practitioners and researchers will find creative ways to study this problem.

Pretreatment Patient Characteristics

Neither age, initial weight, body fat, percentage overweight, mood, nor age of onset of obesity has consistently predicted attrition in programs that have employed conventional reducing diets (Dubbert & Wilson, 1983; Perri, Shapiro, Ludwig, Twentyman, & McAdoo, 1984; Wilson, 1985; Wing, Marcus, Epstein, & Kupfer, 1983). Though fewer in number, studies of very low calorie diets also have failed to find a relationship between attrition and age, initial weight, or age of onset of obesity (Ashwell, Durrant, & Garrow, 1978; Garrow, Durrant, Mann, Stalley, & Warwick, 1978). Somewhat more favorable findings, however, have been reported recently for such patient variables as binge eating, hunger, dietary restraint, and life stress.

Binge Eating

Approximately 25% to 70% of participants in weight reduction programs report that they regularly engage in binge eating for which they do not compensate by purging (Gormally, Black, Daston, & Rardin, 1982; Marcus, Wing, & Lamparski, 1985; Spitzer et al., in press; Wadden, Foster, & Letizia, in press). Investigators have yet to fully agree upon the criteria for this disorder or the best method of assessing it (Wilson, 1991). Nevertheless, two studies reported greater attrition among obese binge eaters than among nonbingers in programs that used either a conventional reducing diet (Marcus, Wing, &

Hopkins, 1988) or a very low calorie diet (Wadden, Foster, & Letizia, in press). Patients' reasons for discontinuing treatment were not identified, but investigators believe that dieting itself may be the problem. Behavioral treatment of obesity requires patients to restrain their eating (i.e., dietary restraint). Laboratory results, in turn, suggest that high levels of dietary restraint precipitate binge eating (Polivy & Herman, 1985). Thus, obese bingers in behavioral weight loss programs may eventually overeat in response to treatment prescriptions to restrict their caloric intake. Distressed by their behavior, they may discontinue treatment.

Further research is clearly needed to determine the best method of treating obese binge eaters (Telch, Agras, Rossiter, Wilfley, & Kenardy, 1990). In the meantime, the practitioner should be alert to these patients' increased risk of attrition and should respond promptly to their absences from treatment sessions, as well as to their reports of troubled eating.

Hunger and Dietary Restraint

LaPorte and Stunkard (1990) observed greater attrition among patients treated by a very low calorie diet who reported high susceptibility to hunger as measured by the Eating Inventory (Stunkard & Messick, 1983). Conversely, patients with high levels of dietary restraint coupled with low susceptibility to hunger were more likely to complete treatment. We (Wadden et al., 1991), however, failed to confirm these findings in a study of 346 men and women who were part of a larger investigation of 517 patients treated by a very low calorie diet and behavior modification (Wadden, Foster, Letizia, & Stunkard, in press). We observed no association between attrition and the three variables measured by the Eating Inventory—cognitive restraint, disinhibition, and hunger. Further investigation is needed to clarify the discrepancy between these studies.

Stress

As part of our investigation described above (Wadden et al., 1991), we asked patients to indicate (by responding yes or no) whether they were currently experiencing significant life changes in the following areas: work, health, relationship with significant other, events related to parents or children, financial or legal difficulties, school, and moving. Each of these variables was examined in relationship to attrition. In addition, we summed the number of stressors that subjects reported to yield a measure of "overall stress." We found that overall stress plus three of the individual variables—financial difficulties, events related to parents, and relationship with significant other—discriminated persons who discontinued treatment from those who remained at each of the periods shown in Table 16.1.

These results confirm our clinical impression that persons who are experiencing unsettling life events should probably wait for a more propitious time

TABLE 16.1. Variables Associated with Attrition in 346 Patients Treated by Very Low Calorie Diet (VLCD) and Behavior Modification

Time of attrition	Variable			
	Overall stress	Relationship with significant other	Events related to parents	Financial or legal difficulties
Prior to 1 month of VLCD	.0001	.001	.001	.001
Prior to 2 months of VLCD	.045	.007	.001	n.s.
Prior to 3 months of VLCD	.054	n.s.	.022	n.s.
Prior to 6 weeks of refeeding	.033	n.s.	n.s.	.023
Prior to end of treatment	.006	n.s.	n.s.	.004

Note. The table presents *p* values for differences between noncompleters and completers on the variables shown. Thus, for example, persons who dropped out of treatment during the first month of VLCD were significantly more likely than those who remained in treatment to experience stress in relationship to their significant others, parents, and financial or legal affairs. They also were more likely to report a greater number of life stresses, as indicated by higher overall stress. Each time period includes cumulative attrition to that date.

to lose weight. Dieting itself is stressful, and patients for whom overeating (or bingeing) is triggered by stress may be at particular risk of attrition. The practitioner may wish to provide the patient a referral to assist in coping with the stressful life event.

Small Weight Losses

Patients work hard to reduce their caloric intake and adhere to program prescriptions. They expect to be rewarded for their efforts when they step on the scale. Yet weight loss frequently slows or stops, even in patients who report that they are fully adherent. The frustration and discouragement resulting from unsatisfactory weight loss may increase patients' risk of attrition.

Few studies report patients' reasons for discontinuing therapy, but in a program that used a conventional reducing diet, 57% of dropouts indicated that slow weight loss was responsible for their discontinuation (Perri, Shapiro, et al., 1984). In our investigation of 407 women and 110 men treated by very low calorie diet (Wadden, Foster, Letizia, & Stunkard, in press), we observed that, among women, patients who dropped out during the first, second, and third months of treatment had significantly smaller weight losses than those who remained in therapy (see Table 16.2). This finding was not true for men but may have been attributable to lack of statistical power resulting from a small sample size.

Thus, patients who are disappointed at the scale require additional counseling, both to determine the cause of their smaller weight losses and to help them through the difficult time. In addition, patients with unrealistic expectations may perceive as unsatisfactory a weekly weight loss that would please others. Such patients also may be at risk of attrition.

Further research is needed to determine precisely how smaller weight losses are related to attrition. While it appears that there is a causal relationship between these variables, small weight losses and attrition from therapy might both instead reflect the patient's lack of interest in treatment or be attributable to some other factor.

Ways to Improve Retention

Wilson and Brownell's (1980) review of 17 behavioral weight loss programs revealed an average rate of attrition of 13.5%. A decade later, Wadden and Bell (1990) observed an average rate of 13.8% in 13 studies. Attrition in behavioral programs conducted in research settings is significantly lower than the 35% to 70% reported in commercial programs that employ conventional reducing diets (Ashwell, 1978; Feuerstein, Papciak, Shapiro, & Tannenbaum, 1989; Volkmar, Stunkard, Woolston, & Bailey, 1981), or the 55% to 76% reported in hospital-based very low calorie diet programs (Blackburn, 1988; Hovell et al., 1988; Kirschner, Schneider, Ertel, & Gorman, 1988). Behavioral treatment is usually delivered in closed groups (in which new members are not admitted after the first few weeks), following a structured, time-limited protocol. The closed-group format is likely to facilitate group interaction and cohesiveness (Yalom, 1985), whereas the structured protocol provides patients a clear beginning and end to treatment, as well as specific goals and methods of achieving weight loss. In contrast, commercial programs often use open-enrollment treatment, in which patients can join an ongoing group at any time. This

TABLE 16.2. Variables Discriminating between 407 Women Who Completed and Did Not Complete Treatment

Week of patients' attrition	n	Variable	Noncompleters	Completers	p
6–9	22	Cumulative weight loss after 1 month of VLCD (kg)	7.0 ± 1.4	9.8 ± 0.3	.0001
10–13	26	Cumulative weight loss after 2 months of VLCD (kg)	12.7 ± 6.5	14.5 ± 0.2	.0001
14–19	64	Cumulative weight loss after 3 months of VLCD (kg)	17.5 ± 0.9	19.1 ± 0.3	.0001

Note. n shows the number of patients dropping out of treatment at each time period. p values are for differences in weight losses between noncompleters and completers as determined by analysis of covariance. Thus, for example, persons who discontinued treatment between the 6th and 9th week lost only 7.0 kg during the first 5 weeks of therapy, as compared with 9.8 kg for persons who remained in treatment through week 9. Values are means ± *SEM*s.

practice prevents group cohesiveness and the development of a structured curriculum, because patients in the same group are at different stages of treatment.

We (Wadden, Foster, Letizia, & Stunkard, in press) investigated 517 patients who were treated in a closed-group, time-limited program that combined a very low calorie diet with behavior modification. Attrition in this study reached 44% after 26 weeks of treatment—a rate that, nevertheless was substantially lower than that observed in programs that used the identical diet but with open-group sessions and open-ended therapy (Blackburn, 1988; Kirschner et al., 1988). These findings await replication in a randomized, clinical trial, but they strongly suggest that attrition is decreased markedly by closed-enrollment, time-limited therapy.

Attrition is also reduced by the use of refundable deposits, in which patients submit a small amount of money before treatment, which is returned to them contingent upon their completing the program. In Wilson and Brownell's (1980) review of behavioral weight loss programs, attrition in the 10 studies that used such deposits averaged 9.5%, whereas in the remaining studies the average was 19.3%. The benefits of refundable deposits were confirmed in a controlled investigation (Hagen, Foreyt, & Durham, 1976).

Patient Factors Predicting Weight Loss

The literature on the prediction of weight loss is substantially greater than that for attrition. Researchers have examined variables that include patients' pretreatment characteristics, as well as process measures that assess patients' behaviors during weight reduction (such as attending treatment sessions or completing homework assignments). We begin by examining pretreatment characteristics, which can be divided into the broad classes of biological, psychological, and behavioral variables.

Biological Factors

Initial Body Weight

Initial body weight is perhaps the most consistent predictor of weight loss; heavier patients tend to lose more weight. The strength of this relationship is modest (i.e., correlation coefficients of .25 to .35), but it holds true whether a conventional reducing diet (Bosello et al., 1980; Dubbert & Wilson, 1984; Jeffery, Wing, & Stunkard, 1978; Murray, 1975; Stein, Hassanein, & Lukert, 1981) or a very low calorie diet is used (Ashwell et al., 1978; Wadden, Bartlett, et al., in press; Wadden, Foster, Wang, et al., in press; Wadden & Stunkard, 1986). Practitioners should use this information to alert group members that lighter individuals may lose less weight than heavier ones. This caveat should help to prevent discouragement among these participants.

The finding of a positive relationship between initial weight and subsequent weight loss could be an artifact of a part–whole correlation (Cohen & Cohen, 1983). The correlation of one variable (i.e., initial weight) with a second one that is partially derived from the first (i.e., weight loss = initial weight − posttreatment weight) frequently produces a spurious correlation. The positive correlation between initial weight and weight loss does not appear to be spurious, however, and is instead based upon the fact that the heavier the individual, the higher the resting metabolic rate (RMR) (Foster et al., 1988; Yang, 1988).

Resting Metabolic Rate

RMR accounts for approximately 70–85% of daily energy expenditure in sedentary individuals (Ravussin & Bogardus, 1989). Thus, when two individuals consume an identical reducing diet, the one with the higher RMR will usually lose more weight as a result of the greater caloric deficit induced in this individual (Yang & VanItallie, Chapter 4, this volume). Several studies have confirmed that RMR is a strong predictor of weight loss in patients treated by both conventional reducing diets (Krotkiewski et al., 1980) and very low calorie diets (Ashwell et al., 1978; Garrow et al., 1978; Wadden, Bartlett, et al., in press). Garrow et al. (1978) found that RMR accounted for a remarkable 64% of the variance in weight loss in patients treated for 3 weeks in a metabolic unit in which food intake was carefully controlled. Less robust results are likely to be obtained in outpatient studies in which patients' dietary adherence and physical activity cannot be controlled to the same degree (Wadden, Bartlett, et al., in press).

RMR is easily and reliably measured by indirect calorimetry (Feurer & Mullen, 1986). This measurement may provide important information concerning the etiology of a patient's obesity (i.e., hypometabolism), but also is one of the best methods of determining the number of calories that a reducing diet should provide. Practitioners, however, without access to indirect calorimetry should know that RMR correlates highly not only with fat-free mass but also with body weight, as noted previously (Garrow et al., 1978; Ravussin & Bogardus, 1989). Thus, initial body weight may predict weight loss almost as well as RMR (Garrow et al., 1978; Wadden, Bartlett, et al., in press).

Fat Cells

In the 1970s, several research teams explored the relationship between weight loss and adipose tissue morphology. A number of studies found that increased fat cell number (i.e., hyperplasia) was positively associated with weight loss; thus, the greater the cell number, the greater the weight loss, as indicated by correlation coefficients ranging from .25 to .45. This finding held in studies that used conventional reducing diets (Krotkiewski et al., 1977; Krotkiewski et al., 1980), as well as very low calorie diets (Ashwell et al., 1978; Wadden,

Foster, Wang, et al., in press). Investigators further found that weight loss slowed and eventually stopped once patients achieved normal fat cell weight, despite the fact that patients frequently remained significantly overweight because of cell hyperplasia (Björntorp et al., 1975). Some studies also found that persons with hyperplastic obesity were more likely to regain weight than were those with hypertrophic obesity (Krotkiewski et al., 1977), although contradictory findings have been reported (Strain, Strain, Zumoff, & Knittle, 1984).

Research on fat cell morphology has waned in recent years. Moreover, measurement of fat cell number is both expensive and inaccessible to most practitioners, which limits its practical value. Measurement of total body fat, as discussed by Yang and VanItallie (Chapter 4, this volume), is a more desirable option that provides important information about the patient's body composition. In addition, initial body fat has been shown to correlate positively with end-of-treatment reductions in both weight and fat (Ashwell et al., 1978; Bosello et al., 1980; Wadden et al., 1988, 1990). Body fat also correlates very strongly with weight, with coefficients typically reaching .90 (Bosello et al., 1980; Wadden, Foster, Wang, et al., in press; Wadden et al., 1990).

Body Fat Distribution

Clinical lore has long held that persons whose excess weight is carried primarily in the lower body (i.e., lower body obesity) are less successful in losing weight than those whose weight is primarily in the upper body (i.e., upper body obesity). The purportedly slower weight loss associated with lower body obesity has been attributed to differences in the lipolytic activity of adipose tissue in the lower and upper body (Björntorp, 1985). In the first controlled study of this issue, however, our research team found that women with lower body obesity actually lost slightly more weight and fat than those with upper body obesity (Wadden et al., 1988). Subsequent studies, with one exception, have either confirmed these findings (Hill et al., 1989) or found no difference in weight losses between patients with lower and upper body obesity (den Besten, Vansant, Weststrate, & Deurenberg, 1988; Lanska et al., 1985; Vansant, den Besten, Weststrate, & Deurenberg, 1988). Pasquali, Casimirri, Colella, and Melchionda (1989), by contrast, observed larger weight losses in persons with upper body obesity. Correlations in all cases have been modest.

In our study, women with upper body obesity achieved a larger percentage reduction in their waist circumference than in their hip circumference (Wadden et al., 1988). Thus, there was a reduction in their degree of upper body obesity, as assessed by the waist-to-hip ratio, and a clear change in the shape of their figures. By contrast, women with lower body obesity achieved virtually identical percentage reductions in their waist and hip circumferences. Thus, neither their waist-to-hip ratio nor the shape of their figures changed, perhaps giving the impression of unsatisfactory weight loss. A patient summarized these findings by noting of her own appearance, "I began treatment with a large pear-shaped figure. At the end of treatment, I'm simply a smaller pear."

Psychological Variables

Numerous studies have investigated the relationship of personality characteristics and psychopathology to weight loss. The Minnesota Multiphasic Personality Inventory (MMPI) has been used to this end more often than any other inventory, and with treatment by conventional reducing diets (McCall, 1973; Penwick, Filon, Fox, & Stunkard, 1971; Wadden & Lucas, 1980), very low calorie diets (Johnson, Swenson, & Gastineau, 1976; Wadden, Foster, Wang, et al., in press), and surgery (Barrash, Rodriquez, Scott, Mason, & Sines, 1987; Blankmeyer et al., 1990; Valley, 1984; Valley & Grace, 1986). We agree fully with Wilson's (1985) conclusion that studies of personality characteristics have yielded inconsistent and contradictory findings. Our own research team, for example, found that depression was negatively correlated with weight loss in one study (Wadden, Stunkard, Brownell, & Day, 1985) but positively in a second (Wadden, Foster, Wang, et al., in press), despite the fact that very similar treatments were used.

Many of the significant findings reported are probably attributable to chance, because investigators frequently run dozens of correlations and fail to control the experiment-wise error rate. Moreover, many of the relationships reported appear to be counterintuitive and to tax investigators' creativity in developing post hoc explanations (Wadden, Foster, Wang, et al., in press). Given these contradictory findings, we cannot recommend the use of personality and psychopathology inventories to predict weight loss. Such inventories, however, may be useful in identifying contraindications to weight loss treatments, as discussed by Wadden and Foster (Chapter 13, this volume).

Self-Efficacy

A possible exception to the conclusion above concerns findings for self-efficacy. Several studies have reported that increased levels of self-efficacy predict greater weight loss in patients undertaking conventional reducing diets (Bernier & Avard, 1986; Forster & Jeffery, 1986; Glynn & Ruderman, 1986; Jeffery et al., 1984) and very low calorie diets (Edell, Edington, Herd, O'Brien, & Witkin, 1987; Oettingen & Wadden, 1991). "Self-efficacy" is defined as confidence in one's ability to perform a behavior required to produce a desired outcome (Bandura, 1977). Thus, patients who report greater confidence in their ability to adhere to treatment prescriptions tend to lose more weight than those who are less confident, with correlation coefficients typically in the range of .25 to .35. Prior to treatment, the practitioner should assess patients' self-efficacy concerning a variety of weight control skills. This can be done through interviews or through the use of scales described in the studies previously cited above. Patient and practitioner should explore the reasons for low efficacy ratings and take steps to improve patient confidence in these areas.

Dietary Restraint

The degree to which patients exercise cognitive control over their eating also may predict weight loss. Two studies using invasive treatments for obesity reported greater weight losses in subjects with high baseline dietary restraint (Björvell, Rössner, & Stunkard, 1986; Kramer et al., 1989). These results, however, were not confirmed in two other investigations of treatment by very low calorie diet (LaPorte & Stunkard, 1990; Wadden et al., 1991). LaPorte and Stunkard (1990) indicated that their results may have been biased by the failure to include data from patients who discontinued treatment; these persons typically have the smallest weight losses. We (Wadden et al., 1991) addressed this issue by including data from dropouts in our analyses, but we still found no association. Thus, further research is needed to determine the conditions under which dietary restraint predicts weight loss.

Behavioral Variables

In this section, we briefly examine two behavioral factors—weight cycling and binge eating—that have been examined for their relationship to weight loss. The influence of additional behaviors such as eating slowly and recording food intake is examined in the section on process variables that follows.

Weight Cycling

Cycles of weight loss and regain have been reported to increase metabolic efficiency, and thus to exacerbate subsequent efforts to lose weight (Brownell, 1988; Brownell, Greenwood, Stellar, & Shrager, 1986; Steen, Opplinger, & Brownell, 1988). Support for this theory was provided by several studies which showed that persons who had participated previously in an organized weight control program lost less weight in a prospective trial than did persons without a history of prior participation (Forster & Jeffery, 1986; Jeffery et al., 1984; Jeffery, Snell, & Forster, 1985). Similarly, Blackburn et al. (1989) reported that obese individuals lost weight at a significantly slower rate the second time that they dieted than the first, despite consuming the same number of calories on each occasion.

These findings, however, are contradicted by results of several studies that found either larger weight losses in cyclers as compared with noncyclers (Bonato & Boland, 1987; Gormally, Rardin, & Black, 1980) or no significant differences between these groups (Beeson, Ray, Coxon, & Kreitzman, 1989; van Dale, Saris, & ten Hoor, 1990; Wadden, Bartlett, et al., in press). Results of our own study, shown in Figure 16.1, revealed that weight cyclers tended, if

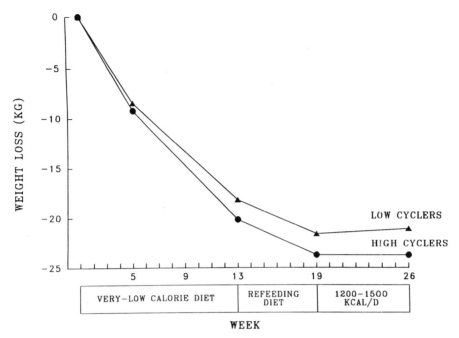

FIGURE 16.1. Weight loss for subjects classified as low versus high weight cyclers, based on the number of diets attempted and lifetime weight loss. Low cyclers reported a mean of 2.8 diets and a lifetime weight loss of 26.4 kg. High cyclers reported a mean of 7.1 diets and a lifetime loss of 78.3 kg. Subjects consumed a diet of 1200 kilocalories (kcal)/day the first week, a very low calorie diet during weeks 2-13, a refeeding diet for weeks 14-19, and a diet of 1000-1500 kcal/day for the remainder of treatment. From "Relationship of Dieting History to Resting Metabolic Rate, Body Composition, Eating Behavior, and Subsequent Weight Loss" by T. A. Wadden, S. J. Bartlett, K. A. Letizia, G. D. Foster, A. J. Stunkard, and A. Conill, in press, *American Journal of Clinical Nutrition*. Copyright by American Society for Clinical Nutrition, Inc. Reprinted by permission.

anything, to lose more weight than noncyclers in a 6-month program that combined very low calorie diet with behavior therapy. We agree with Wing's (in press) conclusion in summarizing this literature that "weight cycling has no consistent effect on metabolic variables, such as energy expenditure, ease of weight loss, or body fat."

Binge Eating

Obese binge eaters have low self-efficacy concerning weight control (Gormally et al., 1982; Marcus et al., 1988) and may be at increased risk of attrition, as previously discussed. Thus, we might expect poorer adherence and smaller weight losses in obese binge eaters than in nonbingers. Studies of this issue, however, have reported contradictory findings. One study found that bingers treated by a conventional reducing diet lost significantly less weight than nonbingers (Keefe, Wyshogrod, Weinberger, & Agras, 1984), whereas another reported that bingers with a history of weight cycling lost significantly more weight than nonbingers (Gormally et al., 1980). In addition, two studies—one that used a conventional reducing diet (Marcus et al., 1988) and the other a very low calorie diet (Wadden, Foster, & Letizia, in press)—found no differences in weight loss between nonbingers and bingers.

In our analyses, we included weight losses of patients who discontinued treatment but still found no differences between bingers and nonbingers (Wadden, Foster, & Letizia, in press). These findings suggest that binge eaters can be successfully treated by a very low calorie diet. We hasten to add, however, that further investigation is needed to determine whether these diets exacerbate binge eating in these patients. Moreover, the possibility of differences in the maintenance of weight loss in bingers and nonbingers needs to be studied further. Marcus et al. (1988) reported that bingers regained weight more rapidly than nonbingers during the first 6 months of follow-up, although there were no significant differences between groups at 1 year.

Process Variables Correlated with Weight Loss

Early Weight Loss

Weight loss during the first few weeks of therapy correlates positively with weight loss at the end of treatment. This finding holds true for conventional reducing diets (Dubbert & Wilson, 1984; Jeffery et al., 1978; Wadden et al., 1990; Wing & Epstein, 1981), very low calorie diets (Wadden, Foster, Letizia, & Stunkard, in press; Wadden, Foster, Wang, et al., in press), and pharmacotherapy combined with a conventional reducing diet (Craighead, Stunkard, & O'Brien, 1981; Rodin, Elias, Silberstein, & Wagner, 1988). Most of these studies controlled for the effect on weight loss of initial weight and obtained correlations ranging from .30 to .50. Thus, patients who achieve large weight losses early in treatment appear to maintain their success, while those with small early losses do not appear to "catch up." Therefore, practitioners should monitor early weight losses closely to identify and assist patients who fail to achieve expected losses.

Attendance

Patients who consistently attend treatment sessions receive more support, counseling, and feedback than persons who frequently miss meetings. Thus, it is not surprising that attendance has been found to correlate positively with weight loss in studies of conventional reducing diets (Jeffery et al., 1984; Wadden et al., 1990) and very low calorie diets (Wadden, Foster, Wang, et al., in press). In our study of 346 patients treated by very low calorie diet and lifestyle modification (Wadden et al., 1991), we found that the number of sessions attended correlated significantly with weight loss in all subjects, including those who dropped out ($r = .50$, $p < .0001$), as well as in only those who completed treatment ($r = .38$, $p < .0001$). Thus, patients who miss sessions are at risk of smaller weight losses.

We hasten to note that the correlation between attendance and weight loss does not prove that attending treatment leads to better weight loss. A third variable, such as motivation or self-efficacy, may be responsible for both weight loss and attendance. Alternatively, patients may choose to attend treatment because they *are* losing weight. Our clinical experience suggests that when patients miss treatment sessions, they are usually having problems with their weight or eating of which they are ashamed. This shame prompts them to avoid treatment, which regrettably only exacerbates their difficulties. As we tell patients, "The time that you least wish to attend treatment is the time that you most need to do so."

Behavior Change

As originally formulated by Stuart (1967), the behavioral treatment of obesity rested upon the assumption that overweight individuals had inappropriate eating and exercise habits, the modification of which would lead to weight loss. Subsequent studies, however, called into question whether the eating habits of obese and nonobese individuals differed significantly (O'Neil & Jarrell, Chapter 11, this volume; Wadden & Bell, 1990). Moreover, Brownell and Stunkard (1978) showed more than a decade ago that changes in eating and other weight-related behaviors frequently did not correlate significantly with weight loss in persons who received behavioral treatment.

The lack of strong findings in this area may be attributable to difficulties in measuring eating behavior. The majority of studies have relied upon patients' self-reports, which may be of limited validity and reliability (Schoeller, 1990). In addition, eating habits displayed in the laboratory may bear little resemblance to those exhibited at home or in private. Finally, the correlation of changes in eating behavior with weight loss may not yield a positive relationship if a significant number of patients report before treatment that they have no difficulty with the behavior in question, such as eating rapidly. Patients may not have room to improve upon the behavior, and thus may lose weight in the apparent absence of behavior change.

With these caveats in mind, we briefly review three behaviors that may be associated with increased weight loss: self-monitoring, goal setting, and slowing the rate of eating. A fourth behavior, exercise, will be discussed in a later section.

Self-Monitoring

Self-monitoring is frequently considered the cornerstone of the behavioral treatment of obesity. Patients record their daily food and caloric intake, times and places of eating, and other information in order to identify and correct inappropriate eating habits. Early studies revealed that patients spontaneously reduced their caloric intake when asked to keep a daily diet diary (Bellack, Rozensky, & Schwartz, 1974; Romanczyk, Tracey, Wilson, & Thorpe, 1973). Additional studies showed that patients who regularly monitored their caloric intake and exercise sessions lost more weight than those who did not use self-monitoring, with correlation coefficients ranging from .45 to .55 (Dubbert & Wilson, 1983; Dubbert & Wilson, 1984; Perri, Nezu, Patti, & McCann, 1989).

Although record keeping may facilitate behavior change and weight loss, it also may simply reflect successful dietary adherence. Many patients report that they do not mind keeping records as long as they are "doing well on the diet." When they have problems with overeating, however, they frequently feel too ashamed and dispirited to record their food intake. Thus, success in keeping a diet diary may be a correlate rather than a cause of successful weight loss. We believe, however, that self-monitoring is a critically important behavior for patients; it can provide an objective assessment of their eating at times when they may severely distort the magnitude of their dietary transgressions.

Appropriate Goal Setting

Two studies using conventional reducing diets reported that patients who set appropriate weight loss goals achieved greater weight losses than persons who did not set goals (Bandura & Simon, 1977; Dubbert & Wilson, 1984). Setting and attaining goals may provide a schedule of reinforcement and self-regulation for continued weight loss. Like self-monitoring, appropriate goal setting may increase weight loss by requiring patients to become more aware of the behaviors that they need to perform to lose weight.

Slowing the Rate of Eating

Patients are frequently encouraged to slow their rate of eating, in order to increase satiety and thus reduce their food intake. Spiegel, Wadden, and Foster (1991) recently showed that patients treated by behavior therapy did slow their rate of eating during treatment, and that this reduction was positively associated with weight loss ($r = .67$). The reduction in eating rate was not sustained during the follow-up period, however.

Treatment Factors Affecting Weight Loss

Efforts to identify patient factors and process variables that predict weight loss have, to a large extent, taken a back seat to efforts to identify treatment interventions that are associated with improved weight loss (or better maintenance of weight loss). We briefly review here three variables that have been shown to improve end-of-treatment weight losses. They include (1) increasing the length of treatment; (2) increasing patients' physical activity; and (3) providing patients with social support.

Increasing the Length of Treatment

Reviews of the literature of behavioral treatment found that mean weight losses increased from 3.8 kg in 1974 to 8.4 kg in 1987 as treatment duration increased from an average of 8.4 sessions to 15.6 (Brownell & Wadden, 1986; Wadden & Bell, 1990). Thus, longer treatment appears to be associated with greater weight losses, as confirmed in a recent controlled study. Perri et al. (1989) found that patients treated by a conventional reducing diet for 20 weeks lost 8.9 kg, whereas those treated for 40 weeks lost 13.6 kg. Perri et al.'s (1989) findings clearly illustrate the benefits of extending treatment. There may, however, be a point of diminishing returns in increasing treatment duration. In Perri et al.'s (1989) study, weekly weight losses slowed from an average of 0.5 kg during the first 20 weeks to 0.2 kg during the last 20 weeks. Thus, patients should beware of expensive treatments that provide limited weight losses over time. In addition, practitioners should watch for patient burnout, which often accompanies long-term therapy.

Increasing Physical Activity

Exercise is now an integral part of weight control programs. It expends calories and has been shown to improve cardiovascular fitness (Fox, Chapter 15, this volume; Pi-Sunyer, Chapter 8, this volume). Research studies, however, are divided over whether exercise increases end-of-treatment weight losses. Three studies found that patients treated by a conventional reducing diet and exercise lost significantly more weight than those who received identical treatment without exercise (Hill et al., 1989; Pavlou, Krey, & Steffee, 1989; Perri, McAdoo, McAllister, Lauer, & Yancey, 1986). Three additional studies, however, reported no effect for exercise at the end of treatment in patients who consumed a conventional reducing diet (Dahlkoetter, Callahan, & Linton, 1979; Harris & Hallbauer, 1973; Stalonas, Johnson, & Christ, 1978), and a fourth found no effect in patients who received a very low calorie diet (Sikand, Kondo, Foreyt, Jones, & Gotto, 1988). These conflicting results, however, should not be interpreted as reason to abandon exercise in weight control programs. Exercise is perhaps the strongest correlate of maintenance of weight loss, as described shortly. Patients who develop a program of regular physical activity during treatment will be more likely to continue exercising, and thus maintain their weight loss.

Social Support

Family interactions are, in some cases, important in the etiology and treatment of obesity (Brownell & Wadden, 1986). Patients who are supported by their families may experience fewer temptations to overeat, be protected from emotional upset, and practice weight control behaviors more regularly. Controlled studies, however, that investigated the effects of spouse support have yielded contradictory findings. Patients treated in several early studies by a conventional reducing diet and spouse involvement lost more weight than those treated by diet alone (Brownell, Heckerman, Westlake, Hayes, & Monti, 1978; Pearce, LeBow, & Orchard, 1981; Rosenthal, Allen, & Winter, 1980; Saccone & Israel, 1978), but not in later investigations (Brownell & Stunkard, 1981; Weisz & Butcher, 1980; Wing, Marcus, Epstein, & Jawad, 1991).

More consistent findings have been reported in studies that investigated the effects of parental participation on children's weight losses. Specifically, children whose parents attended therapy sessions lost significantly more weight than children treated alone (Brownell, Kelmar, & Stunkard, 1983; Epstein, Wing, Koeske, Andrasik, & Ossip, 1981; Wadden et al., 1990). These positive results may be attributable to the greater control that parents have over their children's food intake than spouses can exert over each other.

Factors Affecting Maintenance of Weight Loss

Only during the past decade have researchers begun to seriously study the issues of relapse and weight loss maintenance. The factors that lead a majority of patients to regain their lost weight within 5 years of completing treatment are poorly understood. Similarly, we do not have a clear understanding of how a small minority of patients successfully maintain their weight losses.

More than likely, there are many paths to weight regain. Some persons may suffer from a genetic predisposition toward obesity (Stunkard, Harris, Pedersen, & McClearn, 1990), or from a low metabolic rate (Geissler, Miller, & Shah, 1987) and increased lipoprotein lipase (LPL) levels (Kern, Ong, Saffari, & Carty, 1990) following weight loss, all of which may cause weight gain in the face of exemplary eating and exercise habits. Others may be free of these biological pressures, but regain weight because they suffer from intra- or interpersonal problems that may be associated with binge eating (Grilo, Shiffman, & Wing, 1989; Marcus et al., 1988). Still others may have excellent mental health, but are unable to modify their eating and exercise habits sufficiently to counteract a national lifestyle that favors a high fat diet and minimal physical activity (Brownell & Wadden, 1991). Thus, relapse, like obesity itself, is probably very heterogeneous in nature.

Given this caveat, we briefly review the patient and treatment factors that appear to be associated with the maintenance of weight loss and, alternatively, with weight regain.

Patient Factors

Exercise

Of all of the factors associated with maintenance of weight loss, exercise appears to be the most important. Numerous studies have shown that patients who successfully maintained their weight losses reported exercising more frequently than those who relapsed (Abrams & Follick, 1983; Gormally et al., 1980; Graham, Taylor, Hovell, & Siegel, 1983; Kayman, Bruvold, & Stern, 1990). For example, Kayman et al. (1990) found in studying persons who had reduced their initial weight by 20% or more that 90% of weight maintainers exercised regularly, as compared with only 34% of relapsers (see Figure 16.2).

Despite this strong positive relationship, researchers have yet to determine conclusively how exercise facilitates weight control (Fox, Chapter 15, this volume; Pi-Sunyer, Chapter 8, this volume). It clearly burns calories, but also has been reported to decrease appetite (Brownell & Stunkard, 1980), to spare fat-free mass (Weltman, Matter, & Stamford, 1980), to prevent the fall in RMR that occurs with dieting (Mole, Stern, Schultz, Bernauer, & Holcomb, 1989), and to improve mood and self-esteem (Steptoe & Cox, 1988). All of these findings, however, with the exception of expending calories, have been contradicted by findings from other studies (van Dale, Saris, Schoeffelen, &

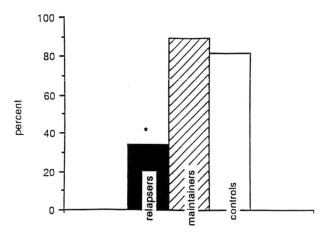

FIGURE 16.2. Percentages of relapsers, maintainers, and control subjects who exercised regularly. Relapsers were 20% or more overweight and had previously lost 20% of their body weight, but regained it. Maintainers were 20% or more overweight, had reduced their body weight, and had maintained the reduced weight for at least 2 years. Control subjects were of average weight and had always remained within 3.6 kg of their current weight. *Denotes significant difference from maintainers and from control subjects, $p < .0001$. From "Maintenance and Relapse after Weight Loss in Women: Behavioral Aspects" (p. 803) by S. Kayman, W. Bruvold, and J. Stern, 1990, *American Journal of Clinical Nutrition, 52*, 800–807. Copyright 1990 by American Society for Clinical Nutrition, Inc. Reprinted by permission.

ten Hoor, 1987; Nieman et al., 1990). Moreover, correlational studies such as that of Kayman et al. (1990) are not methodologically sufficient to prove that exercise is responsible for maintenance of weight loss (as discussed later). Nonetheless, we strongly encourage our patients to develop a program of regular physical activity because of the health benefits alone of exercise, independent of its possible effects on weight.

Self-Monitoring

Persons who maintain their weight losses are also more likely than relapsers to continue to monitor their weight and food intake and to engage in other behaviors typically taught in treatment (Jeffery et al., 1984; Kayman et al., 1990; Perri et al., 1986, 1988) (see Table 16.3). Where reported, correlation coefficients ranged from .25 to .50. Weight maintainers also report recognizing weight regain earlier than relapsers and taking appropriate steps to correct it (Kayman et al., 1990; Marston & Criss, 1984).

Stress and Coping

Several studies have observed that, as compared with weight maintainers, patients who relapse report more negative life events during the same period of time (Dubbert & Wilson, 1984; Gormally et al., 1980; Kayman et al., 1990; Leon & Chamberlain, 1973). In addition, relapsers and maintainers appear to employ different coping styles. Maintainers confront their problems directly and use rational, problem-solving skills to find solutions (Kayman et al., 1990). By contrast, relapsers are more likely to seek ways of reducing the emotional distress that they experience (i.e., emotion-based coping), a search that may well lead to the temporary comfort of food (see Figure 16.3). Not surprisingly, weight maintainers also have more positive thoughts about themselves and their weight control efforts than do relapsers (Bandura & Simon, 1977; Carroll, Yates, & Gray, 1980; Gormally et al., 1980; Kayman et al., 1990).

Physiological Factors

Physiological factors are likely to play a very significant but as yet poorly understood role in the struggle to maintain weight loss. The role of LPL provides a useful example. LPL is an enzyme that mobilizes fatty acids for lipid storage; increased levels of LPL are associated with increased adipose synthesis. Kern et al. (1990) found that, as compared with pretreatment levels, LPL and its messenger RNA were significantly elevated in 9 patients following a mean weight loss of 43 kg. These patients would appear poised to regain weight as a result of the increased LPL activity.

Investigators will not be able to fully determine the contribution of behavior to weight maintenance until they have isolated the effects of LPL and other physiological variables (including genetics and various components of energy expenditure). Thus, it is possible that, immediately following weight loss, many patients continue to exercise and keep diet diaries. Despite these behaviors, some may begin to regain weight because of the influence of LPL or other physiological factors. Such persons are likely to feel unrewarded for their efforts to modify their behavior and eventually abandon them. By contrast, patients free of such physiological factors may continue to exercise, monitor their food intake, and maintain their weight losses. The reader can appreciate

TABLE 16.3. How Maintainers of Reduced-Weight and Always-Average-Weight Women (Control) Subjects Stay at Their Desired Weights

Strategy	Maintainers ($n = 30$)	Control subjects ($n = 34$)
Watches weight on scale (monitors weight)	26 (87)	26 (76)
Is active (more active)	25 (83)	30 (88)
Eats less	25 (83)	25 (73)
Watches intake	18 (60)	18 (50)
Reduces intake of high fat foods	17 (57)	13 (38)
Reduces intake of high sugar foods	17 (57)	17 (50)
Changed to good eating habits	17 (57)[a]	10 (29)
Changed attitude toward food and eating	14 (47)[b]	3 (9)
Eats what she wants and does not feel guilty about what was eaten, deny, or deprive herself; if goes off diet, does not hate herself or feel bad	9 (30)	1 (3)
Knows size by feel of clothes	7 (23)	10 (29)
Does not eat three meals/day	6 (20)	13 (38)
Fantasizes, uses imagery techniques	3 (10)	0 (0)
Avoids snacking by engaging in activity incompatible with eating	3 (10)	1 (3)
Goes to Weight Watchers or other "maintenance program"	3 (10)	1 (3)
Recalls old feelings of how bad she felt	2 (7)	0 (0)
Knows and avoids situations when she would overeat	2 (7)	1 (3)

Note. Values presented are numbers of subjects (with percentages of subjects in parentheses). From "Maintenance and Relapse after Weight Loss in Women: Behavioral Aspects" (p. 803) by S. Kayman, W. Bruvold, and J. Stern, 1990, *American Journal of Clinical Nutrition, 52*, 800–807. Copyright 1990 by American Society for Clinical Nutrition, Inc. Reprinted by permission.

[a]Denotes significant difference from control subjects, $p < .05$.

[b]Denotes significant difference from control subjects, $p < .001$.

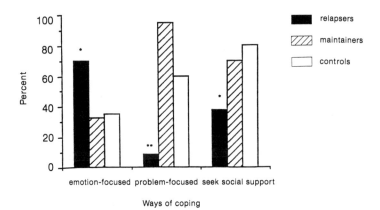

FIGURE 16.3. Percentages of relapsers, maintainers, and control subjects who used emotion-focused or problem-focused ways of coping or who sought social support to aid in coping with problems. Relapsers were 20% or more overweight, and had previously lost 20% of their body weight, but regained it. Maintainers were 20% or more overweight, had reduced their body weight, and had maintained the reduced weight for at least 2 years. Control subjects were of average weight and had always remained within 3.6 kg of their current weight. *Denotes significant difference from maintainers, $p < .01$. **Denotes significant difference from maintainers, $p < .001$. From "Maintenance and Relapse after Weight Loss in Women: Behavioral Aspects" (p. 805) by S. Kaymen, W. Bruvold, and J. Stern, 1990, *American Journal of Clinical Nutrition, 52*, 800–807. Copyright 1990 by American Society for Clinical Nutrition, Inc. Reprinted by permission.

the possible error that exists in inferring that exercise (or other behavior) is responsible for maintenance of weight loss. It may well be that the absence of adverse physiological factors, in addition to appropriate behavior, is responsible for successful weight control.

As indicated earlier, despite the lack of definitive scientific findings, we strongly encourage patients to continue exercising and practicing the other behaviors that they have learned during treatment. Such behaviors may not be sufficient for long-term weight control in all persons, but they are likely to be necessary. Stated differently, these behaviors may not help everyone but they certainly cannot hurt, provided that they are not pursued to excess.

Treatment Factors

Perri (Chapter 19, this volume) has provided an excellent summary of the treatment factors associated with the maintenance of weight loss. In short, persons who maintain contact with their practitioner in the year following treatment are significantly more likely to maintain their weight losses than are persons who discontinue contact. Weight maintenance therapy may be as simple as patients' mailing to the practitioner each week postcards on which they record their weight, caloric intake, exercise, and other relevant information. The practitioner may respond to the card with a brief telephone call (Perri, McAdoo, Spevak, & Newlin, 1984; Perri, Shapiro, et al., 1984). Alternatively, patients may attend group treatment sessions every other week in which they review any weight-related problems that have arisen (Perri et al., 1988). The specific content of these meetings, beyond covering these basics, appears to be less important than the structure and support that patients receive from attending the sessions.

Consistent with the correlational data previously reviewed, results of controlled randomized studies have demonstrated the importance of exercise for long-term weight control (Dahlkoetter et al., 1979; Harris & Hallbauer, 1973; Hill et al., 1989; Perri et al., 1986; Pavlou et al., 1989; Sikand et al., 1988; Stalonas et al., 1978). The most promising findings were reported by Pavlou et al. (1989), who observed excellent maintenance of weight loss at a 3-year follow-up in a group of mildly obese men treated by a program of intensive exercise combined with either a conventional reducing diet or a very low calorie diet.

Summary and Conclusions

This review has yielded a number of findings that should help practitioners improve their care of seriously obese individuals. In assessing patients' dieting readiness (Brownell, 1990), the practitioner should be aware that those who report binge eating or significant life stress (including financial problems) are likely to be at increased risk of discontinuing treatment prematurely. Neither of these research findings is sufficiently strong, however, to justify automatic exclusion of these patients from treatment. Instead, the practitioner should discuss the reported difficulty with each patient, assess its possible effects on treatment, and then carefully monitor the patient's progress during weight reduction, if it is initiated. Patients with small weight losses early in treatment also should be monitored more intensively; this might include brief individual meetings with patients whose treatment otherwise consists of group care.

We do not think that it is useful to attempt to predict weight loss except in the broadest sense of trying to identify persons at risk of not achieving a therapeutic reduction of 10-15% of initial body weight (Kanders & Blackburn, Chapter 9, this volume). We generally attempt to discourage patients' preoccupation with obtaining a specific weight loss (or a particularly large reduction), in favor of focusing their attention on events over which they have greater control. Attending treatment sessions and monitoring eating and exercise habits are two such events, and two that are positively related to weight loss.

While not trying to predict weight loss per se, the practitioner may frequently find it useful to alert lighter patients (and those with low RMRs) who participate in group treatment that they may lose less weight than other participants. This helps to normalize what can be a very frustrating experience.

The practitioner should also meet individually with persons with small weight losses early in treatment, because of their increased risk of attrition and smaller losses throughout therapy.

Weight losses of all patients, whether treated by a conventional reducing diet or a very low calorie diet, are likely to be increased by extending the length of treatment. The practitioner should be aware, however, that there probably will be a point of diminishing returns, at which the high cost of treatment (in terms of work and money) will not be justified by the limited additional weight loss. This is particularly true for patients who have already achieved a 10–20% reduction in initial body weight (Kanders & Blackburn, Chapter 9, this volume).

Maintenance of weight loss is facilitated by patients' developing a regular program of physical activity during treatment (in addition to monitoring food intake and other weight-related behaviors), which they continue thereafter. The best long-term results are likely to be achieved by persons who enroll in a formal program of weight maintenance. This option would appear to be critical for persons with a history of weight loss and regain, as well as advisable for first-time dieters to prevent their acquisition of such a history.

References

Abrams, D. B., & Follick, M. J. (1983). Behavioral weight-loss intervention at the worksite: Feasibility and maintenance. *Journal of Consulting and Clinical Psychology, 51*, 226–233.

Ashwell, M. (1978). Commercial weight loss programs. In G. Bray (Ed.), *Recent advances in obesity research: II. Proceedings of the Second International Congress on Obesity* (pp. 266–276). London: Newman.

Ashwell, M., Durrant, M., & Garrow, J. S. (1978). Does adipose tissue cellularity or the age of onset of obesity influence the response to short-term inpatient treatment of obese women? *International Journal of Obesity, 2*, 449–456.

Bandura, A. (1977). Self-efficacy: Toward a unifying theory of behavior change. *Psychological Review, 84*, 191–215.

Bandura, A., & Simon, K. M. (1977). The role of proximal intentions in self-regulation of refractory behavior. *Cognitive Therapy and Research, 1*, 177–193.

Barrash, J., Rodriquez, E. M., Scott, D. H., Mason, E. E., & Sines, J. O. (1987). The utility of MMPI subtypes for the prediction of weight loss after bariatric surgery. *International Journal of Obesity, 11*, 115–128.

Beeson, V., Ray, C., Coxon, A., & Kreitzman, S. (1989). The myth of the yo-yo trap: Consistent rate of weight loss with successive dieting by very-low-calorie diet. *International Journal of Obesity, 13*, 135–139.

Bellack, A. S., Rozensky, R., & Schwartz, J. S. (1974). A comparison of two forms of self monitoring in a behavioral weight reduction program. *Behavior Therapy, 5*, 523–530.

Bernier, M., & Avard, J. (1986). Self-efficacy, outcome, and attrition in a weight-reduction program. *Cognitive Therapy and Research, 10*, 319–338.

Björntorp, P. (1985). Regional patterns of fat distribution: Health implications. *Annals of Internal Medicine, 103*, 994–995.

Björntorp, P., Carlgren, G., Isaksson, B., Krotkiewski, M., Larson, B., & Sjöström, L. (1975). Effect of an energy-reduced dietary regimen in relation to adipose tissue cellularity in obese women. *American Journal of Clinical Nutrition, 28*, 445–452.

Björvell, H., Rössner, S., & Stunkard, A. J. (1986). Obesity, weight loss, and dietary restraint. *International Journal of Eating Disorders, 5,* 727-734.

Blackburn, G. L. (1988). *Perspectives on obesity: Sandoz OPTIFAST program health and obesity study.* Paper presented at the Sandoz Nutrition Postgraduate Seminar, Orlando, FL.

Blackburn, G. L., Wilson, G. T., Kanders, B. S., Stein, L. J., Lavin, P. T., Adler, J., & Brownell, K. D. (1989). Weight cycling: The experience of human dieters. *American Journal of Clinical Nutrition, 49,* 1105-1109.

Blankmeyer, B. L., Smylie, K. D., Price, D. C., Costello, R. M., McFee, A. S., & Fuller, D. S. (1990). A replicated five cluster MMPI typology of morbidly obese female candidates for gastric bypass. *International Journal of Obesity, 14,* 235-247.

Bonato, D. P., & Boland, F. J. (1987). Predictors of weight loss at the end of treatment and 1-year follow-up for a behavioral weight loss program. *International Journal of Obesity, 11,* 573-577.

Bosello, O., Ostuzzi, R., Rossi, F. A., Armellini, F., Cigolini, M., Micciolo, R., & Scuro, L. A. (1980). Adipose tissue cellularity and weight reduction forecasting. *American Journal of Clinical Nutrition, 33,* 776-782.

Brownell, K. D. (1988). The yo-yo trap. *American Health Magazine,* pp. 78-84.

Brownell, K. D. (1990). The Dietary Readiness Test. *Weight Control Digest, 1,* 6-8.

Brownell, K. D., Greenwood, M. R. C., Stellar, E., & Shrager, E. E. (1986). The effects of repeated cycles of weight loss and regain in rats. *Physiology and Behavior, 38,* 459-464.

Brownell, K. D., Heckerman, C. L., Westlake, R. J., Hayes, S. C., & Monti, P. M. (1978). The effect of couples training and partner cooperativeness in the behavioural treatment of obesity. *Behaviour Research and Therapy, 16,* 323-333.

Brownell, K. D., Kelmar, J. H., & Stunkard, A. J. (1983). Treatment of obese children with and without their mothers: Changes in weight and blood pressure. *Pediatrics, 71,* 515-523.

Brownell, K. D., & Stunkard, A. J. (1978). Behaviour therapy and behavior change: Uncertainties in programs for weight control. *Behaviour Research and Therapy, 16,* 301.

Brownell, K. D., & Stunkard, A. J. (1980). Physical activity in the development and control of obesity. In A. J. Stunkard (Ed.), *Obesity* (pp. 300-324). Philadelphia: W. B. Saunders.

Brownell, K. D., & Stunkard, A. J. (1981). Couples training, pharmacotherapy, and behavior therapy in the treatment of obesity. *Archives of General Psychiatry, 38,* 1224-1229.

Brownell, K. D., & Wadden, T. A. (1986). Behavior therapy for obesity: Modern approaches and better results. In K. D. Brownell & J. P. Foreyt (Eds.), *Handbook of eating disorders: Physiology, psychology, and treatment of obesity, anorexia, and bulimia* (pp. 180-197). New York: Basic Books.

Brownell, K. D., & Wadden, T. A. (1991). The heterogeneity of obesity: Fitting treatments to individuals. *Behavior Therapy, 22,* 153-177.

Carroll, L. J., Yates, B. T., & Gray, J. J. (1980). Predicting obesity reduction in behavioral and nonbehavioral therapy from client characteristics: The self-evaluation measure. *Behavior Therapy, 11,* 189-197.

Cohen, J. & Cohen, P. (1983). *Applied multiple regression/correlation analysis for the behavioral sciences* (2nd ed.). Hillsdale, NJ: Erlbaum.

Craighead, L. W., Stunkard, A. J., & O'Brien, R. M. (1981). Behavior therapy and pharmacotherapy for obesity. *Archives of General Psychiatry, 38,* 763-768.

Dahlkoetter, J., Callahan, E. J., & Linton, J. (1979). Obesity and the unbalanced energy equation: Exercise versus eating habit change. *Journal of Consulting and Clinical Psychology, 47,* 898-905.

den Besten, C., Vansant, G., Weststrate, J. A., & Deurenberg, P. (1988). Resting metabolic rate and diet-induced thermogenesis in abdominal and gluteal-femoral obese women before and after weight reduction. *American Journal of Clinical Nutrition, 47,* 840-847.

Dubbert, P., & Wilson, G. T. (1983). Treatment failures in behavior therapy for obesity: causes, correlates, and consequences. In E. Foa & P.M.G. Emmelkamp, (Eds.), *Treatment failure in behavior therapy* (3rd ed., pp. 127-153). New York: Wiley.

Dubbert, P. M., & Wilson, G. T. (1984). Goal-setting and spouse involvement in the treatment of obesity. *Behaviour Research and Therapy, 22*, 227-242.

Edell, B. H., Edington, S., Herd, B., O'Brien, R. M., & Witkin, G. (1987). Self-efficacy and self-motivation as predictors of weight loss. *Addictive Behaviors, 12*, 63-66.

Epstein, L. H., Wing, R. R., Koeske, R., Andrasik, F., & Ossip, D. J. (1981). Child and parent weight loss in family-based behavior modification programs. *Journal of Consulting and Clinical Psychology, 5*, 674-685.

Feuerstein, M., Papciak, A., Shapiro, S., & Tannenbaum, S. (1989). The weight loss profile: a biopsychosocial approach. *International Journal of Psychiatric Medicine, 19*, 181-192.

Feurer, I. D., & Mullen, J. L. (1986). Measurement of energy expenditure. In J. Rombeau & M. Caldwell (Eds.), *Clinical nutrition* (pp. 224-236). Philadelphia: W. B. Saunders.

Forster, J. L., & Jeffery, R. W. (1986). Gender differences related to weight history, eating patterns, efficacy expectations, self-esteem, and weight loss among participants in a weight reduction program. *Addictive Behaviors, 11*, 141-147.

Foster, G. D., Wadden, T. A., Mullen, J. L., Stunkard, A. J., Wang, J., Feurer, I. D., Pierson, R. N., Yang, M. U., Presta, E., VanItallie, T. B., Lemberg, P. S., & Gold, J. (1988). Resting energy expenditure, body composition, and excess weight in the obese. *Metabolism, 37*, 467-474.

Garrow, J. S., Durrant, M. L., Mann, S., Stalley, S. F., & Warwick, P. M. (1978). Factors determining weight loss in obese patients in a metabolic ward. *International Journal of Obesity, 2*, 441-447.

Geissler, C. A., Miller, D. S., & Shah, M. (1987). The daily metabolic rate of the post-obese and the lean. *American Journal of Clinical Nutrition, 45*, 914-920.

Glynn, S. M., & Ruderman, A. J. (1986). The development and validation of an eating self-efficacy scale. *Cognitive Therapy and Research, 10*, 403-420.

Gormally, J., Black, S., Daston, S., & Rardin, D. (1982). The assessment of binge eating severity among obese persons. *Addictive Behaviors, 7*, 47-55.

Gormally, J., Rardin, D., & Black, S. (1980). Correlates of successful response to a behavioral weight control clinic. *Journal of Consulting and Clinical Psychology, 27*, 179-191.

Graham, L. E., Taylor, C. B., Hovell, M. F., & Siegel, W. (1983). Five-year follow-up to a behavioral weight-loss program. *Journal of Consulting and Clinical Psychology, 51*, 322-323.

Grilo, C. M., Shiffman, S., & Wing, R. R. (1989). Relapse crises and coping among dieters. *Journal of Consulting and Clinical Psychology, 57*, 488-495.

Hagen, R. L., Foreyt, J. P., & Durham, T. W. (1976). The dropout problem: Reducing attrition in obesity research. *Behavior Therapy, 7*, 463-471.

Harris, M. B., & Hallbauer, E. S. (1973). Self-directed weight control through eating and exercise. *Behaviour Research and Therapy, 11*, 523-529.

Hill, J. O., Schlundt, D. G., Sbrocco, T., Sharp, T., Pope-Cordle, J., Stetson, B., Kaler, M., & Heim, C. (1989). Evaluation of an alternating-calorie diet with and without exercise in the treatment of obesity. *American Journal of Clinical Nutrition, 50*, 248-254.

Hovell, M. F., Loch, A., Hofstetter, C. R., Sipan, C., Faucher, P., Dellinger, A., Borok, G., Forsythe, A., & Felitti, V. J. (1988). Long-term weight loss maintenance: Assessment of a behavioral and supplemented fasting regimen. *American Journal of Public Health, 78*, 663-666.

Jeffery, R. W., Bjornson-Benson, W. M., Rosenthal, B. S., Lindquist, R. A., Kurth, C. L., & Johnson, S. L. (1984). Correlates of weight loss and its maintenance over two years of follow-up among middle-aged men. *Preventive Medicine, 13*, 155-168.

Jeffery, R. W., Snell, M. K., & Forster, J. L. (1985). Group composition in the treatment of obesity: Does increasing group homogeneity improve treatment results? *Behaviour Research and Therapy, 23*, 371-373.

Jeffery, R. W., Wing, R. R., & Stunkard, A. J. (1978). Behavioral treatment of obesity: The state of the art 1976. *Behavior Therapy, 9*, 189-199.

Johnson, S. F., Swenson, W. M., & Gastineau, C. F. (1976). Personality characteristics in obesity:

relation of MMPI profile and age of onset of obesity to success in weight reduction. *American Journal of Clinical Nutrition, 29,* 626-632.
Kayman, S., Bruvold, W., & Stern, J. (1990). Maintenance and relapse after weight loss in women: Behavioral aspects. *American Journal of Clinical Nutrition, 52,* 800-807.
Keefe, P. H., Wyshogrod, D., Weinberger, E., & Agras, W. S. (1984). Binge eating and outcome of behavioural treatment of obesity: A preliminary report. *Behaviour Research and Therapy, 22,* 319-321.
Kern, P. A., Ong, J. M., Saffari, B., & Carty, J. (1990). The effects of weight loss on the activity and expression of adipose-tissue lipoprotein lipase in very obese humans. *New England Journal of Medicine, 322,* 1053-1059.
Kirschner, M. A., Schneider, G., Ertel, N. H., & Gorman, J. (1988). An eight year experience with very-low-calorie formula diet for control of major obesity. *International Journal of Obesity, 12,* 69-80.
Kramer, F. M., Stunkard, A. J., Spiegel, T. A., Deren, J. J., Velchik, M. G., Wadden, T. A., & Marshall, K. A. (1989). Limited weight losses with a gastric balloon. *Archives of Internal Medicine, 149,* 411-413.
Krotkiewski, M., Garellick, G., Sjöström, L., Persson, G., Bjurö, T., & Sullivan, L. (1980). Fat cell number, resting metabolic rate, mean heart rate, and insulin elevation while seeing and smelling food as predictors of slimming. *Metabolism, 29,* 1003-1012.
Krotkiewski, M., Sjöström, L., Björntorp, P., Carlgren, G., Garellick, G., & Smith, U. (1977). Adipose tissue cellularity in relation to prognosis for weight reduction. *International Journal of Obesity, 1,* 395-416.
Lanska, D. J., Lanska, M. J., Hartz, A. J., Kalkhoff, R. K., Rupley, D., & Rimm, A. A. (1985). A prospective study of body fat distribution and weight loss. *International Journal of Obesity, 9,* 241-246.
LaPorte, D. J., & Stunkard, A. J. (1990). Predicting attrition and adherence to a very-low-calorie diet: A prospective investigation of the Eating Inventory. *International Journal of Obesity, 14,* 197-206.
Leon, G. R., & Chamberlain, K. (1973). Comparison of daily eating habits and emotional states of overweight persons successful or unsuccessful in maintaining a weight loss. *Journal of Consulting and Clinical Psychology, 41,* 108-115.
Marcus, M. D., Wing, R. R., & Hopkins, J. (1988). Obese binge eaters: Affect, cognitions, and response to behavioral weight control. *Journal of Consulting and Clinical Psychology, 56,* 433-439.
Marcus, M. D., Wing, R. R., & Lamparski, D. M. (1985). Binge eating and dietary restraint in obese patients. *Addictive Behaviors, 10,* 163-168.
Marston, A. R., & Criss, J. (1984). Maintenance of successful weight loss: Incidence and prediction. *International Journal of Obesity, 8,* 435-439.
McCall, R. J. (1973). MMPI factors that differentiate from remediably and irremediably obese women. *Journal of Community Psychology, 1,* 34-36.
Mole, P. A., Stern, J. S., Schultz, C. L., Bernauer, E. M., & Holcomb, B. J. (1989). Exercise reverses depressed metabolic rate produced by severe caloric restriction. *Medicine and Science in Sports and Exercise, 21,* 29-33.
Murray, D. C. (1975). Treatment of overweight: I. Relationship between initial weight and weight change during behavior therapy of overweight individuals: Analysis of data from previous studies. *Psychological Reports, 37,* 243-248.
Nieman, D. C., Haig, J. L., Fairchild, K. S., DeGuia, E. D., Dizon, G. P., & Register, U. D. (1990). Reducing-diet and exercise-training effects on serum lipids and lipoproteins in mildly obese women. *American Journal of Clinical Nutrition, 52,* 640-645.
Oettingen, G., & Wadden, T. A. (1991). Expectation, fantasy, and weight loss: Is the impact of positive thinking always positive? *Cognitive Therapy and Research, 15,* 167-175.
Pasquali, R. Casimirri, F., Colella, P., & Melchionda, N. (1989). Body fat distribution and weight loss in obese women. *American Journal of Clinical Nutrition, 49,* 185-187.

Pavlou, K. N., Krey, S., & Steffee, W. P. (1989). Exercise as an adjunct to weight loss and maintenance in moderately obese subjects. *American Journal of Clinical Nutrition, 49*, 1115–1123.

Pearce, J. W., LeBow, M. D., & Orchard, J. (1981). The role of spouse involvement in the behavioral treatment of obese women. *Journal of Consulting and Clinical Psychology, 49*, 236–244.

Penwick, S., Filon, R., Fox, S., & Stunkard, A. J. (1971). Behavior modification in the treatment of obesity. *Psychosomatic Medicine, 33*, 49–55.

Perri, M. G., McAdoo, W. G., McAllister, D. A., Lauer, J. B., & Yancey, D. Z. (1986). Enhancing the efficacy of behavior therapy for obesity: Effects of aerobic exercise and a multicomponent maintenance program. *Journal of Consulting and Clinical Psychology, 54*, 670–675.

Perri, M. G., McAdoo, W. G., Spevak, P. A., & Newlin, D. B. (1984). Effect of a multicomponent maintenance program on long-term weight loss. *Journal of Consulting and Clinical Psychology, 52*, 480–481.

Perri, M. G., McAllister, D. A., Gange, J. J., Jordon, R. C., McAdoo, W. G., & Nezu, A. M. (1988). Effects of four maintenance programs on the long-term management of obesity. *Journal of Consulting and Clinical Psychology, 56*, 529–534.

Perri, M. G., Nezu, A. M., Patti, E. T., & McCann, K. L. (1989). Effect of length of treatment on weight loss. *Journal of Consulting and Clinical Psychology, 57*, 450–454.

Perri, M. G., Shapiro, R. M., Ludwig, W. W., Twentyman, C. T., & McAdoo, W. G. (1984). Maintenance strategies for the treatment of obesity: An evaluation of relapse prevention training and posttreatment contact by mail and telephone. *Journal of Consulting and Clinical Psychology, 52*, 404–413.

Polivy, J., & Herman, C. P. (1985). Dieting and binging: A causal analysis. *American Psychologist, 40*, 193–201.

Ravussin, E., & Bogardus, C. (1989). Relationship of genetics, age, and physical fitness to daily energy expenditure and fuel utilization. *American Journal of Clinical Nutrition, 49*, 968–975.

Rodin, J., Elias, M., Silberstein, L. R., & Wagner, A.. (1988). Combined behavioral and pharmacologic treatment for obesity: Predictors of successful weight maintenance. *Journal of Consulting and Clinical Psychology, 56*, 399–404.

Romanczyk, R. G., Tracey, D. A., Wilson, G. T., & Thorpe, G. L. (1973). Behavioural techniques in the treatment of obesity: A comparative analysis. *Behaviour Research and Therapy, 11*, 629–640.

Rosenthal, B. S., Allen, G. J., & Winter, C. (1980). Husband involvement in the behavioral treatment of overweight women: Initial effects and long-term follow-up. *International Journal of Obesity, 4*, 165–173.

Saccone, A. J., & Israel, A. C. (1978). Effects of experimenter versus significant other-controlled reinforcement and choice of target behavior on weight loss. *Behavior Therapy, 9*, 271–278.

Schoeller, D. A. (1990). How accurate is self-reported dietary energy intake? *Nutrition Review, 48*, 373–379.

Sikand, G., Kondo, A., Foreyt, J. P., Jones, P. H., & Gotto, A. M. (1988). Two-year follow-up of patients treated with a very-low-calorie diet and exercise training. *Journal of the American Diabetic Association, 88*, 487–488.

Spiegel, T. A., Wadden, T. A., & Foster, G. D. (1991). Objective measurement of eating rate during behavioral treatment of obesity. *Behavior Therapy, 22*, 61–67.

Spitzer, R. L., Devlin, M., Walsh, B. T., Hasin, D., Wing, R., Marcus, M., Stunkard, A. J., Wadden, T., Yanovski, S., Agras, W. S., Mitchell, J., & Nonas, C. (in press). Binge eating disorder: A multisite field trial of the diagnostic criteria. *International Journal of Eating Disorders*.

Stalonas, P. M., Johnson, W. G., & Christ, M. (1978). Behavior modification for obesity: The evaluation of exercise, contingency management, and program adherence. *Journal of Consulting and Clinical Psychology, 46*, 463–469.

Steen, S. N., Opplinger, R. A., & Brownell, K. D. (1988). Metabolic effects of repeated weight loss and regain in adolescent wrestlers. *Journal of the American Medical Association, 260,* 47-50.

Stein, P. M., Hassanein, R. S., & Lukert, B. P. (1981). Predicting weight loss success among obese clients in a hospital nutrition clinic. *American Journal of Clinical Nutrition, 34,* 2039-2044.

Steptoe, A., & Cox, S. (1988). Acute effects of aerobic exercise on mood. *Health Psychology, 7,* 329-340.

Strain, G. W., Strain, J. J., Zumoff, B., & Knittle, J. (1984). Do fat cell morphometrics predict weight loss maintenance? *International Journal of Obesity, 8,* 53-59.

Stuart, R. B. (1967). Behavioural control of overeating. *Behaviour Research and Therapy, 5,* 357-365.

Stunkard, A. J., Harris, J. R., Pedersen, N. L., & McClearn, G. E. (1990). The body-mass index of twins who have been reared apart. *New England Journal of Medicine, 322,* 1483-1487.

Stunkard, A. J., & Messick, S. (1983). *Eating Inventory.* San Antonio, TX: Psychological Corporation.

Telch, C. F., Agras, W. S., Rossiter, E., Wilfley, D., & Kenardy, J. (1990). Group cognitive-behavioral treatment for the non-purging bulimic: An initial evaluation. *Journal of Consulting and Clinical Psychology, 58,* 629-635.

Valley, V. (1984). Pre-operative psychologic assessment in determining outcome from gastric stapling for morbid obesity. *Canadian Journal of Surgery, 27,* 129-130.

Valley, V., & Grace, D. M. (1986). Psychosocial risk factors in gastric surgery for obesity: Identifying guidelines for screening. *International Journal of Obesity, 11,* 105-113.

van Dale, D., Saris, W. H. M., & ten Hoor, F. (1990). Weight maintenance and resting metabolic rate 18-40 months after a diet/exercise treatment. *International Journal of Obesity, 14,* 347-359.

van Dale, D., Saris, W. H. M., Schoeffelen, F. M., & ten Hoor, F. (1987). Does exercise give an additional effect in weight reduction regimens? *International Journal of Obesity, 11,* 367-375.

Vansant, G., den Besten, C., Weststrate, J., & Deurenberg, P. (1988). Body fat distribution and the prognosis for weight reduction: Preliminary observations. *International Journal of Obesity, 12,* 133-140.

Volkmar, F. R., Stunkard, A. J., Woolston, J., & Bailey, R. A. (1981). High attrition rates in commercial weight reduction programs. *Archives of Internal Medicine, 141,* 426-428.

Wadden, T. A., Bartlett, S. J., Letizia, K. A., Foster, G. D., Stunkard, A. J., & Conill, A. (in press). Relationship of dieting history to resting metabolic rate, body composition, eating behavior, and subsequent weight loss. *American Journal of Clinical Nutrition.*

Wadden, T. A., & Bell, S. J. (1990). Obesity. In A. S. Bellack, M. Hersen, & A. E. Kazdin (Eds.), *International handbook of behavior modification and therapy* (2nd ed.) (pp. 449-473). New York: Plenum.

Wadden, T. A., Foster, G. D., & Letizia, K. A. (in press). Response of obese binge eaters to treatment by behavior therapy. *Journal of Consulting and Clinical Psychology.*

Wadden, T. A., Foster, G. D., & Letizia, K. A. (1991). *Predictors of attrition and weight loss in patients treated by very-low-calorie diet and behavior modification.* Unpublished manuscript.

Wadden, T. A., Foster, G. D., Letizia, K. A., & Stunkard, A. J. (in press). A multi-center evaluation of a proprietary weight reduction program for the treatment of marked obesity. *Archives of Internal Medicine.*

Wadden, T. A., Foster, G. D., Wang, J., Pierson, R. N., Yang, M.-U., Moreland, K., Stunkard, A. J., & VanItallie, T. B. (in press). Clinical correlates of short- and long-term weight loss. *American Journal of Clinical Nutrition.*

Wadden, T. A., & Lucas, R. A. (1980). MMPI as a predictor of weight loss. *Psychological Reports, 46,* 984-986.

Wadden, T. A., & Stunkard, A. J. (1986). Controlled trial of very-low-calorie diet, behavior therapy, and their combination in the treatment of obesity. *Journal of Consulting and Clinical Psychology, 54,* 482-488.

Wadden, T. A., Stunkard, A. J., Brownell, K. D., & Day, S. C. (1985). Advances in the treatment of moderate obesity: Combined treatment by behavior modification and very-low-calorie diet. In J. Hirsch & T. B. VanItallie (Eds.), *Recent advances in obesity research: IV. Proceedings of the Fourth International Congress on Obesity* (pp. 312-319). London: John Libbey.

Wadden, T. A., Stunkard, A. J., Johnston, F. E., Wang, J., Pierson, R. N., VanItallie, T. B., Costello, E., & Peña, M. (1988). Body fat deposition in adult obese women: II. Changes in fat distribution accompanying weight reduction. *American Journal of Clinical Nutrition, 47,* 229-234.

Wadden, T. A., Stunkard, A. J., Rich, L., Rubin, C. J., Sweidel, G., & McKinney, S. (1990). Obesity in black adolescent girls: A controlled clinical trial of treatment by diet, behavior modification, and parental support. *Pediatrics, 85,* 345-351.

Weisz, G., & Butcher, B. (1980). Involving husbands in the treatment of obesity: Effects on weight loss, depression, and marital satisfaction. *Behavior Therapy, 11,* 643-650.

Weltman, A., Matter, S., & Stamford, B. A. (1980). Caloric restriction and/or mild exercise: Effects on serum lipids and body composition. *American Journal of Clinical Nutrition, 33,* 1002-1009.

Wilson, G. T. (1985). Psychological prognostic factors in the treatment of obesity. In J. Hirsh & T. B. VanItallie (Eds.), *Recent advances in obesity research: IV. Proceedings of the Fourth International Congress on Obesity* (pp. 301-311). London: John Libbey.

Wilson, G. T. (1991). *Binge-eating in obese patients.* Manuscript submitted for publication.

Wilson, G. T., & Brownell, K. D. (1980). Behavior therapy for obesity: An evaluation of treatment outcome. *Advances in Behavior Research and Therapy, 3,* 49-86.

Wing, R. R. (in press). Weight cycling in humans: A review of the literature. *Annals of Behavioral Medicine.*

Wing, R. R., & Epstein, L. H. (1981). Prescribed level of caloric restriction in behavioral weight loss programs. *Addictive Behaviors, 6,* 139-144.

Wing, R. R., Marcus, M. D., Epstein, L. H., & Jawad, A. (1991). A "family-based" approach to the treatment of obese type II diabetic patients. *Journal of Consulting and Clinical Psychology, 59,* 156-162.

Wing, R. R., Marcus, M. D., Epstein, L. H., & Kupfer, D. (1983). Mood and weight loss in a behavioral treatment program. *Journal of Consulting and Clinical Psychology, 51,* 153-155.

Yalom, I. D. (1985). *The theory and practice of group psychotherapy* (3rd ed.). New York: Basic Books.

Yang, M.-U. (1988). Body composition and resting metabolic rate in obesity. In R. T. Frankle & M.-U. Yang (Eds.), *Obesity and weight control* (pp. 71-96). Rockville, MD: Aspen Systems Corporation.

17

The Challenge of Weight Control: A Personal View

JANET JASPER

It's been over 3½ years since I lost weight on a very low calorie diet (VLCD) program, yet I am not "cured." Weight management is a lifelong challenge. You'll note I did not say "lifelong problem," but "lifelong challenge." It is a challenge that confronts and will confront me for the rest of my life. And every day I get to choose how I will handle that challenge. Do I make the choices that are required for me to maintain my weight? And sometimes the choices entail sacrifice. Am I willing to begin again? A great deal of what I've learned over the past 3 years consists simply of beginning again—not starting yet another diet, but simply beginning again. Old behaviors (and overeating is a behavior) have a way of reasserting themselves in my life. When I recognize this happening, my challenge is to be honest enough to acknowledge the behaviors and to correct unhealthy eating or lack of exercise. My task is to self-correct; to begin again; to be who I am.

I am a weight loss/weight management success. I weigh 165 pounds. In my adult life I have weighed more, as much as 267 pounds, and I have weighed less, as little as 150 pounds. I am 46 years old. I have been younger; I hope to live to a ripe old age. I am 5 feet, 9 inches tall. I have been shorter. I will probably shrink an inch or two if I live to that ripe old age. I have the gray hairs I have. One day I might decide to color my hair, but for today, I like my hair precisely as it is. I have the wrinkles and crow's feet that I have. I have some loose flesh that results from losing almost 100 pounds. One day plastic surgery might be a choice—I haven't ruled it out.

But for today, I love my body with its life scars. I love, accept, and forgive my body—yes, forgive—because as I dieted and came to realize that I would finally attain my long-sought goal weight, the bittersweet realization dawned on me that I would be thin, but that my stretched skin would never be the same again. I would never be young again; I would not have the supple skin of youth, the firm breasts and thighs. The evidence of having been 100 pounds overweight would be with me for the rest of my life, and the thought saddened me. I would not have the body I had envisioned. I would have to come to love and accept the body I did have. It would have to be enough, and this seemed so unfair. After all, I reasoned, I had given up so much—the ability to eat whenever and whatever I so desired in whatever amounts I wanted—and I was only getting a flawed body in return. I wanted the body in the Kellogg's Special K commercial. I wanted more than was humanly possible. My skewed logic told me that I had sacrificed so much on the VLCD in the hopes of attaining "perfect fitness." Now, I was beginning to glimpse what was to become a fundamental truth: that I would have to work hard to maintain even this level of fitness, work hard to maintain this "imperfect" body—and for me the costs incurred just to be "imperfectly" fit and thin seemed high.

I then had to answer these questions: How much fitness is enough, and what price am I willing to pay for it? How thin do I want to be? How thin can I become? What weight can I maintain? How much exercise will I have to do? How much food will I have to forego? In short, what am I willing to sacrifice for thinness? And all of these questions assume that I have answered the most fundamental question for anyone who has been grossly overweight and who loses weight: What is thinness?

There are those who would argue that 165 pounds is not thin. I am here to argue the opposite point: that for me, a tall woman who has weighed as much as 267 pounds in her adult life, 165 pounds is indeed thin. I know what it costs me in terms of exercise and diet to maintain 165 pounds—a reasonable weight for me. I also know that my body fat percentage is normal, that I wear a size 10 dress/suit. For me, 165 pounds is thin enough. So, answering the questions "What is thinness?" and "How thin is thin enough?" is an individual matter. Each person who struggles with weight loss and weight maintenance must come to an answer for himself or herself.

My Weight History

I was a large baby (11 pounds at birth), a normal size toddler, and a normal size child. At puberty I began to put on weight. I am the 6th child of an African-American family of 11 children. My father is 6 feet, 1 inch tall and weighs 170–180 pounds. He is tall and wiry and has never had a weight problem, and at 79 years of age he is still slim and healthy. My mother died from a stroke at 65 years of age. She was 5 feet, 4 inches tall and weighed approximately 220 pounds—a weight I recall seeing once on a physical exam form. She never dieted and only lost weight after she became ill in her 60s.

I used to joke that my dad was tall and thin, my mom was short and fat, and I had inherited tall and fat. At my fattest (267 pounds) I was the heaviest of all my sisters—heavier, in fact, than all of my brothers save one.

As a child and young woman, even as an adult, my dad never criticized or teased me because of my weight, but my mother was merciless. You might think she would have been more understanding, since she had been a fat child and was ridiculed by her very thin stepmother. In retrospect, as a parent, I can better understand her anxiety. She did not want me to suffer as she had suffered because of obesity. She simply did not know what to say and do to help me.

At puberty, when I began to put on weight, I was very self-conscious about being fat. Looking back at old photographs, I realize that I was not fat, just a large girl. The summer I turned 13, between eighth and ninth grades, my oldest sister took me to the first of what would be a long succession of diet doctors. I still remember how excited I felt when I entered his office. I would be thin and pretty. I would be of "normal weight."

The doctor ran an assembly-line operation. The nurse took my medical history, my blood pressure, and my weight. No one seemed to care that I was obviously a 12-year-old child. I was led to a cubicle to await the arrival of the doctor. He appeared, administered a shot, and dispensed a packet of pills and a diet sheet (which told me to eat toast for breakfast, two pieces of fruit for lunch, and a dinner of lean meat and vegetables off a saucer). All of this took about 4 minutes.

During the first week I lost 10 pounds—my first "successful" diet. Even then I knew there was something not quite right about the powerful amphetamine I was taking, but I reasoned that this doctor would not administer anything harmful to me. I lost about 25 pounds and returned to school in September unrecognizably thin. Before the semester was over, all of the weight was regained and all of the stylish new clothes were too small.

This first "successful" weight loss set two precedents for me. It taught me that the only way I could lose weight was with diet pills and that weight loss leads to weight regain. As a consequence, all of my adult life (except for when I was pregnant), I controlled my weight with diet pills. I wasn't always taking pills, but whenever my weight threatened to exceed an acceptable upper limit, I'd run to the latest diet doctor for pills. Meanwhile, my "acceptable upper limit" kept creeping up. Once it was 160 pounds, then 170, then 180. . . .

Intermittently, I tried other methods to lose weight, including Weight Watchers and dieting on my own. On one occasion, around 1977, I tried liquid protein for about 6 or 7 weeks and lost about 35–40 pounds, but stopped because I felt so awful. Lucky me. It was only later that I would learn how dangerous this low quality "liquid protein" was and how indeed it turned out to be the "Last Chance Diet" for several unfortunate people who died as a result of using it.

In 1979 I went to Overeaters Anonymous and lost approximately 50 pounds. I kept it off for about a year before I regained it all. This was a milestone for me. It was the first time in my adult life (aside from the liquid protein) in which I was able to lose weight without taking diet pills. In addition, the regaining of lost weight was slower this time.

After this, there were many half-hearted attempts to lose weight, but nothing significant until 1987, when I began the VLCD.

Before the Diet—Contemplation

Eating is pleasurable! It's right up there with sex—sometimes above sex in my hierarchy of values. So why would someone in her right mind want to give it up for 16 weeks? Why would anyone want to fast?

In my journal under the date April 7, 1987, I wrote, "Can a person be treated for sheer exhaustion? World weariness, nothing left to give? Burnout? I'm not caring about too many things. I'm tired." And one of the major reasons for being so tired was the 260-plus pounds that I carried around at the time.

I was the single parent of a college junior. I had been working a full-time job plus a part-time job for 5 years, and there was never enough money or time for me to do much for myself. So I spent whatever time and money I could steal from the budget on food. I ate a lot. My appetite was gargantuan, and I fed it. I rationalized by saying that I needed more energy to work the grueling schedule that I had set for myself, but the reality was that the large amounts of food I consumed often left me feeling sluggish and lethargic. Is it any wonder that I felt so burned out?

Earlier in the year, I had done a videotaped presentation at work. I knew my stuff. My facts were well ordered and pertinent. My argument was lucid and persuasive. My delivery, speech patterns, and gestures were all on point, and my presentation was instrumental in getting a policy change implemented in my department. At the conclusion of this presentation, I was pleased, even excited by my success. This was short-lived. Later, when I got to view the videotape of the presentation, the shock of recognition was devastating. I was the largest person in the room, men and women included. I was huge. My suit revealed bulges in the most unflattering places, and my sheer bulk surprised and saddened me—so very much so that when the tape was sent to our videotape library, I found occasion to borrow it one day, never to return it. I have it to this day, stashed away in my home. I haven't had the courage to trash it altogether, but I hope that it will never see the light of day again.

Also around this time, I ended a long-term but unsatisfying relationship with a man I'd been dating for several years. I also had been passed over not once but three times for a job that I was eminently qualified to perform and, in fact, had been performing on a temporary basis.

So, in early 1987, I was 43 years old, alone, overworked, fat, lethargic, passed over for yet another job promotion, and in possession of a tape that proved I was immense. At this point, my answer to the question "Who would want to fast?" was very easy. I wanted to, and I wanted to in the worst way. I didn't want to continue living the way I was living, and my weight was one of the things I wanted to change. Why would anyone want to fast? In my case, it was because I was miserable with fat, burned out, sick and tired, angry, and sad. I had had enough of the old behaviors that no longer worked, and I wanted to and was ready to change.

A friend had participated in a weight reduction study at a local hospital a few years earlier, and I had called inquiring about when and if another study might take place and whether I could be considered for it. They apparently kept my name and phone number on file. One Monday evening out of the blue, a staff member from the hospital called and asked if I wanted to participate in a weight loss program. He told me that they were beginning a study and that there would be two groups: one on a liquid VLCD of approximately 450 kilocalories (kcal) daily, and the other on a 1200-kcal diet. He explained that one goal of the study was to compare the long-term results achieved by the two approaches. You bet your life I was interested and enthusiastically agreed to come in for the interview.

This was a ray of hope for me, a life buoy tossed to a drowning woman, something to grasp on to. But I had determined ahead of time that I would not participate unless selected for the VLCD group. This was critical. As desperate as I was, and as much as I wanted to lose weight, I somehow knew that a rapid and dramatic weight loss would be required for me to make any lasting changes in my life. I welcomed the VLCD, as I eagerly anticipated a respite from food. I did not want to have to deal with my nemesis on a daily and ongoing basis while undergoing the weight-losing phase.

I went into the interview with enthusiasm and hope for the first time in a long time. The program was an answered prayer. My weight, my body fat percentage, my cholesterol, my basal metabolic rate, and my heart would be monitored throughout my weight loss. I would be able to chart my progress. I would be rehabilitated. There was so much hope; I knew that I must be selected for this study. Not only would I get to lose weight, but I would learn things about nutrition and exercise that would make it possible for me to maintain my weight loss.

My disappointment was palpable when I was informed that I was not going to be in the VLCD group, that I had been assigned to the 1200-kcal group. Despite all of the excitement about being a part of this study, I could not do the 1200-kcal diet. I felt a strong need to lose weight rapidly and without having to confront food on a daily basis. I'd tried Weight Watchers over 30 times, only to last 5 or 6 weeks. I'd tried diet pills, the Scarsdale Diet, and a host of other approaches with little success. I felt the need to do something as drastic as the VLCD. I felt so strongly about my desire to do the liquid diet that I informed the office that I could not participate at all unless I could do the VLCD. I said thanks, but no thanks. And this was crucial for me.

It was a milestone for a lot of reasons, the most important being that I asked for what I wanted. This was significant for a woman not well versed in asking for what she wanted or needed. Today, after the VLCD, and after losing 90 pounds and maintaining that weight loss for the past 3½ years, I have become better at wanting what I want. It has become easier to want something honestly and openly and to go after it. Certainly, I risk not getting what I want, but I am committed not to lie about what it is that I want. And this was a crucial first step for me.

As it turned out, the program staff allowed me to participate in the VLCD group. They had obtained enough persons in both groups to conduct their study and were offering treatment to a few additional people who, technically, would not be in the study. I had been selected as one of these additional participants. I was pleased and grateful. I got what I wanted.

Since I had been given what I wanted, it was incumbent on me not to squander this opportunity. I recognized that I was being given the chance of a lifetime. I would be monitored and tested and watched over. I would be asked to share my experiences, opinions, and feelings. I would be a guinea pig, for lack of a better term, in an area of utmost interest in my life—obesity. I was determined to take full advantage of everything offered, because at 43, I knew full well that for me "the prognosis was not good." The prognosis for anyone who wants to lose almost 100 pounds and to maintain that loss is indeed not good. Notwithstanding all this, I knew I would give my best efforts to this enterprise.

I began my VLCD in May 1987. I was primed for the diet, and I proceeded on faith that it would work for me, and on faith in the reputation of the local hospital that I would not be harmed in the process. I was willing to do whatever was required of me. I would show up for weekly meetings. I would do the suggested exercises. I would listen and take notes. I trusted our group leaders implicitly. I trusted their expertise, but perhaps over and above their credentials, I had faith in them as people. They engendered a sense of trustworthiness and compassion that I have rarely seen in people working with the obese. Their concern for us as individuals was always apparent. I was about to begin my 16-week period of not eating, and I couldn't have been happier.

The Very Low Calorie Diet

The First Week on the Diet

Before the VLCD began, it was suggested that we moderate our eating. During the 2 weeks prior to beginning the VLCD, I lost 4 or 5 pounds. We were told that during the first week of the VLCD we would lose approximately 4 to 10 pounds. We were advised of some of the possible side effects, including fatigue, feeling cold, constipation, light-headedness, dizziness, and probably fantasies about food. It was suggested that we record the times of our meals and all calories consumed from diet gum, diet soda, and bouillon. We were also told to drink at least 2 quarts of water daily. When we were informed that an average weight loss of 3 to 4 pounds per week was possible on the VLCD, I immediately went home and made up a chart with my projected weight loss at 4 pounds per week. I kept this chart during the entire 16-week VLCD, and my projections were pretty much on target.

On the first day of the fast, I noted in my journal:

Thursday, 5/21/87, first day of VLCD, 9:16 P.M. Not hungry, but several times during the day, I thought of eating. At lunchtime I missed eating. Driving out of the parking lot on deadline day—I usually overeat a great deal on Thursday. Most hungry period during the day was between 5 and 7 P.M. Almost went to Popeye's to get chicken. Decided to go through the motions—to drink my dinner, to wait and see. I waited. I saw. I went for a walk, then came home, had bouillon, bathed, bedtime. A good feeling of tiredness.

I am a sales representative for a large metropolitan newspaper. Thursday is deadline day for Sunday's paper, and it is my busiest day. My job entails talking to advertising agency representatives, processing orders, juggling multiple phones, and putting up with major stressors. Often I would work until 6:30 or 7 P.M., and when I left for home, I anticipated eating a large amount of food. And it was on Thursday that I began my VLCD. I remember the feeling of not being hungry, yet wanting to eat. It is not so unusual that I would miss eating—it was on this day more than on any other that I'd reward myself with food. Others might unwind with a martini or a glass of wine; not me. I'd eat large portions of whatever food I had a taste for. Often I'd have fast foods such as pizza, fried chicken, or burgers; on those occasions when I did cook, I ate large portions. A typical evening's meal might be a steak with a baked potato and vegetable, followed by dessert, and later in the evening assorted snacks such as popcorn or chips. In essence, I ate anything and everything I wanted.

On this first evening of the VLCD, when I got into my car to leave work, it was as though I were on automatic pilot. It was an act of faith that I did not drive to a fast-food restaurant. Instead, I decided to proceed on faith alone. I drank my liquid diet because I had been told that it would satisfy my hunger. It did. On the second day, I wrote:

Didn't eat anything, but spent a lot of time thinking of food ... and missing food; haven't said good-bye to food.

By the second day, I realized that the VLCD would satisfy my hunger and that after drinking my shake and perhaps having a cup of bouillon I was physically satisfied. But it did not satisfy my appetite, or what I call that gnawing desire to eat something, anything, to satisfy an altogether different longing. For me, a person for whom food had assumed paramount importance, I spent a lot of time during the first week thinking of food, missing food, salivating like Pavlov's dog in the presence of food. Food was ubiquitous and inescapable.

Because food is so ubiquitous, I became concerned early on that I would not make it through 16 weeks of the VLCD. Instead of concentrating on one day at a time, I began looking down the long road of "not eating" with a great deal of fear. Sixteen weeks (112 long days) of not eating solid food was incomprehensible to me. I had no experience to prove I could do this VLCD, and it was during these critical first few days that I relied most heavily on the promises made to me in the first meeting. Those promises were that I would lose a considerable amount of weight during the VLCD; that I would feel better in a few days; that I might even begin to feel better than usual after a few weeks on the VLCD; and that I would not damage my health. Also critical, I learned that the desire to eat—even the fear of eating—does not necessarily lead to eating. With each passing day, my ability to withstand the pressures of ever-present food cues became stronger.

I found that I could make it easier on myself in the meantime if I watched less television. I discovered that exercise helped me maintain a better outlook, and my exercise of choice was walking.

On the third day of my VLCD, I went to an evening wedding reception. All day long, I had agonized over whether or not to attend. During the day as I made and remade plans, I thought of possible contingencies: not going, just going to the wedding, or simply dropping the gift off at the home. I decided to attend, and just prior to leaving for the reception, I drank my liquid diet. The food at the wedding was less bothersome than I had anticipated. I reminded myself: "This is not the last food you'll encounter; there will be other eating opportunities, but today is not one of them." I was fine at the reception for about 2 hours, at which time I said my good-byes and left. On Sunday morning, I awoke to the realization that I had successfully completed 3 days of the VLCD.

I had committed myself to exercise at least five times per week, and I began walking and stationary cycling. It was also around this time that I began the practice of giving myself a star for accomplishing any one of several goals: to drink the liquid diet five times daily, to exercise, to record my day's accomplishments in my journal. In short, I found lots of ways to positively reinforce my new behaviors. To some it might appear childish, but for me it was a joy to behold a calendar filled with multicolored stars. It was tangible evidence that I was keeping my word to myself. And it was fun.

There were many, many occasions during the first week when I thought about eating, but I didn't. As much as possible, I kept temptation out of the house. This was Memorial Day weekend, and the air was redolent with charcoal and burgers and chicken. So much food to choose from. In a way, having no choice was a blessing. On a later occasion, I noted in my journal:

There are five pistachio nuts in the kitchen and I've been tempted to eat just one. But I don't want to sabotage my program. If I can justify eating just one nut, that opens the door to God only knows what. So, I didn't succumb to temptation. Give myself a star.

During the first week, when I thought about eating, I thought about the rest of the group and how I would be the goat if I ate. I wondered if it was as hard for them as it had been for me, and I didn't want to embarrass myself if they were able to run the food gauntlet while I was unable to make it through the first week. I did not yet have a sense of responsibility to the rest of the group; that would come later. At this point, it was more a spirit of competitiveness. I did not want to look bad.

During our first group meeting, after week 1 on the VLCD, it was revealed that only one person had gone off the diet. On several occasions, Judy tried to tell everyone about what she had eaten and how, nevertheless, she'd managed to lose over 8 pounds. Our group leader tried, unsuccessfully, to prevent the recitation of pork chops and mashed potatoes and Wendy's and potato salad and grilled hamburgers, but this individual pressed on with her recitation. Finally, the group leader was able to stop her and told her he would like to talk to her after our session. He followed her out to quiet her upset, to talk to her, and to help her get back on track. While they were out of the room, another group member said that she was angry with Judy for eating, and I realized that I was also angry. It was only later that I would understand how critical the group would be in my success. At this early stage of the VLCD, it was imperative that we stick to the protocol as outlined, not to undermine our efforts. And Judy had done what all of us were afraid we might do—eat something not on the diet. More than anything, I was afraid of her. As it turned out, she decided she was not ready for a VLCD at this time in her life and subsequently withdrew from the program. The remainder of the group fasted successfully for the following 15 weeks.

Strategies I Found Helpful

During the first week of the VLCD, I learned firsthand that I needed to do the following:

1. To maintain a social life, notwithstanding the fact that I was not eating solid food.
2. To consume the liquid diet five times daily, spread out over the day.
3. To moderate my exercise schedule and not to overdo it.
4. To make interim goals on a weekly or biweekly basis, and not to project too far into the future.

Maintaining a Social Life

I decided to attend the wedding reception, but made plans beforehand. On another occasion, I declined an invitation to go to Atlantic City to the casinos. I went to a cookout, but declined all invitations to go to restaurants. I found it easier to accept invitations that enabled me to have more flexibility.

Need to Spread Out Consumption of the Diet

On one occasion, I noted in my journal:

> *Am very tired now. Rather lethargic, slightly nauseated, sleepy-eyed. Imagined once again that a little food would help. But no, it's not worth breaking my word for it, so I'll ride out this weakness; it will pass. Perhaps I'll go to the spa.*

Later that same day, I wrote:

> *After the above notes were recorded, it occurred to me that I was hungry and should take my serving of the liquid diet, which I did. I felt fine afterwards, so I went to the spa to exercise. Did the circuit weight training, felt okay. Still slightly lethargic. Swimming and sauna. Now feel a little sleepy. Will take a nap.*

Because we were taking in so very few calories, it was stressed how imperative it was to spread our food intake out over the day and not to allow ourselves to get too hungry. I was to discover firsthand the effects of the "fasting fog"—the wretched, tired, sluggish feeling one gets after going too long without eating. I became more diligent in not allowing this to happen after the first week or two. In addition, I learned the importance of moderate exercise.

Exercise: Don't Overdo It

Looking back, I realize I did too much during the first weeks. I was riding my stationary bicycle, walking, and doing circuit weight training and sometimes swimming and aerobics—not every day, but far too frequently for the limited number of calories I was taking in. We were later advised to avoid anaerobic exercises, such as weight training, and to stick to mild aerobics.

Interim Goals

As mentioned earlier, I made up a chart with my projected weekly weight loss, and I kept a calendar on which I gave myself stars for accomplishing any one of several interim goals. I found this helpful and encouraging. No one else saw the chart and calendar (except for my weight loss group); they were for my eyes only and for my benefit. The only "down side" to setting weekly weight loss goals was my constant jumping on the scale.

We were advised not to weigh ourselves between visits, but this is tantamount to telling a bee not to buzz. Dieters, especially those who are losing weight rapidly, will weigh themselves—or, I should say, I weighed myself. I would reposition the scale around the bathroom floor until I got the most favorable weight, at which point I was satisfied. It was a game I played during the first few weeks of the VLCD, and I do not think it was detrimental. The only other time that I was weighed, aside from at group meetings, was at the health spa I attended. The scales there were different from those at group, yet somehow I felt they were "official" and should be given more authority than my home scale. It was upsetting when the spa's scale registered higher than the scale at our meeting, so I determined that I would not weigh on any other scales besides my home scale (which I could manipulate) and the scale at my group meetings.

Another down side to establishing interim weight loss goals was the feeling that I could not go into the meeting without having lost weight. I knew full well that I was responsible only for maintaining the protocol (five servings of the liquid diet daily, 2 quarts of water, etc.), and that I had no control over the manner in which my body would actually lose the fat. Yet every week, I agonized over going into a meeting without having lost weight.

Going Public with the Fast

Early in the VLCD, I took a week's vacation, during which time I exercised heavily at the health club, walked extensively, and drank my liquid diet. When I returned to work, I noted in my journal:

> *Returned to work today and almost everyone commented on how good I looked. I was pleasantly surprised by the attention. Feel good—not hungry. Keep jumping on scale, but my weight has been staying the same. Can't go in on Wednesday not having lost any weight.*

Although I had lost only 20 pounds by this point, it apparently showed. This began what was to become an ongoing dialogue with my friends, family, and coworkers, who watched while I rapidly lost weight. I opted to go public with my efforts, and I have no regrets about that decision. I got very little negative feedback, and it was as though I invited the support and encouragement of my friends and family. For the most part, that is what I got—encouragement, even admiration. It was a little disconcerting to be the focus of so much attention, but only in the beginning. As every dieter knows, the fear inherent in this kind of attention is fear of the possible displeasure, censure, and even ridicule when weight is regained.

So going public was a leap of faith. I also reasoned that if I planned to lose 100 pounds, there was no way I could keep the attempt a secret. When people asked what I was doing, I told them. I did have ways to protect myself from criticisms of the "Isn't-that-dangerous" type. The line that I found most helpful was "I am under a doctor's supervision; I trust his expertise, and what I eat or do not eat is between me and my doctor. Thank you for your concern."

When a person was downright rude—which I might add only occurred once—I said, "I do not discuss my weight with people whose opinions I do not respect." This worked for me, and the individual in question never brought up the subject again.

Gaining Momentum with the Diet

After a few weeks on the VLCD, I began to feel great. I was still occasionally tired, but overall, I had not felt that good, that energetic in years. When tempted to eat, I'd think of all that I was being given by the program. All that was asked of me in return was that I follow the protocol as outlined. It was the least that I could do.

At this early stage, I knew I could continue on the liquid diet for 16 weeks. The rewards were tangible and immediate. Even though I was not hungry, I must admit I was still occasionally tempted to eat. There was another issue that I had yet to confront; I call it "missing food." One Friday evening, I noted in my journal, "Tired, got my period, missing food."

It had been 2 weeks, actually the beginning of the third week of the VLCD, and I was not physically hungry. In fact, I made a point to emphasize that I was "not hungry," but this was the first time that the issue of "missing food" became so critical. It is no surprise that it came up on a Friday evening when I was tired, alone, perhaps lonely, and beginning a menstrual period. I was missing what probably had been my best friend over the past few years. Food as friend. Food as tranquilizer. Food to assuage loneliness. Food that enabled me to eat myself into the oblivion of sleep. Food the comforter. And I missed the sheer gustatory pleasure of eating whatever I wanted in the amounts that I wanted. Ah, the pleasure of eating. I was missing the gratification of eating. The familiar feeling of my body stuffed to capacity, sated, warm, and somehow less lonely.

Food and food alone brought on those feelings. I could eat what I wanted and then curl up with a good book or fall asleep watching television, secure in the only sure pleasure in my life, or so I had thought. And for someone who grew up in a family where it was not okay to show your needs (or only okay to show this one need—the need for food), I was missing food. Food met my needs. Other unmet needs were not dealt with, having been so deeply buried or denied or distorted. But food and fulfilling the need for food was allowed. And I was missing food. I was mourning the loss of food.

It was around this time that I learned that I would have to be more honest about my needs; that I would have to find out what they were; that I would have to ask openly for what I needed; and that this was risky. During the program, I was encouraged to challenge old assumptions as I relearned and remembered other needs that I had denied or buried under layers of fat. The need to matter, to love, to be loved, to do work that interests me, to accomplish goals, to feel strong, to be able, to learn, to risk, to grow. I would ultimately reclaim all of my emotions: my anger, my sadness, my joy, my sorrow, my sensuality. But at this point, I did not know this. I was mourning the loss of my best friend. I had not yet said good-bye to food.

Food, Ubiquitous Food

Food is ubiquitous. Each day brings pictures of food, radio commercials about food, food smells wafting through the mall to assault unsuspecting dieters as they stroll by. Advertisers know all too well how to play into our predisposition not only to eat, but to overeat. So all throughout my VLCD, I had a real, healthy fear that I might just one day decide to eat and blow the whole thing. I was elated by my early successes but my elation was always tempered. I went to every meeting with the phrase indelibly etched in my mind and spoken just as frequently: "I know the prognosis is not good." Even as I was losing weight rapidly, I knew that the prognosis for maintaining a weight loss was not good. I harbored no illusions that I was being miraculously cured of fat. I knew the damning statistics. I had seen in my own life how I had lost weight only to regain it. Perhaps because of this healthy fear, I developed an appreciation for how difficult weight maintenance would be. In group meetings, I listened and incorporated anything and everything passed out or suggested that might help me maintain my weight. When our group leader told us that studies show that people who exercise have a better chance of maintaining their weight loss, that was enough for me. I made sure that I had an exercise program that I could do forever—and for me that was walking. Exercise has been an integral part of my life for the past 4 years. Today, I still know that the prognosis is not good, but now I know it is not impossible.

Other Issues besides Food

As I continued to lose weight, I came to realize that I wanted to make other changes in my life. Many of these changes had to do with my relationships with friends and family. I began to realize that if I wanted to be treated differently, I would have to behave differently. I realized that it was my responsibility to teach friends and family how I wanted to be treated in the future. I had to let people know that my reasons for behaving a certain way in the past were now changing. On one instance, I wrote in my journal:

> *I allow myself to be treated this way. There's something about my behavior that screams out to other people, "Don't treat Janet special, she can't handle the attention; she doesn't even think she deserves it. She thinks of herself as undeserving, so we'll oblige her. We'll take her for granted." I would not allow this any longer.*

The past 3½ years have included many changes in my life, but perhaps more significant than the weight loss is the fact that I treat myself better in other areas as well. I treat myself better, and as a direct consequence, people treat me better. I am more able to assert myself, to be kind to myself, to forgive myself, and to love myself; I am also more able to love, accept, and forgive my friends and family. I am not responsible for my loved ones, not in the way I imagined I was responsible for them 4 years ago. In a very real sense, losing 90 pounds gave me my freedom.

Handling Food

Because I lived alone, I did not have food in the house, except on those occasions when I entertained at home. On one occasion, I invited my 6-year-old nephew to visit for a week. I had a very real fear of handling food and having it in the house. I thought about my friends in the program who were required to cook every day for their families and wondered if I could do it. It had been relatively easy for me up to now. What if I had to cook every day? How would I handle it? I was soon to find out.

By the eighth week of the VLCD, I had lost 35 pounds, and it was around this time that my nephew came to visit with me. I wrote in my journal:

Hallelujah! Have made it to July. Thank God. This past week I've been to every conceivable type of children's restaurant—to movies, to the theater, to museums, to the Franklin Institute, to Pizza Hut, to see Benji save mountain lion cubs, to cookouts, to swim parties, and through it all, it never occurred to me to eat, that I could have had any of the stuff being eaten. Nor did I want it. But on one occasion I almost slipped. I was offered a drink—rum and Coke—and I'd asked if they had Diet Coke to go with my rum before remembering that I'm not drinking alcohol. That was funny. But food was easy, surprisingly easy, this week.

This was during a week when I had food in the house, when I cooked for my nephew, and when we dined out often, but food was easy. I never thought I'd say that, but not eating was a breeze.

By this time, dining out was not a problem. I could sit in a restaurant and drink my liquid diet or have a cup of tea or bouillon and was fine. I have a blind friend who has a Seeing Eye dog. Once we went to a banquet where this individual was the speaker of the evening. As we drove to the banquet, I asked her how she handled the problem of her dog's being present in a dining room. Did the dog ever beg for food or make a scene? She simply said, "She knows it is not her time to eat." It was so simple. Many times during the VLCD, that phrase recurred to me. When tempted, I had only to remind myself that it was not yet my time to eat. I am not Pavlov's dog. I can restrain myself. I can be in control.

I could be around food and not be bothered by it! I could be sociable with people in the presence of food! I could entertain! I could handle, prepare, and cook food without putting it in my mouth! *What a powerful lesson to learn!*

Transition from Fat Woman to Thin Woman

After having lost around 40 pounds, I began to think of myself as thin. I was far from my goal weight, but due to the exercise and weight loss, I now wore a size 16 dress—a minor miracle, considering that when I started I wore a size 20 or 22. I was enjoying the VLCD and the rapid weight loss, although, in my illogic, the weight loss was never enough. I know this makes no sense. For anyone who has ever dieted successfully, an average weight loss of 4 pounds a week is nothing to disparage. There was, however, an irrational corner in my mind that wanted even more. My more sane and rational mind was very pleased with my progress. It was around this time that I was making the transition to thinking of myself as a thin woman. Once, while walking toward a store window, I saw myself before I recognized myself. And the shock of recognition was "Oh, it's me, and I'm smaller than I remembered." On another occasion, I was out shopping and tried on a size 14 dress that almost fit. I could get into it, and noted:

Boy, was I pleased and shocked. It was a freak. I still wear a size 18 or in the best case scenario a size 16. And I looked great. I can tell I've lost weight when I look at myself in the mirror. Also, I'm acting as if I'm thin.

After losing around 50 pounds, I then began acting like a thin woman. I began to go out more. I felt more attractive. Shopping was absolute joy. Most times I didn't buy anything, but it was exhilarating just trying on clothes. I would try on a dress one week, only to return in a week or two to find that the same dress was too big.

My energy level was high. I was able to do yard work, aerobic walking, dancing, roller skating, just about any activity I could do ordinarily. I did notice that I had less muscle strength, and had long ago stopped the weight training. Also, when carrying groceries from the car into the house, I could not lift and carry as many bags as before. My strength would return to normal after I resumed eating.

Ending the Diet

Toward the end of August, with a little over a week remaining in the VLCD, I went to visit my father in Georgia. In my journal I wrote:

Only a week and a half remaining. Feeling wonderful. Have lost 63 pounds. Want to make it 70 by the 8th of September. That means 7 pounds in 10 days. I can do it.

My sister and I were going to Georgia to visit our dad, and I was looking forward to the trip with a great deal of fear and excitement. I would see relatives I had not seen in quite a long time. And I would see the family farm, perhaps for the last time.

I had been very successful on the liquid diet, and I still wanted to achieve my goal of 70 pounds lost by the end of the VLCD. In order to do that, I reasoned, I would have to step up my exercising to at least 2 hours per day. My calculations told me that 2 hours of walking/cycling would burn up 600–800 kcal/day, and with a resting energy expenditure of approximately 1500 kcal, I could achieve a loss of 2 pounds or more every 3 days. I had 10 days to lose 7 pounds. It would be hard, but I reasoned I just might be able to accomplish it. I was still setting goals.

While we were visiting in Georgia, my Uncle Eddie said, "You've gotten your youthful form back." And my dad said, "Good gosh, girl, I hardly recognized you." He was happy and proud, and he dragged me and my sister around the hamlet of Milledgeville to show us off to every relative and friend. We ate out frequently and cooked a few days. Anyone who is at all familiar with Southern hospitality will confirm that food—high calorie food—is an integral part of that hospitality. I was remarkably okay until the last few days, when I realized that I did not want to sit and watch while others ate. No more. I could handle it; I just didn't want to do it anymore. I think I was anticipating the end of the VLCD and all that it entailed. I had been so successful on this portion of the program, and I was fearful and did not know what to expect in returning to conventional food.

When I returned home, I noted in my journal that I was having more thoughts about food these past few days. I wrote:

I've been thinking about food quite a bit. I won't eat until September 9th or 10th, and even then I'll be eating a very controlled and very limited amount of food. I'm a little afraid.

Refeeding and Stabilization

Finally, finally, after 16 weeks of the VLCD, we were given a suggested menu and the go-ahead to eat solid food. This was on Wednesday, yet I put off the decision to eat until Sunday. I was afraid. Sure, I had to shop and cook and prepare my food, but perhaps more important, I had to prepare myself mentally. More than anything else, I was afraid. I did not eat until Sunday, September 13. I wrote:

I ate food today. Chicken and string beans. It was delicious and consumed rapidly. Eaten quickly and with my fingers on occasion. I left nothing on my plate and could have eaten more, although my physical hunger was sated. I've lost over 70 pounds. I feel and look better than I have in years.

The food, though bland, was delicious. A gourmet feast could not have been more pleasurable for me on the evening of Sunday, September 13, 1987. I ingested solid food. And I was proud of my accomplishment—of following the protocol to the best of my ability. I was not perfect, but I was pretty near perfect in my adherence to the VLCD part of the program. Now I had to confront the fear that I would not do as well on the refeeding part of the program as I had on the liquid diet. On the second day of eating, I wrote:

Ate chicken and string beans again today. Once again, ate rapidly. Was quite hungry. Held off for a while, but ate early 6 P.M. Am quite full now. My body feels sluggish as though trying to digest a large amount of food. Also, I feel tired. The liquid diet was easier—absolutely no choice. I enjoyed my food today, although the necessity of choosing wisely and planning calories does frighten me a lot. I'm upstairs in the bedroom where it seems safer. I feel stuffed.

The recurring themes in my journal during the early days of refeeding were fear, my inability to be perfect, and staying away from food as much as possible. I made a conscious decision to deal with food as little as possible, to stay out of the kitchen as much as possible, and not to re-excite long-dormant taste buds.

But refeeding was "messy." There was no chance to be "perfect." During the 6-week refeeding phase of the program, I continued to lose weight; by Thanksgiving, I had lost an additional 20 pounds. In our group, there were varying degrees of success during refeeding. It was during this time that we were all acutely aware of our task. We were all struggling publicly with the issues of how much weight loss is enough, how much food is enough, how much exercise is enough. Meanwhile, our bodies were going through a physiological readjustment to solid food.

It was around this time—Thanksgiving, to be specific—that I was most fearful. I didn't want to have to cook. I didn't want to have to entertain. I didn't want food in my home. My daughter, whom I had not seen since the summer, was coming home from college, and I wrote in my journal:

I'm afraid that Donna will be disappointed when she sees me after all this dieting. I'm still nothing special—not to anyone.

On Thanksgiving morning, I awoke early and went to the track to race-walk for an hour. I came home and finished the last-minute preparations for the big dinner, and when my daughter walked through the door, she was so pleased with my appearance. She kept smiling and saying over and over again, "Mommy, you look wonderful!" and "I'm so proud of you!"

Yes, refeeding was difficult. The issues we discussed and argued over most during the meetings were the fuzziness of the guidelines, the inability of any governing authority to tell us with 100% certainty what to do and how to do it—what to eat and when to eat it. It was so unlike the VLCD we had all done so well on. We were moving from the liquid diet, where a "perfect" day by definition consisted of drinking five shakes and 2 quarts of water, period. Refeeding, by definition, had no such rigid parameters, nor did it have, by definition, the possibility of perfection. We would have to learn to make choices. And making choices meant sometimes choosing unwisely. We would have to learn, and the learning would go on quite publicly. Unwise food choices could, and in some cases did, lead to weight gain.

As exhilarating as the VLCD part of this comprehensive 18-month program was, it was what happened during the following 14 months that proved critical and most life-changing for me. It was during the weekly and then biweekly meetings that I learned the things that have served me well in my ongoing weight maintenance efforts.

Perhaps the most critical thing that I learned was simply learned through showing up at meetings, especially when I was struggling, doing poorly, or even gaining weight. It was in the meetings that I was to discover that weight gain can be reversed, but that first I must honestly confront it. I learned that my past success was just that, past; in order for me to be an ongoing success, I could not rest on my laurels, on yesterday's accomplishments. I learned to take courage from my successes, but more significantly, I discovered how to learn from my failures.

We were all in transition, and that transition, I believe, was designed to enable us all to function on our own, to become our own experts, to become our own coaches. It was hard. During this time, one individual in particular was struggling with the issue of perfection, and I wrote to her. But I think I was writing more to myself. The letter read:

> *I've wanted to write to you for quite some time, but kept putting it off. You see, I wanted to perfectly express my genuine concern and love for you. Yes, love. In the past when discussing our group with my daughter, she has remarked that I speak of individual group members with such affection that it seems as though I'm talking about family. And in many respects, you are my family. So I want you to know of my admiration for your courage. I want to thank you for your support and encouragement and to acknowledge your perseverance.*
>
> *These past weeks have been fraught with struggle and fear and a desire, if only temporary, to throw in the towel, to pull the sheets up over my head, to bury my head in the sand. It passed, but it terrified me. I've begun to realize more now than ever that I'm socially backward in many situations. My view has been that of a fat woman, so egocentric, and so concerned about how people are going to react to me as a fat woman. And my perspective has not changed. All the energy expended on protecting and defending me as a "fat woman" still insists on doing that same job. Eventually I'll have to learn how to act like a "thin person." And for me that means learning to be more at ease in social settings that I've avoided heretofore. It means stepping into the unknown, or, more accurately, a leap of faith into the unknown. It means fully realizing that what ails me will not be solved by more food, that my existential angst will not be resolved by eating more food, that my life's dilemma does not lend itself to*

> solution by gluttony (stuffing myself into unconsciousness). It means fully knowing, to paraphrase Søren Kierkegaard, that nothing is ever solved once and for all, forever. Every day, I will be faced with the same inexorable dialectic—to overeat or not to overeat. To wallow in self-pity or not to wallow in self-pity. To forgive myself or not to forgive myself. To simply get on with it or not to get on with it. And this frightens me! The word that keeps recurring is "transition." I feel in a state of flux right now, uncertain even of my own physical boundaries, and the most secure place, the most supportive people for me right now, are my fellow group members. It is in these meetings that I have felt accepted at 263 pounds, at 230 pounds, at 170 pounds—at whatever weight. I have felt accepted when I was self-punishing. I have felt accepted when I was judgmental. I have felt accepted when I shared parts of my life that had been buried under layers of shame and fat—things never shared with another human being. I have always felt accepted. And because I was always accepted, notwithstanding my imperfections, it has become a little easier to love and accept myself. It makes it possible for me to tell others that I love them, however imperfectly expressed it may come out.

During the 14 months after the VLCD, my weight stabilized. After a year, I had regained approximately 20 of the 90 pounds I had lost, but—and this is crucial—I had the experience and the information available to me that proved I could maintain a large weight loss. Even though I had regained 20 pounds, my weight remained stable. It was as though my body had decided that this was the weight I was able and willing to maintain at this point in my life. As the formal 18-month program ended, I knew I could and indeed one day would achieve my goal weight of 165 pounds. I was happy with my efforts. I knew I was doing the best I possibly could do with my weight management efforts. I never compromised on my goal weight, and today, 4 years later, I have achieved and am maintaining my goal weight. This is the result of a 4-year learning cycle, and I'm still learning.

Living with Weight Loss

Dealing with Temptation

There are days when every cell in my body cries out to eat—to eat the ice cream, the potato chips, the overstuffed sandwiches, the junk stuff. Nothing healthy, just junk food. It is on these days that I must call on every available tool in my arsenal to get me through the temptation. I believe, after undergoing 3½ years of successful weight management, that I can survive most temptation with a good plan and strategies to keep my eye on my goal.

There have been days when I've actually driven to the pizza parlor or to the convenience store and parked and was about to go inside to place my order, but instead managed to sit quietly in the car and focus my attention on what I was doing and how it would affect my goals. Not only my goals of weight management, but the other goals: What do I want out of life? How do I want to live my life? How do I want to feel? What do I want to look like? If I give in to this particular temptation, will I be less able to face the next temptation? For if there is a surety to weight management, it is this: There will always be another temptation, another time to "go off my eating plan, just this once." For me, the three little words "just this once" had led in the past to a weight just shy of 270 pounds.

There are many days when eating according to my maintenance plan is very easy and requires very little thought and effort. As a matter of fact, most of my days fall into this category. The critical times, however, for me are those days when I am tempted. What do I do then? When I am tempted and caught up in the moment, and when I have not made the final decision to put the food into my mouth and chew (but rather am engaged in a titillating game of food foreplay), there is still hope. When caught up in this game, I begin to imagine what the particular food will taste like, wandering up and down the supermarket aisles, eyeballing it, trying to decide if I should buy it. When I am just being a "food tease" and have not brought the offending food into my home, then there is hope. Once I have made the decision to purchase the food, it is practically a surety that I will eat it. So my first rule in weight management is to stay out of harm's way.

I do the things we are all told to do, but few follow. *Never—I repeat, never—shop when hungry!* An ancillary rule is this: Always, always have a backup meal in the house that may be prepared and eaten at a moment's notice. This cannot be overemphasized. Without a safe meal available at home, I have found myself wandering up and down the supermarket aisles, tired and hungry, searching for something for dinner, perhaps some chicken and fresh vegetables. Strangely, my cart is brimming over with chips and dip, as well as pretzels and peanuts and ice cream. So, I try to stay out of places with tempting foods when I am too hungry to make good food decisions.

After surviving the initial impulse to purchase or eat a food not on my eating plan, and after safely navigating the rocky shoals and siren calls, next I must refocus my attention on what it is I am trying to do. For me, what I am trying to do adds up to more than simply resisting a pint of ice cream. Resisting temptation, although necessary in a successful weight management plan, has a negative connotation. It's about what I'm not getting. It's about deprivation. So I've developed some tools that enable me to refocus on what I'm getting. What am I trying to do? Indeed, what am I getting in return for eating in a rational and balanced manner?

Simply put, I like the way I look and feel when I am thin. I've developed a lifestyle that requires me to be thin to enjoy all its benefits. I do things at a lower weight that I would be unable to do if heavier, or at least would be less able to do (e.g, roller skating, acting in amateur drama productions, participating in and winning racewalks). And I—not my doctor, not my parents, not my lover, not my daughter, but I—have determined what is thin enough for me. I have determined how much fitness I am able and willing to work for.

Focusing on My Goals

As a formerly obese person, how do I keep my memory green? How do I keep my attention focused on my goal of weight maintenance? I reread old "fat journals" to remind myself of how miserable I once was and never want to be again. I look at old pictures and videotapes of myself at a weight in excess of 200 pounds, and I look at my more recent pictures. It is in these new pictures that I have before my eyes tangible evidence of how I look today and how I want to continue looking. I have invested in weight loss and weight maintenance, and I realize that there is a price to pay. For today, I am willing to pay that price.

Don't let anyone lie to you or try to fool you. Yes, there is a price to pay in terms of exercise and moderate eating. I know full well that on any given day I may decide that I no longer wish to pay the price necessary to maintain my lower weight, and that if and when I make that decision, the sure result will be weight gain. I suffer no delusions about that.

I know my obesity is arrested for this day, and I know that it requires zeal and extra effort on my part. Some people who do not understand this point have accused me of becoming a zealot on issues of health and weight management, and somewhat abnormal. Perhaps my efforts are "abnormal." Rather, I'd like to think of my attempts as analogous to the training required of an athlete or a ballet dancer. It is not normal behavior to dance around on the points of one's toes, yet dancers do just that. They train their bodies and minds to perform the pirouettes and arabesques that make up the art of ballet. Nor is it "natural" or the norm for sprinters to run the 100-yard dash in times under 10 seconds; yet it is done. It is done because people, albeit naturally talented, have pushed and trained themselves because they have wanted it enough to make the sacrifices necessary to attain it. For me, the "it" I work to attain is a normal body weight. I walk for 45 minutes at least four times per week—sometimes more, rarely less—and I moderate my eating.

For me and the thousands of other individuals who work hard to lose and maintain that weight loss, there are no accolades, no victor's garland, no curtain calls or encores. As a matter of fact, quite the contrary is true. My quotidian efforts to maintain a large weight loss are often greeted with comments from unknowing friends and associates who wonder, "Are you regaining weight?" Or "Why so much walking; are you training for the Olympics?" Sometimes as I racewalk around my neighborhood, strangers will comment, "Keep it up, you'll lose that weight." And I think to myself, "If they only knew."

On occasion, when a stranger has spoken to me, I've felt compelled to stop long enough to explain that I have lost a substantial amount of weight and that

I'm trying to maintain that weight loss. Often, people who are exercising on an ongoing basis just to maintain a large weight loss get little respect from the general public. Despite public knowledge that weight loss all too often is followed by weight regain, people still don't understand the exercise connection. In addition, because my weight loss on the liquid diet was so public, so too is my struggle to maintain my weight loss.

For the athlete there will be medals and applause. But for the individual working to maintain a large weight loss, the only reward is staying the same. So, being successful at weight maintenance requires that you become an expert on yourself, that you become your own coach and cheerleader. Tom Landry, the former coach of the Dallas Cowboys, was quoted as saying that a coach's job "is to get people to do what they don't want to do to achieve what they want to achieve." Everybody wants to be successful, but not everybody wants to pay the price to be successful. Just substitute the word "thin" for "successful," and you have the definition of the successful weight management coach.

Through the comprehensive 18-month weight loss study, and through my ongoing reading and experience, I have learned some coaching tricks that I can use to motivate myself. I have learned to monitor my efforts—writing down what I eat, keeping an exercise log, shopping tips, dining-out aids—and I have also learned that when my efforts at self-coaching fall short, it is imperative that I look for a coach outside myself to help me get back on track. Otherwise, I fall into "dieter's denial." I continue eating out of control; I shun the scale only to awaken one morning, jump on the scale, and exclaim, "Oh, my God, when did I gain 30 pounds?" I have discovered some people and organizations that help me get a grip when all my efforts are insufficient.

Weight Watchers

I have found Weight Watchers to be the least expensive way to get honest, to be monitored, to be reminded of what I already know—that is, calorie intake and exercise must create a negative caloric balance in order to lose weight. Weight Watchers, because of its structure, affords me an opportunity to eat a regimented, well-balanced, healthy diet.

Overeaters Anonymous

I have found Overeaters Anonymous less helpful to me, because when I am in meetings all I can think of is how I could better use the time for a good walk or a workout at the spa, rather than listening to a lot of talk about losing abstinence. Bear in mind that not all meetings are the same, but those I attended had a disproportionate number of people who were having a great deal of difficulty. Also, I think that in my heart I do not believe I am a compulsive overeater. I do believe I have aberrant eating behavior, but I also know that there are other components to my weight (i.e., genetics, sex, race, basal metabolism, and exercise or the lack thereof), and that these components are as important as the amounts and kinds of food I do or do not eat. Although for me Overeaters Anonymous has been less helpful in my weight maintenance efforts, I do endorse it with an important proviso: Be diligent to find a group in which you feel comfortable. If you feel at all uncomfortable about a group's consciousness, trust your judgment. Find another meeting.

Friends

I have two good friends with whom I can discuss anything, including my weight. One of them went through the liquid diet program, and when I talk to her it's like talking to a sister. We share our feelings and hopes, our despairs and triumphs. I can be as honest with her as with anyone I know. She has given me her friendship, and whether I am up 10 or 15 pounds or down 20, I can talk to her openly and honestly.

My Therapist

When the weight loss program ended after 18 full months, I found that my weight had stabilized, even though it was a little higher than I had hoped for. A family member was in a great deal of distress, and I found my moderate eating and healthy behaviors going out the window. How, I reasoned, could I be so self-absorbed as to worry about my weight at a time like this? Well, I learned through seeing a caring and gifted therapist that times like this will always be with me in one form or another. There is always stress. My choice is how to handle it to minimize its damaging effects.

Prayer and Faith

When times are the hardest, I hold on in faith, simply remembering my track record of success. When I am discouraged or saddened that my efforts have fallen far short of the mark, I press on to the goal anyhow. I love and respect myself. I am gentle and kind to myself. Self-abnegation and mean-spiritedness never worked for me. Today, my faith tells me that God loves me anyhow, and that I am perfectly okay, whether I weigh 165 pounds or whether I weigh 250 pounds. I attempt to be the best person possible, and to utilize the talents God has given me—not to bury them or squander them through misuse, but to do the tasks I have chosen to do to the best of my ability. Outside judgment is inescapable, but my internal judgment is more critical.

Self-Trust

I do not put myself down. Nor am I self-effacing. I am not self-critical, nor do I discount compliments and acknowledgments from people whose opinions I respect. This gentle self-acceptance has sustained me when the outside world has been unkind or critical or mean or uncaring. It enables me to begin again, and as I stated earlier, most of successful weight management is simply beginning again.

I know that my own biology, my genetics, my sex, and even my race affect my weight. I have learned that women, more than men, tend to be obese; that women who have borne children tend to be heavier than those who have not; and that women whose parents (but particularly whose mothers) were obese have a greater chance of becoming obese. I know that African-American women, more than Caucasian women, have a greater tendency toward obesity. Yet, notwithstanding my genetic inheritance, I know it is possible for me to attain and maintain my goal weight—at a price. I know that you can't buy fitness with money. If the answer were money, Oprah Winfrey, Liz Taylor, and Roseanne Barr Arnold would be fat-free for life. You cannot buy fitness, but fitness does cost.

Nor is intellect the answer. I have a brilliant friend with a PhD in psychology who is no more able because of her intellect to conquer her fat than are the rest of us. So if the answer is neither money nor brains, what is it? I think it is willingness. The willingness to investigate what it will cost for you to be thin, and then the willingness to pay that price which sometimes entails sacrifice. It is a willingness to face the unfairness of it all—the genetic crap shoot that perhaps gave you "fat genes." It is a willingness not to be lied to, but to be told the brutal, frank truth: *The prognosis for weight loss/weight maintenance is not good, but it is not impossible. Weight loss/weight maintenance is do-able. It is possible.* So, what will you do to achieve it? I have told you what I will do.

PART FIVE

MAINTENANCE OF WEIGHT LOSS AND ALTERNATIVE THERAPIES

18

Relapse and the Treatment of Obesity

KELLY D. BROWNELL

"95% of the people who lose weight will regain it."
"It is easy to lose weight; keeping it off is the hard part."

These statements appear time and time again in the popular press and are probably the most widely heard refrains about the treatment of obesity. Writers from the national press who contact experts often begin their interview with a statement such as this: "Since 95% of people regain weight, what can be done, or why diet at all?"

This sentiment is also expressed in the scientific literature. In 1959, Stunkard and McLaren-Hume published a paper that declared, "Most obese persons will not stay in treatment. Of those who stay in treatment, most will not lose weight, and of those who do lose weight, most will regain it" (p. 79). This is probably the most often quoted statement in the obesity literature, which led in the 1980s to the paper's designation as a "Citation Classic" by the Institute of Scientific Information.

One would assume from this gloomy picture that nearly all dieters fail, and that scientists and the public alike know the exact extent of the problem. This chapter will deal with several fundamental issues related to this topic. First, the genesis of the commonly used relapse figures will be discussed, and information will be presented to show that the numbers may be incorrect. Second, an approach will be presented for conceptualizing the process and prevention of relapse. Information on determinants and predictors of relapse will be provided, research needs will be identified, and intervention strategies will be discussed. The picture I hope to paint in this chapter is more optimistic than one might predict from the statements above.

Relapse Rates and What They Mean

The Early Reports

The report by Stunkard and McLaren-Hume in 1959 had an enormous impact on the field. They studied 100 patients treated for obesity in a hospital nutrition clinic. Only 12% of the patients lost 20 pounds or more, and only 6% maintained a 20-pound loss a year after treatment. The authors concluded that 95% of dieters regain weight within 5 years of treatment.

When we hear of the 95% failure rate, this is its origin. It is from a study conducted more than three decades ago, using treatments that bear little resemblance to modern-day techniques. At the time, the paper portrayed the state of the art; however, it may be a mistake to persist in using these numbers.

Current Data

A number of reviews and follow-up studies are now available to determine the long-term effectiveness of different diet programs. Very low calorie diets (VLCDs) and behavior therapy have been the most extensively tested approaches.

My colleagues and I (Brownell & Wadden, 1986; Brownell & Kramer, 1989) have summarized the results of behavioral approaches, as shown in Table 18.1. In the studies reviewed from 1986, the average weight loss after treatment of 16.7 weeks was 10 kg. The average loss at an average follow-up of 44 weeks was 6.6 kg, or 66% of the initial weight loss. These studies obtained much greater initial losses and better maintenance than would be suggested by the report of Stunkard and McLaren-Hume (1959).

Wadden and colleagues have done the longest and most extensive follow-up evaluations in their study of VLCDs and behavior therapy (Wadden,

TABLE 18.1. Summary of Data from Controlled Trials of Behavior Therapy Completed before and during 1974, and during 1978, 1984, and 1986

	1974	1978	1984	1986
Number of studies included (%)	15	17	15	6
Sample size	53.1	54.0	71.3	93.3
Initial weight (lb)	163.0	194.0	197.0	210.6
Initial percentage overweight	49.4	48.6	48.1	53.4
Length of treatment (wk)	8.4	10.5	13.2	16.7
Weight loss (lb)	8.5	9.4	15.4	22.0
Loss per week (lb)	1.2	0.9	1.2	1.4
Attrition (%)	11.4	12.9	10.6	20.7
Length of follow-up (wk)	15.5	30.3	58.4	44.0
Loss at follow-up (lb)	8.9	9.1	9.8	14.5

Note. All values are means across studies. Studies are those appearing in *Journal of Consulting and Clinical Psychology, Behavior Therapy, Behaviour Research and Therapy,* and *Addictive Behaviors.* The data are from Brownell and Wadden (1986) and Brownell and Kramer (1989).

TABLE 18.2. Percentage of Patients Losing 5 or 10 kg or More in Trial of Diet and Behavior Therapy

	End of therapy	1-year follow-up	3-year follow-up	5-year follow-up
Diet alone				
Lost 5 kg	96%	52%	33%	11%
Lost 10 kg	74%	14%	27%	11%
Behavior therapy				
Lost 5 kg	96%	55%	29%	13%
Lost 10 kg	64%	23%	7%	0%
Combined therapy				
Lost 5 kg	97%	55%	44%	27%
Lost 10 kg	90%	52%	31%	9%

Note. Data on initial loss and 1-year follow-up are from Wadden and Stunkard (1986). Data on the 3-year follow-up are from Wadden et al. (1988) and for the 5-year follow-up are from Wadden et al. (1989).

Sternberg, Letizia, Stunkard, & Foster, 1989; Wadden & Stunkard, 1986; Wadden, Stunkard, & Liebschutz, 1988). In their primary study, patients were randomly assigned to a VLCD alone, behavior therapy alone, or their combination (Wadden & Stunkard, 1986).

The data from this study and the follow-up papers are summarized in Table 18.2. Several conclusions may be drawn from these data (Wadden et al., 1989). First, initial weight losses and maintenance of loss at a 1-year follow-up are clearly superior to earlier results. In addition, behavior therapy was effective at maintaining some of the loss produced by the VLCD. At the 1-year follow-up, 32% of patients in the combined treatment maintained all of their weight loss, compared to 5% for the VLCD alone. The results deteriorated in the ensuing years, such that by the 5-year evaluation, the mean weight of patients in all three conditions had returned to baseline. Some patients, however, were able to maintain some or all of their weight loss. Of the total sample, 18% maintained a loss of 0.1–5 kg, and 18% maintained a loss greater than 5 kg; 5% of the sample maintained their entire weight loss.

Several other studies have evaluated the long-term results of VLCDs combined with behavior therapy. Hovell et al. (1988) studied patients in a health maintenance organization. Of the patients who completed the program, the average person lost 84% of excess weight. Mean weight losses were 28.6 kg for males and 24.5 kg for females. By a 30-month follow-up, 59–82% of the excess weight had been regained. Andersen, Stokholm, Backer, and Quaade (1988) followed 30 subjects who lost weight on a VLCD. At a 5-year follow-up, only 5 subjects (17%) had not relapsed (had maintained less than a 10-kg loss). In another study with a 2-year follow-up, patients on VLCD alone regained all but 0.8 kg, and subjects on VLCD plus exercise were still 9.1 kg below their starting weight (Sikand, Kondo, Foreyt, Jones, & Gotto, 1988).

Relatively few studies, other than those just mentioned, have had follow-up evaluations of more than 1 year. The findings on initial loss and 1-year maintenance have been replicated in other studies, particularly in the series by Perri and colleagues, which are described in detail in the next chapter (Perri, 1987; Perri et al., 1988; Perri, Lauer, McAdoo, McAllister, & Yancey, 1986; Perri, Shapiro, Ludwig, Twentyman, & McAdoo, 1984). More work is needed to determine whether the 5-year results reported by Wadden et al. (1989) are the rule or the exception.

It does appear that there has been great improvement in initial weight losses and maintenance as long as 1 year, compared to the data of Stunkard and McLaren-Hume (1959). Follow-up evaluations as long as 5 years yield better results, but are still discouraging. It would appear that treatments are improving, but that further improvement is clearly needed. The suggestions given later in this chapter, and the information provided in Chapter 19 by Perri, highlight the new developments that may lead to improved results.

Data on Self-Cure

Relatively little is known about people who change their behavior without the aid of formal programs. Given this fact, combined with the lack of data on the effectiveness of commercial and self-help programs, little can be said about the vast majority of people who lose weight.

Schachter (1982) attempted to address this issue of self-cure in a study of self-quitting smokers and of individuals who had lost weight and kept it off. He interviewed 83 members of the Department of Psychology at Columbia University, and 78 entrepreneurs and working people from a resort community on Long Island. These persons reported substantially higher rates of success with both smoking and obesity than one would expect from the scientific literature. Schachter concluded that the self-cure rate was two to three times higher than that reported for clinic programs. Comparable findings were reported in a replication with 92 members of the Department of Psychology at the University of Vermont (Rzewnicki & Forgays, 1987).

Schachter's methods of data collection were weak and his sample was quite selective, so it is not surprising that his methods have been criticized (Jeffery & Wing, 1983; Prochaska, 1983). Population-based surveys (Jeffery et al., 1984) or prospective studies would provide better means of data collection. As an example, Cohen et al. (1989) reported data from 10 long-term prospective studies with more than 5000 self-quitting smokers, and found that success rates were no better than those for formal treatment programs. Therefore, the rates of self-cure that Schachter described may or may not be accurate. The main contribution of his paper was to emphasize the fact that cure rates derived from clinical studies may be very different from rates for people losing weight with nonclinical methods.

Interpreting Relapse Rates

Interpreting relapse rates and making inferences about treatment effectiveness can be a difficult process. As an example, the cry is now loud for long-term follow-up studies of treatments for obesity. In the 1970s, a 3-month follow-up was sufficient for publication of results, but now a 1-year evaluation is the minimum. Many investigators believe that even longer follow-up evaluations are necessary, because individuals may be able to sustain their losses for 1 year but not longer.

This demand for long-term surveillance creates several problems. In studies where the investigators are fortunate enough to maintain contact for such long periods, patients are brought in for weigh-ins at intervals of 6 or even 12 months. These "snapshot" weights provide little information about what occurs between assessments, so that people may gain or lose weight unknown to investigators.

Another problem lies in interpreting group averages, which can be deceiving if patients are examined only once per year. As an example, let us say that 20% of subjects in a weight reduction study lost at least 20 kg at 1 year, and that the same 20% figure was reported at 2 years. This would suggest good maintenance of the loss among the 20%. However, different subjects might comprise this group at each assessment. Some people might regain and thus drop out of the successful group, while others might lose and drop in.

Attributing long-term results to a specific intervention can also be complicated. Many patients use self-imposed diets, commercial or self-help programs, diet books, exercise programs, and other approaches both during and after the time they may be in a formal research program. Wadden and colleagues reported follow-up data on subjects involved in their study of behavior modification and VLCDs (Wadden & Stunkard, 1986). At a 3-year follow-up, more than 40% of the subjects had received additional therapy for weight reduction; the number increased to 55% at a 5-year follow-up (Wadden et al., 1988; 1989). If a woman begins a program at 80 kg, loses to 65 kg, and then 5 years later is still at 65 kg, is the program responsible? The question is not easily answered if she undertook other programs in the interim, which is likely to have been the case.

Perhaps the most difficult aspect of evaluating long-term results is selecting the appropriate reference point (Brownell & Jeffery, 1987). When many people interpret long-term weight loss figures, they use an unspoken reference point that may not be correct. Let us say that the average weight loss for a particular study is 15 kg after treatment and 5 kg at a 2-year follow-up. This is likely to be viewed as a discouraging result because two-thirds of the lost weight was regained, and the average person was only 5 kg better off because of the program. This assumes, however, that the individuals in the program would have maintained a steady weight if they had never been treated. This assumes an understanding of the natural history of weight loss that cannot be supported by data.

It is quite possible that obese persons gain weight if no intervention occurs. This possible outcome is represented by line A in Figure 18.1. Should this be true, even complete weight regain must be viewed in a more favorable light if the alternative of no treatment would have been associated with substantial weight gain. This is a radical perspective, which also cannot be supported by data. The appropriate studies of the natural history of weight change must be conducted so that we can interpret the effects of treatment over the long term.

Fortunately, these problems in interpreting long-term data can be remedied by methodological improvements. Lack of knowledge of weight changes between infrequent measurements can be remedied by more frequent assess-

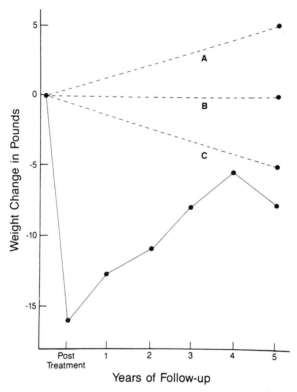

FIGURE 18.1. Mean weight change in weight loss programs plotted against hypothetical outcomes of a reference group consisting of individuals who received no treatment (lines A, B, and C.). Line A represents the natural history of obese persons receiving no treatment as gradual weight gain, line B shows stable weight, and line C shows gradual loss. Interpreting long-term weight loss must be done with an appreciation of the appropriate reference group. From "Improving Long-Term Weight Loss: Pushing the Limits of Treatment" (p. 355) by K. D. Brownell and R. W. Jeffery, 1987, *Behavior Therapy*, *18*, 353–374. Copyright 1987 by Association for Advancement of Behavior Therapy. Reprinted by permission.

ments. Determination of whether individuals embark on other weight loss efforts during follow-up evaluation can be accomplished by more thorough assessment. Having the appropriate reference group can be achieved through population studies of the natural history of weight change.

Conclusions about Relapse Rates

For the reasons mentioned above, relapse rates can be difficult to interpret. It is fashionable to call for follow-up periods of up to 5 years, but without knowledge of what occurs between assessments, and without the proper comparison groups, the figures will have little meaning. Even with this limitation, however, we can draw some conclusions about the prevailing rates of relapse in weight loss programs.

The 95% relapse rate figure that is so frequently cited is from a study conducted in the 1950s, with little confirming evidence in the meantime. Data from reviews of clinical studies show much more encouraging figures, but it is still true that relatively few people achieve sustained weight loss. The advent of comprehensive behavioral programs, along with the increasing recognition that exercise is helpful for maintenance, should continue to improve long-term success rates.

Almost everything known about relapse comes from clinical studies. Such studies use intensive interventions and work with highly selected samples. One can assume that most patients in clinical studies are heavier, more secure financially (because of relatively high fees), and perhaps more desperate about their problem than the average person who diets using other methods.

These data from clinical programs could either underestimate or overestimate success rates in general (Brownell, Marlatt, Lichtenstein, & Wilson, 1986). An underestimation could occur if rates in clinics are low because the most difficult cases are seen. An overestimation could occur if clinic rates are relatively high because the most powerful treatments are used. My belief is that clinic results underestimate rates of success, but this can only be tested with more studies on nonclinic samples.

Conceptualizing the Relapse Process

The Importance of Conceptual Work

Developing theoretical and conceptual frameworks from which to view relapse is important from both clinical and research perspectives. From a clinical perspective, the way we deal with relapse in our patients is driven by why we believe it occurs, and whether we believe it can be prevented or corrected. Researchers, in turn, test interventions that are derived from their conceptual views of relapse.

Since the mid-1980s, important advances have been made in theories on relapse. Three distinct steps in this process can be noted. First, Marlatt and Gordon (1985) published an important book (entitled *Relapse Prevention*), in which they proposed that relapse is a process rather than an outcome, and provided a conceptual framework from which to view this process. This work has had a positive impact on treatment programs for obesity.

The second advance is the work of Prochaska, DiClemente, and colleagues, who developed and refined a model depicting the stages of change individuals undergo as they attempt to modify behavior (DiClemente et al., 1991; Prochaska & DiClemente, 1982; Prochaska, DiClemente, & Norcross, in press; Prochaska, DiClemente, Velicer, Ginpil, & Norcross, 1985; Prochaska, Norcross, Fowler, Follick, & Abrams, in press; Prochaska, Velicer, DiClemente, & Fava, 1988).

The third advance is the increasing recognition of the value of integrating information on relapse from various disorders, including obesity, smoking, alcoholism, and compulsive gambling (Brownell et al., 1986; Marlatt & Gordon, 1985). This has led to interaction across areas and advances in both theory and intervention.

This theoretical and conceptual work will be used throughout the remainder of this chapter to provide a framework for understanding the relapse process. As is the case in various areas of the addictions, treatments and research studies on relapse prevention have, for the most part, not been driven by theory. The situation is changing, however, and the field will proceed more rapidly as a result.

The Process of Relapse

Marlatt and Gordon's (1985) model was among the first to depict relapse as a process that occurs in response to a specific series of cognitions and behaviors. Their model integrates the individual's environment, situational factors, cognitive function, and self-efficacy (Bandura, 1977).

Figure 18.2 shows our (Brownell & Rodin, 1990) adaptation of Marlatt and Gordon's work. The adaptation was made to specify the model to eating problems. The model begins with an individual's exposure to a high risk situation in which overeating is likely to occur. The individual can follow one of two paths, depending on whether coping skills have been learned to deal with the risk. Path 1 in the model shows a positive outcome. The individual has the necessary skills to avoid overeating; this prevents a lapse, which in turn increases confidence (self-efficacy), which leads to long-term control. Path 2 shows a different outcome. In this case, the individual does not possess the skills and thus lapses; this decreases confidence and leads to more eating. Relapse and collapse can be the final result.

The model proposed by Marlatt and Gordon (1985) has had an important impact on the field. It has underscored the fact that relapse occurs as a process,

THE PROCESS OF LAPSE AND RELAPSE

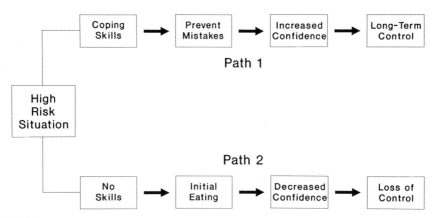

FIGURE 18.2. A cognitive-behavioral model of the relapse process, beginning with exposure to a high risk situation. Path 1 depicts successful coping with risk, leading to increased confidence and decreased probability of relapse. Path 2 depicts increased probability of relapse due to lack of coping skills. This model is adapted to apply to obesity from a model developed by Marlatt and Gordon (1985). From *The Weight Maintenance Survival Guide* (p. 37) by K. D. Brownell and J. Rodin, 1990, Dallas: American Health Publishing Co. Copyright 1990 by American Health Publishing Co. Reprinted by permission.

that there are both cognitive and behavioral components to the process, and that coping skills form the key junction determining whether a person follows a path with a positive or negative outcome. The model has stimulated much research and is also useful for clinical reasons. Showing patients the scheme depicted in Figure 18.2 can be helpful in depicting that risk does not mean inevitable failure and that learning new skills is the key to change.

Stages and Processes of Change

Behavior change in areas such as weight loss and smoking cessation has typically been viewed as a dichotomous outcome. A person either succeeds or fails, maintains weight or relapses. Prochaska, DiClemente, and colleagues have undertaken a series of studies showing that the process of behavior change can be broken down into a series of stages (e.g., DiClemente et al., 1991; Prochaska, DiClemente, & Norcross, in press). They propose two interrelated dimensions by which behavior changes. The first dimension is stages of change. These stages represent the temporal, motivational, and stability aspects of change (Prochaska, DiClemente, & Norcross, in press). The stages are "precontemplation," "contemplation," "action," and "maintenance." The definitions of these stages that follow are adapted from Prochaska, DiClemente, and Norcross (in press):

1. *Precontemplation.* The stage in which people do not intend to change behavior in the near future. Some people are unaware of their problems or deny their problems, while others are simply unwilling to change.

2. *Contemplation.* At this stage, people are aware that a problem exists and are thinking about changing it. Contemplation is necessary for change but may not be sufficient, and people can often remain in this stage for extended periods.

3. *Action.* This is the stage in which individuals modify their behavior and environment to remedy their problem. Much activity and energy is required in this stage, and this is when the efforts to change are most visible.

4. *Maintenance.* This stage occurs when people work to prevent relapse and to consolidate changes made during the action stage. This period can last for months or years.

One key aspect of the stage model is that the stages occur in a cyclic as opposed to a linear fashion (see Figure 18.3). Prochaska, DiClemente, and Norcross (in press) explain this process:

> The cyclical pattern . . . illustrates how most people actually move through the stages of change. In this cyclical pattern, people progress from contemplation to action to maintenance, but most individuals relapse. During re-

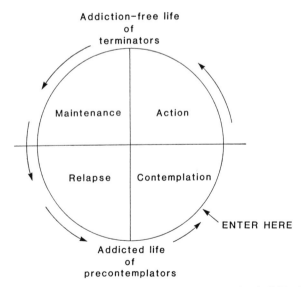

FIGURE 18.3. A cyclic model of stages of change. The model shows that individuals who relapse return to earlier stages of change. This scheme is consistent with the finding that "cures" often occur in people who have changed and relapsed many times previously. From "In Search of How People Change" by J. O. Prochaska, C. C. DiClemente, and J. C. Norcross, in press, *American Psychologist*. Reprinted by permission of the authors.

lapse, individuals regress to an earlier stage. Some relapsers feel like failures—embarrassed, ashamed and guilty. These individuals become demoralized and don't want to think about changing. As a result, they return to the precontemplation stage and can remain there for various periods of time.... Fortunately, our research indicates that the vast majority of relapsers—85% of smokers for example—recycle back to the contemplation stage.... They begin to make plans for their next action attempt and try to learn from their recent efforts.

This cyclic model has implications for both research and treatment. From the research perspective, it is important to examine which stages individuals return to if they do relapse. From a treatment perspective, relapse is not necessarily an end-stage event, if the person cycles back to a stage in which future change is possible. This can influence how professionals deal with patients when they do relapse, and in turn, how the patients feel about themselves and their future.

The second dimension represents processes of change (Table 18.3). In contrast to the stages, which show *when* specific changes occur, the processes show *how* change occurs. The 10 processes shown in Table 18.3 are derived from a "transtheoretical" analysis, in which aspects of behavior change were examined across different types of therapy and across different types of psychological and addictive problems (Prochaska, 1979).

The processes outlined by Prochaska, DiClemente, and Norcross (in press) are thought to exist to different degrees, depending on the target problem.

TABLE 18.3. Stages of Change and Processes of Change for Individuals Changing Personal Behavior

Stages of change
1. Precontemplation
2. Contemplation
3. Action
4. Maintenance

Processes of change
1. Consciousness raising
2. Self-re-evaluation
3. Self-liberation
4. Counterconditioning
5. Stimulus control
6. Reinforcement management
7. Helping relationships
8. Dramatic relief
9. Environmental re-evaluation
10. Social liberation

Note. Adapted from "In Search of How People Change" by J. O. Prochaska, C. C. DiClemente, and J. C. Norcross, in press, *American Psychologist.* Adapted by permission of the authors.

Individuals with psychological distress rely most on helping relationships and consciousness raising, while overweight individuals rely more on self-liberation and stimulus control (Prochaska & DiClemente, 1985).

The stages and processes of change provide a theoretical framework for examining the natural course of behavior change and relapse, and also for developing intervention programs. Much of the application of the model, however, has taken place in the area of smoking. More extensive application to the field of obesity may help improve long-term results. Suggestions for doing this appear later in this chapter, in the sections on research needs and suggestions for intervention.

Can Different Relapse Models Be Integrated?

The two prevailing models in the relapse area are the Marlatt and Gordon (1985) model of the process of relapse, and the work of Prochaska, DiClemente, and Norcross (in press) on stages and processes of behavior change. The models are compatible and address distinctly different aspects of behavior change.

Integration of these two models, and others that may appear in the future, will be important for developing a comprehensive view of relapse and for stimulating work on new interventions. Relatively little work has been done using these models in the obesity field, so it is still early to integrate these models into a single conceptual scheme. As more work appears, this may be possible. It is encouraging that theory and conceptual schemes are being used to direct treatment. This is a positive development that promises to lead to more rapid advances in treatment and prevention.

Determinants and Predictors

There has been a vigorous search for predictors of weight loss. The search has not been fruitful, for the most part. Typically, a predictor that appears promising in one study is shown to have no value in another. This may occur because obesity has multiple origins, and a single treatment is likely to have much different effects on different people (Brownell & Wadden, 1991). For example, psychological measures may explain much of the variance in weight loss in persons whose obesity is attributable to psychological factors, but may explain little in persons whose problem is determined by genetic or metabolic factors.

The exception in this disappointing search is exercise. Kayman, Bruvold, and Stern (1990) studied individuals who had successfully maintained weight loss, and compared them to never-obese controls and to individuals who had lost weight and then relapsed. Among the maintainers, 90% exercised regularly, compared to 82% of the controls and 34% of the relapsers. Several other investigators have also found exercise to be correlated with success (Colvin & Olson, 1983; Miller & Sims, 1981; Pavlou, Krey, & Steffee, 1989). It would appear from these findings that exercise should be one of the central features of a weight control program.

The search for predictors of relapse has been more promising. This work began with a study by Cummings, Gordon, and Marlatt (1980) in which 311 relapse episodes were studied in heavy drinkers, smokers, compulsive gamblers, overweight individuals, and heroin addicts. Several determinants emerged, and then were grouped by the authors into individual (intrapersonal) and situational (environmental) categories. Intrapersonal factors included mood states such as depression and anxiety, whereas the interpersonal factors included negative life events and interactions with others. Negative emotional states accounted for 30% of all relapses, while 48% occurred in association with interpersonal events (one-third of these stemmed from conflict).

Much of the research on relapse has come from studies on smoking (Shiffman, 1984). The application to weight loss has just begun, but is producing interesting findings. Grilo, Shiffman, and Wing (1989) did posttreatment interviews with 57 obese persons with Type II diabetes who had been through a weight loss program. Situations where subjects lapsed were compared with those in which they overcame the temptation to overeat. The analysis yielded three categories of relapse crises: mealtime, low arousal, and emotional upset. The authors reported that situations of emotional upset almost always led to overeating. Situational factors such as exposure to food cues increased risk of relapse. The strongest correlate of positive outcome was the use of coping skills. This is consistent with the focus on coping skills both in conceptual models of relapse (Marlatt & Gordon, 1985) and in intervention programs (Brownell & Rodin, 1990).

Consequences of Relapse

Relapse is considered a negative event in almost all quarters. When a person loses weight and then regains it, the expectation is that the person becomes depressed, embarrassed, and ashamed, and that self-esteem is battered. The experience is thought to be sufficiently negative to decrease the individual's chance of success on a next attempt.

This issue has not been studied in detail, so data cannot be assembled to support intuition. One can argue, in fact, that the outcome of relapse can be positive. Learning can occur, and a person can become more sensitive to the degree of commitment necessary to maintain lost weight and to the events that stimulate relapse. Maintenance studies in other areas have shown than many individuals who finally recover from serious problems do so after many unsuccessful attempts. This has been shown in regard to alcoholism (Vaillant, 1983) and smoking (U.S. Department of Health and Human Services, 1983). The cyclic model of Prochaska, DiClemente, and Norcross (in press) suggests that relapse may send a person back to an earlier stage of change, but that future change is still possible (see Figure 18.3).

Whether relapse is a positive or negative event in the final analysis probably depends on the individual, the circumstances, and the tenacity of the problem. Clinicians can help patients make the experience as constructive as possible by emphasizing that learning occurs and by helping them understand that there is a chance for a positive outcome in the future.

Research Needs

Research on relapse is relatively new, so many unanswered questions remain. Answers to these questions are needed to refine existing theoretical models, to develop new models on the natural history, effects, determinants and predictors of lapse and relapse, and to improve methods for management and prevention. My colleagues and I (Brownell et al., 1986) have described research needs in the area of relapse (Table 18.4); these include both theoretical and practical issues.

Implications for Intervention

A number of interventions have been suggested and tested for improving the maintenance of weight loss. Examples are booster sessions following treatment (Kingsley & Wilson, 1977), spouse involvement (Brownell & Stunkard, 1981; Dubbert & Wilson, 1984), exercise (Perri et al., 1986), relapse prevention training (Perri et al., 1984), posttreatment contact with professionals (Perri et al., 1984), and use of a comprehensive behavioral program in conjunction with VLCDs (Wadden & Stunkard, 1986) or pharmacotherapy (Craighead, 1984; Craighead, Stunkard, & O'Brien, 1981). In some cases these interventions have been derived from theory, and in other cases they are tests of interventions that appear reasonable from clinical experience. A description of several of these interventions, along with a summary of the supporting studies, appears in the chapter by Perri.

Many possible interventions for preventing and managing relapse can be proposed when integrating information from psychology, nutrition, exercise physiology, public health and other fields. Only a fraction of the possible approaches have been tested. We (Brownell & Jeffery, 1987) reviewed the literature on the maintenance of weight loss and proposed a number of interventions, listed in Table 18.5. They include screening prior to treatment, aggressive initial interventions, more emphasis on the social environment and exercise, and public health approaches such as altering mechanisms for food delivery.

TABLE 18.4. Research Needs in the Areas of Lapse and Relapse

Areas	Questions to be answered
Natural history	1. Is a relapse incremental learning or a failure experience? 2. Does the chance of relapse increase or decrease with time? 3. What are the stages of the lapse and relapse processes? 4. Is there a "safe" point beyond which a person will not relapse? 5. How frequent are lapses, and do they precede relapse?
Effects of lapse and relapse	1. What are the effects on mood? 2. Do lapse and relapse influence self-efficacy? 3. Do others' reactions influence lapse and relapse? 4. What are the physiological effects of lapse and relapse? 5. How do professionals deal with relapse in their patients?
Determinants and predictors	1. Do various treatments influence probability of relapse? 2. Does early response to treatment predict relapse? 3. Is past history of success and relapse predictive? 4. What are the roles of withdrawal symptoms, cravings, and urges? 5. What are the roles of conditioning and compensatory responses? 6. What are the mechanisms of social support? 7. Do physiological factors influence risk? 8. Can relapse be predicted after treatment but before maintenance?
Prevention of lapse and relapse	1. What criteria can be used to screen patients? 2. Does screening influence false positive and false negative rates? 3. What is the role of exercise? 4. Are cue extinction procedures helpful? 5. Is there any role for programmed relapse? 6. What are the relevant coping strategies? 7. Can motivation be enhanced at various points in treatment? 8. Is lifelong treatment necessary?

Note. From "Understanding and Preventing Relapse" (p. 778) by K. D. Brownell, G. A. Marlatt, E. Lichtenstein, and G. T. Wilson, 1986, *American Psychologist, 41,* 765-782. Copyright 1986 by American Psychological Association. Reprinted by permission.

Summary and Conclusions

Although relapse is often cited as the most important issue in the management of obesity, surprisingly little is known about how often it occurs, why it occurs, its predictors and consequences, its natural history, and methods for its prevention. The situation is changing, but much, much more work is needed.

The lore in the field, and in the eyes of the public and the press, is that 95% of people who lose weight relapse. These numbers were suggested in a study published in the 1950s and have not been updated. Data from modern-day clinical programs suggest better results, but no matter how the numbers are interpreted, the relapse problem is severe. Very little is known about the long-term effects of self-change efforts, and almost no data are released from the large commercial and self-help programs in which millions of people lose weight.

TABLE 18.5. Suggestions for Methods to Enhance Long-Term Weight Loss

1. Consider other treatments for our patients.
2. Develop criteria to match patients to treatments.
3. Develop criteria for screening patients to determine if there would be a better time to diet or a better program to join.
4. Increase initial weight losses.
5. Increase the length of treatment.
6. Be more aggressive about attaining goal weight. Consider the "initial treatment phase" as the period necessary to reach goal weight. "Maintenance" should not be considered until there is a substantial weight loss to maintain.
7. Increase the emphasis on exercise. Structured, supervised exercise programs need to be tested against current programs in which patients are given only verbal or written advice about exercise.
8. Exploit the social environment as a means to improve long-term adherence. More research is necessary to define the factors in the family, work site, community, etc., that can be used to facilitate weight loss.
9. Financial incentives, which have been effective in producing some of the best losses in behavioral studies, need to be extended for use in the long term.
10. Combine behavioral programs with other treatments, such as commercial and self-help programs, aggressive diets, or surgery.
11. Evaluate the cognitive factors that are included in most programs by consensus, but which have not been studied in detail.
12. Possibly extend stimulus control methods into the dieter's daily life by considering different mechanisms for food delivery and for supervised exercise.
13. Study the use and timing of relapse prevention methods in more detail.

Note. From "Improving Long-Term Weight Loss: Pushing the Limits of Treatment" (p. 370) by K. D. Brownell and R. W. Jeffery, 1987, *Behavior Therapy, 18,* 353-374. Copyright 1987 by Association for Advancement of Behavior Therapy. Reprinted by permission.

Interpreting relapse figures can be difficult. In most follow-up studies, subjects are weighed infrequently, so changes in weight occurring between assessments may go undetected. Another problem is that individuals typically enter other programs during a follow-up phase, so attributing change to the initial intervention is not a straightforward process.

Several advances have been made in conceptualizing relapse. These have come in work on the stages and processes of change, and on the process of relapse itself. These theoretical approaches have suggested interventions, only a few of which have been tested. Some of the interventions that have been tested have shown promising results. The field is ripe for more work on both theory and intervention.

References

Andersen, T., Stokholm, K. H., Backer, O. G., & Quaade, F. (1988). Long-term (5-year) results after either horizontal gastroplasty or very-low-calorie diet for morbid obesity. *International Journal of Obesity, 12,* 277-284.

Bandura, A. (1977). Self-efficacy: Toward a unifying theory of behavior change. *Psychological Bulletin, 84,* 191-215.

Brownell, K. D., & Jeffery, R. W. (1987). Improving long-term weight loss: Pushing the limits of treatment. *Behavior Therapy, 18,* 353-374.

Brownell, K. D., & Kramer, F. M. (1989). Behavioral management of obesity. *Medical Clinics of North America, 73,* 185-201.

Brownell, K. D., Marlatt, G. A., Lichtenstein, E., & Wilson, G. T. (1986). Understanding and preventing relapse. *American Psychologist, 41,* 765-782.

Brownell, K. D., & Rodin, J. (1990). *The weight maintenance survival guide.* Dallas: American Health Publishing Co.

Brownell, K. D., & Stunkard, A. J. (1981). Couples training, pharmacotherapy, and behavior therapy in the treatment of obesity. *Archives of General Psychiatry, 38,* 1224-1229.

Brownell, K. D., & Wadden, T. A. (1986). Behavior therapy for obesity: Modern approaches and better results. In K. D. Brownell & J. P. Foreyt (Eds.), *Handbook of eating disorders: Physiology, psychology and treatment of obesity, anorexia, and bulimia* (pp. 180-197). New York: Basic Books.

Brownell, K. D., & Wadden, T. A. (1991). The heterogeneity of obesity: Fitting treatments to individuals. *Behavior Therapy, 22,* 153-177.

Cohen, S., Lichtenstein, E., Prochaska, J. O., Rossi, J. S., Gritz, E. R., Carr, C. R., Orleans, C. T., Schoenbach, V. J., Biener, L., Abrams, D., DiClemente, C., Curry, S., Marlatt, G. A., Cummings, K. M., Emont, S. L., Giovino, G., & Ossip-Klein, D. (1989). Debunking myths about self-quitting: Evidence from 10 prospective studies of persons who attempt to quit smoking by themselves. *American Psychologist, 11,* 1355-1365.

Colvin, R. H., & Olson, S. B. (1983). A descriptive analysis of men and women who have lost significant weight and are highly successful at maintaining the loss. *Addictive Behaviors, 8,* 287-295.

Craighead, L. W. (1984). Sequencing of behavior therapy and pharmacotherapy for obesity. *Journal of Consulting and Clinical Psychology, 52,* 190-199.

Craighead, L. W., Stunkard, A. J., & O'Brien, R. M. (1981). Behavior therapy and pharmacotherapy for obesity. *Archives of General Psychiatry, 38,* 763-768.

Cummings, C., Gordon, J. R., & Marlatt, G. A. (1980). Relapse: Prediction and intervention. In W. R. Miller (Ed.), *The addictive disorders: Treatment of alcoholism, drug abuse, smoking, and obesity* (pp. 291-322). Elmsford, NY: Pergamon Press.

DiClemente, C. C., Prochaska, J. O., Fairhurst, S., Velicer, W., Velasquez, M., & Rossi, J. (1991). The process of smoking cessation: An analysis of precontemplation, contemplation, and determination stages of change. *Journal of Consulting and Clinical Psychology, 59,* 295-304.

Dubbert, P. M., & Wilson, G. T. (1984). Goal setting and spouse involvement in the treatment of obesity. *Behaviour Research and Therapy, 22,* 227-242.

Grilo, C. M., Shiffman, S., & Wing, R. R. (1989). Relapse crises and coping among dieters. *Journal of Consulting and Clinical Psychology, 57,* 488-495.

Hovell, M. F., Koch, A., Hofstetter, C. R., Sipan, C., Faucher, P., Dellinger, A., Borok, G., Forsythe, A., & Felitti, V. J. (1988). Long-term weight loss maintenance: Assessment of a behavioral and supplemented fasting program. *American Journal of Public Health, 78,* 663-666.

Jeffery, R. W., Folsom, A. R., Luepker, R. V., Jacobs, D. R., Gillum, R. F., Taylor, H. L., & Blackburn, H. (1984). Prevalence of overweight and weight loss behavior in a metropolitan adult population: The Minnesota Heart Survey experience. *American Journal of Public Health, 74,* 349-352.

Jeffery, R. W., & Wing, R. R. (1983). Recidivism and self-cure of smoking and obesity: Data from population studies. *American Psychologist, 37,* 852.

Kayman, S., Bruvold, W., & Stern, J. S. (1990). Maintenance and relapse after weight loss in women: Behavioral aspects. *American Journal of Clinical Nutrition, 52,* 800-807.

Kingsley, R. G., & Wilson, G. T. (1977). Behavior therapy for obesity: A comparative investigation of long-term efficacy. *Journal of Consulting and Clinical Psychology, 45*, 288-298.

Marlatt, G. A., & Gordon, J. (Eds.). (1985). *Relapse prevention: Maintenance strategies in the treatment of addictive behaviors.* New York: Guilford Press.

Miller, P. M., & Sims, K. L. (1981). Evaluation and component analysis of a comprehensive weight control program. *International Journal of Obesity, 5*, 57-65.

Pavlou, K. N., Krey, S., & Steffee, W. P. (1989). Exercise as an adjunct to weight loss and maintenance in moderately obese subjects. *American Journal of Clinical Nutrition, 49*, 1115-1123.

Perri, M. G. (1987). Maintenance strategies for the management of obesity. In W. G. Johnson (Ed.), *Advances in eating disorders: Vol. 1. Treating and preventing obesity* (pp. 177-194). Greenwich, CT: JAI Press.

Perri, M. G., Lauer, J. B., McAdoo, W. G., McAllister, D. A., & Yancey, D. Z. (1986). Enhancing the efficacy of behavior therapy for obesity: Effects of aerobic exercise and a multicomponent maintenance program. *Journal of Consulting and Clinical Psychology, 54*, 670-675.

Perri, M. G., McAllister, D. A., Gange, J. J., Jordan, R. C., McAdoo, W. G., & Nezu, A. M. (1988). Effects of four maintenance programs on the long-term management of obesity. *Journal of Consulting and Clinical Psychology, 56*, 529-534.

Perri, M. G., Shapiro, R. M., Ludwig, W. W., Twentyman, C. T., & McAdoo, W. G. (1984). Maintenance strategies for the treatment of obesity: An evaluation of relapse prevention training and posttreatment contact by mail and telephone. *Journal of Consulting and Clinical Psychology, 52*, 404-413.

Prochaska, J. O. (1979). *Systems of psychotherapy: A transtheoretical approach.* Homewood, IL: Dorsey Press.

Prochaska, J. O. (1983). Self-changers versus therapy changers versus Schachter. *American Psychologist, 37*, 854.

Prochaska, J. O., & DiClemente, C. C. (1982). Transtheoretical therapy: Toward a more integrative model of change. *Psychotherapy: Theory, Research, and Practice, 19*, 276-288.

Prochaska, J. O., & DiClemente, C. C. (1985). Common processes of change in smoking, weight control, and psychological distress. In S. Shiffman & T. Wills (Eds.), *Coping and substance abuse* (pp. 345-364). New York: Academic Press.

Prochaska, J. O., DiClemente, C. C., & Norcross, J. C. (in press). In search of how people change. *American Psychologist.*

Prochaska, J. O., DiClemente, C. C., Velicer, W. F., Ginpil, S., & Norcross, J. C. (1985). Predicting change in smoking status for self-changers. *Addictive Behaviors, 10*, 395-406.

Prochaska, J. O., Norcross, J. C., Fowler, J., Follick, M., & Abrams, D. B. (in press). Attendance and outcome in a work site weight control program: Processes and stages of change as process and predictor variables. *Addictive Behaviors.*

Prochaska, J. O., Velicer, W. F., DiClemente, C. C., & Fava, J. (1988). Measuring processes of change: Applications to the cessation of smoking. *Journal of Consulting and Clinical Psychology, 56*, 520-528.

Rzewnicki, R., & Forgays, D. G. (1987). Recidivism and self-cure of smoking and obesity: An attempt to replicate. *American Psychologist, 42*, 97-100.

Schachter, S. (1982). Recidivism and self-cure of smoking and obesity. *American Psychologist, 37*, 436-444.

Shiffman, S. (1984). Coping with temptations to smoke. *Journal of Consulting and Clinical Psychology, 52*, 261-267.

Sikand, G., Kondo, A., Foreyt, J. P., Jones, P. H., & Gotto, A. M. (1988). Two-year follow-up of patients treated with a very-low-calorie diet and exercise training. *Journal of the American Dietetic Association, 88*, 487-488.

Stunkard, A. J., & McLaren-Hume, M. (1959). The results of treatment for obesity. *Archives of Internal Medicine, 103*, 79-85.

U.S. Department of Health and Human Services. (1983). *The health consequences of smoking:*

Cardiovascular disease. A report of the Surgeon General. Washington, DC: U.S. Government Printing Office.

Vaillant, G. E. (1983). *The natural history of alcoholism: Causes, patterns and paths to recovery.* Cambridge, MA: Harvard University Press.

Wadden, T. A., Sternberg, J. A., Letizia, K. A., Stunkard, A. J., & Foster, G. D. (1989). Treatment of obesity by very low calorie diet, behavior therapy, and their combination: A five-year perspective. *International Journal of Obesity, 13,* 39–46.

Wadden, T. A., & Stunkard, A. J. (1986). Controlled trial of very low calorie diet, behavior therapy, and their combination in the treatment of obesity. *Journal of Consulting and Clinical Psychology, 54,* 482–488.

Wadden, T. A., Stunkard, A. J., & Liebschutz, J. (1988). Three- year follow-up of the treatment of obesity by very low calorie diet, behavior therapy, and their combination. *Journal of Consulting and Clinical Psychology, 56,* 925–928.

19

Improving Maintenance of Weight Loss Following Treatment by Diet and Lifestyle Modification

MICHAEL G. PERRI

Following treatment for obesity, most patients regain weight. Indeed, many regain all of the weight that they had lost in treatment. The literature on dietary and behavioral interventions for weight loss is replete with follow-up studies documenting the existence of a "maintenance problem" (cf. Bennett, 1987). For example, in a review of behavioral treatment studies for obesity that were conducted in 1985–1987, Wadden and Bell (1990) found that during the year following treatment, patients on average regained 37% of the weight they lost in treatment. Moreover, studies with 5-year follow-up evaluations suggest that the *majority* of patients relapse to their pretreatment weights (Stalonas, Perri, & Kerzner, 1984; Wadden, Sternberg, Letizia, Stunkard, & Foster, 1989). Because of such findings, one prominent reviewer of the obesity treatment literature recently concluded that "the most pressing continuing challenge is maintaining weight loss" (Jeffery, 1987, p. 20).

This chapter summarizes six studies that tested the effectiveness of maintenance strategies for the behavioral management of obesity. The weight loss maintenance problem was viewed from a biobehavioral perspective, wherein physiological and psychological factors are assumed to interact to hinder the long-term maintenance of weight loss. Cognitive–social learning theory provided the conceptual framework guiding our development of interventions to maintain behavior change. Thus, this series of randomized, prospective investigations evaluated the following maintenance strategies: (1) continued professional guidance through therapist contacts following initial treatment; (2) skills training to equip patients to cope more effectively with the challenges of the posttreatment period; (3) social influence programs to provide patients with enhanced social support after treatment; (4) aerobic exercise to provide patients with positive physical and psychological effects that may enhance long-term success; and (5) multicomponent interventions marshaling several combinations of strategies to help patients sustain behavior change and maintain weight loss.

Study 1: Continued Professional Contact and Skills Training

Traditionally, the most common weight loss maintenance strategy has been the "booster session" approach. Following treatment, health care professionals schedule their patients to return for additional sessions during the follow-up period. The purpose of these sessions is to review and reinforce the behavioral changes accomplished in treatment, with the expectation that habit changes will persist because of "overlearning." Intuitively, this approach is appealing. It makes sense to believe that additional sessions scheduled after the conclusion of treatment would "boost" patients' adherence to behavioral prescriptions, and thereby enhance maintenance of weight loss. Nonetheless, during the 1970s, the results of several carefully designed studies failed to support the efficacy of booster sessions as a maintenance strategy (Ashby & Wilson, 1977; Beneke & Paulsen, 1979; Hall, Hall, Borden, & Hanson, 1975).

In retrospect, it is easy to see why the booster session approach did not work. The number of sessions was minimal, usually three to six, and they were often scheduled 1 to 3 months apart. Consequently, these sessions may not have provided patients with sufficient advice and support at the times when they most needed it. In addition, the content of booster sessions was limited to a review of weight loss strategies previously used in treatment. Poor maintenance may result, however, from problems specific to the posttreatment period. Therefore, maintaining behavior change may require a different set of strategies from those used to initiate behavior change. In addition, poor maintenance may reflect decreased motivation following treatment. Thus, simply reviewing treatment techniques may not address the specific posttreatment needs of patients. During the posttreatment period, patients may need greater amounts of advice and guidance, as well as training in skills specifically targeted to maintain the behavior change and weight loss accomplished in treatment. The first study in our series (Perri, Shapiro, Ludwig, Twentyman, & McAdoo, 1984) addressed the maintenance problem by evaluating the effects of posttreatment professional contact as well as skills training targeted at preventing relapse following treatment.

Most clinicians recognize that when an initial phase of weight loss treatment concludes, their patients will be faced with a significant challenge in maintaining the behavior change accomplished in treatment. Reversion to the patterns of eating and inactivity that led to weight gain occurs all too easily. For patients, addressing this challenge requires ongoing vigilance, an active awareness about critical aspects of their eating, and exercise. A key function of posttreatment professional contacts is to encourage patients to be continuously mindful of their progress. Such contacts can also serve to enhance motivation by reframing the patients' experiences in a positive, constructive, and hopeful fashion. The contacts can also provide an opportunity for problem solving when difficulties arise.

One method of providing professional support and advice during the follow-up period is the use of posttreatment therapist contacts by telephone and mail. Having patients mail to their therapists self-monitoring data with information about their eating and exercise behavior (and weight) may enhance vigilance and maintenance (Hall, Bass, & Monroe, 1978; Hall et al., 1975), and the use of frequent posttreatment telephone contacts between therapists and patients has shown promise as an effective maintenance strategy across a variety of problem areas (cf. Spevak, 1981). In Study 1, we evaluated posttreatment professional contacts as a maintenance strategy by having patients mail to their therapists weight-related monitoring data, and by having the therapists, in turn, telephone the patients to discuss continued efforts at weight control (Perri, Shapiro, et al., 1984).

Providing frequent therapist contacts and a high degree of social support may help patients to sustain the behavioral changes begun during the initial treatment period, but an effective maintenance program may also need to equip patients with a new set of abilities: the skills to anticipate, avoid, and cope with those circumstances that increase the risk of their experiencing a relapse (Marlatt & Gordon, 1985; Brownell, Marlatt, Lichtenstein, & Wilson, 1986). The relapse prevention model developed by Marlatt and his colleagues provides the most comprehensive conceptual framework for understanding and treating the maintenance problem in addictive behaviors. Let us consider its applicability to obese individuals who have successfully lost weight during therapy. Sometime after treatment, the patients will face situations in which they will be tempted to exceed a prescribed calorie goal or deviate from the techniques taught in treatment. If they do not have the skills to cope with this high risk situation, they may have a slip or lapse in self-control. Moreover, if patients interpret the lapse as evidence that they are failures at self-control, they are likely to experience a sense of hopelessness and a decrease in self-efficacy. This initial slip becomes the start of a full-blown relapse. The individuals then may abandon the habits acquired in treatment, return to previous eating patterns, and regain weight. If, on the other hand, patients are equipped to face high risk situations with an effective coping response, they are likely to experience an increased sense of self-efficacy and are more likely to maintain the positive changes accomplished in treatment.

Marlatt and Gordon (1985) have recommended several specific strategies to prevent or minimize relapse following treatment. First, patients need to be trained to recognize and identify those situations that pose a high risk for relapse. Second, training in problem solving may be used as a means of generating coping strategies for high risk situations. Third, patients need practice in coping with actual high risk situations. Finally, patients need to be trained in cognitive strategies to overcome guilt feelings and the sense of failure often associated with slips. During the posttreatment period, virtually all patients will experience some form of lapse. The therapist can prepare them with appropriate coping techniques to view such slips as learning experiences—independent events to be avoided in the future through appropriate coping responses.

Thus, in Study 1, we examined the effects of posttreatment professional contact and skills training on the maintenance of weight loss (Perri, Shapiro, et al., 1984). More specifically, we evaluated whether providing patients with relapse prevention training or posttreatment therapist contact by mail and telephone would enhance the long-term maintenance of weight loss.

Method

The subjects were 129 mildly to moderately obese volunteers. At pretreatment, they averaged 88.6 kg and 57% over ideal body weight. Subjects were assigned randomly to one of six conditions in a 3 × 2 factorial design. Three treatment conditions (i.e., nonbehavioral treatment, behavior therapy, behavior therapy plus relapse prevention training) were crossed with two posttreatment conditions (i.e., no further contact or posttreatment therapist contact by telephone and mail).

All treatments consisted of 15 weekly group sessions, each 2 hours in duration. The nonbehavioral treatment included exchange plan diets, recommendations for exercise, and group sessions emphasizing the development of insight into the "underlying reasons" for overeating. Behavior therapy consisted of treatment sessions focused on the various self-control techniques typically used in behavioral programs for weight reduction (Johnson & Stalonas, 1981). The behavior therapy plus relapse prevention training condition supplemented the behavior therapy program with exercises designed to minimize or prevent relapse, and to promote the maintenance of habit change and weight loss. Patients were trained to identify those situations and circumstances posing a high risk for slips, and they were taught problem-solving skills (D'Zurilla & Nezu, 1982) as a means of generating appropriate coping strategies for negotiating high risk situations. Patients received *in vivo* practice in coping with two high risk situations: an actual dinner at an Italian restaurant where the availability of low calorie foods was limited, and a "pitch-in party" with high calorie snack foods provided by the therapists. In addition, patients were trained in cognitive strategies to cope with the feelings of guilt and failure associated with slips. Therapists instructed patients to view a slip as a "learning experience," a single independent event to be avoided in the future by use of an appropriate coping response.

After the 15-week treatment phase of the study, participants in three of the experimental cells had no further contact with their therapists except for assessments. Patients in the posttreatment contact condition were instructed to monitor and record daily on postcards information concerning weight-related behaviors. They mailed the cards weekly to their therapist during the first 6 months following the initial treatment. The therapists, in turn, telephoned patients to discuss briefly (approximately 5-10 minutes) the information received. Therapists' support and advice was tailored to each individual, but remained consistent with the patient's initial treatment condition. Therapists made weekly telephone contacts during the first 3 months following treatment and faded their telephone contacts over the second 3-month period. At 6 months posttreatment, patient–therapist contact by telephone and mail was discontinued.

Change in body weight was the major outcome measure for this study. Weight change was assessed at posttreatment and at 3-, 6-, and 12-month follow-up sessions. Subjects' use of behavioral techniques was assessed through questionnaires at posttreatment and follow-up sessions.

Results and Discussion

All treatments produced substantial initial weight losses ($M = 8.5$ kg; see Table 19.1), and there were no significant between-group differences at posttreatment (i.e., week 15). Over the course of the 12-month follow-up, a significant three-way interaction emerged for time $\times$ initial treatment $\times$ maintenance condition ($p < .05$). The effects of posttreatment contact varied according to the type of initial treatment that patients received. Posttreatment patient–therapist contact by telephone and mail enhanced the maintenance of weight loss for groups that received nonbehavioral treatment or behavior therapy plus relapse prevention. However, the posttreatment contact strategy did not improve maintenance for the groups receiving behavior therapy only.

Behavior therapy plus relapse prevention training and posttreatment contact was the only condition in which patients maintained their mean posttreatment weight loss and did not suffer significant relapse over the 12 months of follow-up. This combination of initial treatment and maintenance strategy was the only one in which patients (1) were trained in specific coping strategies to prepare for posttreatment difficulties, and (2) received supervised practice in

TABLE 19.1. Mean Weight Losses (kg) of Groups in Study 1 at Posttreatment and Follow-Up Sessions

Time of assessment	Group					
	B + R + C ($n = 17$)	B + R ($n = 15$)	B + C ($n = 15$)	B ($n = 21$)	N + C ($n = 16$)	N ($n = 15$)
Posttreatment	9.63	8.55	8.72	7.51	8.55	8.13
3-month follow-up	11.76	7.25	10.55	8.49	9.23	7.88
6-month follow-up	10.78	4.90	8.69	7.65	7.25	5.00
12-month follow-up	10.34	2.96	5.77	6.28	6.16	3.16

Note. B, behavior therapy; N, nonbehavioral therapy; R, relapse prevention training; and C, posttreatment contact by mail and telephone. Adapted from "Maintenance Strategies for the Treatment of Obesity" (p. 181) by M. G. Perri, 1987, in W. G. Johnson (Ed.), *Advances in Eating Disorders: Vol. 1. Treating and Preventing Obesity* (pp. 177–194). Greenwich, CT: JAI Press. Copyright 1987 by JAI Press. Adapted by permission.

the application of those strategies during the actual follow-up period. Self-report data suggested that the superior performance of participants in this condition may have resulted from their greater use during follow-up of key strategies including self-monitoring, stimulus control, and exercise.

An interesting finding was the surprisingly poor performance of the group that received behavior therapy plus relapse prevention training *without* post-treatment contact. Perhaps the relapse prevention training conducted during the initial treatment failed to provide patients with sufficient opportunity to master the various cognitive strategies for their own use during the posttreatment period. Alternatively, the relapse prevention training experiences may have in practice given patients "permission" to experiment with deviations from the recommended eating and exercise habits. Some patients may distort the cognitive coping procedures into "rationalizations" for a sustained series of slips (e.g., "My therapist expected that I would slip up once in a while—this doesn't necessarily mean I'm off the program for good!"). Unfortunately, without confronting feedback from a therapist, some patients may never resume the eating and exercise habits needed to sustain weight loss. Thus, as a maintenance package, relapse prevention training may offer little or no benefit unless it is combined with a therapist's posttreatment guidance to ensure appropriate implementation.

The interaction of the posttreatment contact strategy with relapse prevention training suggests that the content of patient-therapist interactions may be a crucial factor in posttreatment success. Therapists' advice about specific coping techniques may have helped patients to negotiate and avoid relapses. Thus, when combined with training targeted at the specific problems of the posttreatment period, therapist contact by mail and telephone appears to have potential as an effective maintenance strategy.

Study 2: Adding Social Support to a Multicomponent Program

Effective maintenance of behavior change may require a *multifaceted* set of posttreatment strategies. In 1980, Stuart suggested that effective maintenance programs would require a combination of strategies, such as continued self-monitoring of positive behaviors, frequent posttreatment patient-therapist contacts, and active patient participation in self-help groups (Stuart, 1980). The posttreatment contact intervention that we employed in Study 1 included two of the three key elements recommended by Stuart: namely, continued self-monitoring of key weight control strategies, and ongoing therapist-patient telephone contacts following initial treatment. In Study 2, we incorporated Stuart's third element into the maintenance package by teaching patients to establish their own self-help groups during the follow-up period (Perri, McAdoo, Spevak, & Newlin, 1984). We then tested the effectiveness of this multicomponent program on the long-term maintenance of weight loss.

Method

Fifty-six patients were randomly assigned to one of two conditions: 26 to a behavior therapy plus booster session condition (M's = 91.1 kg and 51.3% overweight), and 30 to a behavior therapy plus multicomponent maintenance program condition (M's = 84.4 kg and 48% overweight). The two conditions did not differ significantly in initial weight or percentage overweight.

Patients in both conditions received an initial course of behavior therapy for obesity, consisting of 14 weekly group sessions. After the initial treatment phase, patients in the behavior therapy plus booster session condition received six biweekly booster sessions aimed at further review and reinforcement of strategies implemented during treatment. Beyond the six booster sessions, no contacts were scheduled with therapists or other group members, except for five follow-up assessment meetings.

Upon completion of the initial treatment, patients in the behavior therapy plus multicomponent maintenance program condition received six biweekly sessions focused on strategies to enhance weight loss progress during the follow-up period. These patients were instructed in how to form their own peer self-help groups. These "buddy groups" incorporated the structure and procedures of a problem-solving approach (D'Zurilla & Nezu, 1982) within the context of a self-help group. Patients were instructed to monitor each other's weight, to use praise to encourage weight loss progress, and to problem-solve as a group when an individual was experiencing difficulties with weight loss efforts. The buddy groups were encouraged to meet on a regular basis during the year following treatment. In addition, patients in the multicomponent maintenance program were asked to mail weekly postcards to their therapists specifying details of their weight loss progress; the therapists, in turn, made brief weekly phone calls to these patients to provide additional support and guidance during the year following treatment (see Study 1).

Results and Discussion

Of the 56 clients who began the program, 4 in each condition dropped out during the initial treatment. Over the 21-month follow-up period, an additional 5 clients from the behavior therapy plus booster session condition dropped out, but there were no additional dropouts from the multicomponent maintenance program condition. This difference in dropout rates during the follow-up period was statistically significant ($p < .05$). During the year following treatment, patients in the multicomponent program, on average, attended 8.5 self-help group meetings, mailed in 22.5 postcards detailing weight loss progress, and received 26.9 telephone calls from their therapists.

At the conclusion of the initial treatment period, the weight losses for the two conditions were equivalent. Over the course of the 21-month follow-up period, there was a significant interaction effect for time × posttreatment condition ($p < .05$). Post hoc comparisons revealed that between-group differences were not significant at either the 3- or 6-month follow-up sessions. However, at the 9-, 15-, and 21-month follow-up sessions, participants in the multicomponent maintenance program demonstrated significantly greater maintenance of weight loss than patients in the behavior therapy plus booster session condition (see Table 19.2). Thus, the major finding in Study 2 was that over the course of a 21-month follow-up period, a multicomponent program of posttreatment social support combined with continued self-monitoring and patient–therapist contacts significantly enhanced the maintenance of weight loss. This positive finding was tempered by the modest amount of weight loss maintained and the substantial cost of therapist time to provide telephone contacts with patients for an entire year following treatment.

Study 3: Aerobic Exercise and a Multicomponent Maintenance Program

In the next study in our series, we examined whether the efficacy of behavior therapy for obesity might be improved by the additions of an aerobic exercise regimen during treatment and a multicomponent maintenance program following treatment (Perri, McAdoo, McAllister, Lauer, & Yancey, 1986). The two goals of this study were, first, to increase the magnitude of initial weight loss in behavioral treatment; and, second, to improve the maintenance of weight loss by replicating the effects of the multicomponent program developed in Study 2.

Behavioral treatment of obesity typically focuses on habit changes designed to reduce food consumption. Often, the role of energy expenditure

TABLE 19.2. Mean Weight Loss (kg) of Patients in Study 2 at Posttreatment and the Follow-Up Evaluations

	Group	
Time of assessment	Behavior therapy plus multicomponent program ($n = 26$)	Behavior therapy plus booster sessions ($n = 17$)
Posttreatment	6.13	5.64
3-month follow-up	8.15	6.95
6-month follow-up	8.02	5.69
9-month follow-up	7.75	3.10
15-month follow-up	5.82	2.09
21-month follow-up	4.56	0.36

Note. Adapted from "Maintenance Strategies for the Treatment of Obesity" (p. 183) by M. G. Perri, 1987, in W. G. Johnson (Ed.), *Advances in Eating Disorders: Vol. 1. Treating and Preventing Obesity* (pp. 177–194). Greenwich, CT: JAI Press. Copyright 1987 by JAI Press. Adapted by permission.

is acknowledged only to the extent that patients are encouraged to "exercise more." Inactivity may be a major factor contributing to obesity. Recent research has indicated that although obese individuals may not consume more calories than persons of average weight, the obese are significantly less active than the nonobese (Brownell, Stunkard, & Albaum, 1980; Garrow, 1986; Stern & Lowney, 1986). Because of these findings, and the modest effects of dietary interventions, several reviewers have concluded that exercise has the potential to play a more significant role in the management of obesity (Brownell & Stunkard, 1980; Epstein & Wing, 1980; Foreyt, 1987; Thompson, Jarvie, Lahey, & Cureton, 1982). Moreover, post hoc data from several studies have indicated that exercise is one of the few factors consistently correlated with long-term success in weight management (Colvin & Olson, 1983; Gormally & Rardin, 1981; Katahn, Pleas, Thackrey, & Wallston, 1982).

Exercise can enhance the treatment of obesity by increasing the rate at which fat is lost while decreasing the loss of lean body mass. Exercise may also facilitate weight loss by increasing metabolic rate, although contradictory findings have been reported in this area, as discussed by Ravussin and Swinburn in Chapter 7 of this volume. Additional positive effects of aerobic exercise include improvements in coronary efficiency, blood pressure, and glucose tolerance (Björntorp, 1978; Martin & Dubbert, 1982). The psychological benefits of regular exercise include improvements in mood and self-concept, and an increased sense of well-being (Folkins & Sime, 1981).

Prior to 1985, few experiments had evaluated the effects of increasing physical activity during behavior therapy for obesity. One study suggested an additive effect of combining exercise with behavior therapy for obesity (Dahlkoetter, Callahan, & Linton, 1979). Two experiments failed to find an effect for exercise during treatment, but suggested that exercise may contribute to the maintenance of weight loss during the follow-up period (Harris & Hallbauer, 1973; Stalonas, Johnson, & Christ, 1978).

In Study 3, we tested the effect of an aerobic program consisting of two specific types of activity (brisk walking and stationary cycling) with fixed levels of intensity, duration, and frequency (Perri et al., 1986). We selected these particular aerobic activities because they entail high energy output, require minimal equipment, and have low injury rates. In Study 3, we also tested the effectiveness of our multicomponent maintenance program consisting of continued self-monitoring, frequent posttreatment therapist contacts, and active patient participation in peer self-help groups.

Method

Subjects were 90 moderately obese adults who at pretreatment averaged 92.1 kg and 60% over ideal body weight. Subjects were assigned randomly to one of four conditions in a 2 × 2 factorial design. Two treatment conditions (i.e., behavior therapy or behavior therapy plus aerobic exercise) were crossed with two posttreatment conditions (i.e., no posttreatment contact or a multicomponent posttreatment maintenance program). Initial treatments consisted of 20 weekly group sessions. Patients in the behavior therapy condition were encouraged (as is the custom in many behavioral programs) to increase their use of routine physical activity (e.g., use of stairs rather than elevators). Subjects in this condition were not provided with a specific program of exercise, but were given lists of the caloric expenditure of a variety of physical activities. Patients were asked to increase their weekly output by 800 kilocalories (kcal).

For patients in the behavior therapy plus aerobic exercise condition, treatment included therapist-led demonstrations and actual practice of an aerobic regimen in each therapy session. Exercise segments consisted of: (1) a warm-up routine to stretch muscles and gradually increase heart rate; (2) a conditioning bout to stimulate heart rate to the aerobic training range; and (3) a cool-down period to allow the intensity level to gradually diminish following the conditioning phase. Initial levels of exercise were set at a minimum of 32 minutes per week. Weekly increases of an additional 4 minutes were scheduled over 12 consecutive weeks to a target level of 80 minutes per week (i.e., 20 minutes per day, 4 days per week). The additional caloric expenditure of the target level of aerobic exercise was approximately 800 kcal/week.

Following the 20-session treatment phase of the study, patients in two of the conditions had no further contact with their therapists except for assessments (at 3-, 6-, 12-, and 18-month follow-up sessions). Patients in the remaining two groups received the multicomponent maintenance program described in Study 2.

Results and Discussion

Over the course of the initial 20-week treatment period, patients in each condition achieved substantial weight losses ($M = 9.45$ kg). Groups that received the aerobic exercise program lost significantly more weight ($M = 10.6$ kg) than those not receiving the program ($M = 8.2$ kg). The net effect of the aerobic exercise program was an additional loss of 2.4 kg during the 20-week treatment period. This amount represented a 29% improvement beyond what was accomplished in the group receiving behavior therapy only (see Table 19.3).

Over the course of the 18-month follow-up period, a significant time × maintenance condition interaction emerged ($p < .001$). At each follow-up assessment, patients who received the multicomponent maintenance program demonstrated significantly better weight loss than patients receiving no posttreatment contact.

The physical activities employed in the aerobic exercise regimen were walking and/or stationary cycling. The use of these particular activities and the manner in which they were implemented may have contributed to the effectiveness of the aerobic exercise program. Indeed, self-reported adherence to the

TABLE 19.3. Mean Weight Losses (kg) of Patients in Study 3 at Posttreatment and the Follow-Up Evaluations

	Condition			
Time of assessment	B + A + M ($n = 17$)	B + M ($n = 15$)	B + A ($n = 15$)	B ($n = 21$)
Posttreatment	10.96	8.60	10.25	7.85
3-month follow-up	12.30	9.99	9.67	6.28
6-month follow-up	11.45	9.57	8.40	3.98
12-month follow-up	9.67	6.78	5.15	0.66
18-month follow-up	7.59	5.07	3.07	0.95

Note. B, behavior therapy; A, aerobic exercise program; and M, multicomponent maintenance program. Adapted from "Maintenance Strategies for the Treatment of Obesity" (p. 186) by M. G. Perri, 1987, in W. G. Johnson (Ed.), *Advances in Eating Disorders: Vol. 1. Treating and Preventing Obesity* (pp. 177–194). Greenwich, CT: JAI Press. Copyright 1987 by JAI Press. Adapted by permission.

prescribed routine was quite high during the treatment phase, with 80% of the subjects exceeding the recommended routine of 20 minutes per day, 4 days per week. The relatively high degree of adherence may be attributed to several factors. The prescribed regimens consisted of simple activities of moderate intensity and did not involve excessive physical pain or stress. The exercise regimens were phased in very gradually and were tailored to each patient's ability. Every session included a therapist-led exercise bout, and patients were able to gauge their progress through regular monitoring of their heart rate during the in-session routines.

Over the course of the 18-month follow-up period, patients' mean self-reported amount of weekly aerobic exercise decreased from more than 100 minutes per week to less than 30 minutes per week, and 42% of the subjects reported that they were not exercising at all at the 18-month follow-up. Successful maintenance of exercise behaviors may require procedures targeted specifically at adherence during the posttreatment period. For example, routine monitoring of coronary efficiency and ongoing peer group exercise opportunities may improve long-term adherence to aerobic regimens.

During the follow-up period, the general tendency was for subjects to regain weight. However, the multicomponent program facilitated maintenance of weight loss. At the 18-month follow-up evaluation, the groups that received the multicomponent posttreatment program maintained, on average, 84% of their mean posttreatment weight losses, whereas the groups without a posttreatment program maintained only 21% of their mean posttreatment weight losses. The maintenance program appeared to be effective because of its participants' greater adherence to behavioral self-management procedures (cf. Stalonas & Kirschenbaum, 1985). The combination of continued monitoring of key behaviors, frequent phone contacts with therapists, and peer group support appears to increase adherence and to foster maintenance of weight loss.

Study 4: Therapist Contact versus Peer Support

In Studies 2 and 3, we demonstrated the effectiveness of a multicomponent maintenance program designed to provide patients with a high degree of support and advice during the posttreatment period. The multicomponent program consisted of a combination of peer group support meetings and patient–therapist contacts during the follow-up period. In Study 4, we tested the specific effectiveness of peer support versus therapist contact as maintenance strategies for weight loss (Perri et al., 1987). The major question that we addressed was whether maintenance programs of peer support or therapist contact would foster better weight loss progress than would a control condition in which patients received no additional contacts during the period following treatment.

Method

Subjects were 85 moderately obese volunteers. All patients received a 20-week program consisting of the standard behavioral treatment for obesity plus the aerobic exercise regimen described in Study 3. Following the initial treatment phase, patients were assigned randomly to one of two maintenance programs or to a control condition with no further contact.

The peer support group maintenance program consisted of a series of 15 biweekly meetings. These meetings incorporated the structure and procedures of a problem-solving treatment within the context of a self-help group. Patients were taught to monitor each other's weight, to use praise to reinforce weight loss progress, and to utilize group problem solving when member encountered difficulties in weight loss efforts.

In the therapist contact maintenance program, patients also attended 15 biweekly sessions. Therapists met with groups of patients whom they had seen in the initial treatment phase of the study. The biweekly meetings included weigh-ins, reviews of self-monitoring data, and therapist-led problem solving of difficulties in maintaining habit changes in eating and exercise.

Results and Discussion

At the conclusion of the 20-session initial treatment period, the mean weight loss across all subjects was 10.7 kg. There were no statistically significant differences among the three conditions. Over the course of the 18-month follow-up period, a significant time × posttreatment condition interaction was observed ($p < .05$). At the conclusion of the maintenance program (i.e., 30 weeks posttreatment), significant between-group differences were apparent. Pairwise comparisons indicated that the therapist contact group showed significantly better weight loss progress than both the peer support and control

TABLE 19.4. Mean Weight Losses (kg) of Patients in Study 4 at Posttreatment and Follow-Ups

Time of assessment	Condition		
	B + T (n = 27)	B + P (n = 32)	B (n = 16)
Posttreatment	10.70	10.90	10.26
7-month follow-up	11.54	9.31	7.82
18-month follow-up	6.39	6.47	3.07

Note. B, behavior therapy; T, therapist contact program; and P, peer support program. Adapted from "Maintenance Strategies for the Treatment of Obesity" (p. 188) by M. G. Perri, 1987, in W. G. Johnson (Ed.), *Advances in Eating Disorders: Vol. 1. Treating and Preventing Obesity* (pp. 177-194). Greenwich, CT: JAI Press. Copyright 1987 by JAI Press. Adapted by permission.

conditions (p's $< .05$; see Table 19.4). Both the peer support and control groups regained weight during this period, and the amounts regained were not significantly different from each other. From 7-month to 18-month follow-up, subjects in all groups tended to regain weight. However, both the therapist contact and peer support programs showed better maintenance of weight loss than the control group (see Table 19.4).

Adherence data derived from questionnaires administered at posttreatment and follow-up indicated that at the 7-month follow-up evaluation, patients in the therapist contact program reported significantly greater use of behavioral self-control strategies than subjects in the peer support and control conditions (p's $< .05$). By the time of the 18-month follow-up, there were no significant differences in self-reported adherence among conditions, and patients in all groups reported significant decreases in their use of weight control strategies.

The weight maintenance achieved by patients in the therapist-led program was limited to that period of time in which they were under the supervision of their therapist. Following the conclusion of the maintenance program, participants began to regain weight and to experience the same pattern of relapse as patients in the peer support condition. Nonetheless, the results of this study suggest that posttreatment programs consisting of either peer group or therapist contacts foster better maintenance of weight loss than programs that do not include a posttreatment maintenance program.

Study 5: Therapist Contact versus Relapse Prevention Training

In study 5, we tested the effectiveness of relapse prevention training versus frequent therapist contacts as maintenance strategies for weight loss (Perri et al., 1990). The major question that we addressed was whether *year-long* posttreatment maintenance programs consisting of either (1) comprehensive training to prevent and overcome relapse or (2) a high frequency of therapist contacts would foster better weight loss progress than would a no-posttreatment-contact condition.

Method

Eighty-eight mildly to moderately obese individuals who were 25-99% over ideal body weight completed a 20-session behavioral weight loss program. Following this initial treatment, subjects were assigned randomly to one of two maintenance programs or to a no-further-contact control condition. The relapse prevention maintenance program was conducted in 26 biweekly meetings scheduled during the year after initial treatment, and included the following procedures: (1) the identification of situations that posed a high risk for relapse, (2) training in problem-solving skills to deal with high risk situations, (3) actual practice in coping with high risk situations, and (4) the development of cognitive coping strategies for overcoming setbacks. The therapist contact maintenance program was also conducted in 26 biweekly meetings scheduled during the year after initial treatment, and consisted of weigh-ins, reviews of progress, and therapist-led problem solving aimed at helping patients to maintain the behavioral changes accomplished during the initial treatment period.

Results and Discussion

At the conclusion of the initial 20-week treatment period, the mean weight loss across all subjects was 8.7 kg, with no significant differences between groups. At 6- and 12-month follow-up evaluations, significant differences in net weight loss emerged among the conditions ($p < .0001$). Post hoc tests indicated (1) that at the 6- and 12-month follow-up evaluations, both the relapse prevention and therapist contact maintenance conditions showed better weight loss progress than the no-posttreatment-contact condition; and (2) that there were no significant differences in weight loss between the relapse prevention and therapist contact maintenance programs (see Table 19.5).

Collectively, these findings suggest (1) that structured posttreatment programs can facilitate the maintenance of weight loss and (2) that a high frequency of therapist contacts may be as effective as relapse prevention training in helping patients to maintain their weight losses.

Study 6: Therapist Contact, Social Influence, and Exercise

Study 6 evaluated the effectiveness of four year-long maintenance programs for the management of obesity (Perri et al., 1988). The four maintenance programs were extensions of procedures that showed promise in our earlier

TABLE 19.5. Mean Weight Losses (kg) of Patients in Study 5 at Posttreatment and the Follow-Up Evaluations

	Condition		
Time of assessment	B + R (n = 29)	B + T (n = 33)	B (n = 26)
Posttreatment	8.89	7.98	9.32
6-month follow-up	9.65	10.13	7.00
12-month follow-up	7.33	9.42	4.52

Note. B, behavior therapy; T, therapist contact program; and R, relapse prevention program.

studies. They were (1) a therapist contact program involving 26 biweekly posttreatment contacts that included weigh-ins and therapist-led problem solving; (2) an aerobic exercise maintenance program that increased prescribed exercise levels from 80 to 180 minutes per week; (3) a social influence maintenance program that included group contingencies for maintenance program attendance and progress toward weight loss goals; and (4) a combination of the aerobic exercise and social influence maintenance programs.

Method

Subjects for this study were 91 moderately obese volunteers. A constructive treatment research design was used in this study; extra components were added to the basic treatment program to determine whether the additions enhanced the efficacy of the basic treatment. Thus, all patients completed a 20-session behavioral weight loss program that included the aerobic exercise regimen described in Study 3. Following the initial treatment period, patients were assigned randomly to one of four maintenance programs or to a no-further-contact control condition. All four maintenance programs were conducted in biweekly sessions scheduled over the course of the 12-month period following the conclusion of the initial treatment period. Patients in the control condition received no additional therapist contact beyond the initial treatment period.

Patients in the behavior therapy plus posttreatment contact condition received the initial behavioral weight loss program plus a posttreatment maintenance program consisting of 26 biweekly therapist contacts. Maintenance sessions consisted of weigh-ins, reviews of self-monitoring data, and therapist-led problem solving of difficulties in maintaining changes in eating and exercise behavior. Patients were asked to maintain their aerobic exercise levels at 80 minutes per week (i.e., 20 minutes per day, 4 days per week).

Patients in the behavior therapy plus posttreatment contact plus social influence maintenance program condition received the initial behavioral treatment and the posttreatment therapist contact program. In addition, they received a multifaceted program of social influence strategies designed to enhance motivation and to provide incentives for continued weight loss progress. The social influence program included monetary group contingencies for program adherence and continued weight loss, active patient participation in preparing and delivering lectures on maintaining weight loss, and instructions on how to provide peer support for weight loss through ongoing telephone contacts and peer group meetings during the posttreatment period.

Patients in the behavior therapy plus posttreatment contact plus aerobic exercise maintenance program condition received the initial behavioral treatment and the posttreatment therapist contact programs. In addition, they received an aerobic exercise maintenance program consisting of a new set of exercise goals for the posttreatment period and therapist-led exercise bouts during the biweekly posttreatment sessions. During the maintenance program, the prescribed frequency and duration of aerobic exercise was increased gradually from 20 minutes per day, 4 days per week, to 30 minutes per day, 6 days per week (i.e., from 80 to 180 minutes per week).

Patients in a fifth experimental condition received the initial behavioral treatment and the posttreatment therapist contact programs. In addition, these participants also received both the aerobic exercise and social influence maintenance programs previously described.

Results and Discussion

At the conclusion of the initial 20-session treatment period, the mean weight loss across all subjects was 12.45 kg, and there were no significant differences among the five conditions. Over the course of an 18-month follow-up, a significant interaction effect for condition × time was observed ($p < .05$). At the 6-month follow-up, the four conditions with posttreatment maintenance programs demonstrated significantly better weight loss than the condition including behavior therapy only, and the condition including all four programs demonstrated a significant additional weight loss of 4.08 kg (all p's $< .05$). At the 12-month follow-up, all four experimental conditions demonstrated significantly better maintenance of weight loss than the condition including behavior therapy only, which showed a significant relapse from pretreatment, with a weight gain of 5.13 kg. The superiority of the four maintenance conditions was still evident at the 18-month follow-up assessment (see Table 19.6). Moreover, on average participants in the four experimental conditions maintained 82.7% of their mean posttreatment losses, whereas patients receiving behavior therapy alone maintained only 33.3% of their original weight loss. No significant differences among the four experimental conditions were evident at the follow-up evaluations.

These results suggest that year-long maintenance programs can help sustain weight loss and behavior begun during the initial treatment period. Moreover, the magnitude of the weight losses at the 18-month follow-up

TABLE 19.6. Mean Weight Losses (kg) of Patients in Study 6 at Posttreatment and Follow-Up Evaluations

Time of assessment	Condition				
	B + C + A + S (n = 17)	B + C + A (n = 15)	B + C + S (n = 15)	B + C (n = 21)	B (n = 16)
Posttreatment	13.67	13.05	11.34	13.17	10.80
6-month follow-up	17.75	15.19	13.54	15.79	8.94
12-month follow-up	15.70	12.97	13.35	12.88	5.67
18-month follow-up	13.54	9.14	8.43	11.41	3.60

Note. B, behavior therapy; C, posttreatment therapist contact; A, aerobic exercise maintenance program; and S, social influence maintenance program. Adapted from "Maintenance Strategies for the Treatment of Obesity" (p. 190) by M. G. Perri, 1987, in W. G. Johnson (Ed.), *Advances in Eating Disorders: Vol. 1. Treating and Preventing Obesity* (pp. 177-194). Greenwich, CT: JAI Press. Copyright 1987 by JAI Press. Adapted by permission.

($M = 10.65$ kg) sustained by participants in the maintenance programs compares very favorably with results reported in the obesity literature. These findings indicate that an intensive therapist-led program directed toward teaching patients how to overcome the specific problems of the posttreatment period can indeed enhance the long-term maintenance of weight loss.

The therapist contact maintenance programs may have been effective to a large extent because of greater participant adherence to weight loss strategies during the first 6 months following the initial behavior therapy period. Through the problem-solving strategies used in maintenance sessions, patients may have been able to overcome obstacles to maintaining the changes in eating and exercise habits acquired in the initial treatment period (cf. Perri, 1987, 1989). In addition, the continuing therapist demand may have influenced participants' adherence as well. The longer patients remain in contact with their therapists, the longer they adhere to the behaviors required for maintenance of weight loss (cf. Bennett, 1986).

Moreover, the prevention of relapse requires the development of posttreatment strategies that enhance patients' long-term coping skills. Compared with subjects who received initial treatment only, patients who received posttreatment training in cognitive and behavioral coping strategies (i.e., problem solving) exhibited better overall adherence to self-control procedures and demonstrated significantly greater long-term maintenance of weight loss.

The results also showed that the addition of the social influence program improved participant adherence during the year following treatment. However, the higher levels of adherence in the social influence condition were not accompanied by significantly better maintenance of weight loss. Moreover, as the various incentives and social supports for weight loss were withdrawn, the degree of adherence decreased dramatically (cf. Brehm & McAllister, 1980; Kramer, Jeffery, Snell, & Forster, 1986).

Study 6 also evaluated whether the addition of high frequency exercise to the posttreatment therapist contact program would enhance long-term weight loss. At the 6-month follow-up assessment, patients in the high exercise maintenance conditions reported significantly greater weekly amounts of aerobic exercise than did subjects in the low exercise maintenance conditions. However, the higher amounts of self-reported aerobic exercise were not accompanied by significantly greater mean weight losses, and the higher exercise levels were not maintained at the 12- and 18-month follow-ups. The weekly goal of 180 minutes per week of brisk walking or stationary cycling may have been too difficult for patients to maintain on a regular basis, particularly during seasons marked by periods of inclement weather. In failing to meet the program's stringent exercise requirements, many patients may have generated negative self-statements about their ability to maintain other self-management strategies as well (cf. Brownell & Foreyt, 1985). Indeed, from 12 to 18 months posttreatment, participants in the behavior therapy plus contact plus aerobic exercise condition reported a significant decrease in overall adherence, whereas patients in the behavior therapy plus contact condition showed no change in overall adherence during the same period.

Finally, Study 6 examined whether the effectiveness of the posttreatment contact program would be enhanced by the addition of both the aerobic exercise and social influence maintenance programs. From posttreatment to the 6-month follow-up, the condition that included all four programs was the only condition to demonstrate a significant additional weight loss ($M = 4.08$ kg; net mean weight loss from pretreatment = 17.75 kg). At the 18-month follow-up evaluation, this condition maintained 99% of its mean posttreatment weight loss. These findings suggest that the combination of high frequency exercise with intensive support from peers and therapists holds potential as a multifaceted approach to improving the long-term management of obesity.

Summary and Conclusions

What conclusions or implications can we draw from this series of studies? First, the bad news. Unless initial weight loss treatments are supplemented with interventions targeted at the problem of maintenance, the prospects for successful long-term management of obesity are meager. Our results indicate that without a posttreatment program, patients generally abandon the self-management strategies taught in treatment and gradually regain weight.

Now, some good news. When initial therapy is supplemented with posttreatment maintenance strategies, patients exhibit greater adherence to weight loss techniques and better maintenance of weight loss. The most consistent finding in this series of studies was that structured programs of posttreatment therapist contact helped patients to maintain their weight losses. Posttreatment contact appears to be effective because the longer patients work with their therapists, the longer they adhere to the eating and exercise habits needed to sustain weight loss.

Maintenance of weight loss in our studies was limited to those time periods when patients were actively involved in either the treatment or maintenance programs. Thus, it is crucial that therapists help obese patients to understand the long-term implications regarding the management of obesity. Like diabetic or hypertensive patients, obese individuals may never be cured of their "disease." Rather, they must be resigned to keeping their condition under control through active efforts at self-management for the rest of their lives. The long-term implication for health care professionals is as daunting. Beyond acknowledging that obesity is a chronic problem, we must begin to structure treatments that will provide patients with lifelong assistance in managing their obesity (cf. Perri, 1989).

Effective maintenance programs will probably require multifaceted sets of strategies. Continued self-monitoring of eating and exercise behaviors appears to be a prerequisite for maintenance of weight loss. A high frequency of patient–therapist contacts (whether by telephone or in person) following treatment also appears essential to maintenance. After initial treatment, most patients require the help of a therapist to cope with the array of problems they face in maintaining their weight loss progress. Posttreatment contacts that utilize a problem-solving approach can provide a basic structure for therapists to assist patients in coping with the challenges of the posttreatment period.

The results from our studies suggest that skills training and social support strategies by themselves may not be sufficient to help patients sustain their weight losses on their own (see Studies 1 and 4). Moreover, the comprehensive year-long program of relapse prevention training in Study 5 did not yield benefits beyond those accomplished by the simpler program of therapist-led problem solving. Similarly, the social support intervention in Study 4 was less effective than the program of posttreatment therapist contacts. Nonetheless, skills training and social support strategies may be useful as components of multifaceted maintenance programs (see Studies 1, 2, 3, and 6).

Exercise can play a key role in the management of obesity. Study 3 showed that a program of regular physical activity can facilitate initial weight loss. Moreover, the results of Study 6 demonstrated that a maintenance program combining therapist contact with high frequency exercise and social support produced significant additional weight loss during the posttreatment period.

Effective regimens for the management of obesity may require multiple stages spanning very long periods of time. Initial treatments need to incorporate strategies to increase the amount of weight lost by patients. Lengthening initial treatments from 20 to 40 weeks can increase the amount of weight loss achieved by patients (cf. Perri, Nezu, Patti, & McCann, 1989). The use of increased physical activity, particularly supervised exercise, also may be useful in this regard (Craighead & Blum, 1989; Wing et al., 1988). The middle stages of long-term programs should be tailored to helping patients to maintain weight loss and to cope with the array of obstacles to maintenance that arise in the posttreatment period. As noted above, multifaceted maintenance programs that include continued self-monitoring and a high frequency of posttreatment therapist-led problem solving would appear appropriate to this end.

Finally, tertiary phases of long-term obesity management programs need to provide for follow-up care. The therapist and patient need to decide what happens after the maintenance program ends. Many patients will require a formal program of support. In some instances, groups such as Weight Watchers or Overeaters Anonymous may be appropriate for this purpose. In other instances, it may be helpful for therapists to develop programs of "follow-up" care that allow checks on progress several times per year. As therapist contact is faded, patients need to be provided with a way to get help if problems arise or relapse occurs. The availability of telephone contacts with the therapist, additional therapy sessions, or a refresher course in behavior therapy is likely to be necessary for successful long-term management of obesity.

Acknowledgment

The research summarized in this chapter was supported in part by the Department of Veterans Affairs Medical Research Service.

References

Ashby, W. A., & Wilson, G. T. (1977). Behaviour therapy for obesity: Booster sessions and long-term maintenance of weight. *Behaviour Research and Therapy, 14*, 451–464.

Beneke, W. M., & Paulsen, B. K. (1979). Long-term efficacy of behavior modification weight loss programs: A comparison of two follow-up maintenance strategies. *Behavior Therapy, 10*, 8–13.

Bennett, G. A. (1986). Behavior therapy for obesity: A quantitative review of selected treatment characteristics on outcome. *Behavior Therapy, 17*, 554–562.

Bennett, W. (1987). Dietary treatments of obesity. In R. J. Wurtman & J. J. Wurtman (Eds.), *Human obesity* (pp. 250–263). New York: New York Academy of Sciences.

Björntorp, P. (1978). Physical training in the treatment of obesity. *International Journal of Obesity, 2*, 149–156.

Brehm, S., & McAllister, D. A. (1980). Social psychological perspectives on the maintenance of therapeutic change. In P. Karoly & J. J. Steffen (Eds.), *Improving the long-term effects of psychotherapy* (pp. 381–406). New York: Gardner Press.

Brownell, K. D., & Foreyt, J. P. (1985). Obesity. In D. H. Barlow (Ed.), *Clinical handbook of psychological disorders* (pp. 299–345). New York: Guilford Press.

Brownell, K. D., Marlatt, G. A., Lichtenstein, E., & Wilson, G. T. (1986). Understanding and preventing relapse. *American Psychologist, 41*, 765–782.

Brownell, K. D., & Stunkard, A. J. (1980). Exercise in the development and control of obesity. In A. J. Stunkard (Ed.), *Obesity* (pp. 300–324). Philadelphia: W. B. Saunders.

Brownell, K. D., Stunkard, A. J., & Albaum, J. M. (1980). Evaluation and modification of exercise patterns in the natural environment. *American Journal of Psychiatry, 137*, 1540–1545.

Colvin, R. H., & Olson, S. B. (1983). A descriptive analysis of men and women who have lost weight and are highly successful at maintaining the loss. *Addictive Behaviors, 8*, 287–296.

Craighead, L. W., & Blum, M. D. (1989). Supervised exercise in behavioral treatment for moderate obesity. *Behavior Therapy, 20*, 49–59.

Dahlkoetter, J., Callahan, E. J., & Linton, J. (1979). Obesity and the unbalanced energy equation. *Journal of Consulting and Clinical Psychology, 47*, 898–905.

D'Zurilla, T. J., & Nezu, A. M. (1982). Social problem solving in adults. In P. C. Kendall (Ed.), *Advances in cognitive-behavioral research and therapy* (Vol. 1, pp. 202–274). New York: Academic Press.

Epstein, L. H., & Wing, R. R. (1980). Aerobic exercise and weight. *Addictive Behaviors, 5*, 371–388.

Folkins, C. H., & Sime, W. E. (1981). Physical fitness training and mental health. *American Psychologist, 36*, 373–389.

Foreyt, J. P. (1987). Issues in the assessment and treatment of obesity. *Journal of Consulting and Clinical Psychology, 55*, 677–684.

Garrow, J. S. (1986). Physiological aspects of obesity. In K. D. Brownell & J. P. Foreyt (Eds.), *Handbook of eating disorders: Physiology, psychology, and treatment of obesity, anorexia, and bulimia* (pp. 45–62). New York: Basic Books.

Gormally, J., & Rardin, D. (1981). Weight loss and maintenance and changes in diet and exercise for behavioral counseling and nutrition education. *Journal of Counseling Psychology, 28*, 295–304.

Hall, S. M., Bass, A., & Monroe, J. (1978). Continued contact and monitoring as follow-up strategies: A long-term study of obesity treatment. *Addictive Behaviors, 3*, 139–147.

Hall, S. M., Hall, R. G., Borden, B. L., & Hanson, R. W. (1975). Follow-up strategies in the behavioural treatment of overweight. *Behaviour Research and Therapy, 13*, 167–172.

Harris, M. B., & Hallbauer, E. S. (1973). Self-directed weight control through eating and exercise modification. *Behaviour Research and Therapy, 11*, 523–529.

Jeffery, R. W. (1987). Behavioral treatment of obesity. *Annals of Behavioral Medicine, 9*, 20–24.

Johnson, W. G., & Stalonas, P. M. (1981). *Weight no longer*. Gretna, LA: Pelican.

Katahn, M., Pleas, J., Thackrey, M., & Wallston, K. A. (1982). Relationship of eating and activity reports to follow-up weight maintenance in the massively obese. *Behavior Therapy, 13*, 521–528.

Kramer, F. M., Jeffery, R. W., Snell, M. K., & Forster, J. L. (1986). Maintenance of successful weight loss over 1 year: Effects of financial contracts for weight maintenance or participation in skills training. *Behavior Therapy, 17*, 295–301.

Marlatt, G. A., & Gordon, J. R. (Eds.). (1985). *Relapse prevention: Maintenance strategies in the treatment of addictive behaviors*. New York: Guilford Press.

Martin, J. E., & Dubbert, P. M. (1982). Exercise applications and promotion in behavioral medicine: Current status and future directions. *Journal of Consulting and Clinical Psychology, 50*, 1004–1017.

Perri, M. G. (1987). Maintenance strategies for the management of obesity. In W. G. Johnson (Ed.), *Advances in eating disorders: Vol. 1. Treating and preventing obesity* (pp. 177–194). Greenwich, CT: JAI Press.

Perri, M. G. (1989). Obesity. In A. M. Nezu & C. M. Nezu (Eds.). *Clinical decision making in behavior therapy: A problem-solving perspective* (pp. 193–226). Champaign, IL: Research Press.

Perri, M. G., McAdoo, W. G., McAllister, D. A., Lauer, J. B., Jordan, R. C., Yancey, D. Z., & Nezu, A. M. (1987). Effects of peer support and therapist contact on long-term weight loss. *Journal of Consulting and Clinical Psychology, 55*, 615–617.

Perri, M. G., McAdoo, W. G., McAllister, D. A., Lauer, J. B., & Yancey, D. Z. (1986). Enhancing the efficacy of behavior therapy for obesity: Effects of aerobic exercise and a multicomponent maintenance program. *Journal of Consulting and Clinical Psychology, 54*, 670–675.

Perri, M. G., McAdoo, W. G., Spevak, P. A., & Newlin, D. B. (1984). Effect of a multicomponent maintenance program on long-term weight loss. *Journal of Consulting and Clinical Psychology, 52*, 480–481.

Perri, M. G., McAllister, D. A., Gange, J. J., Jordan, R. C., McAdoo, W. G., & Nezu, A. M. (1988). Effects of four maintenance programs on the long-term management of obesity. *Journal of Consulting and Clinical Psychology*, *56*, 529–534.

Perri, M. G., McKelvey, W. F., Schein, R. L., Renjilian, D. A., Viegener, B. J., & Nezu, A. M. (1990, November). *Relapse prevention training versus frequent therapist contacts as weight-loss maintenance strategies.* Paper presented at the annual meeting of the Association for Advancement of Behavior Therapy, San Francisco.

Perri, M. G., Nezu, A. M., Patti, E. T., & McCann, K. L. (1989). Effect of length of treatment on weight loss. *Journal of Consulting and Clinical Psychology*, *57*, 450–452.

Perri, M. G., Shapiro, R. M., Ludwig, W. W., Twentyman, C. T., & McAdoo, W. G. (1984). Maintenance strategies for the treatment of obesity: An evaluation of relapse prevention training and posttreatment contact by mail and telephone. *Journal of Consulting and Clinical Psychology*, *52*, 404–413.

Spevak, P. A. (1981). Maintenance of therapy gains: Strategies, problems, and progress. *JSAS: Catalog of Selected Documents in Psychology*, *11*, 35. (Ms. No. 2255)

Stalonas, P. M., Johnson, W. G., & Christ, M. (1978). Behavior modification for obesity: The evaluation of exercise, contingency management, and program adherence. *Journal of Consulting and Clinical Psychology*, *46*, 463–469.

Stalonas, P. M., & Kirschenbaum, D. S. (1985). Behavioral treatments for obesity: Eating and exercise habits revisited. *Behavior Therapy*, *16*, 1–14.

Stalonas, P. M., Perri, M. G., & Kerzner, A. B. (1984). Do behavioral treatments of obesity last? A five-year follow-up investigation. *Addictive Behaviors*, *9*, 175–184.

Stern, J. S., & Lowney, P. (1986). Obesity: The role of physical activity. In K. D. Brownell & J. P. Foreyt (Eds.), *Handbook of eating disorders: Physiology, psychology, and treatment of obesity, anorexia, and bulimia* (pp. 145–158). New York: Basic Books.

Stuart, R. B. (1980). Weight loss and beyond: Are they taking it off and keeping it off? In P. O. Davidson & S. M. Davidson (Eds.), *Behavioral medicine: Changing health lifestyles* (pp. 151–194). New York: Brunner/Mazel.

Thompson, J. K., Jarvie, G. J., Lahey, B. B., & Cureton, K. H. (1982). Exercise and obesity: Etiology, physiology, and intervention. *Psychological Bulletin*, *91*, 55–79.

Wadden, T. A., & Bell, S. T. (1990). Obesity. In A. S. Bellack, M. Hersen, & A. E. Kazdin (Eds.), *International handbook of behavior modification and therapy* (2nd ed., pp. 449–473). New York: Plenum.

Wadden, T. A., Sternberg, J. A., Letizia, K. A., Stunkard, A. J., & Foster, G. D. (1989). Treatment of obesity by very low calorie diet, behavior therapy, and their combination: A five-year perspective. *International Journal of Obesity*, *13*, 39–46.

Wing, R. R., Epstein, L. H., Paternostro-Bayles, M., Kriska, A., Nowalk, M. P., & Gooding, W. (1988). Exercise in a behavioural weight control programme for obese patients with type 2 (non-insulin-dependent) diabetes. *Diabetologia*, *31*, 902–909.

20
Long-Term Pharmacological Treatment of Obesity

BERNARD GUY-GRAND

Advances in modern medicine and the indisputable progress that has been made over the past 50 years in the treatment of human diseases are based primarily upon the use of drugs, including such Promethean actions as grafting of vital organs and notwithstanding concurrent iatrogenic pathology.

Obesity has reached epidemic proportions in Western countries. Although many efforts have been made to combat this disorder (as discussed in this book), pharmacotherapy of obesity has received relatively little attention and, in fact, is frequently disparaged by the medical community. Among the many reasons likely to foster such an unfavorable attitude are a misconception of obesity itself, lack of commitment to the necessity of treatment, underestimation of its requirements, and undue expectations of drug therapy. Such attitudes have resulted in a lack of investigations in this area, and disappointment in the efficacy and risk-benefit ratio of pharmacological treatments for obesity.

Research on the etiology of obesity has increased dramatically during the past three decades and has led to several important findings. Curiously enough, however, this advancement in knowledge has not led to more successful treatment for the majority of obese patients. There is widespread agreement that the treatment of obesity remains an unsolved challenge. Although some innovative combinations of treatment have been attempted (Björvell & Rössner, 1985; Wadden & Stunkard, 1986), conventional outpatient therapies are still largely unsuccessful in helping people maintain weight losses over time (Bennett, 1987; Stunkard, 1984; Wing & Jeffery, 1979), and have improved only marginally over the last 40 years (Stunkard & McLaren-Hume, 1959). Surgical procedures are appropriate in limited circumstances (Task Force of the American Society for Clinical Nutrition, 1985) and may be associated with untoward consequences. Thus, a re-evaluation of the goals and strategies of the treatment of obesity is warranted.

Strategies for Weight Control

An examination of the history of weight control efforts leads to an appreciation of the need for a long-term managerial strategy (for a full discussion, see

Guy-Grand, 1987b). Body weight results from the complex interplay of genetic factors (mostly involving energy expenditure) and environmental factors (mostly involving food intake) (Bouchard, 1985; Bouchard et al., 1990; Ravussin et al., 1988). An individual's weight cannot be changed without inducing a negative energy balance. Techniques for accomplishing this include the "big five" of (1) various calorie-restrictive diets; (2) behavior and lifestyle modification; (3) drugs; (4) physical exercise; and (5) gastric surgery.

With sufficient external constraints and adequate motivation, most patients will achieve a negative energy balance and begin to lose weight. Counteracting factors progressively begin to intercede, however, and decrease the rate of weight loss. The influence of these factors, which include metabolic, psychological, and behavioral variables, has been discussed elsewhere (Guy-Grand, Waysfeld, & Le Barzic, 1984). With all types of treatment, including gastric surgery, a new state of weight equilibrium is reached after some weeks or months. (The exception, of course, is with starvation or semistarvation, which overrides the adaptive capabilities of the body and can eventually lead to death.) This new weight may or may not be located in the so-called "normal" range, depending on a number of factors; these include the cause of the obesity, the extent to which internal and external changes have been made, and, in some cases, the duration and severity of the constraints themselves. This new weight equilibrium represents the point where the counteracting factors have equaled the impact of the treatment. When the constraint is terminated, or if the patient is able to escape it, the energy balance again becomes positive. The consequence is weight gain as the patient relapses. All too frequently, patients regain all of their lost weight, and occasionally more. Such relapse almost invariably occurs following treatment by diet alone (Atkinson, 1990; Bennett, 1987), after withdrawal of drugs to induce weight loss (see below), and to a lesser extent following behavioral treatment (Foreyt et al., 1982). Approximately three-fourths of the patients presenting at our clinic report a history of such weight loss and regain (i.e., the "yo-yo syndrome"). Such weight cycling may be as harmful as the obesity itself (Lissner et al., 1991).

Hence, there is a clear need for the development of long-term strategies to control body weight in obese individuals. This is a critical issue that was raised some 15 years ago (Bray, 1978; Stunkard & Penick, 1979; Wilson, 1978), but that has only recently been addressed (Brownell, Marlatt, Lichtenstein, & Wilson, 1986; Stalonas, Perri, & Kerzner, 1984). As Rössner (1989) has noted, the majority of efforts have been directed toward short-term weight loss studies instead of long-term results and the prevention of relapse.

Factors Responsible for Poor Outcome

There are many reasons for the poor long-term outcome of treatments for obesity, some of which will be discussed briefly.

1. *View of obesity as a homogeneous disorder.* Garrow (1981) has indicated that the general trend in therapeutic research has been to design a

treatment and test its efficacy with "the obese in general." Most current techniques are well standardized, but have been used among patient populations that vary widely. Obesity, however, is increasingly recognized as a heterogeneous disorder, multifactorial in origin and etiology. Hence, failure of one method with a given patient does not indicate that another method also will fail. Indeed, it should be pointed out that whatever the technique used, it will be successful with some patients (Wing & Jeffery, 1979). Practitioners, however, are generally unable to identify the predictors of success. A more promising approach may be to match individuals to the treatment programs from which they would benefit the most. To achieve this goal, more reliable clinical indicators must be identified and developed (Guy-Grand, 1987b).

2. *Obesity as a chronic condition.* The treatment of obesity cannot be restricted to a standardized program designed to induce short-term weight loss. As in most chronic and disabling diseases (e.g., hypertension, diabetes), it is naive to believe that a short-lived action—mimicking the prescription of antibiotics for infectious diseases or appendicitis—can solve the problem. Indeed, the vast majority of treatments that are available today are mostly palliative, not curative in nature: They are able to alleviate the symptom but not to cure it.

3. *Unrealistic expectations.* The goal weights assigned to patients (or chosen by patients themselves) are often unrealistic. Such goals give little credence to physiological and psychological limitations, and thus establish conditions that encourage relapse or severe malnutrition. Large weight losses do not appear to be possible or even necessary in all patients. Small weight losses of 10–15% of initial body weight are more easily achieved and maintained. They can be beneficial, even in massively obese people. Such patients experience multiple risk factors as a result of their weight, so that even a small decrease in weight may induce a substantial decrease in overall risk.

4. *Weight loss as the focus of obesity treatment.* It should be noted that weight loss is not the *only* goal of obesity therapy. Halting weight gain in rapidly gaining or relapsing patients, achieving weight stability in those with a history of yo-yo dieting, and improving psychological and social functioning (in patients who cannot lose sufficient weight to meet social standards) are worthy tasks for practitioners. Such improvements, however, cannot be evaluated in terms of weight loss, and their achievement is seldom considered in the literature.

It is apparent from this discussion that the long-term control of obesity must include either the cure of a fundamental etiologic disturbance or the lifelong management of this disorder by appropriate symptomatic means. Thus, in the majority of patients, the multifactorial origins of the disorder make an etiological approach to treatment unlikely, and possible only when an irreversible hyperplasia of adipose tissue has not occurred (Sjöström, 1980). On the other hand, few palliative measures are available that provide a favorable long-term outcome. Among other perspectives discussed in this volume, long-term pharmacotherapy may provide a novel approach if not an old temptation. Although it has not been considered favorably (Galloway, Farquhar, & Munro, 1984) or included in routine medical care to date (at least officially), recent data suggest that pharmacotherapy may make an important contribution to the management of some obese patients (Guy-Grand, 1989).

Rationale for Long-Term Pharmacotherapy

According to most current licensing regulations, the pharmacological treatment of obesity is only allowed for short periods, most commonly 12–16 weeks. This practice may reflect, in part, the belief that obesity can be treated successfully on a short-term basis, as well as the fact that clinical trials until recently have been limited to brief periods.

It is well known, however, that most of the weight lost during short-term treatment is fully regained when the drug is discontinued (Bray, 1978; Craighead, Stunkard, & O'Brien, 1981; Munro & Ford, 1982; Wing & Jeffery, 1979). Even our continuous prescription of dexfenfluramine for 1 year was associated with weight regain when the drug was withdrawn (Guy-Grand et al., 1990). Such a finding is hardly surprising. It follows that short-term drug therapy is inappropriate in most instances and of little value when the maintenance over time of a reduced body weight is the goal (Guy-Grand & Waysfeld, 1978; Munro & Ford, 1982). When a large, rapid weight loss is needed for medical or surgical reasons, other procedures such as very low calorie diets (VLCDs) are indicated.

The question of the long-term (eventually lifelong) administration of drug therapy could be raised (Garrow, 1990; Guy-Grand, 1987b, 1989; Munro, 1987) when one considers that (1) obesity is a major health problem; (2) the management of diseases with severe medical and social consequences (e.g., hypertension, diabetes, hyperlipidemia, chronic respiratory disease, arthritis of the hips and knees) is often dependent upon weight loss; (3) only sustained weight loss confers medical benefits; and (4) current therapy too often ends in failure. This proposal reflects the current *Zeitgeist* in the management of most other chronic disabling diseases, such as hypertension, diabetes, hyperlipidemia, and gout, in which palliative drugs with potentially severe side effects are commonly used on a lifelong basis. Unfortunately, obese patients are still frequently considered guilty, self-indulgent gluttons who require moral exhortation (to adhere to punitive diets), rather than such assistance as might be offered by pharmacotherapy. Thus, to employ drug therapy with the obese flies in the face of the usual recommendations.

The question is thus raised as to whether any available drug is ethically usable today in the long-term management of obesity. As proposed some years ago (Guy-Grand, 1988), the main properties that an antiobesity drug must have to be used on a long-term basis are listed in Table 20.1. Similar criteria have been proposed by Garrow (1990).

The first condition, efficacy, is self-evident. It is important, however, that the composition of the weight loss consist predominantly of fat and not of

TABLE 20.1. Characteristics of a Drug for Long-Term Use

1. Potent weight-lowering effect in short-term controlled trials.
2. Acceptable clinical tolerance.
3. No addictive properties.
4. Sustained effects when treatment is continued.
5. Absence of major hazards after years of administration.
6. Known mechanisms of action.

fluids or fat-free mass. Such criteria would thus exclude agents such as diuretics and thyroid hormones (Abraham, Densem, Davies, Davies, & Wynn, 1985).

The second criterion, clinical tolerance, does not necessarily require that the drug be devoid of side effects, but that such side effects be bearable and/or transient in order to facilitate adherence and minimize attrition from therapy.

The third condition, concerning addictive properties of the drug, is particularly important for centrally acting agents, since a toxicomanic predisposition seems quite frequent (although this has not been precisely evaluated) among the obese population.

The fourth condition, long-term efficacy, is essential. Only long-term studies will be able to detect a true pharmacological tolerance to a drug (i.e., weight regain while the drug is still administered, and maintenance of the effect only by an increase in the dose). Presently, long-term trials have been performed with only a few drugs (see below). The duration of such trials must not be less than 1 year (Apfelbaum et al., 1987). Given the difficulties and increased cost of such investigations, it seems unlikely that longer trials will be conducted frequently.

The fifth condition, concerning long-term safety, is essential to ascertain that the risk-benefit ratio remains acceptable. As with all drugs commonly prescribed for extended periods, only extensive follow-up of large numbers of patients will alert investigators to issues concerning long-term safety.

The last condition, an explanation of the mechanisms of action, is also important. Such an understanding will allow practitioners to select patients likely to benefit from the use of the drug, according to the physiopathological features that characterize each specific condition.

Potential Sites of Action of Drugs

Energy metabolism is regulated by a complex and integrated system that controls food intake, energy storage, and energy expenditure. It involves many different and interdependent steps, each of which could be a potential pharmacological target. Only a limited number of theoretical possibilities have been explored so far; some others are in development. (An additional question that can be raised is whether obesity results from definite impairments in this system or from a normal response of the system to changing environmental conditions. However, this discussion is beyond the scope of this chapter.)

Although this is an obvious oversimplification, it is easy to separate (1) peripheral mechanisms involving organs (sensory organs, gastrointestinal tract, liver, muscles, adipose tissue, glands) with their more or less specific biochemical processes and their psychomotor expression (behavior), viewed as effectors of the system; (2) central mechanisms involving the brain, viewed as the controller of the system and integrating biological and psychological information; and (3) mechanisms conveying signals between both levels (metabolic substrates, hormones, and the autonomic nervous system).

Centrally Acting Drugs

Centrally acting drugs promote directly or indirectly (via their metabolites) the release of monoamines, inhibit monoamine reuptake by neuronal endings, and probably have specific actions on some of the subtypes of monoamine receptors. Therefore, such drugs interfere with the complex network of neurochemical pathways of the integrated biopsychological system that controls feeding behavior (Blundell, 1991) and includes different functions (hunger, appetite, satiation, satiety) and operations (food choice, food preferences). Some drugs act via the adrenergic and dopaminergic pathways (e.g., *d*-amphetamine), while others act upon the serotonergic pathways, indicating that different drugs are able to modify different functions. The serotonergic drugs (primarily *dl*-fenfluramine and dexfenfluramine) have given rise to extensive pharmacological investigations (for a review, see Garattini, Bizzi, Caccia, Mennini, & Samanin, 1988). Their actions on feeding behavior are largely different from those of amphetamine-like drugs, as they function by increasing and extending the physiological satiating power of food, postponing hunger. Such drugs also may reduce motivation for eating in different situations and thus may modify eating patterns (Nathan & Rolland, 1987). In animals, a rapid tolerance is shown for the suppression of food intake, but not for weight reduction (Rowland & Carlton, 1986).

In addition, centrally acting drugs can be expected to modify not only behavioral reactions, but also some important metabolic functions as well. Dexfenfluramine, for example, has been shown to partially prevent the decreases in resting metabolic rate and glucose-induced thermogenesis that occur with weight loss (Van Gaal, Vansant, Van de Woorde, & De Leeuw, 1991). Thus, in effect, such drugs may reset body weight at a lower level (Stunkard, 1982) and should no longer be regarded as simply altering quantitative food intake, as indicated by the term of "anorectics" or "appetite suppressants." In addition, they are likely to interfere with functions that are not directly and specifically involved in the physiological regulation of energy metabolism. The stimulation of general psychomotor activity with adrenergic drugs, and the modification of stress reactions with dexfenfluramine (Brindley, 1988), are examples. Moreover, some drugs may have direct peripheral effects on cellular metabolism (Turner, 1979).

Peripherally Acting Drugs

Peripherally acting drugs alter the functioning of effector organs. Such effects, however, may be bypassed by compensatory mechanisms or may achieve efficacy only when the target organ's functioning is severely impaired. For example, drugs to increase thermogenesis through peripheral mechanisms have been tested with unfavorable results. Dinitrophenol, an uncoupler of oxidative phosphorylation, have proved toxic; thyroid hormones induce a loss of fat-free mass. Agonists of β_1- and β_2-adrenergic receptors, particularly ephedrine, have been tested in very short-term trials in humans with unconvincing results (Bray, 1988) and produced tachycardia, a worrisome side effect. Recently, preclinical data have been presented for drugs that are possible agonists of the new β_3-adrenergic receptor. These agents include RO 40-2148 in humans (Jéquier, Munger, & Felber, 1992) and in fatty rats BRL 35 135 and its metabolite BRL 37 344 (Cawthorne, Sennitt, Arch, & Smith, 1992). Drugs that limit nutrient absorption in the gastrointestinal tract have also been investigated. Acarbose, an α-glucidase inhibitor, has been shown to help prevent relapse in severely obese persons (William-Olson, Krotkiewski, & Sjöström, 1985), but it is not commonly used in obesity therapy. Tetrahydrolipstatin, a potent inhibitor of pancreatic lipase, has proven effective in preclinical trials with rats (Meier et al., 1991). The inhibition of fat absorption (or prevention of high fat intake due to steatorrhea) may be important, since fat accumulation correlates with fat ingestion (Jéquier, Schutz, & Flatt, 1991).

Future research may provide new drug therapies, but at present only the so-called anorectics are available. The most widely used of these compounds are listed in Table 20.2. They are structurally related to β-phenylethylamine, except mazindol, which is related to the tricyclic antidepressants.

Drugs Eligible for Long-Term Use

This section will review drugs currently available with respect to the four first conditions listed in Table 20.1—short-term efficacy, clinical tolerance, potential for addiction, and long-term efficacy. A tentative model for the prospective development of future drugs will be offered.

Efficacy in Short-Term Clinical Trials

Many short-term (e.g., 4- to 12-week) controlled trials of appetite suppressants plus various dietary recommendations in obese subjects have shown that these

TABLE 20.2. Centrally Acting Anorectic Drugs

Catecholaminergic[a]	Serotonergic
Diethylpropion	dl-Fenfluramine hydrochloride
Phentermine	Dexfenfluramine
Mazindol	dl-Fluoxetine[b]
Phenylpropanolamine	

[a]Drugs of DEA Classes II and III have been omitted.
[b]Licensed as an antidepressant drug.

drugs produce weight losses two to four times greater than those associated with a placebo (for reviews, see Bray, 1988; Galloway et al., 1984; Munro & Ford, 1982). These drugs include dexfenfluramine (Guy-Grand, 1987a), fluoxetin (Levine, Enas, Thompson, Byymy, & Daver, 1989), and phenylpropanolamine (Greenway, 1989).

These studies, however, have several limitations, including (1) a high level of dropout (up to 60%); (2) the wide use of fractional weight loss (kilograms per week) as an index of success; (3) enormous variability in response to each drug; and (4) better results in unselected patients than in those with refractory obesity (Guy-Grand, 1987a; Munro & Ford, 1982).

1. *High dropout rates.* In some studies, attrition rates reach 60%. Investigators do not report data for those individuals who drop out of the study, thus limiting an assessment of the overall clinical usefulness of the drug.

2. *Fractional weight loss.* Most often, weight loss is reported in fractional form (e.g., kilograms per week). While such an index may be useful in the short term, its relevance is questionable in longer-term studies in which weight maintenance after weight loss is the goal of treatment.

3. *Variability of individual responses.* Frequently, mean weight loss in patients completing the study is reported as the sole end-point variable. Such practice may mask important differences in individual responses to treatment. Differences in adherence may in fact account for the significant variability in weight loss, but is more likely to be related to the heterogeneity in drug metabolism, metabolic states, or physiopathological traits among included patients. Greater variability is also observed with small sample sizes. The same variability also occurs when treatment is limited to diet or behavioral modification. When a single therapy is administered to a heterogeneous disorder of multiple etiology, marked variability of response is to be expected.

A few studies have directly compared the short-term efficacy of two or more drugs and found them to be roughly equivalent. Examples include comparisons of diethylpropion and dl-fenfluramine (Silverstone, Cooper, & Begg, 1970), diethylproprion and mazindol (Allen, 1977), phentermine and dl-fenfluramine (Tuominen & Hietula, 1990), and phenylpropanolamine (plus caffeine) and diethylpropion (Altschuler, Conte, Sebok, Marlin, & Winick, 1982).

Side Effects

The high attrition rates in most clinical studies (with no information reported on patients lost to follow-up) may confound the frequency of adverse experiences and their influence on adherence rates. In studies with few subjects, such differences between the drug and placebo conditions rarely achieve statistical significance.

The drugs that act via catecholamine pathways are typically sympathetic activators and thus often result in insomnia, nervousness, irritability, headaches, sweating, palpitations, and dry mouth. Although euphoria is less common than with amphetamines and phenmetrazines, it can occur with all drugs (with the exception of mazindol). Hence, these drugs are not suitable for all patients. Individuals with psychotic structure are at risk of decompensating. Hypertension and angina pectoris are additional contraindications.

The serotonergic drugs have sedative effects. Unpleasant symptoms include tiredness, diarrhea, nausea, and drowsiness. Depression, especially after acute withdrawal, and mood disorders have been reported with *dl*-fenfluramine. (Depression after withdrawal may be a potential side effect of dexfenfluramine, but has not been evaluated to date.) Dexfenfluramine is not recommended in patients with a history of depression except in those with seasonal affective disorder (O'Rourke, Wurtman, Wurtman, Chebli, & Gleason, 1989). Dose-dependent sweating, asthenia, and somnolence have been reported with fluoxetine (Levine & al., 1989). The combination of phentermine and fenfluramine resulted in fewer adverse effects overall (Weintraub, Hasday, Mushlin, Dean, & Lockwood, 1984). In general, however, the incidence and experience of such side effects do not severely affect the clinical tolerance of these drugs.

Potential for Abuse

It has been shown that *dl*-fenfluramine and dexfenfluramine are unlikely to induce drug addiction (Götestam & Dahl, 1987). The same is probably true for fluoxetine.

With the exception of Drug Enforcement Agency (DEA) Class II and Class III drugs (amphetamine, *d*-amphetamine, phenmetrazine, benzphetamine, phendimetrazine), catecholaminergic drugs have a low potential for abuse. The exception is diethylpropion, for which cases of abuse have been reported infrequently, and mainly in those predisposed by a previous history of addiction (Griffith, Brady, & Bradford, 1979). To date, no long-term data are available on the potential for abuse. Thus, although the risk of addiction is low, careful consideration is warranted before using such drugs.

Maintenance of Action over Time

Only a handful of studies have evaluated the efficacy of drug therapy lasting more than 20 weeks. All of these studies have shown that weight loss plateaued over time—from 8 weeks to 6 months. Munro, McGuish, Wilson, and Duncan (1968) reported that when phentermine was administered continuously or every 2 months to induce weight loss during 24 weeks, a stable weight was maintained until 36 weeks. Enzi, Baritussio, Machion, and Crepaldi (1976) found that with mazindol, weight loss continued beyond 6 months with both the drug and the placebo. The results of this study, however, are clearly atypical. An open study with continuous administration of dl-fenfluramine (80 mg/day) resulted in the maintenance of weight loss for 1 year with low attrition rates and few adverse reactions (Hudson, 1977). More recently, Douglas, Ghough, and Preston (1983), in their study of obese patients who had lost weight during a run-in period, found that 8 of 21 subjects (38%) receiving drug therapy maintained their weight loss over 1 year, as compared with 1 of 21 (4.8%) of patients who were on placebo. In a 52-week trial that used 60 mg fluoxetine (i.e., three times more than the recommended dose for antidepressant action) and included 52 patients (of whom only 21 completed treatment), Marcus, Wing, Ewing, Kern, and McDermott (1990) observed maintenance of body weight after the 20th week. This effect was stronger in nonbingeing than in bingeing patients. Thus, there is evidence that some drugs, including phentermine, mazindol, and dl-fenfluramine, are able to maintain initial weight loss when prescribed over longer periods of time. Such findings, however, remain preliminary.

In an effort to further investigate the feasibility of long-term pharmacotherapy of obesity, a 1-year trial of dexfenfluramine known as INDEX (the International Dexfenfluramine Study) was undertaken (Guy-Grand et al., 1989). Dexfenfluramine was selected for several reasons: (1) its documented short-term efficacy; (2) low risk of addiction; (3) preliminary data demonstrating the efficacy of dl-fenfluramine during long-term administration; (4) efficacy at half the dose of the racemic compounds (Silverstone, Smith, & Richards, 1987); and (5) the findings that the l isomer results in minimal weight loss and is a less specific serotonin agonist than the d isomer (Garattini, 1990; Garattini et al., 1988).

INDEX was a randomized double-blind trial involving 24 centers in nine countries. Designed by an independent scientific committee, INDEX included 822 obese patients who ranged from 120% to 306% over ideal body weight. About half the subjects received dexfenfluramine, 15 mg twice daily, while the other half received the placebo. In addition, all patients were prescribed a balanced-deficit diet because it was judged to be unethical to maintain patients on placebo alone over 1 year. Results of the study are summarized below.

Attrition

By 12 months, 189 subjects (45%) had withdrawn from the placebo, compared to 150 subjects (37%) from dexfenfluramine. Dissatisfaction with the rate of weight loss (84 vs. 49 subjects) was the only reason more frequently reported by the placebo group and, in fact, accounted for almost all of the excess withdrawals. Other reasons, including side effects, were equally distributed between both groups.

Weight Loss

Both absolute and relative weight loss were calculated. Relative weight (i.e., percentage reduction in initial weight) may avoid the bias produced by the fact that weight loss correlates directly with initial body weight. Hence, relative weight may be a more valid measure, since patients vary widely in initial weights. It also allows comparison among studies including cohorts of patients with different mean weights.

The "cohort analysis," which accounts for all patients who achieve a given target weight loss, is probably the least biased way to interpret data. It also addresses the problem of clinical relevance, since it includes data on all patients who enter the study and regards the dropouts as nonlosers. At 12 months, more than twice as many patients on dexfenfluramine as on placebo achieved a weight loss of greater than 10% of their initial weight or more than 10 kg. They represented one-third of the initial cohort. Complete failure (including withdrawals and dropouts) was observed in 36.9% of dexfenfluramine patients.

A comparison of the mean weight loss in the residual cohorts of completing patients—patients attending all the mandatory visits—is a more conventional method of reporting outcome data. However, both weight losers and nonlosers are thus included, and the measures are largely dependent upon attrition. Dexfenfluramine patients lost significantly ($p < .001$) more weight after 12 months (9.82 ± 0.49 kg) than placebo patients (7.15 ± 0.49 kg) (10.26% and 7.18% of initial weight, respectively). This difference may appear to be minimal; however, in reality those individuals who received dexfenfluramine lost 33% to 52% more weight than placebo patients (depending on how weight loss is expressed).

It is important to note that the significant weight loss achieved by the placebo cohort was the likely result of the combined effects of the placebo, dietary changes, and the supportive counseling offered by the investigators. The results achieved with the placebo can be favorably compared with those of programs incorporating diet alone (Wing & Jeffery, 1979; Bennett, 1987). Overall, results achieved with dexfenfluramine fell well within the range of those obtained with behavior therapy (Craighead et al., 1981; Foreyt et al.,

1982) or combined conservative treatment (Björvell & Rössner, 1985; Wadden & Stunkard, 1986).

Time Course of Weight Loss

Another important issue in the INDEX trial was the time course of the weight loss (see Figure 20.1). On average, a weight plateau was reached with dexfenfluramine after 6 months, with maintenance of the weight loss up to 12 months. However, some patients continued to lose, some regained, and some plateaued. Those in the placebo group regained weight significantly ($p < .05$). When dexfenfluramine was withdrawn after completion of the study, a rapid weight gain occurred within 2 months. This regain was twice as large as that which occurred after the withdrawal of the placebo. This clearly indicates that the pharmacological effect of the drug continued during the 6-month plateau phase (Guy-Grand et al., 1990). During this period the action of the drug was not to promote additional weight loss but to prevent weight regain.

Other studies of 6 months' duration with obese patients have confirmed that dexfenfluramine will assist in weight maintenance by preventing weight regain or inducing additional weight loss. Recently, Finer, Finer, and Naoumova (1989) reported a 14-kg weight loss in severely obese patients who participated in an 8-week VLCD program. Upon completion, the patients were randomized blindly into dexfenfluramine or placebo conditions, each of which was associated with a less restrictive diet for a 26-week period. Dexfenfluramine patients continued to lose weight (5.8 kg), whereas placebo patients regained 2.6 kg. Only 3 of 16 patients on dexfenfluramine regained some weight, as compared with 11 of 16 patients who were on placebo. Also, Noble (1990) blindly administered dexfenfluramine or placebo for 24 weeks to obese

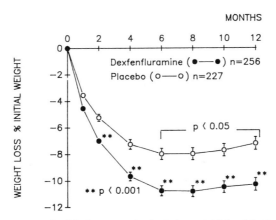

FIGURE 20.1. Time course of weight loss, expressed relative to initial weight, in patients completing the INDEX study. **Denotes significant differences between groups. Data from Guy-Grand et al. (1989).

patients who had lost weight and were weight-stable (although still dieting). Again, dexfenfluramine patients lost 6.2 kg on average ($p < .001$) while placebo patients lost an additional 2.6 kg (n.s.). Taken together, these data indicate that dexfenfluramine in conjunction with a balanced-deficit diet may be useful in helping obese individuals maintain or increase weight loss for longer periods of time.

Dexfenfluramine use was not associated with major health complications in the INDEX study. Tiredness, diarrhea, dry mouth, polyuria, and drowsiness were the only adverse experiences more frequently reported while taking the drug than while taking the placebo. Most of these symptoms were reported during the first month of treatment.

Taken together, these findings show that continuous administration of dexfenfluramine may foster dietary adherence, facilitate further weight reduction without harmful side effects, and enhance maintenance of the initial weight loss.

When one is evaluating the appropriateness of a drug for long-term use (outlined in Table 20.1), dexfenfluramine appears to meet the first four criteria (i.e., short-term efficacy, clinical tolerance, low potential for abuse, and evidence of long-term efficacy). While other drugs have demonstrated short-term efficacy and clinical tolerance, only dexfenfluramine has been adequately evaluated in terms of its long-term efficacy and mechanisms of action. A recent 1-year trial with fluoxetine (Darga, Carroll-Michels, Botsford, & Lucas, 1991) found that drug unable to maintain initial weight loss beyond 6 months. Clearly, a 1-year period (considered lengthy for drug trials) is, in fact, a short period with respect to the lifelong treatment of obesity. The reader is cautioned not to extrapolate the data to longer periods, as rates of compliance, pharmacological action, and safety over years of administration remain to be evaluated by careful follow-up. There is no evidence to suggest that long-term use of dexfenfluramine may be harmful. Thus long-term pharmacotherapy can no longer be considered utopian.

Practical Use of Long-Term Pharmacotherapy

To engage a patient in any lifelong treatment requires serious consideration. This applies to pharmacotherapy as well as to nutritional modification, as addressed by Bennett (1987).

First, obesity is a very complex symptom. No one strategy is effective for all patients, and adapting the treatment program to the specific needs of a given patient is an integral part of any comprehensive approach.

Second, the use of drugs should be restricted to those who are at risk as a result of their obesity, or to those with medical conditions that will be ameliorated by sustained weight loss (e.g., diabetes, hypertension, rheumatology, and respiratory disorders). Dexfenfluramine, which has been shown to have hypotensive properties (Andersson, Zimmerman, Hedner, & Björntorp, 1991) and to improve insulin resistance (Scheen, Paolisso, Salvatore, & Lefebvre, 1991) independent of weight loss, may be of particular interest for individuals with abdominal obesity (Björntorp, 1987).

Third, since drugs are used to help obese individuals reduce their caloric intake below societal norms, they must be included in a program that combines nutritional information, lifestyle changes, careful monitoring, and adequate reinforcement. The use of any drug should not replace other types of interventions when they appear more appropriate.

Long-term pharmacotherapy may be appropriate for consideration under two circumstances. The primary indication would be to induce and maintain weight loss in patients unable to follow a reasonable diet (but this must be tried first) or in those with a lifelong history of weight loss and regain. Serotonergic drugs (mostly dexfenfluramine) are able to decrease the intermeal craving frequently reported by such individuals (Wurtman, Wurtman, Reynolds, Tsay, & Chew, 1987); however, to date there are no data clearly indicating that the presence of such cravings is a predictor of sustained action.

The secondary indication for the use of dexfenfluramine is to increase weight loss and/or avoid relapse in patients who have lost weight with conventional diets, VLCDs, or behavioral programs. Since food restriction has been shown to increase an individual's sensitivity to stress (Halmi, Stunkard, & Mason, 1980) and to increase the urge to eat (Herman & Polivy, 1975), dietary restriction over the long term may have untoward consequences that could be improved by serotonergic drugs. More trials of longer duration than that of Finer et al. (1989) are warranted to identify which drugs are appropriate, when to best include them in the course of therapy, and for which patients.

Some practitioners may consider the efficacy and safety data available thus far on dexfenfluramine as insufficient to allow for use beyond 1 year, although there is no evidence that such sustained use would be harmful. On the other hand, if a drug appears helpful for certain patients in facilitating weight loss, weight maintenance, or metabolic improvement, there is no reason to deprive them of this help.

Conclusion

Given the difficulty that many patients experience in maintaining their initial weight losses achieved with standard dietary and behavior modification programs, the concept of long-term drug therapy to facilitate weight control seems warranted. To date, the drug dexfenfluramine has been studied the most extensively. Evidence indicates that this drug may be effective in this regard and should be considered as part of a long-term strategy to control health-threatening obesity. Future research is likely to identify other pharmacological tools that will help manage this still unsolved challenge.

References

Abraham, R. R., Densem, J. W., Davies, P., Davies, M. W., & Wynn, V. (1985). The effects of triiodothyronine on energy expenditure, nitrogen balance and rates of weight and fat loss in obese patients during prolonged caloric restriction. *International Journal of Obesity, 9,* 433–442.

Allen, G. S. (1977). A double blind trial of diethylpropion hydrochloride, mazindol and placebo in the treatment of exogenous obesity. *Current Therapeutics and Research, 22,* 678–683.

Altschuler, S., Conte, A., Sebok, M., Marlin, R., & Winick, C. (1982). Three controlled trials of weight loss with phenylpropanolamine. *International Journal of Obesity, 6,* 549–556.

Andersson, B., Zimmerman, M. R., Hedner, T., & Björntorp, P. (1991). Hemodynamic, metabolic and endocrine effects of short-term dexfenfluramine treatment in young obese women. *European Journal of Clinical Pharmacology, 40,* 249–254.

Apfelbaum, M., Björntorp, P., Garrow, J., James, W. P. T., Jéquier, E., & Stunkard, A. J. (1987). Standards for reporting the results of treatment for obesity. *American Journal of Clinical Nutrition, 45,* 1035–1036.

Atkinson, R. L. (1990). Usefulness and limits of VLCD in the treatment of obesity. In Y. Oomura, S. Tarui, S. Inoue, & T. Shimazu (Eds.), *Progress in obesity research* (pp. 473–480). London: John Libbey.

Bennett, W. (1987). Dietary treatments of obesity. *Annals of the New York Academy of Science, 499,* 250–263.

Björntorp, P. (1987). The prevalence of obesity: Complications related to the distribution of body fat. In A. E. Bender & L. J. Brookes (Eds.), *Body weight control: The physiology, clinical treatment, and prevention of obesity* (pp. 185–192). Edinburgh: Churchill Livingstone.

Björvell, H., & Rössner, S. (1985). Long-term treatment of severe obesity: Four year follow up of results of combined behavioral modification programme. *British Medical Journal, 291,* 379–382.

Blundell, J. (1991). Pharmacological approaches to appetite suppression. *Trends in Pharmacological Sciences, 12,* 147–157.

Bouchard, C., Tremblay, A., Despres, J. P., Nadeau, A., Lupien, P., Theriault, G., Dussault, J., Moorjani, S., Pinault, S., & Fournier, G. (1990). The response to long-term overfeeding in identical twins. *New England Journal of Medicine, 322,* 1477–1482.

Bouchard, C. (1985). Inheritance of fat distribution and adipose tissue metabolism. In J. Vague, P. Björntorp, B. Guy-Grand, M. Rebuffe-Scrive, & P. Vague (Eds.), *Metabolic complications of human obesity* (pp. 87–96). Amsterdam: Excerpta Medica.

Bray, G. A. (1978). To treat or not to treat—that is the question. In G. Bray (Ed.), *Recent advances in obesity research: II. Proceedings of the Second International Congress on Obesity* (pp. 248–265). London: Newman.

Bray, G. A. (1988). Obesity: Part II. Treatment. *Western Journal of Medicine, 149,* 555–571.

Brindley, J. (1988). Metabolic and hormonal effects of dexfenfluramine on stress situations. *Clinical Neuropharmacology, 11*(Suppl. 1), S86–S89.

Brownell, K. D., Marlatt, G. A., Lichtenstein, E., & Wilson, G. T. (1986). Understanding and preventing relapse. *American Psychologist, 41,* 765–782.

Cawthorne, M. A., Sennitt, M. V., Arch, J. R. S., & Smith, S. A. (1992). BRL 35135, a potent and selective atypical β-adrenoreceptor agonist. *American Journal of Clinical Nutrition, 55,* 252S–257S.

Craighead, L. W., Stunkard, A. J., & O'Brien, R. (1981). Behavior therapy and pharmacotherapy of obesity. *Archives of General Psychiatry, 38,* 763–768.

Darga, L., Carroll-Michels, L., Botsford, S., & Lucas, C. (1991). Fluoxetine's effect on weight loss in obese subjects. *American Journal of Clinical Nutrition, 54,* 321–325.

Douglas, J. G., Ghough, J., & Preston, P. G. (1983). Long-term efficacy of fenfluramine in treatment of obesity. *Lancet, i,* 384–386.

Enzi, G., Baritussio, A., Machion, E., & Crepaldi, G. (1976). Short-term and long-term clinical evaluation of a non amphetamine anorexiant (mazindol) in the treatment of obesity. *Journal of Internal Medicine and Research, 4,* 305-310.

Finer, N., Finer, S., & Naoumova, R. P. (1989). Prolonged use of a very low calorie diet in massively obese patients: Safety, efficacy and additional benefit from dexfenfluramine. *International Journal of Obesity, 13*(Suppl. 1), 91-93.

Foreyt, J. P., Mitchell, R. E., Garner, D. T., Gee, M., Scott, L. W., & Gotto, A. M. (1982). Behavioral treatment of obesity: Results and limitations. *Behavior Therapy, 13,* 153-161.

Galloway, S., Farquhar, D. L., & Munro, J. F. (1984). The current status of antiobesity drugs. *Postgraduate Medical Journal, 60*(Suppl. 3), 19-26.

Garattini, S. (1990). Experimental pharmacology of serotoninergic drugs. *International Journal of Obesity, 14*(Suppl. 2), 32.

Garattini, S., Bizzi, A., Caccia, S., Mennini, T., & Samanin, R. (1988). Progress in assessing the role of serotonin in the control of food intake. *Clinical Neuropharmacology, 11*(Suppl. 1), 8-33.

Garrow, J. S. (1981). *Treat obesity seriously: A clinical manual.* Edinburgh: Churchill Livingstone.

Garrow, J. S. (1990). Drugs for the treatment of obesity. What do we need? *Pharmaceutical Medicine, 4,* 213-218.

Götestam, K. F., & Dahl, C. B. (1987). Fenfluramine and drug addiction. In A. E. Bender & L. J. Brookes (Eds.), *Body weight control: The physiology, clinical treatment and prevention of obesity* (pp. 271-279). Edinburgh: Churchill Livingstone.

Greenway, F. (1989). A double blind clinical evaluation of the anorectic activity of phenylpropanolamine versus placebo. *Clinical Therapeutics, 11,* 584-589.

Griffith, R., Brady, J., & Bradford, L. (1979). Predicting the abuse liability of drugs with animal drug self-administration procedures, psychomotor stimulants and hallucinogens. *Advances in Behavioral Pharmacology, 2,* 163-208.

Guy-Grand, B. (1987a). Therapeutic use of dexfenfluramine. In A. E. Bender & L. J. Brookes (Eds.), *Body weight control: The physiology, clinical treatment and prevention of obesity* (pp. 280-285). Edinburgh: Churchill Livingstone.

Guy-Grand, B. (1987b). A new approach to the treatment of obesity: A discussion. *Annals of the New York Academy of Science, 499,* 313-317.

Guy-Grand, B. (1988). Place of dexfenfluramine in the management of obesity. *Clinical Neuropharmacology, 11*(Suppl. 1), S216-S223.

Guy-Grand, B. (1989). Long-term pharmacotherapy in the management of obesity: From theory to practice. In P. Björntorp & S. Rössner (Eds.), *Obesity in Europe, 88* (pp. 311-318). London: John Libbey.

Guy-Grand, B., Apfelbaum, M., Crepaldi, G., Gries, A., Lefebvre, P., & Turner, P. (1989). International trial of long-term dexfenfluramine in obesity. *Lancet, ii,* 1142-1144.

Guy-Grand, B., Apfelbaum, M., Crepaldi, G., Gries, A., Lefebvre, P., & Turner, P. (1990). Effect of withdrawal of dexfenfluramine on body weight and food intake after a one year's administration. *International Journal of Obesity, 14*(Suppl. 2), S48.

Guy-Grand, B., & Waysfeld, B. (1978). Pharmacologie de l'obésité. In J. P. Giroud, G. Mathe, & G. Meyniel (Eds.), *Traité de pharmocologie clinique* (pp. 924-936). Paris: Expension Scientifique Française.

Guy-Grand, B., Waysfeld, B., & Le Barzic, M. (1984). Resistances à l'amaigrissement. *Revue du Praticien, 34,* 3111-3120.

Halmi, K. A., Stunkard, A. J., & Mason, E. E. (1980). Emotional responses to weight reduction by three methods: Diet, jejuno ileal bypass, and gastric bypass. *American Journal of Nutrition, 33,* 446-451.

Herman, C. P., & Polivy, J. (1975). Anxiety, restraint and eating behavior. *Journal of Abnormal Psychology, 984,* 666-672.

Hudson, K. D. (1977). The anorectic and hypotensive effect of fenfluramine in obesity. *Journal of the Royal College of General Practitioners, 27,* 497-501.

Jéquier, E., Munger, R., & Felber, J. P. (1992). Thermogenic effects of various β-adrenoceptor agonists in humans: Their potential usefulness in the treatment of obesity. *American Journal of Clinical Nutrition, 55,* 249S–251S.

Jéquier, E., Schutz, Y., & Flatt, J. R. (1991). Nutrient balance in body weight regulation: Its importance for the development of obesity in man. *International Journal of Obesity, 14*(Suppl. 2), 22.

Levine, L., Enas, G., Thompson, W., Byymy, R., & Daver, A. (1989). Use of fluoxetine, a selective serotonin-uptake inhibitor in the treatment of obesity: A dose–response study (with a commentary by Michael Weintraub). *International Journal of Obesity, 13,* 635–645.

Lissner, L., Odell, P. M., D'Agostino, R. B., Stokes, J., Kreger, B. E., Belanger, A. J., & Brownell, K. D. (1991). Variability of body weight and health outcomes in the Framingham population. *New England Journal of Medicine, 324,* 1839–1844.

Marcus, M. B., Wing, R. R., Ewing, L., Kern, E., & McDermott, M. (1990). A double-blind, placebo controlled trial of fluoxetine plus behavior modification in the treatment of obese binge-eaters and non-binge eaters. *American Journal of Psychiatry, 147,* 876–881.

Meier, M., Blum-Kaelin, D., Bremer, K., Isler, D., Joly, R., Keller-Rup, P., & Lengsfeld, H. (1991). Preclinical profile of the lipase inhibitor tetrahydrolipstatin (RO 18-06 47), a potential drug for the treatment of obesity. *International Journal of Obesity, 15*(Suppl. 1), 31.

Munro, J. F. (1987). Drug treatment: An overview. *International Journal of Obesity, 11* (Suppl. 3), 13–15.

Munro, J. F., & Ford, M. J. (1982). Drug treatment of obesity. In T. Silverstone (Ed.), *Drugs and appetite* (pp. 125–157). London: Academic Press.

Munro, J. F., McGuish, A., Wilson, E., & Duncan, G. (1968). Comparison of continuous and intermittent anorectic therapy in obesity. *British Medical Journal, i,* 352.

Nathan, C., & Rolland, Y. (1987). Pharmacological treatments that affect CNS activity, serotonin. *Annals of the New York Academy of Sciences, 499,* 277–296.

Noble, R. E. (1990). A six month study of the effects of dexfenfluramine on partially successful dieters. *Current Therapeutics and Research, 47,* 612–619.

O'Rourke, D., Wurtman, J. J., Wurtman, R. J., Chebli, R. N., & Gleason, R. (1989). Treatment of seasonal affective depression with d-fenfluramine. *Journal Clinical of Psychiatry, 50,* 343–347.

Ravussin, E., Lilioga, S., Knowler, W. C., Christin, L., Fremont, D., Abbot, W., Boyce, V., Howard, B., & Bogardus, C. (1988). Reduced rate of energy expenditure as a risk factor for body weight gains. *New England Journal of Medicine, 318,* 467–472.

Rössner, S. (1989). Towards a new policy for obesity treatment. In P. Björntorp & S. Rössner (Eds.), *Obesity in Europe 88* (pp. 29–34). London: John Libbey.

Rowland, N., & Carlton, J. (1986). Disorders of eating behavior, a psychoneuroendocrine approach. In E. Ferrari & F. Brambilla (Eds.), *Advances in the biosciences* (pp. 367–374). Oxford: Pergamon Press.

Scheen, A. J., Paolisso, G., Salvatore, T., & Lefebvre, P. (1991). Dexfenfluramine reduces insulin resistance independently of weight reduction in obese type II diabetic patients. *Diabetes Care, 14,* 325–332.

Silverstone, T., Cooper, R., & Begg, R. (1970). A comparative trial of fenfluramine and diethylpropion in obesity. *British Journal of Clinical Practitioners, 24*(Suppl. 10), 423–425.

Silverstone, T., Smith, G., & Richards, S. (1987). A comparative evaluation of dexfenfluramine and dlfenfluramine. In A. E. Bender & L. J. Brookes (Eds.), *Body weight control: The physiology, clinical treatment and prevention of obesity* (pp. 240–246). Edinburgh: Churchill Livingstone.

Sjöström, L. (1980). Fat cells and body weight. In A. J. Stunkard (Ed.), *Obesity* (pp. 72–100). Philadelphia: W. B. Saunders.

Stalonas, P. M., Perri, M. G., & Kerzner, A. B. (1984). Do behavioral treatments of obesity last? A five year follow up investigation. *Addictive Behaviors, 9,* 175–183.

Stunkard, A. J. (1982). Anorectic agents lower a body weight set point. *Life Sciences, 30,* 2043–2055.

Stunkard, A. J. (1984). The current status of treatment for obesity in adults. In A. J. Stunkard & E. Stellar (Eds.), *Eating and its disorders* (pp. 157-173). New York: Raven Press.

Stunkard, A. J., & McLaren-Hume, M. (1959). The result of treatment for obesity. *Archives of Internal Medicine, 103*, 79-85.

Stunkard, A. J., & Penick, S. B. (1979). Behavior modifications in the treatment of obesity, the problem of maintaining weight loss. *Archives of General Psychiatry, 36*, 801-806.

Task Force of the American Society for Clinical Nutrition. (1985). Guidelines for surgery for morbid obesity. *American Journal of Clinical Nutrition, 42*, 904-905.

Tuominen, S., & Hietula, M. (1990). Double blind trial comparing fenfluramine, phentermine and dietary advice on treatment of obesity. *International Journal of Obesity, 14*(Suppl. 2), 138.

Turner, P. (1979). Peripheral mechanisms of action of fenfluramine. *Current Medical Research and Opinion, 6*(Suppl. 1), 101-106.

Van Gaal, L., Vansant, G., Van de Woorde, K., & De Leeuw, I. (1991). Positive effects of dexfenfluramine on energy expenditure during long-term weight reduction in obese women. *International Journal of Obesity, 15*(Suppl. 1), 70.

Wadden, T. A., & Stunkard, A. J. (1986). Controlled trial of very low calorie diet, behavior therapy and their combination in the treatment of obesity. *Journal of Consulting and Clinical Psychology, 54*, 482-488.

Weintraub, M., Hasday, J., Mushlin, A., Dean, H., & Lockwood, D. (1984). A double-blind clinical trial in weight control: Use of fenfluramine and phentermine alone and in combination. *Archives of Internal Medicine, 144*, 1143-1148.

William-Olson, T., Krotkiewski, M., & Sjöström, L. (1985). Relapse reducing effect of acarbose after weight reduction in severely obese patients. *Journal of Obesity and Weight Regulation, 4*, 20-32.

Wilson, G. T. (1978). Methodological considerations in treatment outcome research in obesity. *Journal of Consulting and Clinical Psychology, 46*, 678-702.

Wing, R. R., & Jeffery, R. W. (1979). Outpatient treatments of obesity: A comparison of the methodology and clinical results. *International Journal of Obesity, 3*, 261-280.

Wurtman, J., Wurtman, R., Reynolds, S., Tsay, R., & Chew, B. (1987). *d*-Fenfluramine suppresses snack intake among carbohydrate cravers but not among non-carbohydrate cravers. *International Journal of Eating Disorders, 6*, 687-699.

21

Surgical Treatment of Obesity

JOHN G. KRAL

The heaviest patients and the most seriously ill should be treated surgically if they are truly motivated to ameliorate their obesity. Other treatments, alone or in combinations, are unsuccessful in the majority of these patients and have almost without exception been attempted before patients request surgery. Safety of performance of the surgery is no longer an issue in most patients. As a consequence, surgical treatment has become more acceptable. The major concerns are maintenance of weight loss and benefits to health beyond 5 years after the operation, and potential side effects of maintaining reduced weight. Optimum amount of total weight loss and the rate of initial weight loss, as well as safety of reoperations and choice of method at reoperation, are also issues in this field.

Indications for surgery are serious diseases such as hypertension, diabetes, thromboembolism or hypoventilation that are treatable by weight loss, in cases where other treatment has failed to achieve or maintain weight loss. In the absence of such manifest diseases, a weight level 45 kg (100 pounds) above life insurance weight standards for height is also considered an indication. Eligibility criteria include the patient's having a clear understanding of the rationale for the surgery and the requirement for lifelong postoperative care. Clearly identifiable self-destructive behavior and emotional instability thought to jeopardize cooperation with postoperative care are contraindications (Task Force of the American Society for Clinical Nutrition, 1985).

The following is a description of currently available techniques, with some critical notes on issues still requiring resolution in the field of antiobesity surgery.

Surgical Methods

Gastric Restriction

Two principally different approaches have dominated the field of surgical treatment of severe obesity: gastric restriction and gastrointestinal bypass (see Table 21.1). The "gastroplasty" operations consist of reducing the receptive capacity of the stomach by creating a small (15-ml) stapled pouch with a small opening (10 mm in diameter), externally reinforced by a ring to prevent stretching (see Figure 21.1). The rationale is that the extreme prolongation of

TABLE 21.1. Major Surgical Techniques for the Treatment of Obesity

Gastric restriction	Gastrointestinal bypass
Gastroplasty • Horizontal[a] • Gastric partitioning[a] • Vertical banded (VBG) • Silastic ring vertical (SRVG)	Intestinal bypass • Jejunoileal[b] with biliointestinal
Gastric banding[b] • Adjustable band	Gastric bypass • "Distal" gastric bypass
Gastric bypass	Biliopancreatic diversion

[a]Obsolete.
[b]Questionable.

emptying of food from the pouch will lead to overdistension, causing "satiety," discomfort, nausea, or pain. The flaws are that (1) liquids and semisolid or easily dissolvable foods of high caloric density (e.g., potato chips, cookies, chocolate) pass virtually unimpeded through the pouch, and can be ingested in excess (the "soft calorie syndrome"; see Table 21.2), and (2) repeated overdistension leads to stretching and increased pouch capacity. This latter problem is

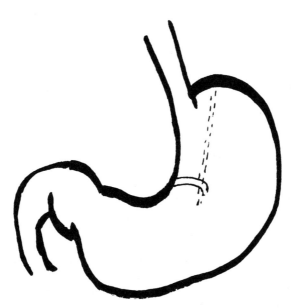

FIGURE 21.1. Gastroplasty. A vertical staple line creates a 15-ml pouch just beyond the gastroesophageal junction. An external band prevents the opening between the pouch and the rest of the stomach from expanding.

TABLE 21.2. Criteria for the Diagnosis of "Soft Calorie Syndrome" after Gastric Restrictive Operations for Obesity

↑ Calorically dense liquids	↑ "Melting" calories
Alcohol	Chips
Sodas	Cookies, cake
↑ Soft calories	Sweet addiction
Ice cream	Chocolate
Cheese	Refined sugar

simplistically being addressed by encircling the pouches with multiple rings. The behavior problem of the soft calorie syndrome cannot be managed by gastroplasty alone (Kral & Kissileff, 1987).

Data on the importance of the size of the outlet are equivocal, though it is clear that weight loss with an external band 5.5 cm in length is less than with a 5.0-cm band. Bands 4.5 cm and shorter seem to cause more disruption of staple lines in gastroplasties, secondary to outlet blockage. An ingenious technique to vary outlet size postoperatively has been developed by L. Kuzmak of New Jersey. A small siliconized reservoir connected to an inflatable gastric band is implanted just beneath the skin. By adding or withdrawing fluid through ultrasound-guided injection into the reservoir, the physician can adjust an appropriately constricting outlet size according to the needs of the patient. Dr. Kuzmak feels that this will diminish maladaptive eating and gastric pouch enlargement. By allowing greater diversity in food choices, it could potentially improve adherence to a "gastroplasty diet" and ultimately lead to healthier food choices. Long-term follow-up is needed to determine whether this indeed is an improvement over other gastric restrictive procedures (Kuzmak, 1989).

Gastrointestinal Bypass

Gastrointestinal bypass operations exclude either 90% of the small intestine ("intestinal bypass") or 90% of the stomach, the whole duodenum, and varying lengths of small intestine ("gastric bypass") (see Figure 21.2). The gastric bypass operation was originally thought to cause gastric restriction, but it is apparent that maldigestive mechanisms as well as complex patterns of peptide release influencing motility and putative satiety receptors participate in causing weight loss (Kellum et al., 1990). By virtue of their superior effectiveness over gastric restriction, bypass operations cause more nutritional deficiencies. These are manageable if patients adhere to follow-up monitoring and prescribed supplements. There are no methods for predicting patients' adherence postoperatively.

Intestinal bypass operations (not involving the stomach) fell into disfavor during the late 1970s owing to large numbers of complications, some of which

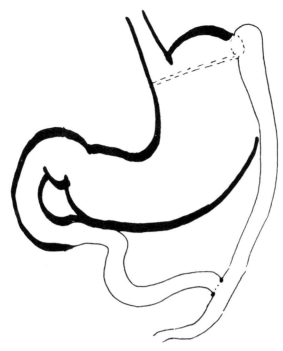

FIGURE 21.2. Gastric bypass. A staple line closes off a 15-ml proximal pouch. A loop of small bowel is joined to the pouch, allowing nutrients to bypass the excluded stomach and the duodenum.

were severe and irreversible. The operations were given the blame, though the management of the patients was clearly suboptimal, resulting from ignorance among physicians and from patients' not complying with surveillance and supplementation of vitamins and minerals. Most complications were caused by bacterial overgrowth, or the "blind loop syndrome," known from other types of small intestinal operations. Several operative strategies for avoiding these problems seem to be fairly successful. Thus, there still seems to be a role for these types of operations in special cases (Kral, 1987).

Gastric bypass has been shown to be consistently more effective than gastroplasty (Hall et al., 1990). Nevertheless, about 25% of patients with gastric bypass either fail to lose more than 40% of their excess weight or regain substantial amounts of weight beyond 3–5 postoperative years. For this reason, modifications of gastric bypass are being performed that either support the restrictive component of the operation by banding the outlet (i.e., banded gastric bypass) or increase the malabsorptive component by bypassing greater lengths of small intestine. The most drastic operation is "biliopancreatic bypass," introduced by N. Scopinaro of Genoa in 1976 (see Scopinaro et al.,

1981). It consists of two-thirds resection of the stomach, closing of the proximal duodenum, and bypass of 50% of the small intestine, diverting the biliopancreatic secretions to the last 50 cm of ileum where absorption ultimately takes place. The "U.S. version" of the operation (i.e., distal gastric bypass) does not resect the stomach, but staples across it, as in conventional gastric bypass. It is likely that observation longer than 5 years is necessary to fully evaluate these operations, because of their potential for causing deficiencies.

In summary, then, there are two generic surgical techniques that are reasonably safe and effective. Just as the 1970s witnessed adjusting the lengths of small bowel in intestinal bypass, and the 1980s saw variations in pouch and outlet size in gastric restriction, it seems that the 1990s will experience "titrating" the optimal proportions among intestinal length, pouch volume, and outlet size. It is possible that a staged approach, with more than one operation, ultimately will prove safest and most efficacious.

Results of Treatment

Complications and Side Effects

Perioperative mortality in severely obese patients having a primary operation to control obesity is below 1% in centers specializing in this type of surgery. The operative complications are similar in type and quantity to those of any other major gastrointestinal surgery. Long-term complications are proportional to the effectiveness of the operation in causing weight loss and reducing obesity comorbidity. Vitamin and mineral deficiencies and anemia occur in 15–30% of patients with gastric bypass, and in somewhat fewer patients with gastroplasty (Halverson, 1987).

Gastric restrictive operations can cause vomiting if the patient does not follow simple rules of eating, such as chewing meticulously, not drinking with meals (only before or at least 2–3 hours after), and recognizing signals of pouch distension. Gastrointestinal bypass operations can cause diarrhea, which is manageable through dietary counseling or antidiarrheal medication. Gastric bypass causes "dumping"—a syndrome of weakness, palpitations, and possible diaphoresis associated with excessive intake of carbohydrate and believed to be responsible for the greater effectiveness of the operation over gastroplasty. Many patients also report intolerance of dairy products, which also might be beneficial for achieving weight loss.

Weight Loss

Weight loss is characteristically between 25% and 35% of preoperative weight. This corresponds to 40–60% of excess weight (the weight exceeding ideal or desirable weight for height, according to life insurance tables). Gastroplasty

Surgical Treatment of Obesity

patients lose the lower percentage, bypass patients the higher one. Though most surgeons require patients to be at least 45 kg (100 pounds) over desirable weight for height, there are considerable differences in mean weights of different surgical series. This is partly due to sex distribution, race, and geographic variations, but may also reflect varying policies among surgeons or differences in referral patterns. Generally, surgical candidates in rural U.S. areas weigh more than those in large U.S. metropolitan areas, where patients are heavier than in Canada, Australia, or Europe.

Patients are reported to lose 80% of excess weight after biliopancreatic bypass, distal gastric bypass, and banded gastric bypass. This degree of weight loss is associated with a greater frequency of nutritional sequelae, which may require hospitalization. It is not known whether very long-term effects of this degree of weight loss may be detrimental to health or longevity. All studies of carefully followed patients have revealed some degree of weight increase beyond 5 postoperative years (Pories, Caro, Flickinger, Meelheim, & Swanson, 1987). It is possible that even patients with extreme weight loss will reach a steady state beyond which they will start to regain.

Comorbidity Reduction

Just as weight loss by nonsurgical methods improves diabetes, hypertension, respiratory insufficiency, sleep apnea, arthritis, and other serious morbidity associated with obesity, so does postoperative weight loss. Table 21.3 is a compilation of the effects of surgery on comorbid conditions. This improvement in health is naturally associated with improved quality of life. One extremely important side effect of severe obesity is a significant impairment in the ability to pursue normal activities of daily living (Sullivan, Sullivan, & Kral, 1987). Weight reduction through surgery is effective in ameliorating

TABLE 21.3. Effects of Surgery on Serious Diseases Associated with Obesity: Pooled Data of More than 1000 Patients Compiled from Published Series

	Prevalence (%)	"Cured"[a] (%)	Improved[b] (%)
Hypertension	30–60	60–65	90
Diabetes	15–20	90–95	100
Dyslipidemia	15–25	70	85
Asthma	10–15	>95	100
Heart failure	10	60	90
Sleep apnea	2–5	100	100

[a]Absence of symptoms with no need for medication.
[b]Reduced dosage of medication.

several aspects of quality of life, though it must be recognized that intrinsic psychosocial problems independent of the obesity will remain unaffected by the loss of weight. For example, marital discord may even be aggravated after surgery and ultimately lead to divorce.

Patient Selection

Just as it is with all forms of treatment of obesity, long-term follow-up is difficult to achieve after surgery. Because of the effectiveness of surgical methods, with risks of developing deficiencies, lifelong surveillance is essential. Furthermore, it is important to ensure that the patients take prescribed supplements to prevent deficiencies. Gastric restrictive operations (i.e., gastroplasty) rely on strict adherence to rules of eating, and in this respect they are no different from other diets. The mechanical component of the operation is effective only until the pouch has stretched or, more commonly, until the patient develops "maladaptive eating" (soft calorie syndrome; see Table 21.2).

Table 21.4 suggests methods for selecting candidates for antiobesity surgery. If the patient understands the severity of the disease, it is expected that motivation is stronger to cooperate in the care plan. Many obese patients exhibit extraordinary denial of the health implications of their condition. By exploring the beliefs and knowledge of the candidate, the practitioner can better tailor preoperative education with a view to increasing the motivation for weight reduction.

Tests for compliance have not been proven to predict or improve outcome of any treatment of obesity, whether surgical or other. Results of diet treatment are *a priori* poor in surgical candidates, so it would seem redundant to use results of diet treatment as a test of compliance. However, in the highly structured and well-defined context of preoperative preparation, it would seem reasonable to use diet performance as a predictor of postoperative cooperation

TABLE 21.4. Methods for Selecting Candidates for Antiobesity Surgery

1. Analysis of health beliefs
    a. Denial of obesity as a disease
    b. Knowledge of health risks
2. Tests of compliance
    a. Diet treatment
    b. Ability to stop smoking
    c. Appointment keeping
3. Assessment of social environment
    a. Secondary gain
    b. Codependency

TABLE 21.5. Subjective Benefits of Being Obese (Secondary Gain)

1. Elicitation of help and pity
2. Excuse for vocational/social failure or lack of competitiveness
3. Compensation for lack of assertiveness
4. Use of food for emotional comfort
5. Protection from unwanted sex
6. Avoidance of physical activity
7. Keeping warm in cold weather

(Charles, 1985). In other fields of medicine, appointment keeping has been shown to be highly correlated with adherence to medication and consequently with the outcome of treatment.

In assessing motivation to lose weight, it is important to recognize numerous mechanisms that patients may have developed to obtain secondary gain from their severely obese state (see Table 21.5). In addition to easily identifiable forms, such as controlling friends and relatives through helplessness, more subtle mechanisms may involve "protection" from sexual experiences or simply coping with exigencies of the workplace or job market. A particularly treacherous pitfall is codependency with spouses or significant others who have an investment in the helplessness of the obese individual. This can be a cause of weight loss failure or of the breakup of relationships after "successful" weight loss.

The same predictors of weight loss or of adherence to a program that have been demonstrated for dieting and other nonsurgical treatment would be expected to apply to gastric restrictive operations. Several studies seeking differences in psychopathology between surgical candidates and other obese patients and normal-weight populations have not detected any significant increases in psychopathology in the obese. However, the Minnesota Multiphasic Personality Inventory and other questionnaires have been able to characterize typical psychological traits in the severely obese population. Personality traits, demographic data, and psychological status have been shown in some studies of patients with gastrointestinal bypass to predict short-term weight loss (maintenance) (Blankmeyer et al., 1989). Long-term data are lacking. Sugerman et al. (1989) demonstrated significantly greater weight loss after gastric bypass than after gastroplasty in patients characterized preoperatively as being "sweets eaters." To date, this is the only study demonstrating any benefit of selective assignment of patients to different types of operations.

Discussion and Summary

Obviously, surgical treatment does not obviate the need for a holistic approach to the patient. It is likely that gastric restrictive operations require active cooperation, with conscious modification of eating behavior, more than the intrinsically aversive bypass operations do. The requisite "behavioral component" of bypass operations involves taking supplements and adhering to surveillance protocols. That such cooperation is easier to achieve than modification of eating behavior is supported by lower dropout rates after bypass surgery than after gastric restriction.

In spite of the shortcomings of surgical treatment and a prevailing disregard for behavioral factors in choice of operations, the results of antiobesity surgery are dramatically superior to those of other forms of treatment. This has not led to complacency on the part of surgeons, who, on the contrary, may be faulted for trying to achieve spectacular and possibly unhealthy weight loss by devising unnecessarily severe operations. To the credit of surgeons, and in sharp contrast to all other groups of professionals treating obesity, surgeons adhere to generally accepted standards of reporting data by requiring 5-year follow-up and showing concern over dropout rates. In those rare exceptions where long-term follow-up data are presented for series of nonsurgical treatments, the failure rate is consistently $\geq 95\%$ (Stunkard, Stinnett, & Smoller, 1986). Although the criteria for success vary and are open to debate, about 50% of severely obese patients undergoing surgical treatment maintain a reduction of greater than 50% of excess body weight 5 years after surgery, with a perioperative mortality of less than 1% in centers experienced in this type of surgery.

"Success" of antiobesity surgery can be measured in different ways, with different implications for determining a procedure of choice or "gold standard." Though it might seem simple to choose longevity or death as an end point, there are several inherent difficulties with this. The natural history of severe obesity, whether treated or not, is not known and is not amenable to study, though it is clear that mortality is significantly increased. Characteristically, the severely obese do not participate in national nutritional or other surveys. With respect to reduction of morbidity, it is not uncommon that obesity comorbidity is exchanged for side effects or complications of the surgery, if it successfully reduces weight. The individual patient is probably the only one capable of choosing which of the risks is preferable. It is obvious that the definition of "success" ultimately must rest with the patient, who best can determine quality of life in terms of physical and psychological well-being; this might include socioeconomic functioning, cosmetic results, or just plain weight loss. Unfortunately, there is often a conflict between the patient's definition and that of the surgeon, which in turn might differ from that of other health professionals (in particular, those without experience in treating obese patients).

Directions for Future Research

1. Accurate and reproducible risk factor profiles should be developed that identify patients who may be treated with gastric restriction without gastro-

intestinal bypass. Special attention should be paid to the importance of formal education, economic status, race, and ethnicity.

2. Further data should be gathered on the long-term safety and efficacy of gastric restriction and gastrointestinal bypass for treating or preventing obesity comorbidity.

3. Methods for reoperation should be determined, with attention to safety and efficacy.

4. The ability of preoperative weight loss to help select patients and to improve safety of the operations should be evaluated.

5. Quality-of-life parameters, particularly regarding functional well-being and psychosocial adaptation after weight loss, need to be assessed.

Summary

The two main types of surgery for obesity—gastric restriction and gastrointestinal bypass—can effectively and safely reduce weight and ameliorate comorbidity, with maintenance for at least 5 years in approximately 50% of patients. In eligible patients, these results are far superior to those of any nonsurgical methods to date. Vomiting and/or diarrhea should not be accepted after these types of operations, but should be treated vigorously, with the understanding that modifiable maladaptive behavior might be the cause. Further improvement in safety and efficacy requires better understanding of motivational factors and selective assignment of patients to specific treatment modalities, surgical or other.

References

Blankmeyer, B. L., Smylie, K. D., Price, D. C., Costello, R. H., McFee, A. S., & Fuller, D. S. (1989). A replicated five cluster MMPI typology of morbidly obese female candidates for gastric bypass. *International Journal of Obesity, 14*, 235-247.

Charles, S. C. (1985). Psychological predictors of obesity surgery outcome. In J. Hirsch & T. B. VanItallie (Eds.), *Recent advances in obesity research: IV. Proceedings of the Fourth International Congress on Obesity* (pp. 254-259). London: John Libbey.

Hall, J. C., Watts, J. M., O'Brien, P., Dunstan, R. E., Walsh, J. F., Slavotinek, A. H., & Elmslie, R. F. (1990). Gastric surgery for morbid obesity: The Adelaide study. *Annals of Surgery, 211*, 419-427.

Halverson, J. D. (1987). Vitamin and mineral deficiencies following obesity surgery. *Gastroenterology Clinics of North America, 16*, 307-315.

Kellum, J. M., Kuemmerle, J. F., O'Dorisio, T. M., Rayford, P., Martin, D., Engle, K., Wolf, L., & Sugerman, H. J. (1990). Gastrointestinal hormone responses to meals before and after gastric bypass and vertical banded gastroplasty. *Annals of Surgery, 211*, 763-771.

Kral, J. G. (1987). Malabsorptive procedures in surgical treatment of morbid obesity. *Gastroenterology Clinics of North America, 16*, 293-305.

Kral, J. G., & Kissileff, H. R. (1987). Surgical approaches to the treatment of obesity. *Annals of Behavioral Medicine, 9*, 15-19.

Kuzmak, L. I. (1989). Gastric banding. In M. Deitel (Ed.), *Surgery for the morbidly obese patient* (pp. 225-259). Philadelphia: Lea & Febiger.

Pories, W. J., Caro, J. F., Flickinger, E. G., Meelheim, H. D., & Swanson, M. S. (1987). The control of diabetes mellitus (NIDDM) in the morbidly obese with the Greenville gastric bypass. *Annals of Surgery, 206*, 316-323.

Scopinaro, N., Gianetta, E., Civalleri, D., Bonalumi, U., Friedman, D., & Bachi, V. (1981). Partial and total biliopancreatic bypass in the surgical treatment of obesity. *International Journal of Obesity, 5*, 421-429.

Stunkard, A. J., Stinnett, J. L., & Smoller, J. W. (1986). Psychological and social aspects of the surgical treatment of obesity. *American Journal of Psychiatry, 143*, 417-429.

Sugerman, H. J., Londrey, G. L., Kellum, J. M., Wolf, L., Liszka, T., Engle, K. M., Birkenbauer, R., & Starkey, J. V. (1989). Weight loss with vertical banded gastroplasty and Roux-Y gastric bypass for morbid obesity with selective versus random assignment. *American Journal of Surgery, 157*, 93-102.

Sullivan, M. B. E., Sullivan, L. G. M., & Kral, J. G. (1987). Quality of life assessment in obesity: Physical, psychological and social function. *Gastroenterology Clinics of North America, 16*, 433-442.

Task Force of the American Society for Clinical Nutrition. (1985). Guidelines for surgery for morbid obesity. *American Journal of Clinical Nutrition, 42*, 904-905.

Index

Abdominal obesity
  coronary artery disease, 138
  dexfenfluramine in, 491
  diabetes risk, 232
  health risks, 6, 7, 14, 25, 26
  and weight loss, 390
Absolute energy deficit, 96, 97
Absolute energy expenditure, 170
Absorption
  and intestinal morphology, animals, 112–114
  species variation, 108, 109
Acarbose, 484
Activity pathway, 365, 366, 370, 372
Adaptation (*see* Metabolic adaptation)
Adherence (*see also* Attrition; Maintenance of weight loss; Relapse)
  exercise programs, 361, 362, 373, 374, 466–473
  group discussion, 315
  posttreatment program, 466
  prediction from initial interview, 306
  refeeding period, 340, 341
  social support effect, 373, 374, 472
  and stimulus narrowing, 317
  therapist contact, value of, 472
Adipose tissue
  lipid metabolism, animals, 114, 115
  refeeding effects, 114, 115
Adolescent-onset obesity
  body image, 258, 263
  fat cell number, 294
Aerobic fitness, 360
  and adherence, 473
  exercise goal, 364, 365
  in multicomponent program, 463–466
Afterload
  in obesity, 142, 143
  weight loss effect, 149

Age
  as attrition predictor, 384
  and risk calculation, 22, 23
Alcohol consumption, 349
Alcoholism
  contraindication for very low calorie diets, 298
  and initial medical evaluation, 277
  and relapse, 444, 449
All-cause mortality, 11–13
"All-or-none thinking," 320
Ambulatory electrocardiogram
  liquid protein diet, 154
  in obesity, 145, 146
American Cancer Society study
  disease-specific mortality, 13
  risk information source, 9, 10
American College of Sports Medicine, 364
American Dietetic Association, 351
Amino acids, liquid protein diet, 121
Amphetamines
  abuse potential, 486
  central actions, 483
Android obesity, 6 (*see also* Abdominal obesity)
Anger, and refeeding, 318
Angina pectoris
  morbidity risk, 18
  and very low calorie diets, 274
  weight loss, effect on, 152
Animal models, 107–131
Anorexia nervosa, cardiac function, 154
Anthropometric indices, 4–7
Antihypertensive medication
  associated risks, 221, 222
  and weight loss benefits, 218, 220–222
Anxiety
  behavioral treatment, 260, 261
  binge eaters, 257

507

Anxiety (*continued*)
  obese persons, 253
  and refeeding, 317, 318
  and very low calorie diets, 259–261, 297
Arterial pressure, 218, 219
Assertiveness, obese persons, 253, 254
Asthma, surgery benefit, 501
Atherosclerosis, 138
Atrial chamber volume, 142
Atrial premature contractions, 120
Atrioventricular block, 120
Attendance, and weight loss, 394, 396
Attributable risk, 9
Attrition, 383–404 (*see also* Adherence)
  binge eaters, 297
  closed-group format, benefit of, 387, 388
  commercial treatment programs, 41, 42
  dexfenfluramine study, 388
  group behavioral treatment, 310, 319
  predictors, 383–404
  rates of, 387
  refeeding period, 319
  and slow weight losses, 386, 387
  very low calorie diets, 56, 60
Availability of food, 202

B

Balance sheet procedure, 371
Balanced-deficit diet, 220
Balanced diet, weight maintenance, 343–345
Basal metabolism (*see also* Resting metabolic rate)
  postexercise period, 192
  semistarvation, effect on, 173, 174
Bazett equation, 146
Beck Depression Inventory, 259, 291
Behavior (*see* Eating behavior)
Behavioral psychologists, 282, 310
Behavioral treatments (*see also* Group behavioral treatment)
  binge eating, impact, 257
  combined modalities, trends, 37
  confidentiality, 313
  contraindications, 299, 300
  diabetes and obesity, 238–244
  and exercise, 278, 315, 371–375
    diabetes, 239–241
  goal setting, 308
  lapses, 243
  long-term effectiveness, 438–440
  maintenance of weight loss, 65, 72
  and mood, 259–261
  patient selection, 310
  posttreatment contact, interaction, 460, 461
  principles, 307, 308
  process orientation, 308
  refeeding period, 316–320
  selection of, 303, 304
  and very low calorie diets, 61–67, 72, 241–243, 278, 310–327
    long-term effectiveness, 438–440
"BEST treatment," 301, 302
Beta-blockers, 280
Bicycling (*see also* Stationary cycling)
Biliopancreatic bypass, 499–501
Binge eating, 256–258
  incidence in weight loss programs, 333
  operational definition, 257, 258
  prevalence in obese, 256
  psychological disturbances, 257
  in refeeding period, 285
  treatment dropouts, 297, 384, 385
  treatment impact, 257
  and very low calorie diets, 53, 54, 297
Binge Eating Scale, 297
Biological impedance analysis
  advantages and limitations, 87
  fat-free mass estimation, 86
Blood pressure, 218–220
Blood sugar
  calorie restriction versus weight loss, 236–238
  monitoring of very low calorie diets, 280
  as predictor of treatment response, 244–246
  self-monitoring, 243, 244
Blood volume, 141–143
Body composition
  and "acceptable" weight loss, 87–89, 149

animal studies, 121, 122
chronic exercise, influence on, 197
definition, 4, 5
energy restriction, effects on, 83–104
measurement, 84–92
terminology of, interpretation, 89, 90
total fasting, effect on, 139
very low calorie diet, effects on, 47, 48, 121, 122
Body fat
and body protein conservation, 101, 102
distribution (*see* Pattern of regional fat distribution)
and energy balance, 172, 173
exercise, benefits of, 355
mass
definition, 4, 5
index, 90, 91
interpretation, 90
measurement, 84, 85
very low calorie diets, rats, 122
Body image
diet effects, 262, 263
exercise benefits, 360
obese persons, 258
video distortion procedure, 262
Body mass index
advantages and disadvantages, 33
and cardiac output, 141, 142
definition, 4, 5
and diabetes, 232–234
mortality risk, 13–15, 28, 29
in obesity workup, 27
Body protein, 101, 102
Body water, 122
Body weight (*see also* Weight loss)
energy balance equation, 164–166
stability of, 165, 166
very low calorie diet criterion, 275, 276
Booster sessions, 450 (*see also* Posttreatment contact)
Borderline personality disorder, 300
Branched-chain amino acids, 99
BRL *35 135*, 484
BRL *37 344*, 484
Buddy groups
and exercise, 374

multicomponent program, 462, 463, 467, 468
Build Study, 9
Bulimia nervosa, 296, 297

C

Cachexia, 155
Calcium
in balanced diet, 346
intestinal transport, animals, 112, 113
liquid protein diet, effect on, 120, 121
Caloric content
variations in very low calorie diets, 335, 336
very low calorie diets, 69, 70, 335, 336
Caloric deficit
treatment measure, 36
very low calorie diets, 45
Caloric intake
measurement problems, 255, 256, 296
obese persons, 255, 256
refeeding period, 340
underestimation, 296
Caloric requirements (*see also* Energy expenditure)
and exercise, 191, 192
Caloric restriction (*see also* Energy deficit)
hyperglycemia benefit, 214, 235–237
and nitrogen balance, 91–104
versus weight loss, diabetes, 236, 237
Calorie counting, 344
Calorie guides, 345
Cambridge diet, 121, 122
Cancer, disease-specific mortality, 13
Carbohydrate
arrhythmia risk, overfeeding, 340
and energy balance, 179, 180
versus fat, protein-sparing, 99
protein-sparing effect, diets, 99
refeeding period, 340
very low calorie diets, 46, 335, 336
Carcass energy, 119
Cardiac arrhythmias
carbohydrate overfeeding, 340
fasting, 153, 154, 281

Cardiac arrhythmias (*continued*)
  liquid protein diet, 154
    rats, 120
  very low calorie diets, 281, 282, 284
  weight loss effect, 150
Cardiac function (*see also* Cardiovascular disease)
  exercise, benefits of, 204
  liquid protein diet, rats, 120, 121
  semistarvation-refeeding effect, 123–130
  very low calorie diets, 51, 52, 156
  weight loss effects, 136–156
Cardiac hypertrophy (*see* Ventricular hypertrophy)
Cardiac output
  in obesity, 140–142
  stroke volume mechanism, 141
  weight loss effect, 149
Cardiac stress test, 278, 281
Cardiac structure, 142–144
Cardiomegaly, 136–138
Cardiovascular disease
  disease-specific mortality, 13
  exercise, benefits of, 357
  morbidity risk studies, 15
  obesity risk, 138
  surgery benefits, 501
  waist-hip circumference ratio, 6, 7
  weight loss, benefits of, 222–224
Catecholaminergic drugs, 483–486
Catecholamines, 179
Cerebrovascular disease, 13
Charles River CD rats, 113
Chemically induced obesity, 110
Childhood-onset obesity
  body image, 258, 263
  exercise, benefits of, 355
  fat cell number, 294
Children, energy expenditure, 191
Cholesterol
  exercise, benefits of, 358
  gallstones
    morbidity risk, 17, 18
    very low calorie diet effect, 52
    weight loss risk, 224, 225
  and hyperinsulinemia, 203
  weight loss, benefits of, 223, 224, 235
Chronic hypoxemia, 138

Cigarette smoking
  confounding effects on risk calculation, 22
  contraindication for very low calorie diets, 298
  and relapse, 444, 449
Closed-group format, 387, 388
Codependency, 503
Cognitive restructuring, 320
Cohort analysis, 488
Cold intolerance, 179
Combined modality treatments
  maintenance of weight loss, 456–475
  in mild obesity, trends, 37
  and very low calorie diets, 61–63
Commercial treatment programs
  attrition rates, 42, 387, 388
  mild obesity, 40–42
Comorbidity (*see* Morbidity)
Compliance (*see* Adherence)
Compulsive gambling, 444
Computerized tomography, 86
"Concentric" cardiac enlargement, 143
Confidentiality, 313
Conservative treatments
  cost-effectiveness, 37, 40
  in mild obesity, 36–40
  selection of, 303, 304
"Convenience" stores, 342
Coping skills
  and relapse, 444, 445, 449, 457–461
  weight loss maintenance, 400, 457–475
Copper concentrations, 120
Coronary artery disease
  exercise, benefits of, 357
  obesity risk, 138, 222, 223
  weight cycling effect, 286
  and weight loss, 152
Cost, very low calorie diets, 336
Cost-benefit ratio, very low calorie diets, 68
Cost-effectiveness
  conservative treatments, 37, 40
  and team treatment, 282, 283
  very low calorie diets, 67–69, 282, 283
"Counterregulation," 255
Creatinine level, 274
Cyclic model, relapse, 446, 447

D

Dating skills, 265
"Deadly quartet," 138
Decision balance sheet procedure, 371
Decision making, and exercise, 371
Depression
  behavioral treatment, 259-261
  contraindication for very low calorie diets, 297
  in diabetics, weight loss, 247, 248
  drug side effect, 486
  and method of assessment, 261
  in obese persons, 252, 253
  and very low calorie diets, 54, 55, 259-261, 297, 298
  weight loss, relationship to, 391
Dexfenfluramine
  central actions, 483
  indications, 491
  long-term weight loss, 487-491
  maintenance of weight loss, 72
  short-term trials, 485
  side effects, 486, 490
  time course of weight loss, 487-491
Diabetes (*see* Type II diabetes)
Diaphragm
  caloric restriction effect, 117
  Syrian hamster model, 117
Diary records (*see* Diet diaries)
Diastolic blood pressure
  exercise, benefits of, 358
  in obesity, 142, 144
  weight loss, benefits of, 149, 218-220
Diet diaries
  as compliance indicator, 333
  safe diet monitoring, 338, 339, 346
  weight loss factor, 395, 396
Diet supplements, 72
Dietary fat intake, 256
Dietary history
  nutritional status, 332, 333
  in obesity evaluation, 293, 295, 332, 333
Dietary Intervention Therapy for Obese Hypertensives, 220
Dietary restraint
  and attrition, 385
  binge eating precipitant, 385
  weight loss predictor, 392
Diethylproprion, 485, 486
Dietitians, 331-351
  monitoring of very low calorie diets, 282
  qualifications, 349, 350
  and refeeding period, 318, 339, 341, 342
  safe diet monitoring, 338, 339
  and weight maintenance, 343-347
Digestion, species variation, 108, 109
Dinitrophenol, 484
Disease-specific mortality, 13
Disinhibition
  binge eaters, 257
  restrained eating consequence, 255
Distal gastric bypass, 500, 501
Distribution of body fat (*see* Pattern of regional fat distribution)
Diuresis, 281
Diuretics, 152, 280
Doubly labeled water technique, 256
Dropout rates (*see also* Attrition)
  commercial treatment programs, 41, 42
Drug abuse, 297
Drug tolerance, 482
Drug treatment (*see* Pharmacologic treatment)
Dry skin, 52
Dual photon absorptiometry, 86
"Dumping," 500
Duodenal morphology, 113, 114
Dynamic energy balance equation, 164-166

E

Early weight loss, 394
Eating behavior
  functional analysis, 307, 308
  normalization of, 312
  obese persons, 255, 256
  in refeeding, 285
  stimulus control, 314, 317, 318
  and weight loss, 395, 396
Eating Inventory, 255
Eating out, 348

Eating slowly, 317, 318, 396
Eating style, 255
"Eccentric" cardiac enlargement
   development in obesity, 143
   electrocardiography, 145, 146
EKG rhythm strips, 284
Electrocardiography
   liquid protein diets, 153
      rats, 120, 121
   in obesity, 145–148
   very low calorie diet monitoring, 284
"Elevator" dieting (*see* Weight cycling)
Emphysema, 117, 118
End-diastolic volume
   in obesity, 142, 144
   weight loss effect, 149
End-systolic volume, 142
Energy balance, 164–183
   dynamic equation, 164–166
   and metabolic adaptation, 174–176
   static equations, 164, 165, 174
   weight loss effect, 171, 172
Energy deficit
   in "acceptable" weight loss, 88, 89
   animal models, 107–131
   definition, 95
   energy expenditure, effect on, 163–183
   fat-free mass as protection, 102
   flaws in experiments, 95, 96
   and nitrogen balance, 91–104
   percentage measure, 96, 97
Energy expenditure, 163–184
   components, 166–170
   cross-sectional studies, weaknesses, 171
   and exercise, 191–193
   longitudinal study, 170, 171
   in obese persons, 190, 191
   and obesity risk, 170, 171
   postexercise period, 192, 193
   in technological societies, 190
   weight loss effect, 171–178
Energy–nitrogen balance
   flaws in studies of, 91, 92
   measurement, 86
Energy substrate balance equation, 180
Ephedrine, 484
Estrogen levels, 224
Estrogen-to-testosterone ratio, 224
Euphoria, initial weight loss, 316

Everted duodenal sacs, 112, 113
Excess death rate, 8
Exchange plan, 343, 344
Exercise, 190–204, 354–377
   acute benefits, 359
   adherence problem, 361, 362, 473
   and behavior modification, 278, 315, 371–375, 463–466
   education component, 370, 371
   energy expenditure, 191–193
   enhanced well-being, 359, 360
   food intake changes, 197–202
   goal setting, 364–366, 372
   groups, 373, 374
   health benefits, 202–204, 357–359
   and identity, 369
   maintenance of weight loss, 356, 357, 403, 463–466
   monitoring of, 372, 466
   in multicomponent program, 463–475
   and nitrogen balance, 99, 100
   program design, 364–368
   physiologists, 282
   rationale, 354–361
   relapse prevention, 374, 375, 466
   resting metabolic rate, interaction, 169
   safety issues, 375, 376
   stereotypes, 369
   stress testing, 375, 376
   support groups, 373, 466
   and thermic effect of food, 169, 193–195
   and very low calorie diets, 278, 279, 315, 355
      diabetics, 239–241
   and weight loss, 178, 354–356, 398, 448, 449
Extracellular fluid, 141
Extracellular protein, 84, 85
Extracellular water
   electrical assessment, 87
   reference values, 85

F

Family history
   initial obesity evaluation, 277, 294, 295
   and prognosis, 294, 295

Index

Family support, 311, 312
Famine victims, 154
Fantasies, 340
Fasting
  electrocardiography, 153
  ventricular arrhythmias, 139, 153, 154
Fat (see also Body fat)
  versus carbohydrate, protein-sparing, 99
  and energy balance, 179, 180
  and nitrogen balance, 99
  very low calorie diets, 335
Fat cell number
  childhood obesity, 294
  obesity, type, 293, 294
  as predictor, 389, 390
Fat cell size, 293, 294
Fat-free mass
  and "acceptable" weight loss, 87–89
  caloric density, 149
  definition, 4, 5, 90
  energy restriction effects, 83–104, 172, 173
  index, 90, 91
  interpretation, 90
  loss in very low calorie diets, 47, 48, 149
  measurement techniques, 84–89
  protective effect of exercise, 169
  and severe caloric restriction, 102
  total starvation effect, 139, 140
Fat intake, obese persons, 256
Femoral–gluteal obesity (see Lower body obesity)
dl-Fenfluramine (see also Dexfenfluramine)
  central action, 483
  long-term use, 487
  short-term trials, 485
  side effects, 486
Financial considerations
  and attrition, 385, 386
  very low calorie diets, 299
Finnish weight study, 12, 13
Fitness testing, 370
Fluid intake, very low calorie diets, 338
Fluoxetine, 485
  efficacy, 485, 490
  long-term use, 487
  side effects, 486
Follow-up studies, 22
Food choice
  refeeding period, 341
  stimulus control, 317, 318
Food cravings, 491
Food cues
  and food intake, 202
  relapse factor, 449
  stimulus control, 314
  very low calorie diets, 262
Food diaries (see Diet diaries)
Food efficiency, 118, 119, 181
Food fantasies, 340
Food intake
  assessment, 296
  lean versus obese women, 199–202
  physical activity effect, 197–204
  self-monitoring, 314
  sensory cues, importance, 202
  thermogenic interaction, exercise, 193–195
  underestimation of, 296
Food labels, 345
Food quotient, 180
Food shopping, 342
"Forbidden" foods, 257
Framingham Heart Study, 15

G

Gallstones (see Cholesterol, gallstones)
Gambian men, 176, 178, 286
Gastric bypass (see Gastrointestinal bypass)
Gastric restriction approaches
  complications/side effects, 500
  versus gastric bypass, 499
  method, 496–498
  outlet size technique, 498
  results, 500–504
  weight loss, 500, 501
Gastric stapling model, 113, 114
Gastrocnemius muscle, 116, 117
Gastrointestinal bypass
  comorbidity benefits, 248, 249, 501, 502

Gastrointestinal bypass (*continued*)
  complications/side effects, 500
  versus gastroplasty, 499
  method, 498–500
  results, 500–504
  weight loss, 500, 501
Gastrointestinal tract
  animal models, diets, 123–130
  morphological change, semistarvation, 112–114
  nutrient absorption, animals, 112–114
  semistarvation–refeeding, 123–130
  species variation, 108, 109
Gastroplasty (*see* Gastric restriction approaches)
Gender differences, and weight loss, 244–246
Genetic obesity, animals, 110, 111
Genetics
  and obesity evaluation, 293, 294
  resting metabolic rate, 167
Glucagon, 281
Gluconeogenesis, 279
Glucose (*see also* Hyperglycemia)
  intestinal transport, animals, 112
  intolerance, 138
  weight loss versus caloric restriction, 236–238
Glycemic control
  diet and exercise, 240, 358
  long-term studies, 238
  predictors, 244–246
  very low calorie diets, 215–217, 235
  weight loss, benefit of, 214–217, 235, 240, 246–249
  weight loss versus caloric restriction, 236–238
Glycosylated hemoglobin, 214, 216, 239–241
Goal setting
  behavioral treatment, 308
  exercise, 364–366, 372
  weight loss, 302, 303, 396
Gout, 275
Grocery shopping, 342
Group behavioral treatment
  advantages, 309
  binge eating, 319, 320
  clinical issues, 312, 313
  confidentiality, 313
  contraindications, 299, 300
  versus individual treatment, 309
  length and structure, 309, 310
  mood changes, 259
  and personality disorders, 300
  refeeding period, 316–320
  weight loss, disappointment with, 315, 316
Growth hormone, 103, 104
Guilt, binge eaters, 257
Gut fill, 280, 281, 285
Gynoid obesity, 6 (*see also* Lower body obesity)

H

Hair loss, 52
"Health worker effect," 10
Heart disease (*see* Cardiovascular disease)
Heart protein
  semistarvation–refeeding, 128
  and weight loss, 149, 150
Heart rate
  exercise goals, 365
  in obesity, 141, 145, 146
  weight loss effect, 149
Heart weight
  high protein, low energy diet, 123
  liquid protein diet, rats, 121
  and obesity, 136, 137
  semistarvation–refeeding cycle, 126
  weight loss effect, 150
Height, 23–25
Height-normalized indices, 90, 91
Hematocrit, 284
Hepatic function, 274
Hepatic glucose output, 235, 236
High blood pressure (*see* Hypertension)
High density lipoprotein
  exercise, benefits of, 203, 204, 357, 358
  and hyperinsulinemia, 203
  weight loss, benefits of, 214, 223, 224, 247
High protein, low energy diet, 122, 123
HMR products, 336
Holidays, 349

Index

Holter monitoring, 281, 284
Home-based exercise, 373, 374
Home glucose monitoring, 280, 283
Hooded male rats, 117, 118
Hospital-based programs, attrition, 387, 388
Human growth hormone, 103, 104
Hunger
  and attrition, 385
  binge eaters, 257
  diabetics, 242
  identification of, 314
  and restrained eating, 255
  and very low calorie diets, 52, 53, 242, 262, 279
Hydrodensitometry, 85
Hypercholesterolemia, 13, 14
Hyperestrogenemia, 224
Hyperglycemia
  calorie restriction versus weight loss, 236–238
  self-monitoring, 243, 244
  weight loss, benefits of, 214–217, 235
Hyperinsulinemia
  exercise, benefits of, 203
  health risks, 203
  weight loss, benefits of, 214–216
Hyperlipidemia, 223, 224
Hyperlipogenesis, and refeeding, 115
Hyperplastic obesity
  childhood-onset, 295
  and dieting history, 295
  exercise effects, 355
  obesity pathology, 293, 294
  weight loss prediction, 389, 390
Hypertension
  and cardiomegaly, 136–138
  exercise, benefits of, 358
  heart function effect, 145, 146
  and hyperinsulinemia, 203
  long-term weight loss, benefits of, 220–222
  morbidity risk, 13, 14, 16, 17, 21
  obesity pathogenesis, 217, 218
  primary prevention, 221
  surgery, benefit of, 501
  weight loss, benefits of, 152, 217–222
Hypertension Prevention Trial, 221
Hypertriglyceridemia, 224

Hypertrophic obesity
  exercise benefits, 355
  prognosis, 293, 390
Hypokalemia, 148
Hypoxemia, 138

I

Ileum, semistarvation effects, 113
Impulse buying, 342
In vivo neutron activation, 84, 86
Incidence rates, 8, 9
INDEX study, 487–491
Indian laborer study, 176
Indirect calorimetry, 389
Initial blood sugar, 245, 246
Initial body weight, 388, 389
Initial interviews, 305–307
Insulin dosage reduction, 215
Insulin–glucose ratio, 242
Insulin-like growth factor I, 103
Insulin resistance
  and blunted thermic response to food, 195
  compensatory hyperinsulinemia, 203
  obesity association, 180
  weight loss, benefits of, 214, 235
Insulin secretion, 241, 242
Insulin sensitivity
  exercise, benefits of, 203, 358
  weight gain predictor, 180
  weight loss, benefits of, 215, 235
International Dexfenfluramine Study, 487–491
Interpersonal relationships, 264, 265
Interviews, behavioral assessment, 305–307
Intestinal bypass, 498, 499
Intestine
  nutrient absorption, animals, 112–114
  morphological change, semistarvation, 113, 114
  semistarvation–refeeding cycle, 123–130
Intracellular protein, 84, 85
Intracellular water, 85, 87
Iron supplements, 284, 346
Ischemic heart disease, 6, 7

J

Jejunal loop perfusion, 112
Jejunal morphology, 113, 114
Junctional escape beats, 120

K

Ketogenesis, and mood, 261
Ketone levels, monitoring, 280
Ketosis, 53, 279
Kidney function (*see* Renal function)
Kidney weight, 123

L

Laboratory tests, very low calorie diets, 277, 278, 283, 284
Lapses
   posttreatment contact, value of, 460, 461
   versus relapse, cognition, 320, 321
   skills training, 457–461
   very low calorie diets, 242, 243
"Last Chance Diet," 152
Lean meat diet, 70, 71
Lean tissue
   exercise, benefits of, 355
   and very low calorie diets, 47, 48
Left ventricular hypertrophy (*see* Ventricular hypertrophy)
Leisure time activities, 368
Length of treatment
   behavioral techniques, 309, 310
   very low calorie diets, 50, 65, 66
   and weight loss, 397
Levodopa, 179
Lewis rats, 113
Life insurance data, 22, 23
Life stress
   and attrition, 385, 386
   maintenance of weight loss factor, 400
   and very low calorie diets, 291, 298
Lifestyle modification
   exercise program, 366
   and very low calorie diets, 61–63, 310–327

Lipid profile, and exercise, 203, 204, 357, 358
Lipofuscin, 153
Lipoprotein lipase
   rebound effects, refeeding, 114, 115
   and weight loss maintenance, 400, 401
Liquid diets
   advantages of, 70, 337
   nutritional content, 336
   versus portion-controlled diets, 71
   preparation and intake, 337, 338
   refeeding, 340
Liquid protein diets
   electrocardiography, rats, 120, 121
   and expected death rate, 276
   metabolic effects, rats, 121, 122
   sudden death syndrome, 152–155
Lithium, 297
Liver
   function, 274
   protein, 128
   weight
      high protein, low energy diet, 123
      liquid protein diet, rats, 121
      semistarvation-refeeding cycle, 124–129
Locus of control, 253
Low calorie diets (*see* Very low calorie diets)
Low density lipoprotein
   and exercise, 203, 204, 358
   high density lipoprotein ratio, 223, 224
   weight loss, benefits of, 223, 224
Lower body obesity
   health risks, 6, 7
   weight loss, 390, 391
Lung structure/function, 117, 118

M

"Magical thinking," 316
Magnesium levels
   initial evaluation, very low calorie diets, 278
   liquid protein, rats, 120
Mail contacts, 458–461
Maintenance energy requirements, 95–97

Maintenance of weight loss, 456–475 (*see also* Relapse)
  behavioral techniques, 65, 321–326
  exercise as benefit, 71, 170, 325, 356, 357, 399, 400
    multicomponent program, 463–466
  long-term follow-up, 438–440
  versus losing weight, 325
  multicomponent program, 456–475
  nutritional counseling, 343–347
  pharmacotherapy, 72, 487–491
  posttreatment contact, value of, 457–461, 468, 469
  self-help groups, 461–463
  therapist contact, value of, 468, 469, 473, 474
  very low calorie diets, 71, 72
Major depression, 297
Marital relationship, 265
Masculinity–femininity, 253
"Matching decision," 304
Mazindol, 485, 487
Meal planning, 345, 346
Medical history-taking, 276, 277
Medical monitoring/evaluation, 273–286
Medifast formulas, 336
Mental health practitioners, 307, 310
Metabolic adaptation
  definition, 174–176
  and exercise, 178
  mechanisms, 179
  resting metabolic rate, 176, 177
  thermic effect of food, 177, 178
  and weight cycling, 180–182
Metabolic complications, very low calorie diets, 55, 56
Metabolic rate (*see also* Resting metabolic rate)
  flexibility, 173, 174
  longitudinal study, 170, 171
  obesity risk, 170, 171
  physical activity role, 190–204
  postexercise period, 192
  very low calorie diets, rats, 122
Methionine, 121
3-*O*-Methyl-glucose, 112
Microangiopathy, 138
Mild obesity
  overweight classification, 33–35
  very low calorie diets, 276
  weight loss measures, 36
MMPI (Minnesota Multiphasic Personality Inventory)
  obese patients, 253
  in psychosocial evaluation, 291
  weight loss relationship, 391
Moderate obesity
  overweight classification, 33–35
  and treatment selection, 35
Moderately restrictive diets, 262
Mood
  behavior modification, 259, 261
  and method of assessment, 261
  very low calorie diets, 259–261
    diabetes, 242
  weight loss, benefits of, diabetics, 247, 248
Morbidity
  assessment of risk, 3–29
  proportional hazards model, 26
  rates, 8, 9
  surgery benefits, 501
Mortality
  assessment of risk, 3–29
  optimal body mass index, 13–15
  proportional hazards model, 26
  rate
    definition, 7
    diabetes, weight loss benefit, 249
    liquid protein diets, 276
    weight cycling, 286
  ratio, 3
    calculation, 8, 28
    diabetes and obesity, 233
    modifying factors, 22–29
Motivation, 291
Multidisciplinary team treatment (*see* Team treatment)
Muscle
  fiber length, 116
  function, 116, 117
  metabolism, 115–117
  protein
    animal models, 115–117
    semistarvation–refeeding, 128
    very low calorie diets, 279
Myocardial ischemia, 138

Myocytes, 116, 117
Myofibers, 153
Myofibrillary fragmentation, 139

N

Narcissistic personality disorder, 300
Natriuresis, 281
Negotiated exercise plan, 364
Nephropathy, 232
Nitrogen balance
  and body fat content, 101, 102
  caloric restriction, effect on, 91–104
  carbohydrate versus fat, 99
  dietary factors, 92–99
  energy restriction, effect on, 83–103
  exercise effects, 99, 100
  fat-free mass as protection, 102
  flaws in studies, 91, 92, 95, 96
  and poor quality protein intake, 98
  protein requirements, 93–95, 97, 98
  rat model, 122–124
  semistarvation-refeeding cycle, 124
  and triiodothyronine levels, 102, 103
  very low calorie diets, 46, 98, 100, 275, 276
No-treatment comparisons, 68, 69
Nonadherence (*see* Adherence)
Non-insulin-dependent diabetes (*see* Type II diabetes)
Noradrenaline, 179
Nurse practitioners, 282
Nurses, diet monitoring, 282
Nurses' Cohort Study, 15
Nutrient absorption (*see* Absorption)
Nutritional education/counseling, 331–351
  versus behavior modification, 239
  behavioral approaches, 37
  information sources, 350
  orientation period, 334
  protein content, 335–337
  refeeding period, 317, 318, 341, 342
  and weight maintenance, 343–347
Nutritional status, 100

O

"Obese eating style," 255
Obese mouse, 110, 111
Obesity workup, 26, 27
Ob/ob mouse, 110
Obsessive–compulsive thinking, 257
Open-enrollment treatment, 387, 388
OPTIFAST Core Program Patient Manual, The, 323
OPTIFAST formulas, 336
Osborne–Mendel rats, 120–123
Overeaters Anonymous, 40, 41, 432, 433
Overeating, recovery technique, 321–324
Overfeeding, metabolic adaptation, 173
Oxygen consumption
  cardiac output effect, 140, 141
  and cardiomegaly, 137
  postexercise period, 192, 193
  semistarvation effect, 173
  very low calorie diets, rats, 121, 122
  weight loss effect, 149

P

P wave, 146
Palatability of food, 202
Pancreatic weight, 126
Parental participation, 398
Parties, 349
Patient–therapist contact (*see* Therapist contact)
Pattern of regional fat distribution
  definition, 4, 6
  diabetes risk, 232–234
  health risks, 6, 7, 25, 26
  and weight loss, 390, 391
Pear shape, 390, 391
Peer self-help groups, 462, 463, 467, 468
Perceived hunger, 255
Percentage energy deficit
  body fat as buffer, 101, 102
  value of as measure, 96, 97
Percentage of weight loss measures, 36
Percentage overweight, 33
Peripheral vascular resistance, 141, 142

Personality
  disorders, 300
  obese persons, 253, 254
  surgery patients, 503
  and weight loss, 391
Pharmacologic treatment, 478–491
  central nervous system action, 483, 484
  long-term use, 487–491
  peripheral action, 484
  rationale, 481, 482
  short-term trials, 484–486
  side effects, 486
Phentermine, 485, 487
β-Phenylethylamine, 484
Phenylpropanolamine, 485
Physical activity, 190–204, 354–377 (see also Exercise)
  adaptation during weight loss, 178
  behavioral programs for, 37, 315
  energy expenditure, 166, 169, 170, 191–193
  and enhanced well-being, 359, 360
  food intake changes, 197–202
  health benefits, 202–204, 357–359
  lifestyle changes, 366
  program design, 364–368
  and resting metabolic rate, 169
  thermic effect of food interaction, 169, 193–195
  and very low calorie diets, 315
  and weight reduction, 171, 172, 178, 398
Physical examination, 277
Physical fitness testing, 370
"Pickwickian syndrome," 138
Pima Indians
  diabetes risk, 16, 232, 234
  low energy expenditure, 170, 171
  weight loss adaptation, 180
Platter method, 199, 202
Portion-controlled diets, 71
Postexercise energy expenditure, 192, 193
Posttreatment contact, 457–461
  multicomponent program, 457–475
  and relapse prevention training, 457–461
  social support, importance of, 462, 463
  therapist contact versus peer support, 467, 468
  value of, 461, 468, 469, 473, 474
Potassium
  deficiency, 148
  levels
    liquid protein diet, rats, 120
    very low calorie diets, 281, 284
Powdered-protein formula diets
  description of, 336
  refeeding, 340
P-R interval, 146, 150
Preload
  in obesity, 142, 143
  weight loss effect, 149
Premature ventricular beats
  obese hypertensive patients, 145
  very low calorie diets, 51
Prevalence rates, 9
Primary prevention
  hypertension, 221
  of relapse, 326
"Problem" foods, 347, 348
Problem solving
  and exercise, 371
  maintenance of weight loss, value of, 472
  in relapse prevention training, 459
  and self-help groups, 462
Proportional hazards model, 26
Protein (see also Heart protein; Muscle, protein)
  and caloric restriction, 101, 102
  catabolism
    animal models, 115–117
    and caloric restriction, 92
    very low calorie diets, 279
    weight loss effect, heart, 150
  efficiency ratio, 98
  intake
    and nitrogen balance, 97, 98
    very low calorie diets, 338
  requirements, 93–95, 97, 98
  in very low calorie diets, 46, 98, 335–337

Protein-sparing modified fast, 336, 337
  advantages of, 70, 71, 337
  nutritional content, 336, 337
  preparation and intake, 337
Psychological hunger, 314
Psychologists, 282, 307
Psychopathology
  binge eaters, 257
  in obese persons, 252, 253
Psychosis, contraindication for very low calorie diets, 297
Psychotherapy, adjunctive use, 305
Pulmonary structure/function, 117, 118
Purging behavior
  contraindication for very low calorie diets, 296
  obese bingers, 257

Q

Q strain (mouse), 116
Quality of life
  exercise benefits, 359, 360
  surgery benefits, 501, 502
QRS complex
  fasting, 153
  liquid protein diets, 153
  obese patients, 146
  and weight loss, 150
QT interval
  liquid protein diets, 153
  obese patients, 146–148
  and potassium deficiency, 148
  and starvation diet, 139, 153
  ventricular arrhythmia risk, 147, 148
  very low calorie diets, 284
  in weight loss, 150, 151
QU interval, 148

R

Rate of weight loss, 89
Rebound effects, 115
Recreational activities, 368
Refeeding
  and anxiety, 318, 319
  and attrition, 319, 340
  basal metabolism, effect on, 174
  behavioral approaches, 316–320
  and binge eating, 53
  cardiac effects, animals, 123–130
  dietitian's role, 339–342
  and food efficiency, 118, 119
  gastrointestinal effects, animals, 123–130
  hyperlipogenesis, rats, 114, 115
  length of, 340
  muscle metabolism, rats, 116
  nutrition education, 317, 318, 341, 342
  psychological problems, 285, 318, 319
  renal effects, animals, 123–130
Refundable deposits, 388
Relapse, 437–452 (*see also* Maintenance of weight loss)
  cognitive-behavioral model, 445
  consequences, 449, 450
  cyclic model, 445–447
  exercise in prevention, 374, 375, 399, 400
  interpretation of studies, 441–443
  versus lapse, cognition, 320, 321
  long-term studies, 438–440
  predictors, 448, 449
  prevention
    drug therapy use, 491
    exercise, 374, 375, 399, 400
    posttreatment contact, value of, 457–461, 468, 469, 474
    skills training, 459–461
    two-step approach, 326
  process of, 444–448
  research needs, 450, 451
Relative energy expenditure, 170
Relative risk ratio, 19–22
Relative weight, 4, 5
Renal function
  semistarvation–refeeding, animals, 123–130
  very low calorie diets, 274
Research settings, 387
Respiratory muscles, 117
Respiratory quotient, 180
Restaurant food, 348
Resting energy expenditure, 45
Resting heart rate, 145, 146

Resting metabolic rate
  adaptation, 174–179
  animal studies, 122
  chronic exercise, influence on, 176
  in energy requirement estimation, 96, 166, 167
  and exercise, 169, 355
  flexibility, 173, 174
  genetics, 167
  indirect calorimetry, 389
  longitudinal study, 170, 171
  obese persons, 256
  obesity risk factor, 170, 171
  postexercise period, 192
  semistarvation effects, 173, 174
  and 24-hour energy expenditure, 176, 177
  and very low calorie diets, 55, 56, 122
  in weight cycling, 181
  and weight loss, 172, 176, 177, 389
Restrained eating, 254, 255
Retinopathy, 232
RO 40-2148, 484
Rotation diet, 182
Rowing machines, 367, 368
R-R interval, 145, 146
Running, 192

S

Sarcomeres, 116
Scapegoating, 265
Secondary gain, 503
Self-consciousness, 253, 254
Self-care, 440
Self-efficacy, 391, 392
Self-esteem
  exercise, benefits of, 359, 360, 369
  weight loss, benefits of, 264
Self-help groups
  multicomponent program, 461–463
  posttreatment value, 463, 468
  versus therapist contact, 467, 468
Self-monitoring
  behavioral treatment phase, 311, 314
  blood sugar, 243, 244
  maintenance of weight loss, 400, 457–461

  posttreatment contact, 457–461
  weight loss factor, 395, 396
Sensory cues
  food intake, 202
  stimulus narrowing approach, 317
  very low calorie diets, 262
Serotonergic drugs, 72, 483, 485, 486, 491 (see also Dexfenfluramine)
Serotonin reuptake inhibitors, 297
Setraline, 72
Serving food, 345, 346
Set point
  body weight control, 166
  and restrained eating, 254
Seventh-Day Adventist study, 12
Severe obesity, 33–35
Sex ratio, weight loss, 244–246
Sexual abuse, 265
Shopping for food, 317
Siblings, metabolic rate, 167
Sinus arrhythmias, 120
Sinus bradycardia, 120
Sitting, energy cost, 196
Skills training
  posttreatment contact, interaction, 460, 461
  relapse prevention, value of, 457–461, 474
  weight loss maintenance, 457–475
Skinfold thickness, 85
Sleep apnea
  initial obesity evaluation, 277
  morbidity risk, 18
  surgery benefit, 501
  weight loss benefit, 264
Sleeping, energy cost, 196
Slips and lapses (see Lapses)
Slow rate of eating, 317, 318, 396
Slow weight losses, 386, 387
Smoking (see Cigarette smoking)
Social relationships, 264, 265
Social support
  exercise, 373, 374
  multicomponent program, 461–475
  posttreatment value, 461–468, 472, 474
  versus therapist contact, 467, 468
  and weight loss, 398, 472

Sodium
  loss, very low calorie diets, 281
  restriction, 218
"Soft calorie syndrome," 497, 498, 502
Soleus muscle, rat, 150
Spouse, support of, 398, 450
Sprague–Dawley rats, 119, 121, 124
S-T segment, 148
"Stairstep" weight loss, 279
Static energy balance equation, 164, 174
Stationary cycling
  adherence problem, 473
  advantages, 367
  in multicomponent program, 463–466
Stature, 23–25
"Stepped care decision," 304
Stimulus narrowing, 317
Stress
  and attrition, 385, 386
  maintenance of weight loss factor, 400
  testing, 278, 291, 375, 376
  and very low calorie diet, 291, 298
Stroke volume, 141, 149
Subscapular skinfold, 25, 26
Substance abuse, 297
Sudden death syndrome
  fasting effect, 153, 154
  liquid protein diets, 152–154
  very low calorie diets, 51, 52
Supermarket shopping, 342
Support systems, exercise, 373, 374
Surgery, 496–505
  complications, 500
  contraindications, 496
  indications, 34, 35, 496, 502, 503
  long-term follow-up, 504
  methods, 496–500
  results, 500–502
"Sweet eaters," 503
Systolic blood pressure
  exercise benefits, 358
  obese persons, 142, 144
  weight loss benefits, 218, 219

T

T-wave changes, 148, 150
Take Off Pounds Sensibly (TOPS), 41

Talking, energy cost, 196
Team treatment
  cost containment, 282, 283
  support role, 279
  very low calorie diets, 48, 49, 279, 282, 283
Telephone contacts, 458–461, 463
Tetrahydrolipstatin, 484
Therapist contact
  and adherence, 472
  versus peer support, 467, 468
  posttreatment value of, 457–475
  versus relapse prevention training, 468, 469
Thermic effect of food, 167–169
  adaptation during weight loss, 177, 178
  and chronic exercise, 195–197
  energy expenditure component, 166–169
  exercise interactions, 172, 177, 178
  and insulin resistance, 195
  measurement difficulties, 168
  and weight loss, 172, 177, 178
Thiazide diuretics, 221
Three-day food record, 333
"Thrifty genotype," 171
Thyroid hormones, 484
Time-limited group treatment, 309, 388
Torsade de Pointes, 148, 153
Total body electrical conductivity, 86, 87
Total body potassium, 85, 86
Total body water, 85, 87
Total peripheral vascular resistance, 141
Treatment dropouts (*see* Attrition)
Treatment duration (*see* Length of treatment)
Treatment selection, 303, 304
Triglycerides
  adipose tissue, rats, 114
  exercise benefits, 203, 358
  and hyperinsulinemia, 203
  very low calorie diets, 235
  weight loss benefits, 224, 235, 247, 248
Triiodothyronine (T_3), 102, 103, 261
Truncal obesity (*see* Abdominal obesity)
Twenty-four-hour energy expenditure, 176–179
Twenty-four-hour recall, 332

Twins, resting metabolic rate, 167
Two-reservoir energy model, 164, 165
Type II diabetes
  behavioral weight control, 239–244
  caloric restriction versus weight loss, 236, 237
  disease-specific mortality, 13
  duration of, 245, 246
  exercise, benefits of, 202, 203, 239–241
  genetic factors, 14, 15
  long-term weight loss, benefits of, 215–217, 238
  microangiopathy, 138
  modest weight loss, benefit of, 246–249
  morbidity risk, 15
  mortality risk, 21, 233
  obesity link, 231–233
  predictors of treatment response, 244–246
  regional fat distribution, 14
  and short-term weight loss, 214, 215
  surgery, benefit of, 501
  very low calorie diets, 63, 64, 231–249
  weight loss, benefits of, 151, 213–217, 236, 237, 246–249

U

University Group Diabetes Program, 238
Unstable angina, 274, 275
Upper body obesity (*see* Abdominal obesity)
Uric acid level, 278, 283, 284

V

Variety of food, 202, 317
Ventricular arrhythmias, 139
Ventricular chamber volume, 142
Ventricular ejection fraction, 144
Ventricular fibrillation, 153
Ventricular function, 144, 149
Ventricular hypertrophy
  electrocardiography, 145, 146
  and obesity, 136, 137, 142, 143
  weight loss effect, 149, 150
Ventricular mass/geometry, 143, 144, 152
Ventricular premature contractions
  liquid protein diet, 154
  morbidity risk, 18
  weight loss effect, 150
Ventricular tachycardia, 153
Ventricular wall
  obesity changes, 142–144
  and weight loss, 149, 150, 152
Very low calorie diets, 44–73
  animal models, 120–130
  attrition, 56, 60, 383–404
  and behavior therapy, 61–67, 72, 241–243, 310–327
    follow-up studies, 438–440
  caloric content importance, 69, 70
  cardiac effects, 148–151, 156
  comparison with conventional diets, 65–67
  complications, 52–56, 281, 282
  composition, 45, 46, 335–337
  contraindications, 48, 274–276, 296–300
  cost-effectiveness, 37, 40, 67–69, 282, 283
  definition, 45, 273, 274
  diabetes, benefit to, 215–217, 231–249
  and exercise, 278, 279, 315, 355, 376
    diabetes, 239–241
  fat-free mass loss in, 47, 48, 148, 149
  guidelines for entrance into, 48, 351
  and hunger, 52, 53, 242, 262
  hypertension, benefit to, 220, 221
  lapses in, 242, 243
  length of treatment, 50, 281, 282
  long-term efficacy, 60–63, 438–440
  maintenance of weight loss, 71, 72
  medical monitoring, 273–286
  metabolic effects, rats, 121, 122
  nitrogen balance, 98, 100
  nutritional counseling, 331–351
  optimizing protein content, 98, 335
  protein recommendations, 335
  psychiatric complications, 53–56
  psychological effects, 258–266
  refeeding period, 55, 56
  safety, 51
  selection of, 335–337

Very low calorie diets (*continued*)
  short-term efficacy, 56–60
  treatment course, 48–51
  versus weight loss, benefit of, 236–238
  weight loss predictors, 383–404
Very low density lipoprotein, 358
Video distortion procedure, 262, 263
Visceral obesity
  diabetes susceptibility, 16
  morbidity risks, 14
Vitamin deficiency, surgery, 500

W

Waist–hip circumference ratio
  health risks, 6, 7
  and weight loss, 390
Walking
  adherence problem, 473
  advantages, 367
  caloric requirements, 192
  in multicomponent program, 463–466
Weigh-in, 315
Weight cycling
  effect on metabolic rate, 181
  energy expenditure effect, 180–182
  and food efficiency, 118, 181, 285, 286
  health effects, 285, 286
  rat models, 118, 119
  and weight loss, 392, 393
Weight gain, reversal of, 326
Weight history, 293
Weight loss (*see also* Maintenance of weight loss)
  behavioral factors, 395, 396
  binge eaters, 393, 394
  versus caloric restriction, 236–238, 246–249
  composition of, 148, 149
  and energy expenditure, 171–184, 389
  exercise, effects on, 354–356, 397
  goal setting, 302, 303
  health benefits, 213–226, 231–249
  and initial body weight, 388, 389
  and length of treatment, 397
  long-term dexfenfluramine, 488–491
  predictors, 388–404
  psychological aspects, 258–266, 391, 392
  resting metabolic rate, role of, 176, 177, 389
  surgery, effect on, 500, 501
  ventricular arrhythmias, 138
  very low calorie diet, 280, 281, 339
  and weight cycling, 392, 393
Weight loss per week measure, 36
Weight maintenance (*see* Maintenance of weight loss)
Weight training, 368
Weight Watchers, 41, 42, 432
Wistar rat model, 112, 113, 116, 117, 119
Wrestlers, weight cycling study, 181

Y

"Yo-yo" dieting (*see* Weight cycling)

Z

Zinc concentrations, 120
Zucker fa/fa rat, 110, 113–115, 119, 121, 122